DATE DUE

D1609642

Cytotoxic Cells:
Basic Mechanisms and
Medical Applications

Cytotoxic Cells: Basic Mechanisms and Medical Applications

Editors

Michail V. Sitkovsky, Ph.D.

Chief, Biochemistry and Immunopharmacology Section
Laboratory of Immunology
National Institute of Allergy and Infectious Diseases
National Institutes of Health
Bethesda, Maryland

Pierre A. Henkart, Ph.D.

Chief, Lymphocyte Cytotoxicity Section
Experimental Immunology Branch
National Cancer Institute
National Institutes of Health
Bethesda, Maryland

LIPPINCOTT WILLIAMS & WILKINS
A **Wolters Kluwer** Company
Philadelphia · Baltimore · New York · London
Buenos Aires · Hong Kong · Sydney · Tokyo

Acquisitions Editor: Jonathan Pine
Developmental Editor: Ellen DiFrancesco
Production Service: Bermedica Production, Ltd.
Supervising Editor: Mary Ann McLaughlin
Manufacturing Manager: Kevin Watt
Cover Designer: Christine Jenny
Compositor: The PRD Group, Inc.
Printer: Edwards Brothers

Figures 14-1 and 14-3 are reproduced from *The Journal of Experimental Medicine*, 1997, 186, pp. 1781–1786, by copyright permission of The Rockefeller University Press; Figure 14-6 is reproduced from *The Proceedings of the National Academy of Sciences*, U.S.A., 1996, 93, 5783–5787, by copyright permission of the National Academy of Sciences, U.S.A.

Library of Congress Cataloging-in-Publication Data

Cytotoxic cells : basic mechanisms and medical applications / [edited
  by] Michail V. Sitkovsky, Pierre A. Henkart.
      p.   cm.
    Includes bibliographical references and index.
    ISBN 0-7817-1603-9
    1. T cells.   2. Killer cells.   3. Cell-mediated cytotoxicity.
  I. Sitkovsky, M. V.   II. Henkart, Pierre.
    [DNLM: 1. Cytotoxicity, Immunologic.   2. Killer Cells—physiology.
  3. T-Lymphocytes, Cytotoxic—physiology.   QW 568 C9971 1999]
  QR185.8.T2C986   1999
  616.07′97+—dc21
  DNLM/DLC
  for Library of Congress   99-34057
                                                                 CIP

10 9 8 7 6 5 4 3 2 1

Contents

V CYTOTOXIC LYMPHOCYTES *IN VIVO*

VI CTL GENERATION AND MEMORY

VII MEDICAL APPLICATIONS OF CYTOTOXIC LYMPHOCYTES

Contributors

Alicia Algeciras-Schimnich, Ph.D.   *Postdoctoral Fellow, Immunology, Mayo Clinic, 221 4th Avenue, Rochester, Minnesota 55902*

James P. Allison, Ph.D.   *Professor, Howard Hughes Medical Institute, Department of Molecular and Cellular Biology, Cancer Research Labs, 415 Life Science Addition, University of California-Berkeley, Berkeley, California 94720-3200*

Sergey G. Apasov, Ph.D.   *Staff Scientist, Biochemistry and Immunopharmacology, National Institute of Allergy and Infectious Diseases, Building 10, Room 11N311, National Institutes of Health, Bethesda, Maryland 20892*

Phillip I. Bird, Ph.D.   *Research Fellow, Department of Medicine, Monash University, Box Hill Hospital, Box Hill, Victoria, 3128 Australia*

Robert V. Blanden, M.D.   *Professor and Head, Division of Immunology and Cell Biology, John Curtin School of Medical Research, Australian National University, Canberra, ACT 2601, Australia*

Reinder L. H. Bolhuis, M.D., Ph.D.   *Head, Department of Clinical and Tumor Immunologies, University Hospital Rotterdam, Daniel Den Hoed Cancer Center, P.O. Box 5021, 3000 CA Rotterdam, The Netherlands*

Doo Hyun Chung, M.D.   *Molecular Biology Section, Laboratory of Immunology, National Institute of Allergy and Infectious Diseases, 9000 Rockville Pike, Building 10, Room 11N311, National Institutes of Health, Bethesda, Maryland 20892-1892*

Francesca Di Rosa, M.D., Ph.D.   *Ghost Lab, National Institute for Allergy and Infectious Diseases, LCMI, Building 4, Room 111, National Institutes for Health, Bethesda, Maryland 20892*

Christopher J. Froelich, M.D.   *Associate Professor, Medicine, Northwestern University Medical Center, 2650 Ridge Avenue, Evanston, Illinois 60201; Research Scientist, Medicine, Evanston Northwestern Healthcare Research Institute, 2650 Ridge Avenue, Evanston, Illinois 60201*

Pierre Golstein, M.D., Ph.D.   *Director of Research, INSERM, Centre D'Immunologie de Marseille-Luminy, Case 906, Avenue de Luminy, 13288 Marseille Cedex 9, France*

Jan W. Gratama, M.D., Ph.D.   *Department of Clinical and Tumor Immunology, University Hospital Rotterdam, Daniel Den Hoed Cancer Center, P.O. Box 5021, 3000 CA Rotterdam, The Netherlands*

Dennis A. Hanson, Ph.D.   *Research Associate, Department of Immunology, Virginia Mason Research Center, 1201 Ninth Avenue, Seattle, Washington 98101-2795*

Hans Hengartner, Ph.D.   *Department of Pathology, University of Zurich, Institute of Experimental Immunology, Schmelzbergstr 12, CH-8091 Zürich, Switzerland*

Pierre A. Henkart, Ph.D.   *Experimental Immunology Branch, National Cancer Institute, Building 10, Room 4B17, National Institutes of Health, Bethesda, Maryland 20892-1360*

CONTRIBUTORS

Stuart W. Hicks, B.S.   *PreIRTA Student, Experimental Immunology Branch, National Cancer Institute, 9000 Rockville Pike, Building 10, Room 4B17, National Institutes of Health, Bethesda, Maryland 20892-1360*

Denis Hudrisier, Ph.D.   *Postdoctoral Fellow, Molecular Immunology, The Ludwig Institute for Cancer Research, Chemin des Boveresses 155, CH-1066 Epalinges, Switzerland*

Arthur A. Hurwitz, Ph.D.   *Assistant Professor, Department of Microbiology and Immunology, State University of New York Health Science Campus, 750 East Adams Street, Syracuse, New York 13210*

Paige L. Jensen, Ph.D.   *Center for Immunology, University of Minnesota Medical School, Box 334 Mayo, 420 Delaware Street SE, Minneapolis, Minnesota 55455; R & D Systems, Inc., 614 McKinley Place NE, Minneapolis, Minnesota 55413*

Dragan Jevremovic, M.D.   *Predoctoral Student, Department of Immunology, Mayo Graduate School, 200 First Street SW, Rochester, Minnesota 55905*

David Kägi, Ph.D.   *Postdoctoral Fellow, Ontario Cancer Institute, 610 University Avenue, Room 8-622, Toronto, Ontario M5G 2M9 Canada*

Kathleen A. Kelly, Ph.D.   *Assistant Professor, Pathology and Laboratory Medicine, Center for Health Sciences, UCLA Medical Center, 10833 Le Conte Avenue, Los Angeles, California 90095-1732*

Hidefumi Kojima, Ph.D.   *Visiting Fellow, Laboratory of Immunology, National Institute of Allergy and Infectious Diseases, 9000 Rockville Pike, Building 10, Room 11N311, National Institutes of Health, Bethesda, Maryland 20892-1892*

Gary A. Koretzky, M.D., Ph.D.   *Kelting Professor of Rheumatology, Internal Medicine, University of Iowa College of Medicine, 540 EMRB, Iowa City, Iowa 52242*

Alan M. Krensky, M.D.   *Shelagh Galligan Professor, Department of Pediatrics, Stanford University School of Medicine, 300 Pasteur Drive, Stanford, California 94305-5208*

Dana R. Leach, Ph.D.   *M&E Biotech A/S, Kogle Allé 6, DK 2970 Hørsholm, Denmark*

Paul J. Leibson, M.D., Ph.D.   *Department of Immunology, Mayo Clinic, 200 First Street SW, Rochester, Minnesota 55905-0001*

Mathias G. Lichtenheld, M.D.   *Associate Professor, Microbiology and Immunology, University of Miami School of Medicine, 1600 NW 10th Avenue, RMSB 3034 (R-138), Miami, Florida 33136*

Judy Lieberman, M.D., Ph.D.   *Associate Professor of Pediatrics, Senior Investigator, Harvard Medical School, Center for Blood Research, 800 Huntington Avenue, Boston, Massachusetts 02115; Consultant in Medicine, Hematology-Oncology, Children's Hospital, 300 Longwood Avenue, Boston, Massachusetts 02115*

Meei Y. Lin, Ph.D.   *Postdoctoral Fellow, Department of Biology, University of California, San Diego, 9500 Gilman Drive, La Jolla, California 92093*

Grayson B. Lipford, Ph.D.   *Research Scientist, Department of Medical Microbiology and Immunology, Technical University Munich, Tvojevstr 9, 81675 Munich, Germany*

Immanuel F. Luescher, Ph.D.   *Ludwig Institute for Cancer Research, Lausanne Branch, Chemin des Boveresses 155, Epalinges-Sur-Lausanne 1066, Switzerland*

David H. Margulies, M.D., Ph.D.   *Chief, Molecular Biology Section, Laboratory of Immunology, National Institute of Allergy and Infectious Diseases, 9000 Rockville Pike, Building 10, Room 11N311, National Institutes of Health, Bethesda, Maryland 20892-1892*

Polly Matzinger, Ph.D.   *Section Head, Ghost Lab, LCMI, National Institute for Allergy and Infectious Diseases, Building 4, Room 111, National Institutes for Health, Bethesda, Maryland 20892*

Alessandra Mazzoni, Ph.D.   *Visiting Fellow, Experimental Immunology Branch, National Cancer Institute, 9000 Rockville Pike, Building 10, Room 4B17, National Institutes of Health, Bethesda, Maryland 20892-1360*

Daniel W. McVicar, Ph.D.   *Principal Investigator, Laboratory of Experimental Immunology, Division of Basic Sciences, National Cancer Institute, NCI-FCRDC Building 560, Room 31-93, Frederick, Maryland 21702-1201*

Matthew F. Mescher, Ph.D.   *Professor and Director, Center for Immunology, University of Minnesota Medical School, Box 334 Mayo, 420 Delaware Street SE, Minneapolis, Minnesota 55455*

Robert L. Modlin, M.D.   *Professor of Dermatology, Microbiology, and Immunology, UCLA School of Medicine, 52-151, 10833 Le Conte Avenue, Los Angeles, California 90095-1750; Chief, Division of Dermatology, UCLA School of Medicine, 52-151 CHS, 10833 Le Conte Avenue, Los Angeles, California 90095-1750*

Arno Müllbacher, Ph.D.   *Senior Fellow, Department of Immunology and Cell Biology, John Curtin School of Medical Research, Australian National University, Canberra, ACT 2601, Australia*

Kannan Natarajan, Ph.D.   *Molecular Biology Section, Laboratory of Immunology, National Institute of Allergy and Infectious Diseases, 9000 Rockville Pike, Building 10, Room 11N311, National Institutes of Health, Bethesda, Maryland 20892-1892*

Lyse A. Norian, M.S.   *Graduate Research Assistant, Program in Immunology, University of Iowa College of Medicine, Iowa City, Iowa 52242*

John R. Ortaldo, Ph.D.   *Chief, Laboratory of Experimental Immunology, Division of Basic Sciences, National Cancer Institute, NCI-FCRDC Building 560, Room 31-93, Frederick, Maryland 21702-1201*

Carlos V. Paya, M.D., Ph.D.   *Professor, Department of Immunology, Mayo Clinic, 200 First Street SW, Rochester, Minnesota 55905*

Eckhard R. Podack, M.D., Ph.D.   *Professor and Chairman, Microbiology and Immunology, University of Miami School of Medicine, 1600 NW 10th Avenue, Miami, Florida 33136*

Barbara Rehermann, M.D.   *Senior Investigator, Liver Diseases Section, NIDOK, National Institutes of Health, 10 Center Driver, Building 10, R9B16, Bethesda, Maryland 20817*

John Paul Ridge, B.S.   *Research Biologist, Ghost Lab, National Institute for Allergy and Infectious Diseases, LCMI, Building 4, Room 111, National Institutes for Health, Bethesda, Maryland 20892*

Paul F. Robbins, Ph.D.   *Biologist, Surgery Branch, National Cancer Institute, Room 7B42, National Institutes of Health, Bethesda, Maryland 20892*

Steven A. Rosenberg, M.D., Ph.D.   *Surgery Branch, National Cancer Institute, Room 7B42, National Institutes of Health, Bethesda, Maryland 20892*

John H. Russell, Ph.D.   *Professor, Molecular Biology and Pharmacology, Washington University School of Medicine, 660 South Euclid Avenue, Box 8103, St. Louis, Missouri 63110*

Kimberly A. Sabelko-Downes, Ph.D.   *Postdoctoral Fellow, Molecular Biology and Pharmacology, Washington University School of Medicine, 660 South Euclid Avenue, Box 8103, St. Louis, Missouri 63110*

David M. Segal, Ph.D.   *Chief, Immune Targeting Section, Experimental Immunology Branch, National Cancer Institute, 9000 Rockville Pike, Building 10, Room 4B36, National Institutes of Health, Bethesda, Maryland 20892-1360*

Liisa K. Selin, M.D., Ph.D.   *Assistant Professor, Department of Pathology, University of Massachusetts Medical School, 55 Lake Avenue North, Worcester, Massachusetts 01655*

Markus M. Simon, Ph.D.   *Senior Fellow, Cell Immunology, Max-Planck-Institut für Immunbiologie, Stübeweg 51, Postfach 1169, D-79108 Freiberg, Germany*

Michail V. Sitkovsky, Ph.D.   *Chief, Biochemistry and Immunopharmacology Section, Laboratory of Immunology, National Institute of Allergy and Infectious Diseases, 9000 Rockville Pike, Building 10, Room 11N311, National Institutes of Health, Bethesda, Maryland 20892-1360*

Steffen Stenger, M.D., Ph.D.   *Clinical Microbiology, Immunology, and Hygiene, University of Erlangen-Nürnberg, Wasserturmstr 3, 91054 Erlangen, Germany*

Fumito Tani, Ph.D.   *Associate Professor, Research Institute for Food Science, Kyoto University, Gokasho, Uji, Kyoto 611, Japan*

Anja R. B. Thilenius, Ph.D.   *Molecular Biology and Pharmacology, Washington University School of Medicine, 660 South Euclid Avenue, Box 8103, St. Louis, Missouri 63110*

Joseph A. Trapani, M.D.   *Associate Professor, John Connell Laboratory, Austin Research Institute, Studley Road, Heidelberg, Victoria 3084, Australia*

Tan Truong, B.S.   *Department of Molecular and Cellular Biology, Cancer Research Laboratory, 415 Life Sciences Addition, University of California-Berkeley, Berkeley, California 94720*

Maries F. van den Broek, Ph.D.   *Institute of Experimental Immunology, University Hospital Zürich, Schmelzbergstr 12, CH 8091, Zürich, Switzerland*

Andrea van Elsas, Ph.D.   *Department of Immunohematology and Bloodbank, Leiden University Medical Center, E3-Q, Albinusdreef 2, 2333 AA Leiden, The Netherlands*

Steven M. Varga, Ph.D.   *Postdoctoral Fellow, Beirne B. Carter Center for Immunology Research, University of Virginia Health Sciences Center, MR-4 Box 4012, Lane Road, Charlottesville, Virginia 22908; Department of Pathology, University of Massachusetts Medical Center, 55 Lake Avenue North, Worcester, Massachusetts 01655*

Jennifer Villasenor, B.S.   *Department of Molecular and Cellular Biology, Cancer Research Laboratory, 415 Life Sciences Addition, University of California-Berkeley, Berkeley, California 94720*

Alberto Visintin, Ph.D.   *Visiting Fellow, Experimental Immunology Branch, National Cancer Institute, 9000 Rockville Pike, Building 10, Room 4B17, National Institutes of Health, Bethesda, Maryland 20892-1360*

Hermann Wagner, M.D., Ph.D.   *Director, Professor, Department of Medical Microbiology and Immunology, Technical University, Trogestrasse 9, D-81675, Germany; Chief, Department of Medical Microbiology and Immunology, Technical University, Trogerstrasse 9, D-81675, Germany*

Rong-Fu Wang, Ph.D.   *Staff Scientist, Surgery Branch, National Cancer Institute, National Institutes of Health, Bethesda, Maryland 20892*

Raymond M. Welsh, Ph.D.   *Professor, Department of Pathology, University of Massachusetts Medical School, 55 Lake Avenue North, Worcester, Massachusetts 01655*

Ralph A. Willemsen, M.Sc.   *Department of Clinical and Tumor Immunology, University Hospital Rotterdam, Daniel Den Hoed Cancer Center, P.O. Box 5021, 3000 CA Rotterdam, The Netherlands*

Jennifer Ziskin, B.S.   *Department of Molecular and Cell Biology, Cancer Research Laboratory, 415 Life Sciences Addition, University of California-Berkeley, Berkeley, California 94720*

Preface

We decided to produce this book on cytotoxic lymphocytes to fill a need for a single source reference in this field. After consulting with numerous colleagues, we thought such a book would be useful to a broad audience, including not only researchers active in this area but those needing an overview of this subject and graduate students or postdoctoral fellows entering this area of research.

Because the *in vitro* measurement of cytotoxicity is a rapid and quantitative functional readout of lymphocyte activation, cytotoxic lymphocytes have long been used for biochemical and pharmacologic studies of lymphocytes. This trend has continued, as can be seen in the chapters of this book on recognition, signaling, and effector molecules. Within the last decade a revolution has occurred in our knowledge of T cell receptors and their recognition of antigen. Even more recently the molecules involved in target recognition by natural killer cells are being illuminated. The extracellular molecules mediating target recognition in turn trigger intracellular signaling cascades, which also have been characterized on a detailed molecular level within the last several years. Finally, the effector molecules that damage target cells have been examined in increasing detail to define not only how the two distinct molecular pathways kill cells but the control elements that regulate their expression at the genetic level.

The current generation of researchers have built on the understanding of how these cells work to assess their biologic roles *in vivo*, and now many groups are examining their role in a variety of clinical situations. From a practical standpoint, the ultimate goal of immunology is to design vaccines that can prevent the infectious diseases still threatening most people on the planet. It is clear that cytotoxic lymphocytes (CTLs) can eliminate many such infections at a preclinical stage, and the generation of a pool of memory CTLs is an important goal for vaccine development. In addition to their protective role, it has become clear that when responding to pathogens CTLs sometimes damage otherwise functional tissue. Thus the term "two-edged sword" often used to describe the immune system as a whole also applies to CTLs. Several examples of immunopathogenicity apparently caused by CTLs are described herein.

Although preventive vaccines do not seem a possibility for most cancers, harnessing the specific and potent activity of CTLs for therapy has long been a goal. After decades of abstract discussions about the nature of tumor antigens we are now at the point of having a number of human tumor antigens defined at the molecular level, and they are being used to generate potent cytotoxic effector cells *in vitro*. These exciting developments are chronicled in the last section of the book, along with the extension of these ideas as a possible means of treating human immunodeficiency virus (HIV) infection.

Reading the summaries of the research groups working with CTLs has stimulated our own thinking about these problems, and we are sure that you will share this response. As you can see, there are numerous areas where a consensus has not yet been reached, but the expression of different viewpoints can only help generate ideas for better experiments to test these concepts. We have found that the chapters in this book are generally excellent in terms of clarity, and we salute our colleagues for the time and effort that went into preparing them.

Michail V. Sitkovsky
Pierre A. Henkart

Cytotoxic Cells: Basic Mechanisms and
Medical Applications, edited by Michail V.
Sitkovsky and Pierre A. Henkart. Lippincott
Williams & Wilkins, Philadelphia © 2000.

I / HISTORICAL OVERVIEW

Chapter 1
Molecular Mechanisms of
T Cell-Mediated Cytotoxicity

Pierre Golstein

*Centre d'Immunologie INSERM-CNRS de Marseille-Luminy, Case 906,
13288 Marseille Cedex 9, France*

By which molecular mechanism(s) is a mammalian cell able to kill another cell? This simple question, especially applicable to the professional killer cells known as cytotoxic T lymphocytes (CTLs), was raised during the early 1960s and received definitive, though still incomplete, answers only during the late 1990s. This quarter-of-a-century hunt has been, in its limited way, a collective venture, as are almost all scientific advances, made most often of painfully acquired and at times exciting and ultimately useful results. Several tens of thousands of publications reflect these efforts, many of which struggled to establish phenomenologic basics in premolecular times.

Why have results crystallized into coherent pathways so rapidly within the last few years, and what are the reasons for acceleration (compared, say, to the initial slow pace of the field, or to the many tens of years required to work out the complement cascade)? The field has benefited not only from the tremendous contribution of molecular biology but also from the convergence in recent years of several independently progressing lines of research. The latter are described here, knowing that convergence may be only apparent and sometimes arguably reconstructed only too easily after the event.

Clearly only a few references can be quoted here out of all the published papers. Being fully aware of the contribution of my many colleagues in the field, I deeply apologize to those who are not (or not sufficiently) quoted owing to mistake, omission, or mere lack of space.

CYTOTOXICITY PATH

The demonstration during the early 1940s of *in vivo* transfer of specific immunity by immune lymphocytes led during the 1940s and 1950s to a number of unsuccessful attempts to demonstrate specific immunity in vitro (1,2). The breakthrough came at the end of the 1950s, when a few papers began to report some toxic effects of immune cells on target cells *in vitro* (3). The best known is the report of Govaerts in 1960 (4), who showed that cells from a dog bearing a kidney homotransplant were able to lyse *in vitro* cells explanted from the second kidney of the donor dog. Cytotoxicity was assessed by morphology and trypan blue exclusion. Effector cells were recipient cells taken from the thoracic duct. However, cytotoxicity was observed only if immune serum was added, suggesting, in retrospect, antibody-dependent cell-mediated rather than T cell-mediated cytotoxicity.

Several reports ensued between 1960 and 1965, also establishing part of the basic methodology for investigating cell-mediated cyto-toxicity *in vitro*. Two main systems were explored. First, allo- or xenoimmunized lymphoid cells were shown specifically to lyse monolayers of relevant target cells. Thus spleen cells from alloimmune BALB/c anti-C3H mice, but not from nonimmune mice, clustered onto target L cells and lysed them (1,5). Similar findings allowing better dem-onstration of immune specificity were ob-tained using, as target monolayers, freshly explanted macrophages (2) or fibroblasts (6). Spleen cells from mice preimmunized with HeLa cells were more cytotoxic to HeLa cells *in vitro* than spleen cells from nonimmune mice (7). The expanding use of combinations of tumor target cells made experiments pro-gressively less cumbersome and improved the definition of the experimental systems. Thus in a then ongoing debate on whether soluble or "cellular" antibodies were at play, it could be shown that the cytotoxicity of alloimmune mouse lymph node cells for the relevant tumor cells in culture (8) could be partially blocked, rather than enhanced, with alloantibodies (9). Similar observations of cytotoxicity that required close proximity and that could be blocked by immune serum were made in a carefully parametered study using cells from alloimmune rats (10).

Among these early reports, a second line of study dealt with cytotoxic cells *in vitro* as revealing possible components of autoim-mune reactions. Thus it was shown that lymph node cells from rats immunized with guinea pig spinal cord in Freund's adjuvant were able to recognize and destroy glial cells *in vitro* (11). Similarly, white blood cells from rabbits with experimental autoimmune en-cephalitis (EAE) exerted cytotoxicity on neonatal rat glial cells cultured *in vitro* (12). Also, white blood cells from patients with ulcerative colitis were cytotoxic to human fetal colon cells *in vitro* (3).

The exact nature of the immunologically specific effector cells was not firmly estab-lished in these early years, although lympho-cytes were the prime suspects, as suggested in particular by the effect of lymph node cells.

Still, macrophages were believed to exert spe-cific cytotoxicity. Alloimmune peritoneal macrophages, in fact peritoneal cells collected 10 days after an intraperitoneal injection of allogeneic tumor cells, comprising "3% to 5% lymphocytes," were able to induce plaques of clearing in monolayers of fibroblasts in an im-munospecific way (13). In retrospect, the cy-totoxicity may have been due to the contami-nating peritoneal exudate lymphocytes (14). Identification of T lymphocytes (15) soon led to the demonstration that these cells were the major effectors of antigen-specific cell-medi-ated lysis *in vitro* (16–18).

During these and subsequent years a con-siderable amount of work dealt with pheno-menologic studies and have been often and extensively reviewed (19–29). Only a few of these advances are mentioned here. Super-natants from activated mouse lymphocytes were shown to be toxic to L cells (30), likely an early description of tumor necrosis factor (TNF)/lymphotoxin effects *in vitro*. Intro-duction of the ^{51}Cr release test in cell-medi-ated cytotoxicity studies (31,32) provided a widely used, convenient, quantitative, and objective, although late, indicator of target cell death. Specific depletion of cytolytic ac-tivity after incubation on relevant cell mono-layers (14,33,34) strongly indicated that spe-cific surface receptors were at play, a forerunner indication of the existence of T cell receptors (TCRs).

Three stages could be identified in the cy-tolytic process (21,35): target cell recognition by the effector cell: lethal hit (35,36), also called programming for lysis (37); and target cell disintegration. Staging was to some ex-tent helped by work on the differential re-quirement of these stages for extracellular divalent cations. Although most of the cytol-ysis by CTL populations or clones requires extracellular Ca^{2+} at the lethal hit stage (21–23), part of the cytotoxic activity they exert can be independent of extracellular Ca^{2+} (38–42), which turned out much later to be of significant help in distinguishing the mech-anisms at play (see below). Also, in the infre-quent studies dealing with the morphology of effector and target cells, interestingly dying target cells were shown to have a "boiling" appearance, "similar" to that seen during "natural cell death" (43), and showed other apoptotic features as well (44). It took several years for the mechanistic implications of these results to be fully appreciated.

GRANULE EXOCYTOSIS/PERFORIN/ GRANZYME B PATH

Granules that could be "secretory" were detected in CTLs (45–48), together with a number of other structural elements then considered in line with a secretory mechanism for cytotoxicity (49–51). These granules purified from rat large granular leukocyte (LGL) tumors or from some T cell lines were shown during the mid-1980s to be cytotoxic to nucleated and nonnucleated target cells, interestingly in a Ca^{2+}-dependent manner (52–54). From subsequent attempts to extract cytotoxic moieties from these granules, a molecule emerged, called perforin or cytolysin, a 60-kD calcium-dependent pore-forming protein (26,55,56) that was structurally homologous to complement components (for reviews on perforin see 57–60). Considering in particular the subcellular localization of perforin in granules, the putative role of perforin in T cell-mediated cytotoxicity was incorporated within the framework of a granule-exocytosis model (26). This model hypothesized that "target cell binding to a membrane receptor induces a secretory process in the effector cell in which the contents of cytoplasmic granules are released by local exocytosis between the effector cell and its bound target" (26), had the potential to encompass granule proteins other than perforin, suggested a delivery system to target cell membranes of effector molecules, and was in agreement with the presence in the target cell membrane of pore-looking structures (49,51), perhaps reflecting the existence of perforin channels, somehow involved in target cell death.

About 10 years of experimental doubts and sometimes bitter arguments elapsed from the discovery of perforin to an unambiguous demonstration of its role in a major mechanism of cytotoxicity. This demonstration was finally provided through the use of perforin "knockout" mice (i.e., mice in which both alleles of the perforin gene had been crippled) (61). Compared to control mice, these mice had lost about 90% of the cytotoxicity induced in viral systems (leukocyte choriomeningitis virus, LCMV) *in vivo* and in antiallogeneic model systems *in vitro* (mixed leukocyte culture cells) or *in vivo* (peritoneal exudate cells). They had also lost the ability to eliminate the virus during LCMV infection.

Perforin, although clearly required for a major mechanism of cytotoxicity, was not sufficient to account for it. This conclusion stemmed in particular from comparisons between the mode of death induced by CTLs and that induced by purified perforin. Indeed, CTLs can cause morphologic events (43,44,62) in the target cell similar to the condensation/fragmentation features often seen with developmental cell death and usually designated apoptosis (see below). Although there are differences between apoptosis occurring in developmental circumstances and in CTL-mediated cell death (e.g., for CTL-mediated death, usually faster kinetics and the absence of block by inhibitors of macromolecular synthesis for "bypass" reasons that are now clear; see below), clearly the morphologic traits are similar. In contrast, treatment of nucleated cells with purified perforin led to dilation of the endoplasmic reticulum, a prominent increase in volume and other alterations of the mitochondria, flocculation (but not condensation) of the nuclear chromatin, and cell swelling (63,64). Also, in target cells attacked by antibody and complement or by perforin, again in contrast to what could be observed in cells undergoing apoptosis, DNA is not cleaved into discrete fragments (65–68), with some reported exceptions (69,70). The gross morphologic features and the usual absence of DNA fragmentation define this type of death as necrosis (63).

The observation that cell death induced by CTLs was mostly apoptotic, whereas cell death induced by purified perforin was mostly necrotic, seemed to exclude a mechanism of lysis based *exclusively* on perforin; it led to a search for alternative molecular mechanisms (see below) and for other molecules, eventually completing a perforin-based mechanism. Serine esterases were likely candidates. Serine esterase inhibitors were found to inhibit T cell-mediated cytotoxicity (71–73), and they could be isolated from CTLs (74–79); moreover, serine esterase genes could be cloned as cDNAs (80–82) and were found to be expressed with relative specificity in CTLs or at least in activated T cells (83,84). These proteins were found in granules of CTLs—hence their designation as granzymes (85). So far, eight granzymes (A–G, M) have been described in the mouse and five (A, B, H, M, tryptase 2) in humans (86,87). Granzyme A was initially cloned as CTLA-3 (80,88) and hanuka factor (81), and granzyme B was initially cloned as CTLA-1 (80) and CCP1 (82).

It took a few more years to demonstrate a role for granzymes at the effector stage of T cell-mediated cytotoxicity. Suggestive lines of evidence stemmed in particular from experiments by Henkart and his colleagues, showing that more DNA fragmentation was induced in target cells by perforin plus granzyme A than by perforin alone (89) and that co-transfection of granzyme A "helps" a perforin-transfected mast cell to perform apoptotic-type cell killing (90,91). Similarly, Greenberg and colleagues showed that perforin plus fragmentins (rat granzymes) induce DNA fragmentation and cell death in target cells (92,93). It was the use of gene knockout technology that led to the formal demonstration that granzyme B was largely required in a mechanism of cytotoxicity (94). The assumption, which has not been thwarted, is that perforin and granzyme B operate in the same mechanism of cytotoxicity, and that perforin somehow helps granzyme B alter target cell components, as further discussed in a later section.

CELL DEATH PATH

The occurrence of cell death in animal tissues has been known for more than a century (95). Cell death occurs as a normal component of the development of multicellular eukaryotes. Classic examples of developmental cell death are the embryonic tissue deletions required for proper morphogenesis (96–101), elimination of neurons failing to establish adequate trophic connections at the appropriate time (102–106), and in immunology particularly the negative selection of thymocytes bearing inappropriate antigen receptors (107,108).

Developmental cell death is programmed, not only for its occurrence in the organism but also for its course within the dying cell. The notion of a programmed course of events in a dying cell came to some extent as a corollary to the description of a given set of morphologic features in a dying cell, called apoptosis (109). This set associates cytoplasmic and nuclear condensation and fragmentation, DNA fragmentation (110–113), and sometimes a requirement for macromolecular synthesis (114,115). In most of the models studied so far, programmed cell death follows an apoptotic pattern, but other cell death patterns have been described (116–119).

The modern history of the cell death field is dominated first by the description of the "apoptotic" morphologic set of features and second by the notion that the programmed course of events within a dying cell that leads to apoptotic features is under genetic control. Thus, the *ced-3* and *ced-4* genes were found to govern developmental cell death in the nematode *Caenorhabditis elegans* (120–122). In the mouse a homolog of *ced-3* was found to be the ICE cysteine protease (123), a finding that led to the description of a series of members of the same "caspase" family (124).

Current understanding of the programmed cell death cascade can be schematized as shown in Figure 1-1. A central stage includes activation of caspases. This activa-

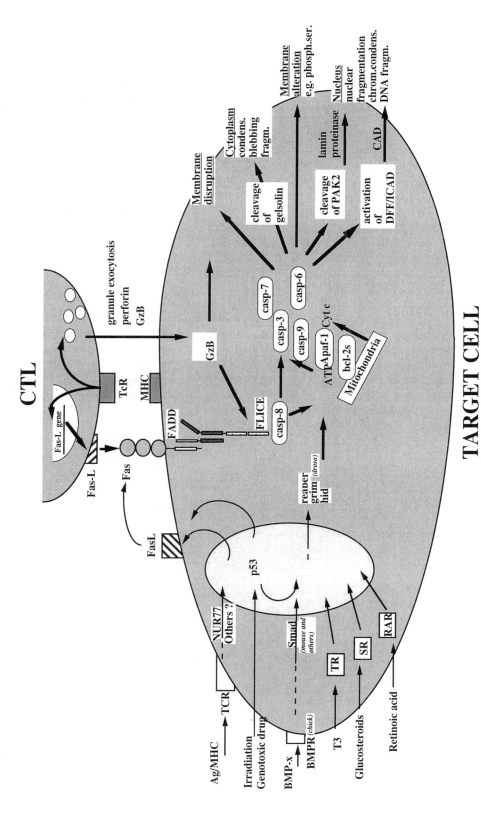

FIG. 1-1. Intersection of cytotoxicity mechanisms and cell death cascade. **Top:** Cytotoxic lympho-cyte, with both Fas-based and granule exocytosis/perforin/granzyme B (*GzB*)-based mechanisms vertically aiming at the target cell. **Bottom:** Target cell, with a cell death cascade oriented horizon-tally, from extracellular death-inducing signals (*left*) to apoptotic morphologic lesions (*right*). Both cytotoxicity mechanisms encounter the cell death cascade mostly by signaling the activation of caspases. Details and references can be found in the text.

tion is under the control of Ced-4 in *C. elegans* (125,126) and its homolog Apaf-1 in mammals (127), which interacts with Ced9 in *C. elegans* (122,128) and the corresponding members of the *bcl-2* family in mammals (129–132) in a mitochondrial context (133). Downstream of caspase activation, the cleavage of caspase substrates leads to systematic dismantling of cell structures, which translates into apoptotic morphologic lesions (134).

Upstream of caspase activation, a complex series of steps leads from extracellular death signals to caspase activation (135). First, extracellular ligands engage membrane or cytoplasmic receptors. These receptors are part of, or activate, transcription factors, which translocate into the nucleus. Second, these transcription factors induce the synthesis of molecules, which govern pathways leading to caspase activation and subsequent cell death. Two such pathways are known. A cytoplasmic pathway has been defined in *Drosophila*. It includes molecules such as reaper (136) and hid and grim (137,138). A membrane pathway, defined in mammals, includes ligands and receptors of the Fas/TNF-R1/NGF family (see below) (139). There might be some evolutionary relationship between the two pathways (140). The membrane pathway, especially Fas, is, as described below, at a crossroad between cell death and one of the mechanisms of T cell-mediated cytotoxicity.

FAS PATH

As shown above, there were indications as early as the mid-1980s that a major mechanism of T cell-mediated cytotoxicity requires perforin and, it later turned out, granzymes. It had long been suspected that in addition to this mechanism there must be at least another mechanism not based on perforin. Among several arguments against an exclusive role of a perforin-based mechanism in T cell-mediated cytotoxicity, a major one was the existence of Ca^{2+}-independent cytotoxicity (see above). A perforin-based mechanism

seems to require Ca^{2+} at several levels (55,141,142), even more so if it involves granule exocytosis. These considerations led, in parallel with further developments on the perforin-based mechanism, to a search for a non-perforin-based mechanism(s).

An immediate methodologic problem was that these mechanisms may, and in fact as we now know do, often coexist in any given CTL, blurring the search for molecules required for only one of these mechanisms. Attempts were therefore made to prune a cytotoxic cell to expressing only one cytotoxicity mechanism and more precisely to prune it of its perforin-based mechanism, as follows. Nabholz and his colleagues in Lausanne a number of years ago constructed a rat × mouse hybridoma called PC60 that is constitutive for growth and inducible for cytotoxicity upon addition of interleukins (143). Interestingly, this hybridoma was functionally unstable, presumably reflecting some genetic instability related to the loss of genetic material from these interspecific hybrids. This finding suggested the possibility of pruning these cells of as much genetic material as possible while preserving some cytotoxic activity. For several years these cells were serially cloned with systematic selection of the most cytotoxic clones (144). It resulted in cell clones exhibiting considerable chromosome loss but still significant cytotoxicity upon activation with phorbol myristic acetate (PMA) and ionomycin. Remarkably, preactivated d10S cells (one of the late clones derived from PC60 cells) exerted lysis without a need for extracellular Ca^{2+} and importantly, as shown below, lysed thymocytes at particularly low effector/target cell ratios (145,146).

In completely unrelated experiments, a cell surface molecule called Fas (Apo-1 or CD95) had been shown to transduce a cell death signal when engaged with the corresponding antibody (147,148). Its cloning indicated that Fas belongs to the TNF-R1 family (149). Fas thus mediates cell death and has been shown to be abundantly expressed on thymocytes (150), which led us to wonder whether Fas accounts for the sensitivity of thymocytes to d10S-mediated cytotoxicity.

To investigate whether Fas at the surface of target thymocytes might be causally involved in their lysis by d10S effector cells, thymocytes from *lpr* mutant mice exhibiting a lymphoproliferative disorder (151) that do not express Fas (152) were used. Whereas MRL thymocytes were sensitive, MRL-*lpr* thymocytes were resistant to d10S cells. Thus thymocytes from mice not expressing Fas were resistant to d10S cells (145). In contrast, thymocytes from *gld* mice (153), which express Fas although having the same cellular phenotype as *lpr* mice (151), were sensitive to d10S. This indicated that *lpr* resistance was directly related to the absence of Fas at the target MRL-*lpr* thymocyte surface, not to a secondary consequence of this mutation on thymocyte development (145). This was the first demonstration of a Fas-based mechanism in T cell-mediated cytotoxicity and of a role for Fas at the cellular level (soon leading to publications from many laboratories considerably extending these results). The key to this demonstration was the availability of target cells bearing or not bearing Fas. Indeed, Fas-positive cells, such as wild-type thymocytes or L1210-Fas transfectant tumor cells, were lysed by d10S effector cells, whereas Fas-negative cells, such as *lpr* thymocytes or L1210 tumor cells, were not (145).

To show that not only d10S cells but also other cytotoxic T cells use the Fas-based mechanism, another essential tool was an absence of the requirement for extracellular Ca^{2+} in this mechanism. The cytotoxicity by preactivated d10S cells was indeed Ca^{2+}-independent (144). Addition of EGTA-Mg^{2+} into cytotoxicity tests chelated Ca^{2+} in the presence of excess Mg^{2+}, suppressing the perforin-based mechanism and enabling us to study the Fas-based mechanism (145), even in the common situations where both mechanisms operate simultaneously. In the presence of EGTA-Mg^{2+}, the residual antigen-specific cytotoxicity by in vivo-raised alloimmune peritoneal exudate lymphocytes

(PELs) (145) and virus-immune spleen cells (154) could be shown to be Fas-based. Not only PELs but *in vitro*-raised alloimmune mixed leukocyte culture cells (MLCs) (145,154–157) and clones (158–162) showed Fas-based antigen-specific cytotoxicity. Antigen specificity demonstrated that with this mechanism of cytotoxicity TCRs must be involved.

The requirement for Fas at the surface of the target cell implied the existence of a Fas ligand at the surface of the effector T cell and thus of d10S cells. Starting from the latter, enriched in relevant surface molecules through FACS sorting using Fas-Fc labeling, the Fas ligand (FasL) was cloned (163) and was shown to belong to the same family as, for instance, TNF. Expression of the Fas ligand is inducible in T lymphocytes. Induction can be antigen-nonspecific using PMA and ionomycin (145,154,158,160,161,164, 165) or concanavatin A, which, at variance with PMA and ionomycin, also induced the perforin-based mechanism (154,155). FasL expression can also be induced through direct stimulation of the TCR with antigen or anti-TCR/CD3 antibodies (156–159,161, 162,164,166). Although extracellular Ca^{2+} is not required for Fas-based cytotoxicity or cell death as such (145), extracellular Ca^{2+} is required for induction of expression of Fas ligand on effector cytotoxic T cells (154,164).

Which cells are able to exert Fas-based cytotoxicity? In a general way, most if not all activated T lymphocytes, both CD4$^+$ and CD8$^+$ cells can do so. T-helper (Th1) CD4 cells do not usually express the perforin-based mechanism of lysis; that is, they seem to lyse only or mostly via the Fas-based pathway. In contrast, CD8$^+$ cells usually express both the Fas-based and the perforin-based mechanisms (145,158,160–162). Most of these experiments made use of T cell clones or activated cell populations, reflecting the fact that the Fas ligand is expressed best and quickest under "reactivation" conditions (161,164). However, even resting peripheral CD4$^+$ T cells could be induced to lyse via the Fas-based mechanism, provided an over-night induction period was used (158,159).

Interestingly, transfection of Fas ligand cDNA into fibroblast-like recipient cells was enough to render these cells cytotoxic (163), suggesting that expression of the Fas ligand may be sufficient to make even a non-lymphoid cell cytotoxic. This was to be con-firmed later, in experiments showing (a) that effector cells expressing FasL can induce the death of Fas-bearing cells, including them-selves, so the Fas pathway can work in *trans* (as in cytotoxicity) or in *cis*; and (b) that using the Fas pathway nonlymphoid cells can even induce the death of lymphoid cells, thus fighting the immune system and demonstra-ting that the Fas pathway does not belong exclusively to the realm of immunology.

WHERE ALL PATHS MEET

The results summarized above, obtained over more than 20 years, converged during the mid and late 1990s to provide at least an overall picture of the ways a CTL is able to affect a target cell (Fig. 1-1). By 1994 two molecular mechanisms (based on granule ex-ocytosis–perforin–granzyme B and on Fas, respectively) of T cell-mediated cytotoxicity had been formally demonstrated. It was im-portant to determine if other mechanisms might also be at play. This point was investi-gated by cytotoxicity tests using effector cells from perforin −/− mice, which could not lyse via the perforin pathway, and target cells not bearing Fas, which could not be lysed via the Fas pathway. Both known mechanisms were thus ablated. No residual cytotoxicity was observed in these experiments, demon-strating that no cytotoxicity mechanism other than the perforin-based and the Fas-based ones could be evidenced in short-term in vitro cytotoxicity tests (154,157,167). The situation may be different for long-term *in vitro* assays or *in vivo*, where in particular other molecules of the Fas/FasL families (139), such as TNF/TNF-R1 (168), may also be involved.

How does the perforin/granzyme B mech-anism lead to target cell death? That is, is this effector cell mechanism related to the target cell death cascade and, if so, how? Granzyme B, which is a serine esterase, shows an enzymatic specificity similar to that of some caspases (169). Accordingly, it is able to cleave and therefore activate caspase 3 (170) and a number of other caspases, and it can cleave some of the known caspase sub-strates (171). These properties probably ac-count for observations that granzyme B can trigger both caspase-dependent and caspase-independent signs of cell death (172–174). Interestingly, granzyme B ends up in the tar-get cell nucleus (175,176). It seems that gran-zyme B can, by itself, cross the target cell membrane and move to some cytoplasmic compartment from which perforin might in-duce its release and thus allow its localization to the nucleus (177,178). It is not entirely clear yet how, when, and where granzyme B acts on its various caspase and noncaspase substrates, leading to cell death. In any case, this mechanism of cytotoxicity reaches the cell death cascade at least at the level of caspases and caspase substrates.

How does the Fas pathway lead to target cell death? In this case as well, how is this effector mechanism molecularly linked to the cell death cascade? Two groups (179,180) showed that, upon engagement by effector cell FasL, target cell Fas recruits an adaptor molecule called FADD, which in turn re-cruits FLICE. Strikingly, the latter is itself a caspase, also called caspase-8, the activation of which leads directly or indirectly to the activation of downstream caspases and to cell death. Thus it is also at the level of caspases that the Fas-based mechanism of cytotoxicity reaches the target cell death cascade.

In Figure 1-1, it is clear that the Fas path-way and the perforin/granzyme B pathway, from the point of view of the effector cell, are mechanisms of cytotoxicity; but from the point of view of the target cell, more pre-cisely of its cell death cascade, they are "just" cell death signals. To emerge in evolution, cell-mediated cytotoxicity apparently made use of the cell death cascade (i.e., a molecular mechanism of developmental cell death) and invented novel signals to activate it. This fulfills in part a prediction that "the immune system might, during evolution, have made opportunistic use of a preexisting mechanism for the controlled elimination of cells through lymphocytes acquiring the capacity to secrete proteins that mediate apoptosis" (64). Moreover, both "cytotoxicity" signals bypass the nucleus (i.e., directly reach the effector segment of the cell death cascade) and involve only posttranslational steps. This accounts at least partially for the relative rapidity and insensitivity to macromolecular synthesis inhibitors of cell death when caused by CTLs versus some other signals.

Thus from the early 1960s, when there was no hint as to how a cell was able to "kill" another cell, we have now reached a situation where the basic molecular mechanisms of T cell-mediated cytotoxicity are known at least in broad terms. Of course much remains to be done in the cytotoxicity field. Present and future investigations might focus, for instance at the effector cell level, on the molecular links and switches between engagement of the TCR and the effector mechanisms (181,182), the precise functioning of CTL degranulation, and the modulation by inhibitory and activatory receptors (183), keeping some specificity for cytotoxicity as a distinct domain of research. Research and researchers might also focus, at the target cell level, on the downstream steps leading to and including the cell death cascade, thereby joining the mainstream research on cell death.

Acknowledgments

I owe much to those who contributed to the cytotoxicity field in my laboratory, in particular Marie-Françoise Luciani, Jean-François Brunet, and Eric Rouvier. I thank INSERM, CNRS, ARC, and LNFCC for their support.

REFERENCES

1. Rosenau W, Moon HD. Lysis of homologous cells by sensitized lymphocytes in tissue culture. *J Natl Cancer Inst* 1961;27:471–483.
2. Brondz BD. Interaction of immune lymphocytes in vitro with normal and neoplastic tissue cells. *Folia Biol* 1964;10:164–175.
3. Perlmann P, Broberger O. In vitro studies of ulcerative colitis. II. Cytotoxic action of white blood cells from patients on human fetal colon cells. *J Exp Med* 1963;117:717–733.
4. Govaerts A. Cellular antibodies in kidney homotransplantation. *J Immunol* 1960;85:516–522.
5. Taylor HE, Culling CFA. Cytopathic effect in vitro of sensitized homologous and heterologous spleen cells on fibroblasts. *Lab Invest* 1963;12:884–894.
6. Vainio T, Koskimies O, Perlmann P, Perlmann H, Klein G. In vitro cytotoxic effect of lymphoid cells from mice immunized with allogeneic tissue. *Nature* 1964;204:453–455.
7. Stuart AE. The cytotoxic effect of heterologous lymphoid cells. *Lancet* 1962;2:180–182.
8. Möller E. Contact-induced cytotoxicity by lymphoid cells containing foreign isoantigens. *Science* 1965;147:873–875.
9. Möller E. Antagonistic effects of humoral isoantibodies on the in vitro cytotoxicity of immune lymphoid cells. *J Exp Med* 1965;122:11–23.
10. Wilson DB. Quantitative studies on the behavior of sensitized lymphocytes in vitro. I. Relationship of the degree of destruction of homologous target cells to the number of lymphocytes and to the time of contact in culture and consideration of the effects of isoimmune serum. *J Exp Med* 1965;122:143–166.
11. Koprowski H, Fernandes MV. Autosensitization reaction in vitro: contactual agglutination of sensitized lymph node cells in brain tissue culture accompanied by destruction of glial elements. *J Exp Med* 1962;116:467–476.
12. Berg O, Kallen B. White blood cells from animals with experimental allergic encephalomyelitis tested on glia cells in tissue culture. *Acta Path Microbiol Scand* 1963;58:33–42.
13. Granger GA, Weiser RS. Homograft target cells: specific destruction in vitro by contact interaction with immune macrophages. *Science* 1964;145:1427–1429.
14. Berke G, Sullivan KA, Amos B. Rejection of ascites tumor allografts. I. Isolation, characterization, and in vitro reactivity of peritoneal lymphoid effector cells from BALB/c mice immune to EL4 leukosis. *J Exp Med* 1972;135:1334–1350.
15. Roitt IM, Greaves MF, Torrigiani G, Brostoff J, Playfair JH. The cellular basis of immunological responses: a synthesis of some current views. *Lancet* 1969;2:367–371.
16. Cerottini J-C, Nordin AA, Brunner KT. Specific in vitro cytotoxicity of thymus-derived lymphocytes sensitized to alloantigens. *Nature* 1970;228:1308–1309.
17. Golstein P, Wigzell H, Blomgren H, Svedmyr EAJ. Cells mediating specific in vitro cytotoxicity. II. Probable autonomy of thymus-processed lymphocytes (T cells) for the killing of allogeneic target cells. *J Exp Med* 1972;135:890–906.
18. Golstein P, Blomgren H. Further evidence for autonomy of T cells mediating specific in vitro cyto-

toxicity: efficiency of very small amounts of highly purified T cells. *Cell Immunol* 1973;9:127–141.

19. Perlmann P, Holm G. Cytotoxic effects of lymphoid cells in vitro. *Adv Immunol* 1969;11: 117–193.

20. Cerottini J-C, Brunner KT. Cell-mediated cytotoxicity, allograft rejection, and tumor immunity. *Adv Immunol* 1974;18:67–132.

21. Golstein P, Smith ET. Mechanism of T cell-mediated cytolysis: the lethal hit stage. *Contemp Top Immunobiol* 1977;7:273–300.

22. Henney CS. T-cell-mediated cytolysis: an overview of some current issues. *Contemp Top Immunobiol* 1977;7:245–272.

23. Martz E. Mechanism of specific tumor-cell lysis by alloimmune T lymphocytes: resolution and characterization of discrete steps in the cellular interaction. *Contemp Top Immunobiol* 1977;7:301–361.

24. Berke G. Interaction of cytotoxic T lymphocytes and target cells. *Prog Allergy* 1980;27:69–133.

25. Sanderson CJ. The mechanism of lymphocyte-mediated cytotoxicity. *Biol Rev* 1981;56:153–197.

26. Henkart PA. Mechanism of lymphocyte-mediated cytotoxicity. *Annu Rev Immunol* 1985;3:31–58.

27. Sitkovsky MV. Mechanistic, functional and immunopharmacological implications of biochemical studies of antigen receptor-triggered cytolytic T-lymphocyte activation. *Immunol Rev* 1988;103: 127–160.

28. Berke G. Functions and mechanisms of lysis induced by cytotoxic T lymphocytes and natural killer cells. In: Paul WE (ed) *Fundamental Immunology*. New York, Raven, 1989, pp 735–764.

29. Young JD-E. Killing of target cells by lymphocytes: a mechanistic view. *Physiol Rev* 1989;69:250–314.

30. Granger GA, Williams TW. Lymphocyte cytotoxicity in vitro: activation and release of a cytotoxic factor. *Nature* 1968;218:1253–1254.

31. Holm G, Perlmann P. Quantitative studies on phytohaemagglutinin-induced cytotoxicity by human lymphocytes against homologous cells in tissue culture. *Immunology* 1972;12:525–536.

32. Brunner KT, Mauel J, Cerottini J-C, Chapuis B. Quantitative assay of the lytic action of immune lymphoid cells on ^{51}Cr-labelled allogeneic target cells in vitro; inhibition by isoantibody and by drugs. *Immunology* 1968;14:181–196.

33. Brondz BD. Complex specificity of immune lymphocytes in allogeneic cell cultures. *Folia Biol* 1968;14:115–131.

34. Golstein P, Svedmyr EAJ, Wigzell H. Cells mediating specific in vitro cytotoxicity. I. Detection of receptor-bearing lymphocytes. *J Exp Med* 1971; 134:1385–1402.

35. Wagner H, Röllinghoff M. T cell-mediated cytotoxicity: discrimination between antigen recognition, lethal hit and cytolysis phase. *Eur J Immunol* 1974;4:745–750.

36. Golstein P, Smith ET. The lethal hit stage of mouse T and non-T cell-mediated cytolysis: differences in cation requirements and characterization of an analytical "cation pulse" method. *Eur J Immunol* 1976;6:31–37.

37. Martz E. Early steps in specific tumor cell lysis by sensitized mouse T-lymphocytes. I. Resolution and characterization. *J Immunol* 1975;115:261–267.

38. MacLennan ICM, Gotch FM, Golstein P. Limited specific T-cell mediated cytolysis in the absence of extracellular Ca^{++}. *Immunology* 1980;39:109–117.

39. Tirosh R, Berke G. T lymphocyte-mediated cytolysis as an excitatory process of the target. I. Evidence that the target may be the site of Ca^{++} action. *Cell Immunol* 1985;95:113–123.

40. Trenn G, Takayama H, Sitkovsky MV. Exocytosis of cytolytic granules may not be required for target cell lysis by cytotoxic T-lymphocytes. *Nature* 1987;330:72–74.

41. Ostergaard HL, Kane KP, Mescher MF, Clark WR. Cytotoxic T lymphocyte mediated lysis without release of serine esterase. *Nature* 1987;330:71–72.

42. Young JD-E, Clark WR, Liu C-C, Cohn ZA. A calcium- and perforin-independent pathway of killing mediated by murine cytolytic lymphocytes. *J Exp Med* 1987;166:1894–1899.

43. Sanderson CJ. The mechanism of T cell mediated cytotoxicity. II. Morphological studies of cell death by time-lapse microcinematography. *Proc R Soc Lond* 1976;192:241–255.

44. Don MM, Ablett G, Bishop CJ, et al. Death of cells by apoptosis following attachment of specifically allergized lymphocytes in vitro. *Aust J Exp Biol* 1977;55:407–417.

45. Matter A, Lisowska-Bernstein B, Ryser JE, Lamelin JP, Vassalli P. Mouse thymus-independent and thymus-derived lymphoid cells. II. Ultrastructural studies. *J Exp Med* 1972;136:1008–1030.

46. Zagury D, Bernard J, Thiernesse N, Feldman M, Berke G. Isolation and characterization of individual functionally reactive cytotoxic T lymphocytes: conjugation, killing, and recycling at the single cell level. *Eur J Immunol* 1975;5:818–822.

47. Bykovskaya SN, Rytenko AN, Rauschenbach MO, Bykovsky AF. Ultrastructural alteration of cytolytic T lymphocytes following their interaction with target cells. I. Hypertrophy and change of orientation of the Golgi apparatus. *Cell Immunol* 1978; 40:164–174.

48. Bykovskaya SN, Rytenko AN, Rauschenbach MO, Bykovsky AF. Ultrastructural alteration of cytolytic T lymphocytes following their interaction with target cells. II. Morphogenesis of secretory granules and intracellular vacuoles. *Cell Immunol* 1978;40:175–185.

49. Dourmashkin RR, Deteix P, Simone CB, Henkart P. Electron microscopic demonstration of lesions in target cell membranes associated with antibody-dependent cellular cytotoxicity. *Clin Exp Immunol* 1980;42:554–560.

50. Simone CB, Henkart P. Permeability changes induced in erythrocyte ghost targets by antibody-dependent cytotoxic effector cells: evidence for membrane pores. *J Immunol* 1980;124:954–963.

51. Podack ER, Dennert G. Assembly of two types of tubules with putative cytolytic function by cloned natural killer cells. *Nature* 1983;302:442–445.

52. Henkart P, Millard PJ, Reynolds CW, Henkart MP. Cytolytic activity of purified cytoplasmic granules from cytotoxic rat large granular lymphocyte tumors. *J Exp Med* 1984;160:75–93.

53. Podack ER, Konigsberg PJ. Cytolytic T cell granules. Isolation, structural, biochemical, and functional characterization. *J Exp Med* 1984;160: 695–710.

54. Criado M, Lindstrom JM, Anderson CG, Dennert G. Cytotoxic granules from killer cells: specificity of granules and insertion of channels of defined size into target membranes. *J Immunol* 1985;135: 4245–4251.

55. Podack ER, Young JD-E, Cohn ZA. Isolation and biochemical and functional characterization of perforin 1 from cytolytic T-cell granules. *Proc Natl Acad Sci USA* 1985;82:8629–8633.

56. Masson D, Tschopp J. Isolation of a lytic, pore-forming protein (perforin) from cytolytic T lymphocytes. *J Biol Chem* 1985;260:9069–9072.

57. Tschopp J, Nabholz M. Perforin-mediated target cell lysis by cytolytic T lymphocytes. *Annu in Rev Immunol* 1990;8:279–302.

58. Griffiths GM, Mueller C. Expression of perforin and granzymes in vivo: potential diagnostic markers for activated cytotoxic cells. *Immunol Today* 1991;12:415–419.

59. Podack ER, Hengartner H, Lichtenheld MG. A central role of perforin in cytolysis? *Annu Rev Immunol* 1991;9:129–157.

60. Yagita H, Nakata M, Kawasaki A, Shinkai Y, Okumura K. Role of perforin in lymphocyte-mediated cytolysis. *Adv Immunol* 1992;51:215–242.

61. Kägi D, Ledermann B, Bürki K, et al. Cytotoxicity mediated by T cells and natural killer cells is greatly impaired in perforin-deficient mice. *Nature* 1994;369:31–37.

62. Matter A. Microcinematographic and electron microscopic analysis of target cell lysis induced by cytotoxic T lymphocytes. *Immunology* 1979;36: 179–190.

63. Wyllie AH, Kerr JFR, Currie AR. Cell death: the significance of apoptosis. *Int Rev Cytol* 1980; 68:251–306.

64. Kerr JFR, Searle J, Harmon BV, Bishop CJ. Apoptosis. In: Potten CS (ed) *Perspectives on Mammalian Cell Death*. Oxford, Oxford University Press, 1987, pp 93–128.

65. Russell JH, Masakovski VR, Dobos CB. Mechanisms of immune lysis. I. Physiological distinction between target cell death mediated by cytotoxic T lymphocytes and antibody plus complement. *J Immunol* 1980;124:1100–1105.

66. Russell JH, Masakovski V, Rucinsky T, Phillips G. Mechanisms of immune lysis. III. Characterization of the nature and kinetics of the cytotoxic T lymphocyte-induced nuclear lesion in the target. *J Immunol* 1982;128:2087–2094.

67. Gromkowski SH, Brown TC, Masson D, Tschopp J. Lack of DNA degradation in target cells lysed by granules derived from cytolytic T lymphocytes. *J Immunol* 1988;141:774–778.

68. Duke RC, Persechini PM, Chang S, Liu C-C, Cohen JJ, Young JD-E. Purified perforin induces target cell lysis but not DNA fragmentation. *J Exp Med* 1989;170:1451–1456.

69. Bachvaroff RJ, Ayvazian JH, Skupp S, Rapaport FT. Specific restriction endonuclease degradation of DNA as a consequence of immunologically mediated cell damage. *Transplant Proc* 1977;9: 807–812.

70. Hameed A, Olsen KJ, Lee M-K, Lichtenheld MG, Podack ER. Cytolysis by Capermeable transmembrane channels: pore formation causes extensive DNA degradation and cell lysis. *J Exp Med* 1989;169:765–777.

71. Chang TW, Eisen HN. Effects of N-α-tosyl-L-lysyl-chloromethylketone on the activity of cytotoxic T lymphocytes. *J Immunol* 1980;124:1028–1033.

72. Redelman D, Hudig D. The mechanism of cell-mediated cytotoxicity. I. Killing by murine cytotoxic T lymphocytes requires cell surface thiols and activated proteases. *J Immunol* 1980;124:870–878.

73. Utsunomiya N, Nakanishi M. A serine protease triggers the initial step of transmembrane signalling in cytotoxic T cells. *J Biol Chem* 1986;261:16514–16517.

74. Pasternack MS, Eisen HN. A novel serine esterase expressed by cytotoxic T lymphocytes. *Nature* 1985;314:743–745.

75. Kramer MD, Binninger L, Schirrmacher V, et al. Characterization and isolation of a trypsin-like serine protease from a long-term culture cytolytic T cell line and its expression by functionally distinct T cells. *J Immunol* 1986;136:4644–4651.

76. Masson D, Nabholz M, Estrade C, Tschopp J. Granules of cytolytic T-lymphocytes contain two serine esterases. *EMBO J* 1986;5:1595–1600.

77. Pasternack MS, Verret CR, Liu MA, Eisen HN. Serine esterase in cytolytic T lymphocytes. *Nature* 1986;322:740–743.

78. Simon MM, Hoschützky H, Fruth U, Simon H-G, Kramer MD. Purification and characterization of a T cell specific serine proteinase (TSP-1) from cloned cytolytic T lymphocytes. *EMBO J* 1986;5: 3267–3274.

79. Young JD-E, Leong LG, Liu C-C, Damiano A, Wall DA, Cohn ZA. Isolation and characterization of a serine esterase from cytolytic T cell granules. *Cell* 1986;47:183–194.

80. Brunet J-F, Dosseto M, Denizot F, et al. The inducible cytotoxic-T-lymphocyte-associated gene transcript CTLA-1 sequence and gene localization to mouse chromosome 14. *Nature* 1986;322:268–271.

81. Gershenfeld HK, Weissman IL. Cloning of a cDNA for a T cell-specific serine protease from a cytotoxic T lymphocyte. *Science* 1986;232:854–858.

82. Lobe CG, Finlay BB, Paranchych W, Paetkau VH, Bleackley RC. Novel serine proteases encoded by two cytotoxic T lymphocyte-specific genes. *Science* 1986;232:858–861.

83. Simon MM, Fruth U, Simon H-G, Gay S, Kramer MD. Evidence for multiple functions of T-lymphocytes associated serine proteinases. *Adv Exp Med Biol* 1990;247A:609–613.

84. Hudig D, Ewoldt GR, Woodard SL. Proteases and lymphocyte cytotoxic killing mechanisms. *Curr Opin Immunol* 1993;5:90–96.

85. Masson D, Zamai M, Tschopp, J. Identification of granzme A isolated from cytotoxic T lymphocyte granules as one of the proteases encoded by CTL-specific genes. *FEBS Lett* 1986;208:84–88.

86. Jenne DE, Zimmer M, Garcia-Sanz JA, Tschopp J, Lichter P. Genomic organization and subchro-

mosomal in situ localization of the murine granzyme F, a serine protease expressed in CD8$^+$ T cells. *J Immunol* 1991;147:1045–1052.

87. Trapani JA, Jans DA, Sutton VR. Lymphocyte granule-mediated cell death. *Springer Semin Immunopathol* 1998;19:323–343.

88. Brunet J-F, Denizot F, Suzan M, et al. CTLA-1 and CTLA-3 serine-esterase transcripts are detected mostly in cytotoxic cells, but not only and not always. *J Immunol* 1987;138:4102–4105.

89. Hayes MP, Berrebi GA, Henkart PA. Induction of target cell DNA release by the cytotoxic T lymphocyte granule protease granzyme A. *J Exp Med* 1989;170:933–946.

90. Shiver JW, Henkart PA. A noncytotoxic mast cell tumor line exhibits potent IgE-dependent cytotoxicity after transfection with the cytolysin/perforin gene. *Cell* 1991;64:1175–1181.

91. Shiver JW, Su L, Henkart PA. Cytotoxicity with target DNA breakdown by rat basophilic leukemia cells expressing both cytolysin and granzyme A. *Cell* 1992;71:315–322.

92. Shi L, Kraut RP, Aebersold R, Greeberg AH. A natural killer cell granule protein that induces DNA fragmentation and apoptosis. *J Exp Med* 1992;175:553–566.

93. Shi L, Kam C-M, Powers JC, Aebersold R, Greenberg AH. Purification of three cytotoxic lymphocyte granule serine proteases that induce apoptosis through distinct substrate and target cell interactions. *J Exp Med* 1992;176:1521–1529.

94. Heusel JW, Wesselschmidt RL, Shresta S, Russell JH, Ley TJ. Cytotoxic lymphocytes require granzyme B for the rapid induction of DNA fragmentation and apoptosis in allogeneic target cells. *Cell* 1994;76:977–987.

95. Clarke PGH, Clarke S. Historic apoptosis. *Nature* 1995;378:230.

96. Saunders JW Jr. Death in embryonic systems. *Science* 1966;154:604–612.

97. Hammar SP, Mottet NK. Tetrazolium salt and electron-microscopic studies of celluar degeneration and necrosis in the interdigital areas of the developing chick limb. *J Cell Sci* 1971;8:229–251.

98. Kerr JFR, Harmon B, Searle J. An electron-microscope study of cell deletion in the anuran tadpole tail during spontaneous metamorphosis with special reference to apoptosis of striated muscle fibres. *J Cell Sci* 1974;14:571–585.

99. Hinchliffe JR. Cell death in embryogenesis. In: Bowen ID, Lockshin RA (eds) *Cell Death in Biology and Pathology.* London, Champman & Hall, 1981, pp 35–78.

100. Lockshin RA, Zakeri Z. Programmed cell death and apoptosis. In: Tomei LD, Cope FO (eds) *Apoptosis. The Molecular Basis of Cell Death.* Cold Spring Harbor, NY, Cold Spring Harbor Laboratory Press, 1991, pp 47–60.

101. Zakeri ZF, Quaglino D, Latham T, Lockshin RA. Delayed internucleosomal DNA fragmentation in programmed cell death. *FASEB* 1993;7:470–478.

102. Cowan WM, Fawcett JW, O'Leary DDM, Stanfield BB. Regressive events in neurogenesis. *Science* 1984;225:1258–1265.

103. Catsicas S, Thanos S, Clarke PGH. Major role for

104. Oppenheim RW. Cell death during development of the nervous system. *Annu Rev Neurosci* 1991;14:453–501.

105. Martin DP, Johnson EM Jr: Programmed cell death in the peripheral nervous system. In: Tomei LD, Cope FO (eds) *Apoptosis: The Molecular Basis of Cell Death.* Cold Spring Harbor, NY, Cold Spring Harbor Laboratory Press, 1991, pp 247–261.

106. Johnson EM Jr, Deckwerth TL. Molecular mechanisms of developmental neuronal death. *Annu Rev Neurosci* 1993;16:31–46.

107. Cohen JJ. Programmed cell death in the immune system. *Adv Immunol* 1991;50:55–83.

108. Golstein P, Ojcius DM, Young JD-E. Cell death mechanisms and the immune system. *Immunol Rev* 1991;121:29–65.

109. Kerr JFR, Wyllie AH, Currie AR. Apoptosis: a basic biological phenomenon with wide-ranging implications in tissue kinetics. *Br J Cancer* 1972;26:239–257.

110. Williamson R. Properties of rapidly labelled deoxyribonucleic acid fragments isolated from the cytoplasm of primary cultures of embryonic mouse liver cells. *J Mol Biol* 1970;51:157–168.

111. Williams JR, Little JB, Shipley WU. Association of mammalian cell death with a specific endonucleolytic degradation of DNA. *Nature* 1974; 252:754–755.

112. Appleby DW, Modak SP. DNA degradation in terminally differentiating lens fiber cells from chick embryos. *Proc Natl Acad Sci USA* 1977;74:5579–5583.

113. Wyllie AH. Glucocorticoid-induced thymocyte apoptosis is associated with endogenous endonuclease activation. *Nature* 1980;284:555–556.

114. Cohen JJ, Duke RC. Glucocorticoid activation of a calcium-dependent endonuclease in thymocyte nuclei leads to cell death. *J Immunol* 1984; 132:38–42.

115. Wyllie AH, Morris RG, Smith AL, Dunlop D. Chromatin cleavage in apoptosis: association with condensed chromatin morphology and dependence on macromolecular synthesis. *J Pathol* 1984;142:67–77.

116. Clarke PGH. Developmental cell death: morphological diversity and multiple mechanisms. *Anat Embryol* 1990;181:195–213.

117. Schwartz LM, Smith SW, Jones MEE, Osborne BA. Do all programmed cell deaths occur via apoptosis? *Proc Nat Acad Sci USA* 1993;90: 980–984.

118. Vaux DL. Toward an understanding of the molecular mechanisms of physiological cell death. *Proc Natl Acad Sci USA* 1993;90:786–789.

119. Schwartz LM, Osborne BA. Programmed cell death, apoptosis and killer genes. *Immunol Today* 1993;14:582–590.

120. Hedgecock EM, Sulston JE, Thomson JN. Mutations affecting programmed cell death in the nematode *Caenorhabitis elegans. Science* 1983;220:1277–1279.

121. Ellis HM, Horvitz HR. Genetic control of pro-

grammed cell death in the nematode *C. elegans*. *Cell* 1986;44:817–829.

122. Ellis RE. Negative regulators of programmed cell death. *Curr Opin Gen Dev* 1992;2:635–641.

123. Miura M, Zhu H, Rotello R, Hartwieg EA, Yuan J. Induction of apoptosis in fibroblasts by IL-1 b-converting enzyme, a mammalian homolog of the *C. elegans* cell death gene *ced-3*. *Cell* 1993; 75:653–660.

124. Thornberry NA, Lazebnik Y. Caspases: enemies within. *Science* 1998;281:1312–1316.

125. Ellis HM, Horvitz HR. Genetic control of programmed cell death in the nematode *C. elegans*. *Cell* 1986;44:817–829.

126. Yuan J, Horvitz HR. The *Caenorhabditis elegans* cell death gene *ced-4* encodes a novel protein and is expressed during the period of extensive programmed cell death. *Development* 1992;116: 309–320.

127. Zou H, Henzel WJ, Liu X, Lutschg A, Wang X. Apaf-1, a human protein homologous to *C. elegans* CED-4, participates in cytochrome c-dependent activation of caspase-3. *Cell* 1997;90:405–413.

128. Hengartner MO, Ellis RE, Horvitz HR. *Caenorhabditis elegans* gene *ced-9* protects cells from programmed cell death. *Nature* 1992;356:494–499.

129. Vaux DL, Cory S, Adams JM. *Bcl-2* gene promotes haemopoietic cell survival and cooperates with *c-myc* to immortalize pre-B cells. *Nature* 1988; 335:440–442.

130. Boise LH, González-García M, Postema CE, et al. *bcl-x*, a *bcl-2*-related gene that functions as a dominant regulator of apoptotic cell death. *Cell* 1993;74:597–608.

131. Oltvai ZN, Milliman CL, Korsmeyer SJ. Bcl-2 heterodimerizes in vivo with a conserved homolog, Bax, that accelerates programmed cell death. *Cell* 1993;74:609–619.

132. Adams JM, Cory S. The bcl-2 protein family: arbiters of cell survival. *Science* 1998;281:1322–1326.

133. Green D, Kroemer G. The central executioners of apoptosis: caspases or mitochondria? *Trends Cell Biol* 1998;8:267–271.

134. Depraetere V, Golstein P. Dismantling in cell death: molecular mechanisms and relationship to caspase activation. *Scand J Immunol* 1998;47: 523–531.

135. Depraetere V, Golstein P. Fas and other cell death signaling pathways. *Semin Immunol* 1997;9: 93–107.

136. White K, Grether ME, Abrams JM, Young L, Farrell K, Steller H. Genetic control of programmed cell death in *Drosophila*. *Science* 1994;264:677–683.

137. Grether ME, Abrams JM, Agapite J, White K, Steller H. The head involution defective gene of *Drosophila melanogaster* functions in programmed cell death. *Genes Dev* 1995;9:1694–1708.

138. Chen P, Nordstrom W, Gish B, Abrams JM. *grim*, a novel cell death gene in *Drosophila*. *Genes Dev* 1996;10:1773–1782.

139. Golstein P. Cell death: TRAIL and its receptors. *Curr Biol* 1997;7:R750–R753.

140. Golstein P, Marguet D, Depraetere V. Homology between Reaper and the cell death domains of Fas

and TNFR1 [letter to the editor]. *Cell* 1995; 81:185–186.

141. Young JD-E, Damiano A, Dinome MA, Leong LG, Cohn ZA. Dissociation of membrane binding and lytic activities of the lymphocyte pore-forming protein (perforin). *J Exp Med* 1987;165:1371–1382.

142. Ishiura S, Matsuda K, Koizumi H, Tsukahara T, Arahata K, Sugita H. Calcium is essential for both the membrane binding and lytic activity of pore-forming protein (perforin) from cytotoxic T-lymphocyte. *Mol Immunol* 1990;27:803–807.

143. Conzelmann A, Corthésy P, Cianfriglia M, Silva A, Nabholz M. Hybrids between rat lymphoma and mouse T cells with inducible cytolytic activity. *Nature* 1982;298:170–172.

144. Golstein P, Mattéi M-G, Foa C, Luciani M-F. Molecular mechanisms of T lymphocyte cytotoxicity, with emphasis on the Fas pathway. In: Gregory CD (ed) *Apoptosis and the Immune Response*. New York, Wiley, 1995, pp 143–168.

145. Rouvier E, Luciani M-F, Golstein P. Fas involvement in Ca^{++}-independent T cell-mediated cytotoxicity. *J Exp Med* 1993;177:195–200.

146. Luciani M-F, Golstein P. Fas-based d10S-mediated cytotoxicity requires macromolecular synthesis for effector cell activation but not for target cell death. *R Soc Philos Trans B* 1994;345:303–309.

147. Yonehara S, Ishii A, Yonehara M. A cell-killing monoclonal antibody (anti-Fas) to a cell surface antigen co-downregulated with the receptor of tumor necrosis factor. *J Exp Med* 1989;169:1747–1756.

148. Trauth BC, Klas C, Peters AMJ, et al. Monoclonal antibody-mediated tumor regression by induction of apoptosis, *Science* 1989;245:301–305.

149. Itoh N, Yonehara S, Ishii A, et al. The polypeptide encoded by the cDNA for human cell surface antigen Fas can mediate apoptosis. *Cell* 1991;66: 233–243.

150. Watanabe-Fukunaga R, Brannan CI, Itoh N, et al. The cDNA structure, expression, and chromosomal assignment of the mouse Fas antigen. *J Immunol* 1992;148:1274–1279.

151. Davidson WF, Dumont FJ, Bedigian HG, Fowlkes BJ, Morse HC III. Phenotypic, functional, and molecular genetic comparisons of the abnormal lymphoid cells of C3H-*lpr/lpr* and C3H-*gld/gld* mice. *J Immunol* 1986;136:4075–4084.

152. Watanabe-Fukunaga R, Brannan CI, Copeland NG, Jenkins NA, Nagata S. Lymphproliferation disorder in mice explained by defects in Fas antigen that mediates apoptosis. *Nature* 1992;356:314–317.

153. Roths JB, Murphy ED, Eicher EM. A new mutation, *gld*, that produces lymphoproliferation and autoimmunity in C3H/HeJ mice. *J Exp Med* 1984;159:1–20.

154. Kägi D, Vignaux F, Ledermann B, et al. Fas and perforin pathways as major mechanisms of T cell-mediated cytotoxicity. *Science* 1994;265:528–530.

155. Vignaux F, Golstein P. Fas-based lymphocyte-mediated cytotoxicity against syngeneic activated lymphocytes: a regulatory pathway? *Eur J Immunol* 1994;24:923–927.

156. Ramsdell F, Seaman MS, Miller RE, Tough TW, Alderson MR, Lynch DH. *gld/gld* mice are unable

to express a functional ligand for Fas. *Eur J Immunol* 1994;24:928–933.

157. Lowin B, Hahne M, Mattmann C, Tschopp J. Cytolytic T-cell cytotoxicity is mediated through perforin and Fas lytic pathways. *Nature* 1994; 370:650–652.

158. Stalder T, Hahn S, Erb P. Fas antigen is the major target molecule for CD4$^+$ T cell-mediated cytotoxicity. *J Immunol* 1994;152:1127–1133.

159. Hanabuchi S, Koyanagi M, Kawasaki A, et al. Fas and its ligand in a general mechanism of T-cell-mediated cytotoxicity. *Proc Natl Acad Sci USA* 1994;91:4930–4934.

160. Ju S-T, Cui H, Panka DJ, Ettinger R, Marshak-Rothstein A. Participation of target Fas protein in apoptosis pathway induced by CD4$^+$ Th1 and CD8$^+$ cytotoxic T cells. *Proc Natl Acad Sci USA* 1994;91:4185–4189.

161. Anel A, Buferne M, Boyer C, Schmitt-Verhulst A-M, Golstein P. T cell receptor-induced Fas ligand expression in cytotoxic T lymphocyte clones is blocked by protein tyrosine kinase inhibitors and cyclosporin A. *Eur J Immunol* 1994;24:2469–2476.

162. Ramsdell F, Seaman MS, Miller RE, Picha KS, Kennedy MK, Lynch DH. Differential ability of Th1 and Th2 T cells to express Fas ligand and to undergo activation-induced cell death. *Int Immunol* 1994;6:1545–1553.

163. Suda T, Takahashi T, Golstein P, Nagata S. Molecular cloning and expression of the Fas ligand: a novel member of the tumor necrosis factor family. *Cell* 1993;75:1169–1178.

164. Vignaux F, Vivier E, Malissen B, Depraetere V, Nagata S, Golstein P. TCR/CD3 coupling to Fas-based cytotoxicity. *J Exp Med* 1995;181:781–786.

165. Walsh CM, Glass AA, Chiu V, Clark WR. The role of the *Fas* lytic pathway in a perforin-less CTL hybridoma. *J Immunol* 1994;153:2506–2514.

166. Alderson MR, Tough TW, Braddy S, et al. Regulation of apoptosis and T cell activation by Fas-specific mAb. *Int Immunol* 1994;6:1799–1806.

167. Kojima H, Shinohara N, Hanaoka S, et al. Two distinct pathways of specific killing revealed by perforin mutant cytotoxic T lymphocytes. *Immunity* 1994;1:357–364.

168. Ando K, Hiroishi K, Kaneko T, et al. Perforin, Fas/Fas ligand, and TNF-alpha pathways as specific and bystander killing mechanisms of hepatitis C virus-specific human CTL. *J Immunol* 1997;158:5283–5291.

169. Thornberry NA, Rano TA, Peterson EP, et al. A combinatorial approach defines specificities of members of the caspase family and granzyme B: functional relationships established for key mediators of apoptosis. *J Biol Chem* 1997;272:17907–17911.

170. Darmon AJ, Nicholson DW, Bleackley RC. Activation of the apoptotic protease CPP32 by cytotoxic T-cell-derived granzyme B. *Nature* 1995; 377:446–448.

171. Andrade F, Roy S, Nicholson D, Thornberry N, Rosen A, Casciola-Rosen L. Granzyme B directly and efficiently cleaves several downstream caspase substrates: implications for CTL-induced apoptosis. *Immunity* 1998;8:451–460.

172. Shi L, Chen G, MacDonald G, et al. Activation of an interleukin 1 converting enzyme-dependent apoptosis pathway by granzyme B. *Proc Natl Acad Sci USA* 1996;93:11002–11007.

173. Darmon AJ, Ley TJ, Nicholson DW, Bleackley RC. Cleavage of CPP32 by granzyme B represents a critical role for granzyme B in the induction of target cell DNA fragmentation. *J Biol Chem* 1996;271:21709–21712.

174. Sarin A, Williams MS, Alexander-Miller MA, Berzofsky JA, Zacharchuk CM, Henkart PA. Target cell lysis by CTL granule exocytosis is independent of ICE/Ced-3 family proteases. *Immunity* 1997;6:209–215.

175. Trapani JA, Browne KA, Smyth MJ, Jans DA. Localization of granzyme B in the nucleus: a putative role in the mechanism of cytotoxic lymphocyte-mediated apoptosis. *J Biol Chem* 1996; 271:4127–4133.

176. Pinkoski MJ, Winkler U, Hudig D, Bleackley RC. Binding of granzyme B in the nucleus of target cells: recognition of an 80-kilodalton protein. *J Biol Chem* 1996;271:10225–10229.

177. Froelich CJ, Orth K, Turbov J, et al. New paradigm for lymphocyte granule-mediated cytotoxicity: target cells bind and internalize granzyme B, but an endosomolytic agent is necessary for cytosolic delivery and subsequent apoptosis. *J Biol Chem* 1996;271:29073–29079.

178. Shi L, Mai S, Israels S, Browne K, Trapani JA, Greenberg AH. Granzyme B (GraB) autonomously crosses the cell membrane and perforin initiates apoptosis and GraB nuclear localization. *J Exp Med* 1997;185:855–866.

179. Muzio M, Chinnaiyan AM, Kischkel FC, et al. FLICE, a novel FADD-homologous ICE/CED-3-like protease, is recruited to the CD95 (Fas/APO-1) death-inducing signaling complex. *Cell* 1996;85:817–827.

180. Boldin MP, Goncharov TM, Goltsev YV, Wallach D. Involvement of MACH, a novel MORT1/FADD-interacting protease, in Fas/APO-1- and TNF receptor-induced cell death. *Cell* 1996;85: 803–815.

181. Wei S, Gamero AM, Liu JH, et al. Control of lytic function by mitogen-activated protein kinase/extracellular regulatory kinase 2 (ERK2) in a human natural killer cell line: identification of perforin and granzyme B mobilization by functional ERK2. *J Exp Med* 1998;187:1753–1765.

182. Holmstrom TH, Chow SC, Elo I, et al. Suppression of Fas/APO-1-mediated apoptosis by mitogen-activated kinase signaling. *J Immunol* 1998;160:2626–2636.

183. Vella A, Teague TK, Ihle J, Kappler J, Marrack P. Interleukin 4 (IL-4) or IL-7 prevents the death of resting T cells: stat6 is probably not required for the effect of IL-4. *J Exp Med* 1997;186:325–330.

Cytotoxic Cells: Basic Mechanisms and Medical Applications, edited by Michail V. Sitkovsky and Pierre A. Henkart. Lippincott Williams & Wilkins, Philadelphia © 2000.

II / TARGET CELL RECOGNITION

Chapter 2

MHC Class I Interactions in T Cell and Natural Killer Cell Immunity

David H. Margulies, Doo Hyun Chung, *Fumito Tani, and Kannan Natarajan

*Molecular Biology Section, Laboratory of Immunology, National Institute of Allergy and Infectious Diseases, National Institutes of Health, Bethesda, Maryland 20892-1892, USA; *Research Institute for Food Science, Kyoto University, Gokasho, Uji, Kyoto 611, Japan*

Cytotoxic lymphocytes kill cells that have been infected with cellular pathogens, such as viruses, or that are phenotypically transformed, as tumor cells. The recognition of such infected or aberrant cells is based on interactions of receptors on the effector T cells with ligands on the targets. Cytotoxic T lymphocytes (CTLs) employ their $\alpha\beta$ immunoglobulin-like T cell receptors (TCRs) to engage major histocompatibility complex (MHC) class I molecules bound to peptide antigens derived from the pathogen or the dysregulated cell to initiate a cascade of signaling events leading to activation of the cytolytic pathway. Natural killer (NK) cells, immune effector cells that lack the immunoglobulin-like T cell receptors, use other NK activating and inhibitory receptors to sense the metabolic state of their targets before killing them. Like CTLs, these NK cells engage MHC class I molecules, though the rules of interaction are very different. In this review we explore the similarities and differences of TCR–MHC and NKR–MHC interactions and speculate on the origin and evolution of these systems that exploit the same family of target receptors.

INTRODUCTION

During the course of their lifetime, vertebrates are repeatedly challenged by infec-

tious agents such as viruses and other cellular parasites and also by their own cells that have succumbed to the cellular dysregulation of oncogenesis. To deal with these threats to survival, cellular recognition systems have evolved that permit the host to identify such aberrant cells and destroy them. The elegant recognition systems that have developed for this purpose are those of both the innate and the adaptive immune systems: coordinated armies of cells and their expressed proteins that first recognize and then react to the nonself and foreign invaders.

The major effector arms of the adaptive immune system, T and B lymphocytes, which express cell surface receptors that result from somatic recombination of distinct variable (V) and constant (C) segments, have been the focus of functional and detailed molecular and genetic studies for years. Based on these analyses, we now understand a great deal about the nature of antigen recognition by antibodies (1,2) and the way TCRs identify target cells or antigen presenting cells bearing specific MHC–peptide complexes (3,4). For the purposes of this review, the focus of our discussion is the TCR, most specifically the $\alpha\beta$ receptor, which binds to MHC class I or class II molecules complexed with specific peptide antigens. Because the subject of this book is cytotoxic cells, we concern our discussion primarily with $\alpha\beta$

TCRs of CD8$^+$ T cells that see classic MHC class I molecules bound to viral or self peptides. Because there has been significant recent progress in several areas of adaptive immune recognition, we also discuss the recognition of peptides bearing carbohydrate antigens, recognition of formyl-methionyl antigens (representative of mitochondrially expressed proteins or bacterial proteins), and lipid antigens presented by the MHC I-related molecule CD1.

The other major advance of the past several years has been the discovery of the important role MHC-I molecules play in the recognition by effector cells of the innate immune system (5), the NK cells (6–8). We now know that receptors on NK cells fall into two major categories: activating receptors and inhibitory receptors. Strong evidence supports the view that some of the inhibitory receptors interact with MHC-I molecules on target cells and that the resulting negative signals modulate the constitutive propensity of the NK effector cell to lyse a cell. The contribution of carbohydrates and of MHC-bound peptides in the functional outcome of this recognition is summarized.

The last major topic we discuss here is the general notion that MHC-I molecules have evolved, and likely continue to evolve, as ligands for a wide variety of molecules. As mentioned above, they serve to interact with T cell $\alpha\beta$ receptors, and they bind NK receptors. Members of the MHC-I family bind peptides, glycopeptides, lipids, and heavy metals. In addition to interacting with TCRs and NK receptors, other members of the MHC-I family can serve as Fc receptors (9), and they can interact with transferrin receptors (10,11) and insulin receptors (12).

BASIC RULES OF PRESENTATION OF PEPTIDES TO THE TCR OF CD8$^+$ T CELLS

A major function of CD8$^+$ T cells is to serve as the cytolytic effectors that recognize specific MHC molecules bound to specific peptides. These peptides are generated from the endogenous peptide pathway, which depends on the normal expression of classic MHC-I molecules (e.g., HLA-A and HLA-B family molecules in humans, and H-2K, D, and L molecules of the mouse), normal function of cytoplasmic proteasomes, normal function of transporters associated with antigen processing (TAP) genes that encode molecules critical to the transfer of peptides from the cytosol to the lumen of the endoplasmic reticulum, and normal expression of the light chain of the MHC-I molecule, β_2-microglobulin (β2-m) (13,14). Thus the usual scenario of antigen presentation to T cells via the MHC-I pathway is that the classic MHC-I molecules, during the course of their biosynthesis, folding, and assembly in the endoplasmic reticulum (ER), gather available peptide fragments that have arisen in the cytosol and have been delivered to the lumen of the ER by TAP molecules. The assembled MHC-I molecules are thus not a homogeneous species but, rather, a population decorated with different peptides. When these MHC-I–peptide complexes arrive at the cell surface, they are available for recognition by surveying T cells.

T cells bearing clonally distributed $\alpha\beta$ receptors, selected in the thymus for weak reactivity against self MHC-I molecules, then identify the particular set of cells bearing the cognate MHC-I–peptide complex; and the binding reaction of the TCRs for the MHC–peptide complex initiates activation of the T cell. A range of affinities of TCRs for MHC–peptide complexes have been measured in both MHC-I-restricted and MHC-II-restricted systems. By and large, the affinities of the specific TCRs for the MHC-I–peptide complex are characterized by a moderate kinetic association rate constant and relatively rapid dissociation rate constants, and they show equilibrium constants ranging from 0.1 μM to more than 10 μM (15–18). That these parameters represent relatively low affinities compared to the intrinsic affinities of most antibodies for their antigens has been the basis of speculation concerning the mechanism of T cell activation (19). Recently, approaches for measuring the affinity of TCRs for MHC–peptide complexes on living cells have raised questions about whether molecules in addition to the MHC–peptide and the TCRs are critically involved in these recognition events (20).

AGONISTS, ANTAGONISTS, PARTIAL AND WEAK AGONISTS

For a particular T cell, a molecular complex of the appropriate MHC-I molecule and bound peptide is sufficient for activation (assuming of course that other needs, such as that of co-stimulation, are provided). Minimal systems, using engineered MHC-I molecules and synthetic peptides made multivalent by attachment to the surface of a tissue culture plate, have been used to evaluate some of the quantitative details of the initial recognition step in T cell activation (21,22).

Recently, the MHC–peptide complex has been more precisely described as an agonist, antagonist, or partial and weak agonist. Variant peptides have been identified that form MHC–peptide complexes that are less potent (weak agonist complexes) than the agonist. Remarkably, other peptide variants have been identified that form complexes with the MHC-I molecule that stimulate some but not all other effector functions in the T cell. These complexes are known as "partial agonists" (23,24). Such partial agonists may stimulate the production of one lymphokine by the T cell and not another, whereas the full agonist peptide–MHC complex effectively stimulates production of several. In some cases peptides in complex with the MHC molecule have been identified that fail to stimulate the T cell but paralyze it, precluding it from responding to a perfectly good agonist–MHC complex during a subsequent exposure. These peptide–MHC complexes are known as "antagonists"; a general name assigned to any peptide–MHC complex that stimulates the T cell in a less than full agonist manner is "altered peptide ligand," or APL (25). Although this nomenclature seems convenient, it simplistically directs attention to the peptide alone as the ligand for the TCR, whereas the biochemical and physiologic ligand is indeed the MHC–peptide complex. Several laboratories have attempted to explain the different functions of different MHC–peptide complexes with respect to agonism, partial and weak agonism, and antagonism in terms of the affinity or the kinetics of the interaction of the MHC–peptide complex with the TCR. Models that include "kinetic proofreading" and "receptor reengagement" have been proposed (26,27). In addition, some evidence of the differential ability of different MHC–peptide complexes to bind the TCR and promote multimeric interactions has been obtained (28–31). It has been proposed that agonist peptides form complexes with the MHC that are capable of multimerizing, but antagonist peptides fail to promote the multimerization. Not all data are consistent with this view (32,33). This remains an area of active investigation. Whatever the mechanistic explanation, it remains clear that different peptides, as part of an MHC complex, may generate TCR ligands that result in different signals being delivered to the T cell (34,35).

STRUCTURES OF MHC–PEPTIDE COMPLEXES

Our knowledge of MHC–peptide structure is detailed owing to the success of many laboratories in determining x-ray crystallographic structures of MHC molecules of the MHC-I (36), MHC-Ib (37,38), and MHC-II (39–42) families. For illustrative purposes, we show the structure of the murine MHC-I molecule, H-2D^d, complexed with a viral decamer peptide derived from the human immunodeficiency virus-1 (HIV-1) envelope glycoprotein 120 (43,44) (Fig. 2-1). This structure illustrates the major canonical features of the MHC-I family. In this case, the decamer peptide, RGPGRAFVTI, is bound tightly in the peptide binding groove, which consists of two antiparallel α-helices supported on a platform of eight strands of anti-

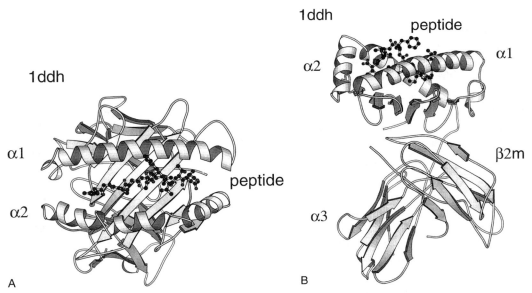

FIG. 2-1. Three-dimensional structure of H-2D^d complexed with a viral antigenic peptide. **A:** Murine MHC-I molecule H-2D^d complexed with a viral decamer peptide, RGPGRAFVTI, derived from the human immunodeficiency virus (HIV) IIIB envelope glycoprotein 120 [protein data bank (45) entry 1ddh] is shown in a side view. The cell surface is expected to be at the bottom of the picture. **B:** Top view of the same molecule, emphasizing the positions of the α1 and α2 helices and the bound peptide (illustrated in a ball-and-stick format). This figure was made with MOLSCRIPT 2.02 (49). Protein structure coordinates are now maintained by The Research Collaboratory for Structural Bioinformatics (http://www.rcsb.org/pdb/). The H-2D^d structure shown has been reported (43), as has an independently determined x-ray structure of the same complex (44).

parallel β-sheet. The platform is supported by the membrane proximal α3 domain and the light chain of the MHC-I molecule, β-2m. Some side chains of the bound peptide are deeply embedded in the binding cleft of the MHC molecule and serve as "anchor" residues to hold the peptide in place (with high affinity), and other amino acid side chains are exposed to the solvent, available for interaction with the TCR. These amino acids are called "epitopic," as they define the major contact sites of the TCR.

STRUCTURES OF MHC–TCR COMPLEXES

In addition to the structure of MHC molecules complexed with their respective peptides, several laboratories have successfully crystallized TCR-bound MHC–peptide (46–48). For illustrative purposes, we show the complex between a human TCR specific for HLA-A2 bound to the Tax peptide of human lymphotropic virus-1 (HTLV-1) (Fig. 2-2). This structure reveals the juxtaposition of the immunoglobulin-like TCR Vα and Vβ domains with the surface of the face of the MHC–peptide complex that includes the α1 helix, the bound peptide, and the α2 helix. The pairing of the Vα and Vβ domains of the TCR generates a molecular surface composed of the complementarity determining regions (CDRs) −1, −2, and −3 of each of the two chains. This surface then interacts with the MHC–peptide surface, with the CDR3 of Vα and Vβ contiguous and focused on the center of the bound peptide. Structures of the same TCR in isolation and bound to its MHC–peptide ligand reveal some local structural adjustments, but there are no major rearrangements observed (50,51). To date, the orientation of α and β chains of the

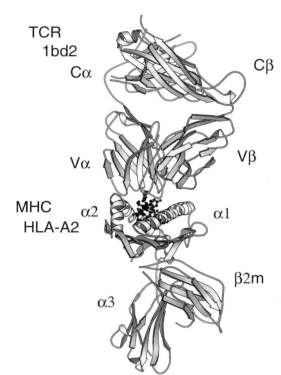

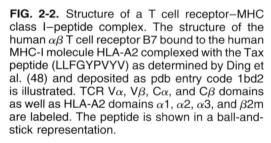

FIG. 2-2. Structure of a T cell receptor–MHC class I–peptide complex. The structure of the human αβ T cell receptor B7 bound to the human MHC-I molecule HLA-A2 complexed with the Tax peptide (LLFGYPVYV) as determined by Ding et al. (48) and deposited as pdb entry code 1bd2 is illustrated. TCR Vα, Vβ, Cα, and Cβ domains as well as HLA-A2 domains α1, α2, α3, and β2m are labeled. The peptide is shown in a ball-and-stick representation.

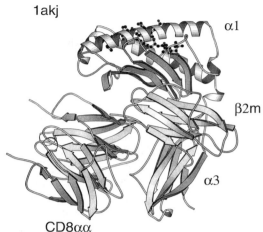

FIG. 2-3. Structure of the complex of the CD8αα homodimer bound to the HLA-A2 MHC-I molecule. The x-ray structure of HLA-A2 bound to the human CD8α domain homodimer has been reported (54) and is deposited as protein data bank entry number 1akj. The positions of the MHC-I domains α1, α3, and β2m, the and the CD8αα homodimer are indicated.

TCR with α toward the amino-terminus of the bound peptide, and β toward the carboxyl-terminus has been conserved in all structures of complexes examined.

STRUCTURES OF MHC–CD8 COMPLEXES

The αβ TCR-expressing T cells that recognize MHC-I–peptide complexes are predominantly of the CD8 class. Recent efforts to understand the interaction of the CD8 with MHC-I derive from affinity labeling experiments (52), CD8 mutagenesis experiments (53), and structure determination of both murine and human MHC molecules with CD8 αα homodimers (54,55). Also, binding studies with soluble CD8 preparations have been useful for understanding the contributions of this co-receptor (56). In Figure 2-3 we show the structure of the human CD8 αα complexed with HLA-A2. This structure is remarkable in that it shows that the immunoglobulin-like CD8 amino terminal domains form an antibody-like interface that is focused on the exposed loop of the HLA α3 domain. In addition, one domain of the CD8αα homodimer makes contact with the α2 helix of the MHC. Whether CD8 is involved in MHC multimerization is an open question at this time.

MHC–NK RECEPTOR INTERACTIONS

In addition to serving as the ligand for αβ T cell recognition by cytolytic cells, members of the MHC-I family interact with receptors on NK cells (57,58). Although the first identification of the interaction of NK receptors with MHC-I molecules was of the interaction of NK inhibitory receptors (59), it is becoming clear that both NK inhibitory and activating receptors are capable of interaction with MHC-I molecules. Members of the NK receptor superfamily belong to both the immunoglobulin superfamily and the C-type lectin family. In humans the predominant group of functional NK receptors are of the immunoglobulin (Ig) superfamily, whereas in the mouse the predominant functional receptors are of the C-type lectin family (60). A full review of this blossoming area of immune recognition is beyond the scope of this brief chapter, but it is important to understand that cytotoxic NK cells employ recognition of MHC-I molecules during both activation and inhibition. In the mouse the members of the Ly49 family of C-type lectin-like receptors have been shown to interact with the MHC-I molecule H-2D^d (Ly49A, Ly49D, and Ly49G2) (61–65) and H-2K^b (Ly49C) (66). Interactions of Ly49A, an inhibitory receptor, with H-2D^d have been shown to be dependent on the MHC-I molecule being peptide-bound, but no peptide specificity has been demonstrated (67,68). In humans the best characterized NK inhibitory receptors are those that have two Ig-like domains, known as KIR2DL2 and KIR2DL3. These domains show specificity for different alleles of HLA-C and discriminate between HLA-Cw3 and HLA-Cw4, which are polymorphic at positions 77 and 80 of the MHC-I molecule. In humans and the mouse, the activation receptors need to associate with a signal transducing chain, known as p12 or DAP-12, to convey the activating signal (69).

Of particular interest is the inhibitory receptor of the C-type lectin family, a heterodimer of CD94 and NKG2, found in both humans and the mouse. This heterodimer interacts with the human MHC-Ib molecule HLA-E (70,71), and in the mouse with the MHC-Ib molecule Qa-1 (72). It is provocative that the peptide required for this binding specificity is derived from an MHC-I leader peptide sequence.

THOUGHTS AND SPECULATION ON MHC-I EVOLUTION

In addition to the classic antigen-presenting function of the MHC-I molecules, by which peptides derived from the intracellular milieu are captured, co-assembled, and displayed at the cell surface for recognition by $\alpha\beta$ T cells with exquisite specificity, we now recognize the ability of MHC-I and MHC-Ib molecules to interact with more restricted families of effector ligands, such as NK receptors. In addition, there are several clear functions that other MHC-I-like molecules perform: They serve as receptors for the Fc portion of Igs to effect the transport of maternal Ig across the gut for delivery to the serum (9); they serve to bind nonpeptide ligands, such as mycobacterial lipids, for presentation to a restricted family of T cells (73–75); as the HLA-HFE protein and its murine homolog, they are involved in iron homeostasis (11); and as a ligand for the insulin receptor, they may play a role in carbohydrate metabolism (12). In addition, the demonstration that a serum protein, zinc α_2-globulin, a molecule with an MHC-I fold, may be a fat-binding protein suggests that the MHC fold has great potential for ligand and receptor binding.

A superficial and speculative scenario of the evolution of immune recognition would be as follows: (a) With the need for protection from parasites and infections that accompanied evolution of the multicellular organisms, a set of primitive immune cytolytic cells developed with receptors of the C-type lectin family, perhaps originally being activated by interaction with carbohydrates on the parasites themselves. (b) Further evolution, with the arrival of MHC-I-like molecules as surface molecules, permitted the development of cytotoxic cells that interacted with these MHC-I-like molecules. Perhaps early cytolytic receptors were predominantly influenced by carbohydrates rather than peptide. (c) Then came the evolution of recombinatorial immune receptors, such as T and B cell receptors. They show finer specificity than that observed with the lectins and reveal an ability to distinguish MHC molecules bound to different peptides, glycopeptides, or lipids. (d) Finally, modulation of the function of both NK cell lineages may have developed with the refinement of NK receptors as both inhibitory and activating molecules, employing interactions with both classic and nonclassic MHC-I molecules. In parallel with this immune strategy, the MHC-I molecules and their extended family are exploited for a wide variety of additional receptor and signaling functions. Further study of MHC-I molecules will certainly disclose more varied functions as a window on the evolution of these complex organisms.

REFERENCES

1. Wilson IA, Stanfield RL. Antibody-antigen interactions: new structures and new conformational changes. *Curr Opin Struct Biol* 1994;4:857.
2. Padlan EA. X-ray crystallography of antibodies. *Adv Protein Chem* 1996;49:57.
3. Ysern X, Li H, Mariuzza RA. Imperfect interfaces [news]. *Nat Struct Biol* 1998;5:412.
4. Garboczi DN, Biddison WE. Shapes of MHC restriction. *Immunity* 1999;10:1.
5. Medzhitov R, Janeway CA Jr. Innate immunity: the virtues of a nonclonal system of recognition. *Cell* 1997;91:295.
6. Lanier LL, Corliss B, Phillips JH. Arousal and inhibition of human NK cells. *Immunol Rev* 1997; 155:145.
7. Lanier LL, Phillips JH. Inhibitory MHC class I receptors on NK cells and T cells. *Immunol Today* 1996;17:86.
8. Yokoyama WM. Natural killer cells. In: Paul WE (ed) *Fundamental Immunology,* 4th ed. Lippincott-Raven Publishers, Philadelphia, 1999, p 575.
9. Simister NE, Ahouse JC. The structure and evolution of FcRn. *Res Immunol* 1996;147:333.
10. Wilson IA, Bjorkman PJ. Unusual MHC-like molecules: CD1, Fc receptor, the hemochromatosis gene product, and viral homologs. *Curr Opin Immunol* 1998;10:67.
11. Feder JN, Penny DM, Irrinki A, et al. The hemochromatosis gene product complexes with the transferrin receptor and lowers its affinity for ligand binding. *Proc Natl Acad Sci USA* 1998;95:1472.
12. Ramalingam TS, Chakrabarti A, Edidin M. Interaction of class I human leukocyte antigen (HLA-I) molecules with insulin receptors and its effect on the insulin-signaling cascade. *Mol Biol Cell* 1997;8:2463.
13. Germain RN, Margulies DH. The biochemistry and cell biology of antigen processing and presentation. *Annu Rev Immunol* 1993;11:403.
14. Pamer E, Cresswell P. Mechanisms of MHC class I-restricted antigen processing. *Annu Rev Immunol* 1998;16:323.
15. Matsui K, Boniface JJ, Steffner P, Reay PA, Davis MM. Kinetics of T-cell receptor binding to peptide/I-Ek complexes: correlation of the dissociation rate with T-cell responsiveness. *Proc Natl Acad Sci USA* 1994;91:12862.
16. Khilko SN, Jelonek MT, Corr M, Boyd LF, Bothwell AL, Margulies DH. Measuring interactions of MHC class I molecules using surface plasmon resonance. *J Immunol Methods* 1995;183:77.
17. Corr M, Slanetz AE, Boyd LF, et al. T cell receptor-MHC class I peptide interactions: affinity, kinetics, and specificity. *Science* 1994;265:946.
18. Davis MM, Boniface JJ, Reich Z, et al. Ligand recognition by alpha beta T cell receptors. *Annu Rev Immunol* 1998;16:523.
19. Margulies DH. Interactions of TCRs with MHC-peptide complexes: a quantitative basis for mechanistic models. *Curr Opin Immunol* 1997;9:390.
20. Sykulev Y, Vugmeyster Y, Brunmark A, Ploegh HL, Eisen HN. Peptide antagonism and T cell receptor interactions with peptide-MHC complexes. *Immunity* 1998;9:475.
21. McCluskey J, Boyd L, Highet P, Inman J, Margulies D. T cell activation by purified, soluble, class I MHC molecules. requirement for polyvalency. *J Immunol* 1988;141:1451.
22. Brower RC, England R, Takeshita T, et al. Minimal requirements for peptide mediated activation of CD8+ CTL. *Mol Immunol* 1994;31:1285.
23. Evavold BD, Allen PM. Separation of IL-4 production from Th cell proliferation by an altered T cell receptor ligand. *Science* 1991;252:1308.
24. Racioppi L, Ronchese F, Schwartz RH, Germain RN. The molecular basis of class II MHC allelic control of T cell responses. *J Immunol* 1991; 147:3718.
25. Evavold BD, Sloan-Lancaster J, Allen PM. Tickling the TCR: selective T-cell functions stimulated by altered peptide ligands. *Immunol Today* 1993; 14:602.
26. McKeithan TW. Kinetic proofreading in T-cell receptor signal transduction. *Proc Natl Acad Sci USA* 1995;92:5042.
27. Lanzavecchia A, Iezzi G, Viola A. From TCR engagement to T cell activation: a kinetic view of T cell behavior. *Cell* 1999;96:1.
28. Reich Z, Boniface JJ, Lyons DS, Borochov N, Wachtel EJ, Davis. MM. Ligand-specific oligomerization of T-cell receptor molecules. *Nature* 1997;387:617.
29. Alam SM, Travers PJ, Wung JL, et al. T cell receptor affinity and thymocyte positive selection. *Nature* 1996;381:616.
30. Alam SM, Davies GM, Lin CM, Zal T, et al. Qualitative and quantitative differences in T cell receptor binding of agonist and antagonist ligands. *Immunity* 1999;10:227.
31. Monks CR, Freiberg BA, Kupfer H, Sciaky N, Kupfer A. Three-dimensional segregation of supra-

molecular activation clusters in T cells. *Nature* 1998;395:82.

32. Al-Ramadi BK, Jelonek MT, Boyd LF, Margulies DH, Bothwell AL. Lack of strict correlation of functional sensitization with the apparent affinity of MHC/peptide complexes for the TCR. *J Immunol* 1995;155:662.

33. Willcox BE, Gao GF, Wyer JR, et al. TCR binding to peptide-MHC stabilizes a flexible recognition interface. *Immunity* 1999;10:357.

34. Sloan-Lancaster J, Shaw AS, Rothbard JB, Allen PM. Partial T cell signaling: altered phospho-zeta and lack of zap70 recruitment in APL-induced T cell anergy. *Cell* 1994;79:913.

35. Madrenas J, Wange RL, Wang JL, Isakov N, Samelson LE, Germain. RN. Zeta phosphorylation without ZAP-70 activation induced by TCR antagonists or partial agonists. *Science* 1995;267:515.

36. Madden DR. The three-dimensional structure of peptide-MHC complexes. *Annu Rev Immunol* 1995;13:545.

37. Wang CR, Lindahl KF, Deisenhofer J. Crystal structure of the MHC class Ib molecule H2-M3. *Res Immunol* 1996;147:313.

38. Zeng Z-H, Castaño AR, Segelke B, Stura EA, Peterson PA, Wilson IA. The crystal structure of murine CD1: an MHC-like fold but with a large hydrophobic antigen binding groove. *Science* 1997; 277:339.

39. Stern LJ, Brown JH, Jardetzky TS, et al. Crystal structure of the human class II MHC protein HLA-DR1 complexed with an influenza virus peptide. *Nature* 1994;368:215.

40. Brown JH, Jardetzky TS, Gorga JC, et al. Three-dimensional structure of the human class II histocompatibility antigen HLA-DR1. *Nature* 1993; 364:33.

41. Jardetzky TS, Brown JH, Gorga JC, et al. Three-dimensional structure of a human class II histocompatibility molecule complexed with superantigen. *Nature* 1994;368:711.

42. Fremont DH, Hendrickson WA, Marrack P, Kappler J. Structures of an MHC class II molecule with covalently bound single peptides. *Science* 1996; 272:1001.

43. Li H, Natarajan K, Malchiodi EL, Margulies DH, Mariuzza RA. Three-dimensional structure of H-2Dd complexed with an immunodominant peptide from human immunodeficiency virus envelope glycoprotein 120. *J Mol Biol* 1998;283:179.

44. Achour A, Persson K, Harris RA, et al. The crystal structure of H-2D^d MHC class I complexed with the HIV-1-derived peptide P18-I10 at 2.4 A resolution: implications for T cell and NK cell recognition. *Immunity* 1998;9:199.

45. Bernstein FC, Koetzle TF, Williams GJ, et al. The Protein Data Bank: a computer-based archival file for macromolecular structures. *J Mol Biol* 1977; 112:535.

46. Garcia KC, Degano M, Pease LR, et al. Structural basis of plasticity in T cell receptor recognition of a self peptide-MHC antigen. *Science* 1998;279:1166.

47. Garboczi DN, Ghosh P, Utz U, Fan QR, Biddison WE, Wiley DC. Structure of the complex between human T-cell receptor, viral peptide and HLA-A2. *Nature* 1996;384:134.

48. Ding YH, Smith KJ, Garboczi DN, Utz U, Biddison WE, Wiley DC. Two human T cell receptors bind in a similar diagonal mode to the HLA-A2/Tax peptide complex using different TCR amino acids. *Immunity* 1998;8:403.

49. Kraulis PJ. MOLSCRIPT: a program to produce both detailed and schematic plots of protein structures. *J Appl Crystallogr* 1991;24:946.

50. Garcia KC, Degano M, Pease LR, et al. Structural basis of plasticity in T cell receptor recognition of a self peptide-MHC antigen. *Science* 998;279:1166.

51. Garcia KC, Degano M, Stanfield RL, et al. An ABT cell receptor structure at 2.5 A and its orientation in the TCR-MHC complex. *Science* 1996;274:209.

52. Luescher IF, Vivier E, Layer A, et al. CD8 modulation of T-cell antigen receptor-ligand interactions on living cytotoxic T lymphocytes. *Nature* 1995;373:353.

53. Devine L, Sun J, Barr MR, Kavathas PB. Orientation of the Ig domains of CD8$\alpha\beta$ relative to MHC class I. *J Immunol* 1999;162:846.

54. Gao GF, Tormo J, Gerth UC, et al. Crystal structure of the complex between human CD8$\alpha\alpha$ and HLA-A2. *Nature* 1997;387:630.

55. Kern PS, Teng M-K, Smolyar A, et al. Structural basis of CD8 coreceptor function revealed by crystallographic analysis of a murine CD8$\alpha\alpha$ ectodomain fragment in complex with H-2K^b. *Immunity* 1998;9:519.

56. Wyer JR, Willcox BE, Gao GF, et al. T cell receptor and coreceptor CD8$\alpha\alpha$ bind peptide-MHC independently and with distinct kinetics. *Immunity* 1999;10:219.

57. Yokoyama WM. Recognition structures on natural killer cells. *Curr Opin Immunol* 1993;5:67.

58. Lanier LL. NK cell receptors. *Annu Rev Immunol* 1998;16:359.

59. Karlhofer FM, Ribaudo RK, Yokoyama WM. MHC class I alloantigen specificity of Ly-49$^+$ IL-2-activated natural killer cells. *Nature* 1992;358:66.

60. Long EO. Regulation of immune responses through inhibitory receptors. *Ann Rev Immunol* 1999;17:875.

61. Karlhofer FM, Ribaudo RK, Yokoyama WM. The interaction of Ly-49 with H-2Dd globally inactivates natural killer cell cytolytic activity. *Trans Assoc Am Physicians* 1992;105:72.

62. Mason LH, Ortaldo JR, Young HA, Kumar V, Bennett M, Anderson SK. Cloning and functional characteristics of murine large granular lymphocyte-1: a member of the Ly-49 gene family (Ly-49G2) [see comments]. *J Exp Med* 1995;182:293.

63. Tay CH, Yu LY, Kumar V, Mason L, Ortaldo JR, Welsh RM. The role of LY49 NK cell subsets in the regulation of murine cytomegalovirus infections. *J Immunol* 1999;162:718.

64. George TC, Mason LH, Ortaldo JR, Kumar V, Bennett M. Positive recognition of MHC class I molecules by the Ly49D receptor of murine NK cells. *J Immunol* 1999;162:2035.

65. Nakamura MC, Linnemeyer PA, Niemi EC, et al. Mouse Ly-49D recognizes H-2Dd and activates natural killer cell cytotoxicity. *J Exp Med* 1999;189:493.

66. Yu YY, George T, Dorfman JR, Roland J, Kumar V, Bennett M, The role of Ly49A and 5E6(Ly49C)

molecules in hybrid resistance mediated by murine natural killer cells against normal T cell blasts. *Immunity* 1996;4:67.

67. Correa I, Raulet DH. Binding of diverse peptides to MHC class I molecules inhibits target cell lysis by activated natural killer cells. *Immunity* 1995;2:61.

68. Orihuela M, Margulies DH, Yokoyama WM. The natural killer cell receptor Ly-49A recognizes a peptide-induced conformational determinant on its major histocompatibility complex class I ligand. *Proc Natl Acad Sci USA* 1996;93:11792.

69. Lanier LL, Corliss BC, Wu J, Leong C, Phillips JH. Immunoreceptor DAP12 bearing a tyrosine-based activation motif is involved in activating NK cells [see comments]. *Nature* 1998;391:703.

70. Braud VM, Allan DS, O'Callaghan CA, et al. HLA-E binds to natural killer cell receptors CD94/NKG2A, B and C. *Nature* 1998;391:795.

71. Braud V, Jones EY, McMichael A. The human major histocompatibility complex class Ib molecule HLA-E binds signal sequence-derived peptides with primary anchor residues at positions 2 and 9. *Eur J Immunol* 1997;27:1164.

72. Bai A, Broen J, Forman J. The pathway for processing leader-derived peptides that regulate the maturation and expression of Qa-1^b. *Immunity* 1998;9:413.

73. Porcelli SA, Brenner MB. Antigen presentation: mixing oil and water. *Curr Biol* 1997;7:R508.

74. Moody DB, Sugita M, Peters PJ, Brenner MB, Porcelli SA. The CD1-restricted T-cell response to mycobacteria. *Res Immunol* 1996;147:550.

75. Melian A, Beckman EM, Porcelli SA, Brenner M. Antigen presentation by CD1 and MHC-encoded class I-like molecules. *Curr Opin Immunol* 1996;8:82.

Cytotoxic Cells: Basic Mechanisms and Medical Applications, edited by Michail V. Sitkovsky and Pierre A. Henkart. Lippincott Williams & Wilkins, Philadelphia © 2000.

Chapter 3

Antigen Recognition by CD8⁺ CTLs

Denis Hudrisier and Immanuel F. Luescher

The Ludwig Institute for Cancer Research, Lausanne Branch, University of Lausanne, 1066 Epalinges, Switzerland

The cytotoxic lymphocytes (CTLs) of the CD8$^+$ type recognize peptides bound to major histocompatibility complex (MHC) class I molecules. These peptides usually are endogenously produced and are eight to ten residues long. In contrast to CD4$^+$ cells, MHC class I-restricted T cells cannot be activated by superantigens because the latter bind only to MHC class II molecules. Crystallographic studies showed that T cell receptors (TCRs) bind MHC-I–peptide complexes in a canonical diagonal orientation in which the MHC-bound peptide runs diagonally between the CDR3 loops, extending from CDR1α to CDR1β. The efficiency of antigen recognition by CTLs is significantly increased by the co-receptor CD8. CD8 increases the avidity of TCR–ligand binding by coordinate binding of TCR-associated MHC-I–peptide complexes and brings the tyrosine kinase p56^{lck} to the TCR–CD3 complex. Antigen recognition by CTLs generally elicits perforin- and Fas-dependent cytotoxicity as well as cytokine production, i.e., interferon gamma (IFNγ) and tumor necrosis factor alpha (TNFα). As for CD4$^+$ T cells, modifications of the peptide or the MHC molecule can affect CTL functions in a diverse manner. For example, they can abolish perforin-dependent killing or cytokine production (or both) while leaving Fas-dependent cytotoxicity unimpaired. Here we review the current knowledge of structural and thermodynamic aspects of TCR and TCR– ligand interactions and discuss how they are related to CTL activation and functional responses. We also discuss the various mechanisms relating to aberrant CTL functional responses.

INTRODUCTION

Adaptive cellular immunity is mainly mediated by T lymphocytes expressing α/β TCRs. In contrast to B lymphocytes, α/β TCRs expressing T lymphocytes recognize antigen in the form of antigen-derived peptides bound to MHC molecules. Mature α/β T cells express either CD4 or CD8 as co-receptor. The former are helper T (Th) cells, which recognize antigenic peptides in the context of MHC-II molecules, and the latter are mainly CTLs, which recognize peptides presented by MHC-I molecules. We first describe molecular and thermodynamic aspects of TCR and TCR–ligand interactions and those of CD8 and then relate this knowledge to antigen recognition by CD8$^+$ CTLs. Finally, we discuss aberrant functional responses of CTLs and their underlying mechanisms.

STRUCTURE OF TCRs AND TCR–LIGAND COMPLEXES

T cell receptors belong to the immunoglobulin superfamily and are composed of disulfide-linked, approximately equally sized α- and β-chains, both of which span the cell membrane (1,2). Their genes are formed by rearrangements of germline-encoded gene segments. Genes encoding for the TCR α-chain are formed by recombinations of variable (V), junctional (J), and constant (C) gene elements; and those encoding the TCR β-chain are produced by recombinations of V, J, diversity (D), and C gene elements (1, 2). The ligand binding site of TCR is formed by two Vα- and two Vβ-encoded CDR loops (CDR1α, CDR2α, CDR1β, and CDR2β) and two junctional, CDR3 loops (CDR3α and CDR3β). In the mouse there are 75 Vα and 23 Vβ and in humans 32 Vα and 138 Vβ. The junctional, or CDR3, loops are highly polymorphic, as they are encoded by recombinations of Vα/Jα and Vβ/Dβ/Jβ gene elements, respectively; and diversity is further increased by additional N-inserts in J and D sequences (1). Based on the limited number of TCR Vα and Vβ gene elements, it has been postulated that the V-encoded CDR1 and CDR2 loops primarily interact with the α-helices of MHC-molecules, which also have limited diversity, and that the hypervariable CDR3 loops primarily interact with residues of MHC bound peptides (1,2). Numerous observations indeed demonstrated that CDR3 residues interact with MHC bound peptides (3–6). More controversial was the orientation in which TCRs interact with MHC–peptide complexes, with different studies suggesting different orientations (3,5,7).

X-ray Crystallography of TCRs

Determination of the three-dimensional structures of TCR confirmed the expected anticipated immunoglobulin-like structure but also revealed several structural features that differentiate TCRs from antibodies. The main differences include the following: (a) The hinge region of TCR β-chains are much more rigid than those of V_L chains of immunoglobulins (8). (b) The TCR Cβ-chains have a unique surface exposed loop of 13 residues (residues 219–232) (Fig. 3-1C) (8).

(c) TCR Cα lacks a β-pleated sheet, compared to the immunoglobulin C_H, and therefore has a poorly ordered structure (9). This site may be a contact region for a CD3 component (see below). (d) In TCR Vα there is strand switch; that is, the C″ strand pairs with the D-strand and not with the C′-strand, as in other members of the immunoglobulin family (10). This implies a reorientation of CDR2α compared to CDR2 of immunoglobulin V_H and flattening of the outer surface of Vα. This finding led to the speculation that TCRs may dimerize via Vα–Vα pairing, as has been observed in Vα crystals (10). Moreover, in TCR CDR1 the loops are typically shorter and hence structurally more conserved than CDR2 loops, and the CDR3 loops on average are shorter and less heterogeneous in length than the immunoglobulins.

Three-Dimensional Structure Analysis of TCR–Ligand Complexes

Crystallographic studies revealed a "diagonal" TCR–ligand orientation in which the MHC-bound peptide runs diagonally between the two CDR3 loops, extending from CDR1α to CDR1β (9–14) (Fig. 3-1). In this orientation the CDR3 loops can interact extensively with the peptide side chains, which are mainly located in the center of the MHC molecules, and with residues of the MHC α-helices. The α-helices of MHC-I molecules are elevated at the N-terminal portions; therefore the approximately planar surface of the TCR–ligand binding site can realize the best contact with the ligand in this orientation (11). This orientation is conserved in all known TCR–MHC-I–peptide complexes, with a few degrees of rotational variability, pivoting or sliding the TCR ligand binding site along the MHC helices. The existence of conserved atomic interactions between TCR and MHC class I molecules, mainly between TCR Vα and residues of the MHC class I α-helices, in part define the observed canonical diagonal orientation of TCR-ligand binding. The existence of a universal orientation of TCR–ligand binding may fa-

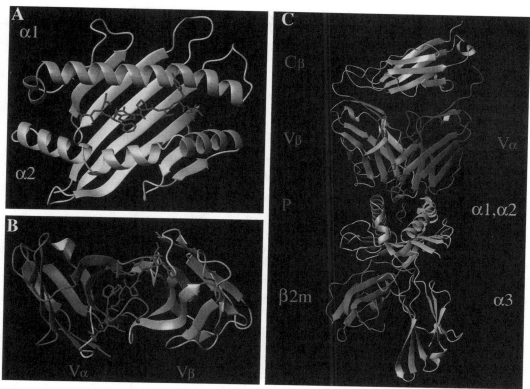

FIG. 3-1. A: Crystal structure of an MHC-I molecule (HLA-A2) presenting an antigenic peptide (tax peptide). **B, C:** A6 TCR–HLA-2–tax peptide complex (11). **B:** Of the complex only the TCR ligand binding site (in backbone ribbon representation) with the tax peptide (backbone with side chains) is shown. **C:** Ribbon diagram of the overall structure of the complex between the A6 TCR (*top*) and the tax peptide-HLA-A2 complex (*bottom*). The Cα domain is not shown. [From the published PDB file (11), using the MOLMOL program. **A** Courtesy of Olivier Michielin.]

cilitate the formation of TCR aggregates and in this sense may be relevant to TCR signaling (13). Because CD8 interacts with TCR-associated MHC-I molecules, the orientation of TCR–ligand interactions is expected to have implications for CD8 coreceptor functions (see below). Whereas CDR2 primarily contacts the MHC molecule, CDR3 interacts mainly with the peptide; CDR1 interacts with both the MHC molecule and the peptide (Fig. 3-1B) (11–13).

TCR–CD3 Complex

T cell receptors can reach the cell surface only after correct assembly with CD3 and ζ chains (15). The CD3 complex is composed of two ε-chains, one δ-chain, one γ-chain, and two ζ-chains (Fig. 3-2) (16). All are membrane spanning proteins consisting of a small unglycosylated extracellular portion, a transmembrane region, and a long cytoplasmic tail. All have membrane proximal cysteines that form disulfide-linked dimers: ε-δ and ε-γ heterodimers and a ζ-chain homodimer. The precise manner by which the various CD3–ζ components associate with TCRs is not known, but the association is strong; and TCR–CD3 complexes can be isolated from cell membranes or can be assembled *in vitro* (17). The TCR–CD3 association involves in part ionic interactions within the cell mem-

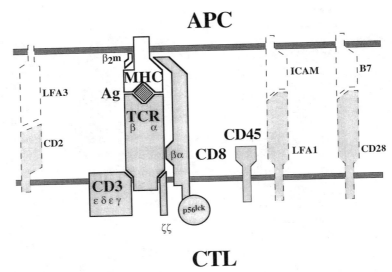

FIG. 3-2. Molecular interactions in CTL–target cell conjugates. Molecules on the antigen presenting cells (APCs) and CTL cell surface are represented in white and gray, respectively. Accessory molecules that play a role as integrins or in co-stimulation (not discussed here) are shown with *dashed lines. Filled circles* at the CD3 cytoplasmic tails indicate ITAM motifs, and *filled bars* on the CD8 stalk regions O-linked, often negatively charged carbohydrates.

brane (TCR spanning regions have positive charges and those of the CD3 components negative ones) and in part dipole–dipole interactions between α-helices (18). In addition, there are interactions of the extracellular portions of CD3 components with the TCR that are still not fully defined. The nine-residue-long extracellular parts of ζ-chains seem to interact in part with the connecting peptide of the TCR; indeed, modifications of these domains had deleterious effects for TCR signaling (19). A recent study suggested that an extracellular portion of CD3ε docks onto Cβ in a cavity formed by the unique surface exposed loop of TCRβ and an array of carbohydrates (20). Moreover, the unique and poorly ordered structure of Cα may also be a docking site for a CD3 component (9). CD3 component and ζ-chain have long cytoplasmic tails, that contain immunoreceptor tyrosine based activation motifs (ITAMs) [i.e., sequences expressing as consensus motif YXX(L/I)X6-8YXX(L/I)], which upon TCR engagement become tyrosine-phos-

phorylated and bind other molecules involved in TCR signaling. CD3 chains have one ITAM each, and the ζ-chains have three (16).

CO-RECEPTOR CD8

CD8 and CD8–MHC-I Structures

The co-receptor of CD8$^+$ CTLs is a disulfide-linked CD8α/β heterodimer (Fig. 3-2) (21). Each chain consists of two extracellular domains, an immunoglobulin (Ig)-folded globular domain that binds to the constant domain of MHC-I molecules, and a stalk region that has a flexible, highly extended structure, spanning the TCR and the variable domain of the MHC-I molecule (22). Remarkably, this distance of approximately 100 Å is spanned by only 45 residues of the α-chain and 32 residues of the β-chain. The stalk regions are rich in prolines and threonines/serines, with frequent O-linked, negatively charged carbohydrates, which by charge repulsion keep these sequences in an extended conformation (23). Interestingly, upon activation of resting CD8⁺ cells the sialic acid content of the CD8β stalk region changes, which is likely to alter its spacer length and hence the avidity of CD8 binding to TCR-associated MHC molecules (24). Both CD8 chains span the cell membrane and have cytoplasmic tails (25). Whereas for CD8β this tail is 19 residues long and not known to interact with other molecules, the tail of CD8α is 26 residues long and contains two cysteines (C200 and C202) that are involved in binding the kinase p56[lck] (22,25,26). Moreover, upon cell activation, the tail of CD8α is phosphorylated at S195 and S216, whereas the tail of CD8β remains unchanged (27,28).

The Ig domain of human CD8α/α homodimers have been crystallized alone as well as complexed with HLA-A2 (29,30). The latter study showed that the contact region between the two molecules is highly extended. From the MHC-I molecule residues in the floor of the α2 domain in various regions of the α3 domain and in β₂-microglobulin all interact with CD8α, mainly with its CDR loops (30–32). The acidic loop 222–229 in the α3 domain is located in the center of the two CD8α units, one of which extends to the α2 domain and the other to the lower part of α3 (29,33–35). From this structure it is clear that the Ig portion of CD8α/α does not interact with TCRs. Thus if TCRs interact with CD8, such contacts must be with the stalk regions. At present there are no crystallographic data on CD8α/β; and because CD8β has only about 30% sequence homology with CD8α and is shorter than CD8α, significant structural differences are possible. This might explain some of the significant differences between CD8α/α, and CD8α/β in terms of co-receptor function.

CD8 Co-Receptor Function

Using cloned CTLs specific for a photoreactive peptide derivative and that permit assessment of TCR–ligand interactions on living cells, we have shown that CD8 substantially increases the avidity of the TCR–ligand interaction (36). It was mainly accounted for by a decrease in TCR–ligand complex dissociation rates. Later, essentially the same findings were obtained using soluble recombinant molecules and surface plasmon resonance (37). This study also showed that CD8α/β has a three- to four-fold higher affinity for MHC-I molecules than CD8α/α (K_D values of about 11–14 μM and 30–39 μM, respectively). The observation that CD8 increases TCR–ligand binding on soluble molecules suggests that either CD8 also interacts with TCRs or that CD8 binding to MHC-I molecules increases their affinity for TCRs. Although CD8 binding induces conformational changes in the constant domain of MHC molecules, a crystallographic study showed that the carbon backbones of α1 and α2 of HLA-A2 are essentially the same, regardless of whether it is bound to CD8α/α (30). We have observed that the CD8-mediated increase of TCR–ligand binding on cells is largely accounted for by the coordinate binding of two membrane proteins (TCR and CD8) to the same MHC–peptide complex because it was barely detectable upon detergent solubilization of cell membranes (unpublished data). Thus the nature of the CD8-mediated increase of TCR–ligand binding, especially in cell-free systems, is still enigmatic.

An important consequence of the coordinate binding of co-receptor to TCR-associated MHC molecules is to bring co-receptor-associated p56[lck] to the TCR–CD3 complex (38,39). Because this kinase plays a key role in the phosphorylation of CD3 and CD3-associated ZAP-70, this co-receptor-mediated recruitment of lck plays an important role in TCR signaling. For CD4⁺ T cells it has been demonstrated to be a major function of the co-receptor (40,41). Indirect evidence suggests that this is also true in the CD8 system. However, because CD8 interacts with MHC-I molecules more avidly than CD4 with MHC-II molecules, CD8 (in contrast to CD4) directly influences TCR–ligand binding by increasing the avidity of TCR–ligand binding and decreasing TCR–ligand complex dissociation (36).

It is interesting to note that some CTL clones are CD8-dependent and others are not; that is, the functional response of some CTL clones is effectively blocked by anti-CD8 monoclonal antibody, whereas other clones are indifferent to such antibodies (42–44). It has been proposed that the TCR–ligand binding is weaker for CD8-dependent CTLs than for CD8-independent ones, and therefore the contribution of CD8 to TCR–ligand binding is more critical. This "rule," however, seems not to be always true, and factors other than TCR–ligand binding affinity can play a role as well (45). For example, it has been observed that CTLs derived from mice expressing transgene TCRs from CD8-dependent clones are more frequently CD8-dependent than CTLs derived from mice expressing transgene TCRs from CD8-independent clones (46). Moreover, it has been observed that the contribution of CD8 to TCR–ligand binding, and hence recruitment of CD8 to the TCR–CD3 complex, can vary among CTL clones and among altered peptide ligands (47,48). It is thus conceivable that the structural properties of TCR–ligand complexes determine in part the avidity of cooperative binding of TCR-associated MHC molecules by CD8. It is also possible that activation of CD8-independent CTL clones is less dependent on CD8-associated p56^{lck} and requires for example p56^{lck} that is not associated with CD8 or p59^{fyn}.

Although CD8^{+} T cells in the periphery express only CD8α/β, it is noteworthy that heterodimeric CD8 is a more efficient co-receptor than homodimeric CD8α/α, which is expressed on intestinal T cells or on natural killer (NK) T cells. Using CD8 transfected T cell hybridomas, it has been shown that cells expressing CD8α/β recognize peptide more efficiently than CD8α/α-expressing ones, especially at low concentrations or in the case of low-affinity peptide variants (49,50). One study showed that CD8α/α supports TCR–ligand binding more avidly than

CD8α/α (49). It has also been demonstrated that CD8α/β associates more extensively with p56^{lck} than CD8α/α, suggesting that the cytoplasmic tail of CD8 directly or indirectly contributes to this association (51). That the CD8β chain is not merely a surrogate α–chain also emerged from experiments where the gene of CD8β was knocked out in mice or the tail of CD8β was deleted (52,53). Even though these animals can still express homodimeric CD8α/α, the frequency of CD8^{+} T cells in the periphery was dramatically reduced in both situations (52,53). It is tempting to speculate that CD8β directly or indirectly couples CD8 to the TCR–CD3 complex. Although it has been observed that CD8 (and CD4) couples with TCR–CD3 following cell activation via p56^{lck} and ZAP-70 (i.e., p56^{lck} binds to the SH2 domains of CD3/ζ-associated ZAP-70) (39,54), the finding that CD8 increases TCR–ligand binding in the absence of these molecules suggests that CD8 may directly interact with TCR. The finding that CD8α/β co-caps more efficiently with the TCRs than CD8α/α is consistent with this view (55). Another possibility is that CD8, especially CD8α/β, can promote and modulate TCR aggregation, which according to some evidence is vital for T cell activation (see Concepts of T Cell Activation, below).

CD8-Dependent Adhesion

As shown by Mescher and coworkers, CD8 can also bind to MHC-I molecules that are not interacting with TCR and thus can act as an adhesion molecule. Similar to integrins (e.g., LFA1 or CD2), this adhesion is induced, (i.e., takes place) only following TCR–CD3 engagement (56–58). For example, CTL adhere to plates coated with purified MHC class I molecules when their TCR is engaged by low concentrations of soluble anti-TCR or anti-CD3 mAb, or specific MHC class I-peptide complexes (57). This induced adhesion is mediated by CD8 and can be completely blocked by anti-CD8 mAbs (57). Interestingly, different anti-CD8 mAbs can affect the CD8-dependent adhesion and CD8–mediated increase in TCR–ligand binding (CD8 co-receptor function) in different ways (36). Often anti-CD8β mAbs dramatically affect CD8 co-receptor function, and anti-CD8α mAbs affect CD8 adhesion function. Similarly, it has been shown that E227K mutation in the acidic loop 222–229 of α3 of MHC-I molecules profoundly impairs CD8 co-receptor function but has no effect on CD8-mediated adhesion (36,59). There is presently no explanation for these findings, but they suggest that CD8 interacts with MHC-I molecules differently for CD8 co-receptor and adhesion function.

CD8-dependent adhesion is blocked by various kinase inhibitors, both tyrosine and serine/threonine kinase-specific ones, indicating that probably several signaling cascades are involved (57). The cytoskeleton is also important for CD8-mediated adhesion; both cytochalasin D and colchicine block this adhesion completely but have little effect on CD8 co-receptor function (58,60). This suggests that CD8⁻-mediated adhesion requires CD8 clustering at the contact site and that significant adhesion relies on an avidity increase by focusing CD8 in the contact site. Moreover, it has been shown that induced CD8-dependent adhesion of CTLs to immobilized MHC-I molecules results in CTL activation (e.g., release of esterases, or granzymes) and is transient. This adhesion is transient, and there are signaling cascades that first activate and later deactivate CD8-dependent adhesion (57). Protein kinase C (PKC) has been found to play an important role in the deactivation of this adhesion because depletion of PKC by phorbol myristic acetate (PMA) treatment impairs CD8 de-adhesion (61). Taken together, these findings indicate that CD8 clearly plays multiple roles in CTL activation that all occur simultaneously during CTL-target cell interactions such as participating in TCR-ligand binding, mediating adhesion, and providing signaling (61). Much still has to be learned about CD8 co-receptor function, which is likely to be more complex than that of CD4. In view of the fact that MHC-I molecules are constitutively expressed on most cells of an organism, whereas the expression of MHC-II molecules is limited to specialized antigen-presenting cells and is induced transiently by cytokines, it is tempting to speculate that CD8 has more regulatory functions than CD4.

AFFINITY AND KINETICS OF TCR–LIGAND INTERACTION

Several difficulties have hampered the analysis of TCR–ligand interactions. For example, both the ligand and the TCR are integral membrane glycoproteins, and both are oligomeric structures. Moreover, TCRs on cells are integrated in the membrane and associated with CD3, which may alter their ligand-binding properties.

Assessment of TCR–Ligand Interactions

The first measurements of TCR–ligand interaction were based on functional competition assays in which soluble MHC–peptide complexes or soluble TCRs were used to inhibit T cell function (62,63). Although these studies suggested a low TCR–ligand affinity, the measurements were indirect and hence not accurate. More recently other measurements of TCR–ligand binding were used. First, Matsui et al. developed a binding assay based on competition between soluble MHC–peptide complexes and a radiolabeled anti-TCR Fab fragment (64). The TCRs studied were 5C.C7 and 2B4, which bind to an I-E^k-cytochrome c peptide. Using a similar assay, ligand binding has been assessed for the H-2L^d-restricted 2C TCR or the ovalbumin/H-2K^b-specific 42.12 TCR (65–67). However, this technique is also indirect and does not allow kinetic measurements. Sykulev et al. introduced a direct binding assay in which cloned 2C CTLs were incubated with radioiodinated peptide–MHC-I complex, and cell-associated and free ligand were separated by centrifugation through density gradients (66)

Presently the most commonly used TCR–ligand binding assay is surface plasmon resonance (SPR), which allows precise measurement of rapid binding and dissociation kinetics (68–71). First used by Corr et al. for the 2C TCR, soluble TCR was immobilized on a dextran layer and reacted with soluble ligand (70). More recently, soluble MHC–peptide complexes were immobilized on the sensor chip and reacted with soluble TCR in solution (37). This technique has a few drawbacks. First, it requires soluble recombinant TCR molecules, which may not be identical to cell-associated TCRs in terms of ligand binding. In one case, however, it has been shown that essentially the same binding values are obtained on intact cells and by SPR measurements (64,69). Moreover, for technical reasons SPR measurements are usually performed at ambient temperature (i.e., at nonphysiologic temperatures). Another potential caveat is that at least in some cases MHC–peptide complex dissociation is not negligible, which complicates accurate quantification of TCR–ligand-binding properties. In one study this problem has been solved by using genetically engineered, covalent peptide–MHC complexes (72).

We have developed another assay to assess TCR–ligand binding that circumvents these difficulties. To this end, bifunctional peptide derivatives were prepared that contain two photoreactive groups, one of which was positioned to be in close contact with the MHC molecule in the MHC-I–peptide derivative complex. Selective photoactivation of this group resulted in efficient crosslinking of the peptide derivative to the MHC-I molecule (60). The other photoreactive group was introduced in a position known to be important for T cell recognition. As this modification impaired or abolished recognition by CTLs specific for the parental peptide, CTLs were generated by immunization with the modified peptide (73,74). Peptide derivative-specific CTLs were readily induced and displayed all the hallmarks of conventional

antigen recognition by CTLs, including MHC restriction and the dependence on auxiliary molecules (60,75). Incubation of these CTLs with covalent MHC-I–peptide complexes and photoactivation resulted in TCR photoaffinity labeling (60,73,74). Because TCR photoaffinity labeling is proportional to TCR–ligand binding and takes place in a few milliseconds, it allows assessment of TCR–ligand binding affinities and kinetics on living cells, detergent lysates, or purified molecules in solution. This unique feature permitted a comparison of the TCR–ligand binding events taking place on living cells with those taking place on purified molecules in solution. This allowed the first direct analysis of CD8 participation in TCR–ligand binding (36). In addition, by mapping the photoaffinity labeled site(s), mutational analysis, and computer modeling, these systems provided the first significant insights in the structural basis of T cell recognition of hapten-modified peptides (the hapten being the photoreactive group) (73,74; Kessler et al., submitted).

Soluble TCRs

The TCR–ligand binding studies and crystallographic studies require soluble TCRs in large quantities. The preparation of soluble TCR molecules turned out to be a much more difficult task than the production of soluble MHC–peptide complexes (76). The main problems were low expression of correctly paired α- and β-chains and the difficulty of assessing the functional integrity of the soluble TCR produced (77). Soluble TCRs have been produced in mammalian expression systems (CHO cells or myelic cell lines), in Sf9 insect cells infected with baculovirus, in stably transfected *Drosophila* cells, or by refolding α- and β-chains produced in bacteria (76). To promote efficient αβ-chain pairing, several strategies have been used. For example, the extracellular domains of TCRs were fused to a variety of molecules, such as phosphatidylinositol glycan membrane anchor (64), ζ-chain (78), immunoglobulin domains (69), or CD3 components (79). An attractive strategy involves C-terminal fusion of TCR α- and β-chains with acidic and basic leucine zippers, respectively, which efficiently promotes correct chain pairing and thus significantly increases the yields of expression (80). Finally, soluble TCRs have been prepared as single-chain Fv molecules using strategies previously developed for immunoglobulins (81–83). The various strategies to produce soluble TCRs have been reviewed by Fremont et al. (76).

Affinities and Kinetics of TCR–Ligand Interactions

Regardless of the technique used, most studies agree that, in general, TCR–ligand binding is of low affinity. Using a competition assay, Matsui et al. found that the interaction between the TCR and c/IE^k cytochrome complex has an equilibrium dissociation constant (K_d) of about 50 μM (64), which was later confirmed by SPR measurements (69). Analysis of the interaction of the alloreactive 2C TCR with various ligands showed K_d values of 10^{-4} to 10^{-7} M (65). The highest affinity was observed for the p2Ca peptide bound to H-2L^d. In general, allegeneic ligands exhibited a higher binding affinity than syngeneic ligands, suggesting that the affinity plays a critical role in thymic selection of T cells (66). One study indicated an inverse relation between the number of ligands required for recognition and the number of ligands on target cells (i.e., the higher the affinity of the TCR–ligand interaction, the lower the number of TCRs required) (67). Taken together, these studies show that TCR–ligand binding affinities are low, comparable to low-affinity antibodies in primary humoral immune responses. It is noteworthy, however, that TCR–ligand binding on cells may be more avid—on one hand, due to participation of the co-receptor in the binding (36) and on the other hand due to conformational changes related to CD3 association with TCRs or integration of the TCRs in the cell membrane (our unpublished observation).

Kinetic studies revealed that the association of TCRs with ligand was fast, the equilibrium being reached in a matter of 1 to 2 minutes at 25°C (64). SPR real time studies showed that for 2C TCR association to H-2L^d-p2Ca peptide the association constant was 2.1×10^5 M^{-1} s^{-1} at 25°C (70). Other studies also using SPR found a slower association rate, although still relatively rapid (84). These differences probably reflect intrinsic properties of each TCR–ligand pair. One study described the interesting observation that association kinetics of the 2C TCR could be fitted better with two simultaneous binding events rather than one bimolecular reaction (70). Whether this may be explained by conformational changes related to the binding event remains to be clarified.

One important point of consensus of all these studies is that TCR–ligand complex dissociation is extremely fast. For example, the half-life of 2C TCR–H-2L^d–p2Ca peptide complex is 27 seconds at 25°C (70). Similar rapid dissociation kinetics have been observed for other TCR–ligand complexes, with half-lives usually less than 1 minute at 25°C (36,47,85). Using TCR photoaffinity labeling, we observed that TCR–ligand complex dissociation was approximately ten-fold faster at 37°C (half-life of 7 seconds) than at 0°C (36,47). Furthermore, measurements of dissociation kinetics on various CTL clones specific for the same MHC–peptide complex revealed significant differences (half-lives ranging from 15 to 60 seconds) and that these differences determined the clone-specific susceptibilities to antagonism (47,48). Similarly, peptide antagonists and partial agonists have been shown to have faster TCR–ligand complex dissociation rates than agonists, although the association rates were comparable (68).

The finding that TCR–ligand interactions have low affinities and rapid dissociation kinetics is in accordance on one hand with the ability of TCRs to interact with different peptides or even with different MHC molecules and on the other hand with the dynamic reading of MHC–peptide complexes on other

cells. Both of these properties are vital for
TCR function and are hardly compatible
with stable high-affinity interactions, which
typically have slower dissociation rates and
high specificity.

NORMAL AND ABERRANT
ANTIGEN RECOGNITION BY CTLs
CTL Recognition of Agonists

The two main functions of CD8$^+$ T cells are
to kill target cells and produce cytokines.
As a rule, epitopes recognized by CTLs are
derived from endogenously produced proteins (i.e., proteins synthesized by the cell),
such as viral-encoded antigens, tumor antigens, or mutant self proteins (86). Nevertheless, CTLs can also recognize target cells
presenting endogenous antigenic peptides;
although the physiologic significance of this
pathway may be small. CTLs (and CD4$^+$ T
cells) can also be readily elicited and specifically recognize epitopes containing nonpeptidic moieties, such as carbohydrates or haptens (6,73,74,86).

Antigen recognition by CTLs generally
elicits three effector functions. First, the most
prominent mechanism by which CTLs kill
target cells is perforin-dependent lysis. CTLs
are rich in granules containing pore-forming
perforin and various esterases called granzymes, which when released into the CTL–
target cell contact region induce cell death
in a synergistic manner (87,88). Second, upon
activation CTLs express Fas ligand (FasL),
which binds to Fas (CD95 or APO1), the
receptor for FasL, which is present on most
cells; this action induces apoptosis via a well
characterized signaling mechanism (89). To
exert its activity FasL can be cell-associated
or secreted in soluble form. Third, CTL activation usually results in the production and
secretion of cytokines, such as TNFα, IFNγ,
and various interleukins (88). TNFα is a cytolytic agent and by binding to CD40 receptor
on cells can induce apoptosis in a manner
similar to FasL. The kinetics and activation
requirements of these three CTL functions

are markedly different. Perforin-dependent
killing is rapid (a few minutes to a few hours)
and can be elicited by TCR signaling too
weak to induce cytokine production, cell proliferation, or TCR down-modulation (89).
Few MHC–peptide complexes on target
cells, perhaps only one, are sufficient to induce perforin-dependent killing. By contrast,
cytokine production and FasL synthesis involve gene transcription, which requires sustained TCR signaling for extended periods
of time. Fas-dependent cytolysis is clearly
slower than perforin-dependent cytolysis
(about 6–18 hours), and TNFα-mediated
killing is slower still (peaks after 16 hours).
In some cases Fas-dependent cytotoxicity involves translocation of preformed, intracellular FasL to the cell surface, which may act
faster (90).

CTL Recognition of Altered
Peptide Ligands

Although TCR–ligand interactions are remarkably specific, it is now well established
that given ligands can interact with various
TCRs (91). Conversely, a given TCR can
interact with different peptide–MHC-I complexes. The structural basis for these cross-
reactivities is only now emerging from crystallographic studies (13,14), but it has long
been noted that modifications of peptide epitopes (altered peptide ligands) or mutations
in the MHC molecule can have diverse effects on T cell effector functions. As first
discovered for CD4$^+$ cells, peptide modifications can alter the pattern of lymphokines
secreted (partial agonists), abolish cell proliferation, or antagonize T cell responses to
agonists (antagonists) (92–94). Epitope
modifications can also affect CD8$^+$ CTL
functional responses in a diverse manner.
For example, epitope modification can selectively impair perforin-dependent killing or
cytokine production, or it can increase or
decrease functional CTL responses (cytotoxicity and cytokine production) (strong and
weak agonists, respectively) (47,48). Interestingly, in most but not all cases strong pep-

tide agonists exhibited rapid, and weak agonists slow, TCR–ligand complex dissociation (47,48). However, if TCR–ligand complex dissociation rates exceed a critical value, antagonism is observed. Consistent with this we observed that blocking of CD8, which accelerates TCR–ligand complex dissociation, either increased the efficiency of antigen recognition or resulted in antagonism (47,48).

Various forms of partial antagonism have been reported for CTLs (95–97). For example, for some altered peptide ligands, perforin-dependent killing is lost whereas Fas-mediated killing or cytokine production is maintained (95). We recently observed a case in which an altered peptide ligand activated cloned CTLs only for Fas-dependent killing in the absence of any other functional response (89). Analogous cases have been described in CD4 systems (98). Selective activation of Fas-dependent cytotoxicity in the absence of other T cell responses may play a role in lymphoid homeostasis (see below).

Several observations indicate that altered peptide ligands have physiologic significance. For example, it has been shown that fast-mutating viruses, such as human immunodeficiency virus (HIV), can give rise to variant CTL epitopes that antagonize virus-specific cytotoxic responses, allowing the virus to evade CTL-mediated eradication (99,100). Although in many *in vitro* systems antagonists must be used in rather large molar excess to be effective, in some of these studies altered viral epitopes effectively inhibited CTL responses at low concentrations (99,100).

Moreover, endogenously produced peptides, often of unrelated sequences, can cross-react with TCRs specific for given antigens. Such peptides play an instrumental role in the positive selection of T cells and hence in shaping the repertoire of peripheral T cells (101–105). Remarkably, these epitopes are often either partial agonists or antagonists for the mature T cells, whereas strong peptide agonists typically negatively select these specificities (106). Likewise, precursors for

mature CD4⁺ and CD8⁺ T cells recognizing peptides modified with carbohydrates or haptens are most likely positively selected by unrelated natural endogenous peptides. Such T cells can be readily elicited *in vivo* and recognize a vast diversity of nonpeptidic moieties, including highly artificial structures (73–75,87,88,107). Some of these T cells play a role in disorders such as allergies, eczema, or delayed-type hypersensitivity (108). On the other hand, in some cases epitopes from foreign antigen can stimulate proliferation of T cells that cross-react with endogenously produced epitopes, which may result in autoimmune disorders (101–103).

TCR Signaling in CTLs

TCR Signaling Induced by Agonists

Although the functional properties of altered peptide ligands are well characterized, the signaling mechanisms accounting for aberrant T cell function are only partially elucidated. Upon TCR engagement by agonists, the src protein tyrosine kinases (PTKs) p56^{lck} and p59^{fyn} are activated, resulting in phosphorylation of ITAMs of the CD3 complex (15,109,110). Activation of these kinases is mediated by the tyrosine-specific phosphatase CD45, which dephosphorylates regulatory tyrosine residues of src PTK (111). This is crucial; indeed T cells lacking functional CD45 cannot be activated via the TCRs (112). The phosphorylated ITAMs are docking sites for various other signaling molecules, importantly for SH2 domains of PTK of the Syk family, (i.e., ZAP-70 and Syk) (110,111). In contrast to src kinases, which are membrane-associated, Syk kinases are cytosolic and as shown for ZAP-70 can be found to a significant extent also in the nucleus (113). CD3/ζ-associated ZAP-70 (and Syk) upon phosphorylation/activation by src PTK (mainly p56^{lck}) phosphorylate various other signaling molecules, such as ras, phospholipase C-γ (PLCγ), and LAT (linker for T cell activation). Importantly, phosphorylated LAT associates with various important signaling molecules, such as (PLCγ), phosphoinositide 3-kinase, Grb2, and glycosylphosphatidylinositol (GPI)-anchored proteins (114). Many of these molecules link the TCR to various signaling cascades, each giving rise to the production of different transcription factors and hence ultimately different cellular responses. For example, phosphorylated/activated PLCγ cleaves phosphatidyl inositol biphosphate (PIP2) to yield diacylglycerol (DAG) and inositol triphosphate (IP3). DAG in turn activates PKC, a serine/threonine kinase that phosphorylates various intracellular proteins, resulting in activation of transcription factors such as NF-JCB, AP-1, and NFAT. On the other hand, IP3, by binding to specific receptors, stimulates an increase in intracellular Ca^{2+} concentrations, which in turn activates calcium-sensitive enzymes such as calcineurin, another serine/threonine kinase, which activates transcription factors, namely a different form of NFAT. Alternatively, activated Ras activates Raf, another serine/threonine kinase, which then phosphorylates MEK and MAPK kinases, ultimately resulting in the activation of Jun, Fos, and other transcription factors (109,110).

TCR Signaling Induced by Altered Peptide Ligands

In CTLs, TCR signaling by peptide agonists initiates several signaling cascades, resulting in the production of various transcription factors that initiate the transcription of genes, encoding lymphokines, Fas-ligand, or molecules involved in cell-cycle control (109,110). How can altered peptide ligands activate some but not other activation events (partial agonists) or impair activation induced by agonists (peptide antagonists)? An important first observation was that partial agonists and antagonists elicit different patterns of ζ-chain phosphorylation. ζ-Chain has three ITAMs, which upon phosphorylation give rise to three electrophoretically distinguishable phosphorylation products, mi-

grating on sodium dodecyl sulfate polyacrylamide gel electrophoresis (SDS-PAGE) with apparent Mr values of 17, 21, and 23 kDa (115,116). Although the 17-kDa species is constitutive (i.e., also observed on resting T cells), agonists mainly induce pp23 phospho-ζ, and partial agonists and antagonists induce predominantly or exclusively the pp21 phospho-ζ form. This is true for $CD4^+$ and $CD8^+$ T cells (48,115–117). These studies also showed that significant phosphorylation/activation of ZAP-70 occurs only after binding of ZAP-70 to pp23-phosphorylated ζ-chain (115–117). ZAP-70, however, can also bind to other forms of ζ-chain, (e.g., pp21 phospho-ζ). Therefore one way TCR antagonists may inhibit T cell activation is by eliciting selective production of pp21 phospho-ζ, which binds ZAP in an unproductive manner, thereby interfering with binding of ZAP-70 to the pp23 phospho-ζ elicited by agonists. This view is consistent with the observation that usually inhibition of T cell responses to agonists requires a large excess of antagonist. The finding that in some cases peptide antagonists can inhibit CTL killing induced by agonist at very low concentrations, however, indicates that there are other ways by which peptide antagonists can inactivate T cells (99,100).

Another important observation was that different ITAMs of the CD3 complex, which all have different sequences, upon phosphorylation are not equivalent in terms of binding other signaling molecules. Thus the ten ITAMs present in a TCR–CD3 complex are not redundant but, rather, diversify TCR signaling by eliciting different signaling cascades upon TCR engagement (118–121). Recently it has been shown that upon TCR engagement the ζ-chain undergoes a series of ordered phosphorylation events. Completion of the phosphorylation steps is dependent on the nature of the TCR ligand. Thus the phosphorylation steps establish thresholds for T cell activation and, depending on the nature of the ligand that engages the TCRs, different specific ζ-chain phosphorylation products are formed (122). In view of the potential of the CD3 complex to initiate different downstream signaling cascades, such differential phosphorylation reactions constitute an important means by which altered peptide ligands (and altered MHC molecules) can induce selectively different cell effector T cell functions. Alternatively, it has been proposed that altered peptide ligands may recruit and differentially activate phosphatases, which then may dephosphorylate/inactivate intermediates critical for the initiation of different signaling cascades (123,124). For example, it has been demonstrated that SHP-1 can bind to phosphorylated ZAP-70, which activates its phosphatase activity (123). However, the role and significance of SHP-1 and phosphatases in aberrant T cell function, if any, remain to be elucidated.

Concepts of T Cell Activation

Conceptually, three models have been suggested to demonstrate how altered peptide ligands can elicit aberrant T cell function. Each of these concepts has been subsequently reformulated in different versions.

Kinetic Proofreading Concept

The kinetic proofreading concept postulates that the half-life of TCR engagement by ligand is of key importance for T cell activation (68,125,126). As described in the previous section, TCR engagement initiates phosphorylation of ITAMs of CD3 by src kinases, mainly p56^{lck}. According to this concept, the nature of this and subsequent phosphorylation reactions is primarily determined by the time of TCR engagement (i.e., by the average time these phosphorylation reactions proceed). In view of the recent finding that phosphorylation of ζ-chain proceeds in an ordered manner, (i.e., that phosphorylation of given tyrosines of ITAMs is dependent on the phosphorylation of other tyrosines) (122), it implies that the time of TCR engagement determines not only the extent but also the pattern of CD3 phosphorylation. This concept has been substantiated

by several observations. For example, it has been demonstrated that partial agonists and peptide antagonists, which elicit limited CD3 phosphorylation and mainly of the pp21 phospho-ζ form, typically have shorter TCR–ligand complex half-lives than agonists (47,48,68,69). Thus in both CD4 and CD8 systems it has been shown that rapid TCR–ligand dissociation gives rise to limited CD3 phosphorylation and hence limited or no activation of ZAP-70, which in turn initiates limited or no functional T cell responses.

Conformational Concepts

According to the conformational concept, epitope modifications invoke conformational changes in TCRs that are transmitted to CD3 and can qualitatively influence the signaling events they initiate (127). In support of this concept is the observation that anti-TCR mAbs and their Fab fragments can influence T cell responses in a diverse and often dramatic manner (128). Although x-ray crystallographic studies so far have provided no evidence that altered peptide ligands induce conformational changes in TCR constant domains, it is still possible that such changes occur in membrane-integrated TCR–CD3 complexes, as they may have a higher conformational fluidity than truncated and deglycosylated TCRs packed in a crystal. Thus the observation that altered peptide ligands give rise to ordered and distinct patterns of ζ-chain phosphorylation could also be accounted for by conformational changes in ITAMs or by subtle differences in the association of CD3 with TCRs, as a result of which the kinases phosphorylate different tyrosines.

As an extension of the conformational model we propose that conformational changes in TCR or MHC–peptide can affect quantitatively and qualitatively CD3 phosphorylation by co-receptor-associated p56^{lck}. The co-receptor CD8 (and CD4) plays a vital role in antigen recognition by T cells. The recruitment of co-receptor-associated p56^{lck} to the TCR–CD3 complex significantly reduces the number of specific MHC–peptide complexes required for cell activation (28,44,48). Assessment of TCR–ligand binding for various altered peptide ligands, in the absence or presence of CD8-blocking reagents, revealed that peptide modifications can alter the avidity of CD8 participation in TCR—ligand binding (44,48). From crystallographic studies it emerged that TCRs bind ligand in a conserved orientation but that there is a certain degree of rotational and lateral variability, not only among different TCR–ligand pairs but among different ligands binding to the same receptor (11–14,129). Because CD8 interacts with defined and conserved regions of MHC class I molecules, CD8 has to follow these movements of the MHC molecule relative to TCRs. Because CD8 (and CD4) is associated with p56[lck], changes in the topology and avidity of docking of CD8 to TCR–ligand complex seem likely to impart qualitative and quantitative changes in p56[lck]-mediated phosphorylation of various ITAMs of CD3.

Concept of Serial TCR Engagement

A third concept is one of serial TCR engagement. As initially shown by Valitutti and coworkers, TCRs serially engage ligand during T cell–APC encounters (130,131). This is so because the half-life of TCR–ligand complexes is several orders of magnitude smaller than that of T cell–APC conjugates. TCRs, after having engaged some 100 ligands, are down-modulated (i.e., are endocytosed and degraded) (131). In support of this concept it has been shown that CTLs can kill target cells that express low ligand densities, perhaps only one per cell (132). Such CTL activation seems difficult to explain on the grounds of TCR aggregation (see below). By measuring TCR–ligand binding, TCR–ligand complex dissociation kinetics, and functional CTL responses, we observed that in most but not all cases weak agonists exhibited slow, and strong agonists rapid, TCR–ligand complex dissociation (44,48). These findings are inconsistent with the kinetic proofreading concept but are in accordance with the concept of serial TCR engagement (i.e., that the magnitude of functional T cell response is related to the frequency of serial TCR engagement). The observation that blocking of TCR–ligand complex dissociation results in rapid and complete loss of TCR signaling also supports this concept (48) and, in addition, indicates that serial TCR engagement is a requirement for antigen-driven T cell activation. It is presently not known why blocking of serial TCR engagement abolishes TCR signaling. Our preliminary results suggest that TCR–ligand cross-linking interferes with activation of p56[lck].

TCR Aggregation

Receptor-mediated activation of various cell types (e.g., B cells, mast cells, basophils, blood platelets, neutrophils, macrophages) has been demonstrated to require receptor crosslinking (i.e., receptor aggregation) (133). There is circumstantial, though strong, evidence that this is also true for TCR-mediated activation of T cells. For example, it has been shown in various systems that T cell activation by soluble MHC–peptide complexes requires that they are at least dimers and that monovalent complexes fail to activate cells (134). The findings that TCRs bind ligand in a canonical diagonal orientation and that the strand switch in $V\alpha$ creates a potential aggregation site support models of TCRs aggregation (10,11,13,129). Also in support of this concept is the observation that TCRs, upon incubation with ligand at high concentrations (near or above the equilibrium constant), form dimers and then larger aggregates (135). It is not known whether this aggregation is two- or three-dimensional (i.e., if it is physiologically relevant). There is also evidence indicating that TCR–CD3 complexes in cell membranes form dimers and that CD3 components are involved (15). For CD4[+] T cells there is good evidence indicating that the co-receptor, by binding to two MHC-II molecules, indirectly promotes TCR dimerization (136). Although according to current knowledge CD8 interaction with MHC-I molecules is monovalent (30), it is still possible that CD8 promotes TCR dimerization/aggregation. For example, the observation that soluble CD8 increases the binding of soluble TCR to immobilized MHC–peptide complexes may be accounted for by CD8 induced TCR aggregation (37), which is consistent with the observations that CD8 at up to 20-fold lower concentrations still increased TCR–ligand binding. This effect is not seen when the TCRs instead of the MHC–peptide complexes are immobilized (37).

The finding that CTLs can recognize target cells expressing few specific MHC-I–peptide complexes, perhaps only one, seems difficult to reconcile with TCR aggregation models— more so because according to all available knowledge MHC-I molecules on cells are monomeric (30,132). There is, however, evidence indicating that specific MHC–peptide complexes concentrate in the T cell–APC contact site, a phenomenon that requires cytoskeleton function (137). Importantly, initial TCR crosslinking, however weak, results in phosphorylation of LAT, which greatly favors TCR aggregation by the formation of microdomains (rafts) containing glycosylphosphatidylinositol (GPI)-anchored proteins (e.g., Thy1), glycolipids, and Src family protein tyrosine kinases (137–140).

REFERENCES

1. Davis MM, Bjorkman PJ. T-cell receptor genes and T-cell recognition. *Nature* 1988;334:395–402.
2. Chothia C, Boswell DR, Lesk AM. The outline structure of the TCRαβ receptor. *EMBO J* 1988;7:3745–3755.
3. Sant' Angelo DB, Waterbury G, Preston-Hurlburg P, et al. The specificity and orientation of a TCR to its peptide-MHC class II ligand. *Immunity* 1996;4:367–376.
4. Katayama CD, Eidelman FJ, Duncan A, Hooshmand F, Hedrick SM. Predicted complementary determining regions of the T cell antigen receptor determine antigen specificity. *EMBO J* 1995;14:927–938.
5. Jorgensen JL, Esser U, de St. Groth BF, Reay PA, Davis MM. Mapping of T cell receptor-peptide contacts by variant peptide immunization of single-chain transgenics. *Nature* 1992;355:224–230.
6. Luescher IF, Anjuére F, Peitsch MC, Jongeneel CV, Cerottini JC, Romero P. Structural analysis of TCR–ligand interactions studied on H-2Kd-restricted cloned CTL specific for a photoreactive peptide derivative. *Immunity* 1995;3:51–63.
7. Sun R, Shepherd SE, Geier SG, Thomas CT, Sheil JM, Nathenson SG. Evidence that the antigen receptors of cytotoxic T lymphocytes interact with a common pattern on the H-2Kb molecule. *Immunity* 1995;3:573–582.
8. Bentley GA, Boulot G, Karjalainen K, Mariuzza RA. Crystal structure of the β chain of a T cell antigen receptor. *Science* 1995;267:1984–1987.
9. Garcia KC, Degano M, Stanfield RL, et al. An alphabeta T cell receptor structure at 2.5 A and its orientation in the TCR–MHC complex. *Science* 1996;274:209–219.
10. Fields BA, Ober B, Malchiodi EL, et al. Crystal structure of the Va domain of a T cell antigen receptor. *Science* 1995;270:1821–1824.
11. Garboczi DN, Ghosh P, Utz U, Fan QR, Biddison WE, Wiley DC. Structure of the complex between human T-cell receptor, viral peptide and HLA-A2. *Nature* 1996;384:134–141.
12. Garcia KC, Degano M, Pease LR, et al. Structural basis of plasticity in T cell receptor recognition of self peptide-MHC antigen. *Science* 1998;279:1166–1172.
13. Ding Y, Smith K, Garboczi D, Utz U, Biddison W, Wiley D. Two human T cell receptors bind in a similar diagonal mode to the HLA-A2/Tax peptide complex using different TCR amino acids. *Immunity* 1998;8:403–411.
14. Speir JA, Garcia KC, Brunmark A, et al. Structural basic of 2C TCR allorecognition of H-2Lᵈ peptide complexes. *Immunity* 1998;8:553–562.
15. Carson G, Kuestner R, Ahmed A, Pettey C, Concino M. Six chains of the human T cell antigen receptor CD3 complex are necessary and sufficient for processing the receptor heterodimer to the cell surface. *J Biol Chem* 1991;266:7883–7887.
16. Wange RL, Samelson L. Complex complexes: signaling at the TCR. *Immunity* 1996;5:197–205.
17. Huppa JB, Ploegh HL. In vitro translation and assembly of a complete T cell receptor-CD3. *J Exp Med* 1997;186:393–403.
18. Hall C, Berkhout B, Alarcon B, Sancho J, Wileman T, Terhorst C. Requirements for cell surface expression of the human CD3/TCR complex in non-T cells. *Eur J Immunol* 1991;3:359–368.
19. Backstrom B, Milia E, Peter A, Jaureguiberry B, Baldari C, Palmer E. A motif within the T cell receptor a chain constant region connecting peptide domain controls antigen responsiveness. *Immunity* 1996;5:437–447.
20. Ghendler Y, Smolyar A, Chang H, Reinherz E. One of the CD3 epsilon subunits within a T cell receptor complex lies in close proximity to the Cbeta FG loop. *J Exp Med* 1998;187:1529–1536.
21. Norment AM, Littman DR. A second subunit of CD8 is expressed in human T cells. *EMBO J* 1988;7:3433–3439.
22. Leahy DJ. A structural view of CD4 and CD8. *FASEB J* 1995;9:17–25.
23. Boursier J, Alcover A, Herve F, Laisney I, Acuto

O. Evidence for an extended structure of the T-cell co-receptor CD8 alpha as deduced from the hydrodynamic properties of soluble forms of the extracellular region. *J Biol Chem* 1993;268:2013–2020.

24. Casabo LG, Mamalaki C, Kioussis D, Zamoyska R. T cell activation results in physical modification of the mouse CD8 beta chain. *J Immunol* 1994;152:397–404.

25. Turner JM, Brodsky MH, Irving BA, Levin SD, Perlmutter RM, Littman DR. Interaction of the unique N-terminal region of tyrosine kinase p56lck with cytoplasmic domains of CD4 and CD8 is mediated by cysteine motifs. *Cell* 1990;60:755–765.

26. Veillette A, Bookman MA, Horak EM, Bolen JB. The CD4 and CD8 T cell surface antigens are associated with the internal membrane tyrosine-protein kinase p56lck. *Cell* 1988;55:301–308.

27. Acres RB, Conlon PJ, Mochizuki DY, Gallis B. Phosphorylation of the CD8 antigen on cytotoxic human T cells in response to phorbol myristate acetate or antigen-presenting B cells. *J Immunol* 1987;139:2268–74.

28. Williams O, Vukmanovic S, Zamoyska R. Phosphorylation of murine CD8 alpha is not essential for responses of T cell hybridomas to antigen. *Int Immunol* 1991;3:785–792.

29. Leahy DJ, Axel R, Hendrickson WA. Crystal structure of a soluble form of the human T cell coreceptor CD8 at 2.6 A resolution. *Cell* 1992;68:1145–1162.

30. Gao G, Tormo J, Gerth U, et al. Crystal structure of the complex between human CD8alpha and HLA-A2. *Nature* 1997;387:630–634.

31. Sun J, Leahy DJ, Kavathas PB. Interaction between CD8 and major histocompatibility complex (MHC) class I mediated by multiple contacts surfaces that include the a2 and a3 domains of MHC class I. *J Exp Med* 1995;182:1275–1280.

32. Giblin PA, Leahy DJ, Mennone J, Kavathas PB. The role of charge and multiple faces of the CD8 alpha/alpha homodimer in binding to major histocompatibility complex class I molecules: support for a bivalent model. *Proc Natl Acad Sci USA* 1994;91:1716–1720.

33. Salter RD, Benjamin RJ, Wesley PK, et al. A binding site for the T-cell co-receptor CD8 on the alpha 3 domain of HLA-A2. *Nature* 1990;345:41–46.

34. Connolly JM, Hansen TH, Ingold AL, Potter TA. Recognition by CD8 on cytotoxic T lymphocytes is ablated by several substitutions in the class I alpha 3 domain: CD8 and the T-cell receptor recognize the same class I molecule. *Proc Natl Acad Sci USA* 1990;87:2137–41.

35. Potter TA, Rajan TV, Dick RFD, Bluestone JA. Substitution at residue 227 of H-2 class I molecules abrogates recognition by CD8-dependent, but not CD8-independent, cytotoxic T lymphocytes. *Nature* 1989;337:73–75.

36. Luescher IF, Vivier E, Layer A, et al. CD8 modulation of T-cell antigen receptor-ligand interactions on living cytotoxic T lymphocytes. *Nature* 1995;373:353–356.

37. Garcia KC, Scott CA, Brunmark A, et al. CD8 enhances formation of stable T-cell receptor/MHC class I molecule complexes. *Nature* 1996;384:577–581.

38. Zamoyska R. The CD8 coreceptor revisited: one chain good, two chains better. *Immunity* 1994;1:243–246.

39. Thome M, Germain V, DiSanto JP, Acuto O. The p56lck SH2 domain mediates recruitment of CD8/p56lck to the activated T cell receptor/CD3/zeta complex. *Eur J Immunol* 1996;26:2093–2100.

40. Madrenas J, Chau LA, Smith J, Bluestone JA, Germain RN. The efficiency of CD4 recruitment to ligand-engaged TCR controls the agonist/partial agonist properties of peptide-MHC molecule ligands. *J Exp Med* 1997;185:219–230.

41. Hampl J, Chien YH, Davis M. CD4 augments the response of a T cell to agonist but not to antagonist ligands. *Immunity* 1997;7:379–385.

42. Maryanski JL, Pala P, Cerottini JC, MacDonald HR. Antigen recognition by H-2-restricted cytolytic T lymphocytes: inhibition of cytolysis by anti-CD8 monoclonal antibodies depends upon both concentration and primary sequence of peptide antigen. *Eur J Immunol* 1988;18:1863–1866.

43. McCarthy SA, Kaldjian E, Singer A. Induction of anti-CD8 resistant cytotoxic T lymphocytes by anti-CD8 antibodies: functional evidence for T cell signaling induced by multi-valent cross-linking of CD8 on precursor cells. *J Immunol* 1988;141:3737–3746.

44. Kessler BM, Bassanini P, Horvath C, Cerottini JC, Luescher IF. Effects of epitope modification on TCR-ligand binding and antigen recognition by seven H-2Kd-restricted CTL clones specific for a photoreactive peptide derivative. *J Exp Med* 1996;185:629–640.

45. Kwan-Lim GE, Ong T, Aosai F, Stauss H, Zamoyska R. Is CD8 dependence a true reflection of TCR affinity for antigen? *Int Immunol* 1993;5:1219–1228.

46. Auphan N, Curnow J, Guimezanes A, et al. The degree of CD8 dependence of cytolytic T cell precursors is determined by the nature of the T cell receptor (TCR) and influences negative selection in TCR-transgenic mice. *Eur J Immunol* 1994;24:1572–1577.

47. Kessler B, Hudrisier D, Cerottini JC, Luescher IF. Role of CD8 in aberrant of cytotoxic T lymphocytes. *J Exp Med* 1997;186:2033–2038.

48. Hudrisier D, Kessler B, Valitutti S, Horvath C, Cerottini JC, Luescher IF. The efficiency of antigen recognition by CD8+ CTL clones is determined by the frequency of serial TCR engagement. *J Immunol* 1998;161:553–562.

49. Renard V, Romero P, Vivier E, Malissen B, Luescher IF. CD8 beta increases CD8 coreceptor function and participation in TCR-ligand binding. *J Exp Med* 1996;184:2439–2444.

50. Wheeler C, Chen J, Potter T, Parnes J. Mechanisms of CD8beta-mediated T cell response enhancement: interaction with MHC class I/beta2-microglobulin and functional coupling to TCR/CD3. *J Immunol* 1998;161:4199–4207.

51. Irie HY, Mong MS, Itano A, et al. The cytoplasmic domain of CD8 beta regulates Lck kinase activation. *J Immunol* 1998;161:183–191.

52. Itano A, Cado D, Chan FKM, Robey E. A role for the cytoplasmic tail of the β chain of CD8 in thymic selection. *Immunity* 1994;1:287–290.

53. Crooks ME, Littman DR. Disruption of T lymphocyte positive and negative selection in mice lacking the CD8β chain. *Immunity* 1994;1:277–285.

54. Anel A, O'Rourke AM, Kleinfeld AM, Mescher MF. T cell receptor and CD8-dependent tyrosine phosphorylation events in cytotoxic T lymphocytes: activation of p56^{lck} by CD8 binding to class I protein. *Eur J Immunol* 1996;26:2310–2319.

55. Kwan Lim GE, McNeill L, Whitley K, Becker DL, Zamoyska R. Co-capping studies reveal CD8/TCR interactions after capping CD8 beta polypeptides and intracellular associations of CD8 with p56^{lck}. *Eur J Immunol* 1998;28:745–754.

56. Kane KP, Mescher MF. Activation of CD8-dependent cytotoxic T lymphocyte adhesion and degranulation by peptide class I antigen complexes. *J Immunol* 1993;150:4788–4797.

57. O'Rourke AM, Rogers J, Mescher MF. Activated CD8 binding to class I protein mediated by the T-cell receptor results in signalling. *Nature* 1990; 346:187–189.

58. O'Rourke A, Apgar J, Kane K, Martz E, Mescher M. Cytoskeletal function in CD8- and T cell receptor-mediated interaction of cytotoxic T lymphocytes with class I protein. *J Exp Med* 1991; 173:241–249.

59. Shen L, Potter TA, Kane KP. Glu227 → Lys substitution in the acidic loop of major histocompatibility complex class I alpha 3 domain distinguishes low avidity CD8 coreceptor and avidity-enhanced CD8 accessory functions. *J Exp Med* 1996;184:1671–1683.

60. Luescher IF, Cerottini JC, Romero P. Photoaffinity labeling of the T cell receptor on cloned cytotoxic T lymphocytes by covalent photoreactive ligand. *J Biol Chem* 1994;269:5574–5582.

61. O'Rourke A, Mescher M. The roles of CD8 in cytotoxic T lymphocyte function. *Immunol Today* 1993;14:183–188.

62. Weber S, Traunecker A, Oliveri F, Gerhard W, Karjalainen K. Specific low affinity recognition of major histocompatibility complex plus peptide by soluble T-cell receptor. *Nature* 1992;356:793–796.

63. Schneck J, Maloy W, Coligan J, Margulies D. Inhibition of an allospecific T cell hybridoma by soluble class I proteins and peptides: estimation of the affinity of a T cell receptor for MHC. *Cell* 1989;56:47–55.

64. Matsui K, Boniface J, Reay P, et al. Low affinity interaction of peptide-MHC complexes with T cell receptors. *Science* 1991;254:1788–1791.

65. Sykulev Y, Brunmark A, Jackson M, Cohen RJ, Peterson PA, Eisen HN. Kinetics and affinity of reactions between an antigen-specific T cell receptor and peptide-MHC complexes. *Immunity* 1994;1:15–22.

66. Sykulev Y, Brunmark A, Tsomides T, et al. High-affinity reactions between antigen-specific T-cell receptors and peptides associated with allogeneic and syngeneic major histocompatibility complex class I proteins. *Proc Natl Acad Sci USA* 1994;91:11487–11491.

67. Schodin BA, Tsomides TJ0, Kranz DM. Correlation between the number of T cell receptors required for T cell activation and TCR-ligand affinity. *Immunity* 1996;5:137–146.

68. Lyons DS, Lieberman SA, Hampl J, et al. A TCR binds to antagonist ligands with lower affinities and faster dissociation rates than agonists. *Immunity* 1996;5:53–63.

69. Matsui K, Boniface J, Steffner P, Reay P, Davis M. Kinetics of T-cell receptor binding to peptide/I-Ek complexes: correlation of the dissociation rate with T-cell responsiveness. *Proc Natl Acad Sci USA* 1994;91:12862–12866.

70. Corr M, Slanetz AE, Boyd LF, et al. T cell receptor-MHC class I peptide interactions: affinity, kinetics and specificity. *Science* 1994;265:946–949.

71. Alramadi BK, Jelonek MT, Boyd LF, Margulies DH, Bothwell ALM. Lack of strict correlation of functional sensitization with the apparent affinity of MHC/peptide complexes for the TCR. *J Immunol* 1995;155:662–673.

72. Crawford F, Kozono H, White J, Marrack P, Kappler J. Detection of antigen-specific T cells with multivalent soluble class II MHC covalent peptide complexes. *Immunity* 1998;8:675–682.

73. Luescher IF, Anjuere F, Peitsch MC, Jongeneel CV, Cerottini JC, Romero P. Structural analysis of TCR-ligand interactions studied on H-2Kd-restricted cloned CTL specific for a photoreactive peptide derivative. *Immunity* 1995;3:51–63.

74. Anjuére F, Kuznetsov D, Romero P, Cerottini JC, Jongeneel CV, Luescher IF. Differential roles of T cell receptor α and β chains in ligand binding among H-2K^d-restricted cytolytic T lymphocyte clones specific for a photoreactive *Plasmodium berghei* circumsporozoite peptide derivative. *J Biol Chem* 1997;272:8505–8514.

75. Romero P, Maryansky JL, Luescher IF. Photoaffinity labeling of the T cell receptor on living cytotoxic T lymphocytes. *J Immunol* 1993;150:3825–3831.

76. Fremont DH, Rees WA, Kozono H. Biophysical studies of T-cell receptors and their ligands. *Curr Opin Immunol* 1996;8:93–100.

77. Traunecker A, Dolder B, Oliveri F, Karjalainen K. Solubilizing the T-cell receptor—problems in solution. *Immunol Today* 1989;10:29–32.

78. Engel I, Ottenhoff TH, Klausner RD. High-efficiency expression and solubilization of functional T cell antigen receptor heterodimers. *Science* 1992;256:1318–1321.

79. Seth A, Stern JL, Ottenhoff TH, et al. Binary and ternary complexes between T-cell receptor, class II MHC and superantigen in vitro. *Nature* 1994;369:324–327.

80. Chang HC, Bao ZZ, Yao Y, et al. A general method for facilitating heterodimeric pairing between two proteins: application to expression of alpha and beta T-cell receptor extracellular segments. *Proc Natl Acad Sci USA* 1994;91:11408–11412.

81. Kurucz I, Jost CR, George AJ, Andrew SM, Segal DM. A bacterially expressed single-chain Fv construct from the 2B4 T-cell receptor. *Proc Natl Acad Sci USA* 1993;90:3830–3834.

82. Hoo WF, Lacy JM, Denzin LK, Voss EW, Hardman KD, Kranz DM. Characterization of a single-chain T-cell receptor expressed in *Escherichia coli. Proc Natl Acad Sci USA* 1992;89:4759–4763.

83. Gregoire C, Lin SY, Mazza G, Rebai N, Luescher IF, Malissen B. Covalent assembly of a soluble T cell receptor-peptide-major histocompatibility class I complex. *Proc Natl Acad Sci USA* 1996;93:7184–7189.

84. Alam S, Travers P, Wung J, et al. T cell receptor affinity and thymocyte positive selection. *Science* 1996;381:616–620.

85. Davis M, Boniface J, Reich Z, et al. Ligand recognition by ab T cell receptor. *Annu Rev Immunol* 1998;16:523–544.

86. Hudrisier D, Gairin JE. Peptide-major histocompatibility complex class I complex: from the structural and molecular basis to pharmacological principles and therapeutic applications. *Curr Top Microbiol Immunol* 1998;232:75–97.

87. Berke G. The CTL's kiss of death. *Cell* 1995; 81:9–12.

88. Depraetere V, Goldstein P. Fas and other cell death signaling pathways. *Semin Immunol* 1997; 9:93–107.

89. Nagata S, Golstein P. The Fas death factor. *Science* 1995;267:1449–1456.

90. Kessler B, Hudrisier D, Schroeter M, Tschopp J, Cerottini JC, Luescher I. Peptide modification or blocking of CD8, resulting in weak TRC signaling, can activate CTL for Fas- but not perforin-dependent cytotoxicity or cytokine production. *J Immunol* 1998;161:6939–6946.

91. Evavold BD, Sloanlancaster J, Wilson KJ, Rothbard JB, Allen PM. Specific T cell recognition of minimally homologous peptides: evidence for multiple endogenous ligands. *Immunity* 1995;2: 655–663.

92. Evavold BD, Allen PM. Separation of IL-4 production from Th cell proliferation by an altered T cell receptor ligand. *Science* 1991;252:1308–1310.

93. DeMagistris MT, Alexander J, Coggeshall M, et al. Antigen analog-major histocompatibility complexes act as antagonists of the T cell receptor. *Cell* 1992;68:625–634.

94. Jameson SC, Carbone FR, Bevan MJ. Clone-specific T cell receptor antagonists of major histocompatibility complex class I-restricted cytotoxic T cells. *J Exp Med* 1993;177:1541–1550.

95. Brossart P, Bevan MJ. Selective activation of Fas/Fas ligand-mediated cytotoxicity by a self peptide. *J Exp Med* 1996;183:2449–2458.

96. Cao W, Tykodi SS, Esser MT, Braciale VL, Braciale TJ. Partial activation of CD8⁺ T cells by a self-derived peptide. *Nature* 1995;378:295–298.

97. Martin S, Kohler H, Weltzien HU, Leipner C. Selective activation of CD8 T cell effector functions by epitope variants of lymphocytic choriomeningitis virus glycoprotein. *J Immunol* 1996;157:2358–2365.

98. Combadière B, Reis e Sousa C, Germain RN, Lenardo MJ. Selective induction of apoptosis in mature T lymphocytes by variant T cell receptor ligands. *J Exp Med* 1998;187:349–355.

99. Klenerman P, Rowland-Jones S, McAdam S, et al. Cytotoxic T-cell activity antagonized by naturally occurring HIV-1 Gag variants. *Nature* 1994;369: 403–407.

100. Bertoletti A, Sette A, Chisari FV, et al. Natural variants of cytotoxic epitopes are T-cell receptor antagonists for antiviral cytotoxic T cells. *Nature* 1994;369:407–410.

101. Wucherpfennig KW, Strominger JL. Molecular mimicry in T cell-mediated autoimmunity: viral peptides activate human T cell clones specific for myelin basic protein. *Cell* 1995;80:695–705.

102. Hemmer B, Fleckenstein B, Vergelli M, et al. Identification of a high potency microbial and self-ligands for a human autireactive class II-restricted T cell clone. *J Exp Med* 1997;185:1651–1659.

103. Salemi S, Caporossi AP, Boffa L, Longobardi MG, Barnaba V. HIVgp120 activates autoreactive CD4-specific T cell responses by unveiling of hidden CD4 peptides during processing. *J Exp Med* 1995;181:2253–2257.

104. Hu Q, Bazemore Walker C, Girao C, et al. Specific recognition of thymic self-peptides induces the positive selection of cytotoxic T lymphocytes. *Immunity* 1997;7:221–231.

105. Hogquist K, Tomlinson A, Kieper W, et al. Identification of a naturally occurring ligand for thymic positive selection. *Immunity* 1997;6:389–399.

106. Jameson SC, Bevan M. T cell receptor antagonists and partial agonists. *Immunity* 1995;2:1–11.

107. Kohler J, Hartmann U, Grimm R, Plugfelder U, Weltzien HU. Carrier-independent hapten recognition and promiscuous MHC restriction by T cells induced by trinitrophenylated peptides. *J Immunol* 1997;158:591–597.

108. Hess DA, Rieder MJ. The role of reactive drug metabolites in immune-mediated adverse drug reactions. *Ann Pharmacother.* 1997;31:1378–1387.

109. Alberola-Ila J, Takaki S, Kerner J, Perlmutter R. Differential signaling by lymphocyte antigen receptors. *Annu Rev Immunol* 1997;15:125–154.

110. Cantrell D. T cell antigen receptor transduction pathways. *Annu Rev Immunol* 1996;14:259–274.

111. Justement LB. The role of CD45 in signal transduction. *Adv Immunol* 1997;66:1–65.

112. Stone JD, Conroy LA, Byth KF, et al. Aberrant TCR-mediated signaling in CD45-null thymocytes involves dysfunctional regulation of Lck, Fyn, TCR-zeta and ZAP-70. *J Immunol* 1997;158:5773–5782.

113. Sloan-Lancaster J, Zhang W, Presley J, et al. Regulation of ZAP-70 intracellular localization: visualization with the green fluorescent protein. *J Exp Med* 1997;186:1713–1724.

114. Zhang W, Sloan-Lancaster J, Kitchen J, Trible R, Samelson L. LAT: the ZAP-70 tyrosine kinase substrate that links T cell receptor to cellular activation. *Cell* 1998;92:83–92.

115. Madrenas J, Wange RL, Wang JL, Isakov N, Samelson LE, Germain RN. ζ Phosphorylation without ZAP-70 activation induced by TCR antagonists or partial agonists. *Science* 1995;267:515–518.

116. Sloan-Lancaster J, Shaw AS, Rothbard JB, Allen PM. Partial T cell signalling: altered phospho-ζ and lack of ZAP70 recruitment in APL-induced T cell anergy. *Cell* 1994;79:913–922.

117. Reis e Sousa C, Levine EH, Germain RN. Partial signaling by CD8+ T cells in response to antagonist ligands. *J Exp Med* 1996;184:149–157.

118. Jensen W, Pleiman ACM, Beaufils P, Wegener AM, Malissen B, Cambier JC. Qualitatively distinct signaling through T cell antigen receptor subunits. *Eur J Immunol* 1997;27:707–716.

119. Kimura T, Kihara H, Bhattacharyya S, Sakamoto H, Appella E, Siraganian RP. Downstream signaling molecules bind to different phosphorylated immunoreceptor tyrosine-based activation motif (ITAM) peptides of the high affinity IgE receptor. *J Biol Chem* 1996;271:27962–27968.

120. Sunder-Plassmann R, Lialios F, Madsen M, Koyasu S, Reinherz EL. Functional analysis of immunoreceptor tyrosine-based activation motif (ITAM)-mediated signal transduction: the two YxxL segments within a single CD3/ζ-ITAM are functionally distinct. *Eur J Immunol* 1997;27:2001–2009.

121. Zenner G, Vorherr T, Mustelin T, Burn P. Differential and multiple binding of signal transducing molecules to the ITAMs of the TCR-z chain. *J Cell Biochem* 1996;63:94.

122. Kersh EN, Shaw AS, Allen PM. Fidelity of T cell activation through multistep T cell receptor zeta phosphorylation. *Science* 1998;281:572–575.

123. Plas D, Johnson R, Pingel J, et al. Direct regulation of ZAP-70 by SHP-1 in T cell antigen receptor signaling. *Science* 1996;272:1173–1176.

124. Racioppi L, Matarese G, D'Oro H, et al. The role of CD4-lck in T cell receptor antagonsim: evidence for negative signaling. *Proc Natl Acad Sci USA* 1996;93:10360–10365.

125. McKeithan T. Kinetic proofreading in T-cell receptor signal transduction. *Proc Natl Acad Sci USA* 1995;92:5042–5046.

126. Rabinowitz J, Beeson C, Lyons D, Davis M, McConnell H. Kinetic discrimination in T-cell activation. *Proc Natl Acad Sci USA* 1996;93:1401–1405.

127. Janeway C. Ligands for the T cell receptor: hard times for avidity models. *Immunol Today* 1995;16:223–225.

128. Yoon ST, Dianzani U, Bottomly K, Janeway CA. Both high and low avidity antibodies to the T cell receptor can have agonist or antagonist activity. *Immunity* 1994;1:563–569.

129. Teng MK, Smolyar A, Tse AGD, et al. Identification of a common docking topology with substantial variation among different TCR-peptide-MHC complexes. *Curr Biol* 1998;8:409–412.

130. Valitutti S, Dessing M, Aktories K, Gallati H, Lanzavecchia A. Sustained signaling leading to T cell activation results from prolonged T cell receptor occupancy. *J Exp Med* 1995;181:577–584.

131. Valitutti S, Muller S, Cella M, Padovan E, Lanzavecchia A. Serial triggering of many T-cell receptors by a few peptide-MHC complexes. *Nature* 1995;375:148–151.

132. Sykulev Y, Joo M, Vturina I, Tsomides T, Eisen H. Evidence that a single peptide-MHC complex on a target cell can elicit a cytolytic T cell response. *Immunity* 1996;4:565–571.

133. Ullrich A, Schlessinger J. Signal transduction by receptors with tyrosine kinase activity. *Cell* 1990;61:203–212.

134. Abastado J, Lone Y, Casrouge A, Boulot G, Kourilsky P. Dimerization of soluble major histocompatibility complex-peptide complexes is sufficient for activation of T cell hybridoma and induction of unresponsivenes. *J Exp Med* 1995;182:439–447.

135. Reich Z, Boniface J, Lyons D, Borochov N, Wachtel E, Davis M. Ligand specific oligomerization of T cell receptor molecules. *Nature* 1997;387:617–620.

136. Wu H, Kwong PD, Hendrickson WA. Dimeric association and segmental variability in the structure of human CD4. *Nature* 1997;387:527–530.

137. Monks CRF, Freiberg BA, Kupfer H, Sciaky N, Kupfer A. Three-dimensional segregation of supramolecular activation clusters in T cells. *Nature* 1998;395:82–86

138. Brdicka T, Cerny J, Horejsi V. T cell receptor signalling results in rapid tyrosine phosphorylation of the linker protein LAT present in detergent-resistent membrane microdomains. *Biochem Biophys Res Commun* 1998;248:356–360.

139. Zhang W, Trible RP, Samelson LE. LAT palmitoylation: its essential role in membrane microdomain targeting and tyrosine phosphorylation during T cell activation. *Immunity* 1998;9:239–246.

140. Friedrichson T, Kurzchalia TV. Microdomains of GPI-anchored proteins in living cells revealed. *Nature* 1998;394:802–805.

Cytotoxic Cells: Basic Mechanisms and
Medical Applications, edited by Michail V.
Sitkovsky and Pierre A. Henkart. Lippincott
Williams & Wilkins, Philadelphia © 2000.

Chapter 4

Murine NK Receptors: Ly-49 Expression, Function, and Intracellular Signaling

John R. Ortaldo and Daniel W. McVicar

*Laboratory of Experimental Immunology, Division of Basic Sciences,
National Cancer Institute-FCRDC, Frederick, Maryland 21702, USA*

Natural killer (NK) cells were discovered by virtue of their ability to lyse selected tumor cell lines in the absence of prior sensitization or immunization. Early studies demonstrated that NK cells could lyse tumor cells regardless of their major histocompatibility antigens (MHC), even lysing tumor lines that lacked detectible MHC. Therefore NK cells were defined as "CD3−, T cell receptor (α, β, γ, δ)- and recombinase negative lymphocytes" that "mediate cytolytic reactions that do not require expression of class I or class II MHC molecules on the target cell" (1). NK cells, because of their prevalence in the circulation and their ability to clear circulating tumor cells, were generally thought to provide surveillance against tumors and virally infected cells. Until recently the surface receptors that NK cells utilized to mediate cytotoxic reactions against tumor targets were not well understood. However, an inverse correlation between the expression of surface MHC class I (MHC-I) molecules on selected targets and their susceptibility to NK-mediated lysis led Kärre to propose the "missing self hypothesis." This hypothesis predicts that upon interrogation of a potential target NK cells spare the target only when they detect self MHC. Exploration of this hypothesis has led to the discovery of a new class of receptors initially described on NK cells (2–4), but also present on other leukocytes, that regulate cellular

function by muting otherwise activating signals. The basis of this regulation appears to be MHC-I recognition. We term the newly discovered molecules leukocyte regulatory receptors (LRRs). Evidence is mounting which suggests that these receptors play a unique role in immunity by regulating effector cell functions in response to various levels of MHC-I expression.

The LRRs are now known to be involved in both positive and negative regulation of immune cell function. Although originally characterized as inhibitory receptors, LRRs can contain either inhibitory or activation motifs within their cytoplasmic domains and include membrane receptors of both the immunoglobulin (Ig)- and C-type lectin superfamilies. LRR expression is broad, with family members being found on a variety of leukocyte associated Ig-like receptor 1 (LAIR) (5), including natural killer and T cells [killer cell inhibitory receptors, KIR (2–4), Ly-49 (6–10), CD94 (11,12), gp49 (13,14), NKG2 (15,16)], B cells [paired Ig-like receptors (17,18)], mast cells [gp49 (13), mast cell function-associated antigen (MAFA) (19,20)], and monocyte/macrophage and dendritic cells [Ig-like transcripts (21,22), leukocyte Ig-like receptor (LIR) (23,24), PIR (17,25)]. This review focuses on the biology of the mouse Ly-49 family of NK cell receptors. We first review Ly-49 expression and biologic functions and then discuss their biochemical mode of action and signal transduction.

EXPRESSION OF LY-49 NK RECEPTORS

Members of the Ly-49 gene family encode type II integral transmembrane proteins that are primarily expressed on the surface of murine NK cells. Most members (Ly-49A, B, C, E, F, G, I, J, and M) of the Ly-49 family of receptors contain inhibitory motifs within their cytoplasmic domains (see below), bind MHC-I, and transmit inhibitory signals that prevent NK cells from mediating cytotoxicity. In addition to these inhibitory Ly-49s, Ly-49s that lack inhibitory motifs and apparently activate NK cells have been described (Ly-49D, H, K, L, and N) (26). The prototype inhibitory receptor, Ly-49A, has been shown to recognize the class I molecules H2-D^d and H2-D^k (27,28). The interaction of Ly-49A with H2-D^d has been shown to transmit a negative signal to the NK cell, the nature of which is discussed later in the chapter (9).

Expression of Inhibitory Receptors

Most studies have examined Ly-49 expression in a few selected strains of mice (e.g., Balb/c or C57BL/6 mice). Our recent study of expression of Ly-49s in 11 strains of mice yielded a complex and interesting pattern of expression. These findings are summarized in Table 4-1. Ly-49G2 was expressed at varying degrees on the NK cells of all strains of mice examined. As seen with Ly-49A, levels of Ly-49G2 expression are lower on strains that express its proposed class I ligand, H2-D (29). Ly-49A was analyzed using numerous anti-Ly-49A antibodies, including A1, YE1/48, and YE1/32. Using these reagents, Ly-49A-expression was found on a low percentage of NK cells from most strains of mice tested, the exceptions being 129/J and SJL/J (28,29). Using SW5E6 (an antibody reactive with both Ly-49C and Ly-49I), we found that, similar to Ly-49A and G,

most strains expressed Ly-49C/I. AKR mice, however, completely lacked Ly-49C/I. Unfortunately, specific reagents are not yet available to identify Ly-49B, E, F, J, or M.

Expression of Activating Receptors

With the recent report of McQueen et al. (26), there are now five putative activating Ly-49s: Ly-49D, H, K, L, and N. Unfortunately, antibodies are currently available only for Ly-49D. Based on two anti-Ly-49D antibodies, 4E5 and 12A8 (12A8 cross-reacts with Ly-49A, but 4E5 is specific for Ly-49D), we have found that NK cells from only certain strains of mice express Ly-49D (30), including SJL/J and 129/J. In C57B1/6 mice nearly 50% of NK cells are Ly-49D-positive (Ly-49D$^+$). Data on the expression of activating and inhibitory KIRs has suggested that regardless of the complexity of the inhibitory repertoire all human NK cells express at least one noninhibitory KIR (31,32). Why each human NK cell would require at least one noninhibitory KIR is, at present, an open question. Confirmation of this observation in murine NK cells through the demonstration of at least one activating Ly-49 on the NK cells of all strains of mice would highlight the potential importance of the activating MHC class I binding receptors. Development of reagents specific for Ly-49H, K, L, and N is undoubtedly underway, so we should have an answer soon.

Although Ly-49s are predominantly expressed on NK cells, a small subset of T cells in the mouse express these NK receptors. Whereas all NK cells express at least one Ly-49, only 2% to 5% of total T cells are Ly-49 positive (Ly-49$^+$). We have detected Ly-49s on both CD4$^+$ and CD8$^+$ T cells and found that most Ly-49$^+$ T cells expressed the NK marker NK1.1 as well. Interestingly, the strain expression pattern for the inhibitory Ly-49s was identical between NK cells and T cells. That is, if the NK cells of a given mouse strain expressed a given Ly-49, that molecule could also be detected

TABLE 4-1. *Strain summary of NK and T cells of Ly-49 expression by flow cytometry: percentage expression from normal spleen lymphocytes*

Strain	Haplotype	CD3⁻ Ly-49A⁺	CD3⁺ Ly-49A⁺	CD3⁻ Ly-49C/I⁺	CD3⁺ Ly-49C/I⁺	CD3⁻ Ly-49D⁺	CD3⁺ Ly-49D⁺	CD3⁻ Ly-49G⁺	CD3⁺ Ly-49G⁺
C57B1/6	b	+	+	+	+	+	−	+	+
DBA/2	d	+	+	+	+	−	−	+	+
AKH2	d/k	+	+	+	+	−	−	+	+
AKR	k	+	+	−	−	−	−	+	+
CBA/J	k	+	+	+	+	−	−	+	+
129/J	b	−	−	−	−	+	−	+	+
Balb/c	d	+	+	+	+	−	−	+	+
CC57B1/6F1	b/d	+	+	+	+	+	−	+	+
C3H/HeJ	k	+	+	+	+	−	−	+	+
Athymics	?	+	+	+	+	−	−	+	+
SJL/J	s	−	−	−	−	+	−	+	+

Freshly isolated spleen cells were analyzed with the indicated antibodies based on a lymphocyte gate (forward and side scatter).

+, > 1% specific expression; −, no specific expression.

on the T cells of that strain (33). These data suggest that whatever force is regulating the Ly-49 repertoire is at work in both NK cells and T cells, seemingly ruling out NK-specific nuclear factors or selection processes that would affect NK cells but not T cells. There was, however, one important exception to the match in expression patterns in T cells and NK cells. In our hands, T cells did not express Ly-49D, the only activating Ly-49 for which specific antibodies are available. Perhaps T cells express one of the newer putative activating Ly-49s (26). Another possible explanation for this finding is centered on the biochemical actions of Ly-49D (see below). Because many of the biochemical pathways activated by Ly-49D, and presumably by other activating Ly-49s as well, are similar to those induced by the T cell receptor (TCR), perhaps expression of a functional TCR precludes the requirement for activating Ly-49s. Elucidation of the biologic role of the activating Ly-49s through genetic or biochemical means may help us understand why T cells sometimes express inhibitory Ly-49s but not activating Ly-49s.

To date, little is known regarding the regulation of Ly-49 expression. Neonatal NK cells lack Ly-49, but expression becomes evident soon after birth (2–3 weeks) and is maximal by 5 to 7 weeks (34). Both *in vitro* and *in vivo* studies have demonstrated that, once established, Ly-49 expression patterns are stable, not being inducible or repressible with various treatments (9,34). The formation of the repertoire of Ly-49 NK cell receptors was investigated by Dorfman and Raulet (34) after in vivo transfer. They found that when NK cells lacking specific Ly-49s were transferred these cells could give rise to cells that expressed those same Ly-49s. In addition, they found that NK cells that expressed some Ly-49s at the time of transfer could give rise to cells expressing others. These developments in the Ly-49 repertoire occurred within 10 days of transfer; after that time the expression patterns were stable. Therefore after Ly-49 receptor expression occurs, it appears to be stable *in vivo*. The one exception noted was that Ly-49A expression did not occur *in vivo* if Ly-49A⁻ NK cells were transferred. The explanation for this finding is currently unclear, although these authors postulated that the expression order of Ly-49s might be nonrandom (34). Further analysis of Ly-49 expression and dissection of their promoters should elucidate the regulatory events taking place in such models.

FUNCTION OF LY-49s

Inhibition of Cytotoxicity

Ly-49A has been shown to recognize the class I molecules H2-D^d and H2-D^k (27,28,35). Early studies examining the interaction of Ly-49A with H2-D^d postulated transmission of a negative or inhibitory signal to the NK cell. This hypothesis was based on the observation that targets expressing class I molecules, either natively or via transfection, were not lysed by Ly-49A expressing NK cells (27,28). When similar studies were performed with Ly-49G2-expressing NK cells, killing was inhibited by target cells expressing H-2D^d and/or H-2L^d (36). Studies with Ly-49$^+$ NK cells have relied primarily on the reversal of target cell inhibition by monoclonal antibodies (mAbs) specific for MHC-I haplotypes or Ly-49s and more recently class I transfected target cell lines (29). The Ly-49C$^+$ subset (defined by SW5E6 antibodies) of NK cells has been shown to bind the class I molecules H-2^b, H-2^d, H-2^k, and H-2^s (37–39). However, recent data indicating that SW5E6 reacts with both Ly-49C and Ly-49I raises concerns regarding which Ly-49 is responsible for these reported class I effects (37). Ly-49G2 and Ly-49A, which mediate strong inhibitory effects on NK cell functions, appear to function similarly in T cells, regulating NK-like cytolytic activity. As a percentage of the total T cell population, however, Ly-49 expression is low (<5%), and the functional role of these unique cells in vivo is not understood. Regardless, the selection and expansion of NK1.1$^+$ or DX5$^+$ T cell populations that co-express Ly-49s demonstrate that the spontaneous lytic process of these cells can be regulated by interactions with class I molecules (33).

Regulation of Noncytotoxic Functions

In addition to the lytic event, effector–target interaction results in NK-mediated production of cytokines. Purified murine NK cells cultured in the presence of targets expressing specific class I molecules produce less interferon gamma (IFN-γ), tumor necrosis factor alpha (TNF-α), and granulocyte/macrophage-colony-stimulating factor (GM-CSF) than those exposed to class I negative targets (33). Cytokine induction with phorbol myristic acetate (PMA) and ionomycin is not modulated by Ly-49 ligation. These results indicate that, in addition to regulation of cytotoxic activity, class I interactions with these inhibitory NK receptors can regulate the production of physiologically important cytokines. Ly-49s inhibit T cell target-induced cytokine production in a manner similar to that displayed by NK cells (40). Interestingly, the addition of targets expressing class I molecules that normally inhibit NK cell function to Ly-49$^+$ T cells had no effect on CD3-induced cytokine production or on pharmacologically induced cytokines. These findings suggest that Ly-49s serve as a regulatory control for T cells under some circumstances but not during CD3-mediated responses.

Ly-49-mediated regulation of NK cytokine production is likely to be an important physiological event in a number of settings. For example, IFN-γ production by NK cells is critical for antiviral effects against leukocyte choriomeningitis virus (LCMV) (41,42). Moreover, studies have demonstrated important marrow-regulating effects of NK cells in perforin and Fas knockout mice (43). These data support the hypothesis that cytokine production by NK cells, and perhaps by T cells, might be paramount in the regulation of hybrid resistance and marrow transplantation. The abilities of Ly-49 molecules to regulate NK cytokine production could therefore have dramatic influences on stem cell repopulation.

Activation of Cytotoxicity

Murine Ly-49D and Ly-49H represent putative activating NK receptors. Our initial studies with antibodies to Ly-49D (using antibody 12A8) demonstrated Ly-49D activation of NK cells by virtue of its ability to mediate reverse antibody-dependent cell-mediated cytotoxicity (ADCC) of FcR$^+$ targets (30). Furthermore, similar to CD16 crosslinking in human NK, cells, Ly-49D ligation results in apoptosis (30). In addition studies from several laboratories have indicated that Ly-49D recognizes class I in a positive manner, resulting in increased killing of selected class I-expressing targets (29). Both Ly-49D and Ly-49H mediate biochemical activation (44,45) (see below), but the functional recognition of, and cellular activation by, Ly-49H awaits the development of anti-Ly-49H antibodies.

IN VIVO FUNCTION OF LY-49s

Bone marrow transplantation (BMT) is used to treat a variety of cancers. Significant obstacles limit its use, however, such as the occurrence of graft-versus-host disease (GVHD) and relapse of the cancer. Attempts to reduce the relapse rate often result in increased GVHD. The use of NK cells during BMT is attractive, as NK cells exhibit direct antitumor effects (46–48) and may promote graft-versus-tumor (GVT) effects by removing minimal residual disease. NK cells also have been shown to promote hematopoietic engraftment (46,47).

In contrast to their beneficial effects, NK cells also can mediate the specific rejection of bone marrow cell (BMC) allografts in lethally irradiated mice. Previous studies have proposed novel ligands such as Hh to explain marrow engraftment. However, the Ly-49 family of molecules present on subsets of murine NK cells appears capable of binding MHC-I molecules, resulting in transmission of a regulatory (inhibitory or activating) signal to the NK cell. Ly-49 NK receptors appear to be the major mechanism for this phenomenon. Studies performed by a variety of laboratories have demonstrated class I recognition patterns in hematopoietic engraftment that parallel, and substantiate, in vitro recognition of class I (Table 4-2) (38,39,48–52). These initial studies indicated that inhibitory receptors turning off NK cell functions seemed to explain the pattern of marrow engraftment. For example, the ability of H-2^b mice to reject H-2^d marrow was not altered by ablation of Ly-49G2-bearing NK cells, as they were inhibited by H-2^d. However, Ly-49C/I-bearing NK cells were a major effector in this rejection, as these cells are inhibited by H-2^b class I but not by H-2^d. The role of the activating NK receptors was elucidated by studies demonstrating that Ly-49D$^+$ NK cells (from H-2^b mice) were also responsible for the rejection H-2^d BMC allografts because Ly-49D is positively engaged by H-2^d (50). These Ly-49D-bearing NK cells therefore could function additively with Ly-49C$^+$ NK cells in the rejection of H-2^d BMCs. These data collectively indicate that both subsets play a role in the rejection

TABLE 4-2. *Summary of Ly-49s*

Ly-49	Ligand	Motif	mAb	Function	Cytokines	Cell type
A	D^d	ITIM	AI, YE1/48	Blocks	↓ IFN-γ	NK, T
	D^k		YE1/32		↓ GM-CSF	
B		ITIM				
C	H2^{d,k,s}	ITIM	5E6, 4LO3311	Blocks		NK, T
	K^b					
D	D^d	ITAM	12A1	Activates	↑ IFN-γ	NK
			12A8			
			4E5			
E		ITIM				
F		ITIM				
G2	D^d	ITIM	4D11	Blocks	↓ IFN-γ	NK, T
	L^d (weak)				↓ GM-CSF	
H		ITAM		Activates	↑ Ca^{+2} flux	
I	D^b	ITIM	5E6	Blocks		

of allogeneic H-2-homozygous H-2^d BMCs. Therefore NK subsets demonstrate a differential ability to reject H-2 homozygous and heterozygous BMCs by combinatorial use of their array of Ly-49 NK receptors, both activating and inhibitory.

SIGNALING BY LY-49 RECEPTORS

Significant increases in our understanding of the biochemical events involved in multichain immune recognition receptor function have occurred over the last several years. This, together with the recent development of reagents specific for several members of the Ly-49 family, have allowed, for the first time, detailed study of the biochemical mechanisms of Ly-49 function. This analysis has broadened to include detailed biochemical, molecular, and genetic studies. As mentioned above, the Ly-49 family is a group of type II transmembrane proteins that includes both positively and negatively signaling receptors. Below we review the evolution of the current models to explain both the positive and negative actions of various Ly-49 family members.

Inhibitory Receptors

Most Ly-49s described to date appear to be negative regulators of receptor-mediated signaling in murine NK cells. Although the phenomenon of inhibition of NK cytolytic activity by class I molecules of the major histocompatibility complex had been documented for some time, the associated biochemical events did not begin to become apparent until the description of FcγRIIB-mediated inhibition of B cell activation in 1992 (53). Mutagenesis suggested that a 13-amino-acid stretch within the cytoplasmic tail of FcγRIIB was required for its inhibitory activity (54). Examination of the sequence revealed a tyrosine-based motif similar to that utilized by activating receptors, YxxV/L, where the tyrosine is in configuration for phosphorylation. However, in activating receptors the YxxV/L is followed

six to eight amino acids later by a second YxxV/L, forming a motif known as an immunoreceptor tyrosine-based activation motif (ITAM) (55). In fact, mutagenesis has demonstrated the importance of the spacing of these tyrosines for positive signaling (56,57). FcγRIIB has only one YxxL, suggesting it would not mediate positive signals. Further study demonstrated that this YxxL became tyrosine-phosphorylated upon co-ligation of FcγRIIB and the B cell antigen receptor; and the operational term immunoreceptor tyrosine-based inhibitory motif (ITIM) was assigned (58). In 1995 Burshtyn et al. demonstrated the existence of functional ITIMs in the carboxyterminal tails of killer cell inhibitory receptors (KIRs), the human counterparts of Ly-49s, modified the definition of the motif to I/VxYxxL and noted the existence of these motifs in proteins of the Ly-49 family (59). All of the inhibitory Ly-49s known to date have a single cytoplasmic ITIM only six or seven amino acids from the translational start site in their cytoplasmic tail (60). The sequences of the Ly-49 ITIMs (Table 4-3) hold well to the consensus suggested by Burshtyn et al. (59). However, Ly-49s most often contain Val at position +3 relative to the phosphotyrosine. Interestingly, the KIR cytoplasmic tails usually carry two-ITIMs, whereas Ly-49 has only one (2). Ly-49s exist as homodimeric receptors resulting in a two-ITIM functional unit (61). This receptor configuration is likely critical given the stoichiometry of the interactions between Ly-49s and their downstream ef-

TABLE 4-3. *Comparison of the Ly-49 ITIMs*

Ly-49	ITIM
Ly-49A	VTYSMV
Ly-49B	VTYTTL
Ly-49C	VTYSTV
Ly-49E	VTYSTV
Ly-49F	VTYSTV
Ly-49G	VTYSTV
Ly-49I	VTYSTV
Ly-49J	VTYSTV
Ly-49M	VTYSTV

fector molecules (see below). It should be noted, however, that no study to date has determined the effectiveness of an Ly-49–receptor complex bearing only one ITIM.

Multiple studies have now demonstrated the effector mechanisms of the Ly-49 ITIMs. Early studies again followed in the footsteps of the biochemical dissection of the KIR mechanisms. Phosphorylated KIR ITIMs bind and activate the protein tyrosine phosphatase SHP-1 in an Src homology (SH2) domain-dependent fashion (59). Early evidence from a study by Olcese et al. (62) showed that phosphopeptides derived from the Ly-49 ITIMs could bind SHP-1 from stimulated Jurkat T cell lysate, suggesting that Ly-49-mediated inhibition might parallel that seen with the KIR (62). We and others have demonstrated this to be the case. The ITIMs of Ly-49s are heavily phosphorylated on tyrosine residues following treatment of the cells with inhibitors of protein tyrosine phosphatases (63). Moreover, once phosphorylated, these receptors recruit the phosphatase SHP-1 (63). The functional connection between recruitment of SHP-1 and Ly-49-mediated inhibition was made by the demonstration that Ly-49A inhibition is severely compromised in mice deficient in SHP-1 (64). Notably, however, these receptors still have some inhibitory activity, possibly through the recruitment of SHP-2 or the inositol phosphatase SHIP.

The dominant effector molecule of Ly-49-mediated inhibition, SHP-1, is one of a family of SH2 domain-containing protein tyrosine phosphatases (65). SHP-1 contains two carboxyl-terminal SH2 domains and an amino-terminal catalytic domain. SH2 domains have a high affinity for phosphotyrosine-containing peptides, and the amino acids flanking the phosphotyrosine residue are critical in determining which SH2 domains bind which tyrosine phosphoproteins and therefore which receptor complexes (66,67). Thus the ITIM is defined not only by a tyrosine in consensus for phosphorylation but also by the flanking residues that favor interaction with the appropriate effector molecule; a hy-

drophobic residue at -2 relative to the phosphotyrosine in the case of SHP-1 (68). Specific binding of the SHP-1 SH2 domains by ITIM phosphopeptides dramatically enhances the phosphatases catalytic activity, presumably by relieving stearic inhibition (68–70). Therefore the engagement of SHP-1 by the ITIMs of Ly-49 serves at least two distinct purposes: activation of the phosphatase and recruitment of the enzyme to the receptor complex where it comes into proximity with its substrates. In fact, it has been speculated that binding of one SH2 domain of SHP-1 activates its catalytic activity, and the second SH2 domain is involved primarily in localization of the phosphatase to the appropriate receptor complex (70). The requirement for binding both of the SHP-1 SH2 domains may be the basis for the homodimeric nature of the single ITIM containing Ly-49 proteins.

Binding studies employing Ly-49 phosphopeptides demonstrated that, in addition to SHP-1, ubiquitously expressed SHP-2 could also be captured from lysates (62). Moreover, binding studies with ITIM peptides derived from FcγRIIB have detected binding of the SH2 domain containing inositol phosphatase SHIP, raising the possibility that phosphatases other than SHP-1 are involved in Ly-49-mediated inhibition (71). In fact, as mentioned above, Ly-49A-mediated inhibition is reduced but not absent in mice lacking SHP-1 (24,64). More detailed study of the recruitment of phosphatases to ITIM-containing receptors has suggested an interesting dichotomy. The phospho-ITIMs of the KIR (and therefore presumably those of Ly-49s) functionally associate preferentially with SHP-1, whereas the ITIM-containing receptors of B cells (FcγRIIB) preferentially bind SHIP-1 (72,73). The functional consequence of binding SHIP versus SHP-1 is that these phosphatases interject at different points in the activation pathways. Protein tyrosine phosphorylation is an early, requisite event in leukocyte signaling by a variety of receptor systems. Therefore through their recruitment of SHP-1, Ly-49s and KIRs are able to prevent effectively even the earliest biochemical events associated with activation (74). In contrast, SHIP functions to dephosphorylate phosphotidylinositol 3,4,5-trisphosphate (PIP3) and inositol 1,3,4,5,-tetrabisphosphate (IP4), themselves products of the action of phosphoinositol 3-kinase, an enzyme activated during earlier events within the activation pathway (75,76). The result is normal intracellular calcium mobilization early in the B cell activation pathway even when FcγRIIB is co-engaged (58). Extracellular influx of calcium later in B cell activation, a function dependent on the targets of SHIP, is impaired when FcγRIIB is co-ligated (54,58,71,73). Why does NK cell inhibition require blockage so early in the pathway, whereas B cells have selected a block further downstream? Gupta et al. speculated that the difference may lie in the requirement for deletion of B cells exposed to antigen–antibody complexes, signifying the presence of ample amount of soluble antibody (72). In contrast, normal cells expressing the ligands for Ly-49 molecules must be spared from NK lysis and the lytic machinery shut down completely, but the NK cells need not be deleted. Cited as evidence for this model is the fact that co-engagement of the B cell receptor and FcγRIIB results in accelerated entry of B cells into apoptosis as they are diverted from activation to deletion (72,77). Compare this to NK cells, a cell type that is biochemically constitutively activated and more likely to respond to partial stimuli than other lymphocytes (78). Perhaps for complete and successful shutdown of NK effector functions, no aspect of the activation pathway may be allowed to proceed. This model would prevent the delivery of partial agonist signals to the NK cells and prevent their deletion.

If one assumes that the recruitment of SHP-1 mediates a near total shutdown of the NK cell activation program, one must assume that the biochemical events that initiate SHP-1 recruitment would be tightly regulated. Clearly, the determination of when Ly-49-mediated inhibition will occur is regulated

by the availability of ligand, but what are the biochemical events that direct the initiation of an inhibitory signal? As with other aspects of Ly-49 biochemistry, there are few data directly addressing this issue. Even within the study of KIRs there are few data to date. Like Ly-49s, many activating receptor systems are also dependent on the initial phosphorylation of tyrosine-containing motifs (the ITAMs). Data from activating systems suggest that this phosphorylation is mediated by members of the Src family of proto-oncogenes (79). These tyrosine kinases are myristoylated and therefore localized to the plasma membrane in proximity with the receptor chains they must phosphorylate (80). In fact, co-immunoprecipitation of Src family kinases has been reported with a number of receptor systems, including the T cell receptor, B cell receptor, and various Fc receptors (81–87). Receptor engagement results in activation of these associated kinases and, as a result, phosphorylation of the receptor chains. In fact, crosslinking of Ly-49s alone does lead to their tyrosine phosphorylation, although, we found the SHP-1 levels within these complexes to be below the level of detection, suggesting that crosslinking alone may not be sufficient to initiate the Ly-49 inhibitory pathway (63). Similarly, crosslinking of KIR has been reported to result in their phosphorylation (88). Here, however, co-immunoprecipitation studies did detect SHP-1. Genetic analysis of the KIR pathway in the Jurkat T cell line demonstrated that the Src family kinase Lck is required for KIR phosphorylation (88). This is in contrast to kinases of the Syk/Zap-70 family, which although critical for TCR and NK cell function are dispensable for KIR phosphorylation. Further evidence for Src family involvement is the fact that overexpression of active Src kinases with KIR results in KIR phosphorylation even in the absence of crosslinking (59). Even though the evidence for Src-mediated phosphorylation is good, no one has reported the physical association of any tyrosine kinase with inhibitory Ly-49s or KIRs. This fact supports a model requiring the recruitment of ITIM-containing receptors, such as Ly-49s, into close proximity with activating receptors (Fig. 4-1). The tyrosine kinases activated by the positive receptors can then phosphorylate the ITIMs of the inhibitors, which in turn down-regulate the positive response. This type of suicide receptor function, a positive receptor being directly responsible for inhibition of its own signal, is supported by reports demonstrating enhanced tyrosine phosphorylation of ITIM containing receptors upon co-ligation of activating and inhibitory receptors (88–90). More direct support of this model comes from studies where mast cells expressing KIRs were stimulated through FcεRI. Independent cross-linking of FcεRI and KIRs results in no inhibition of the FcεRI signal (91). However, if the two were co-ligated, the KIR profoundly inhibited FcεRI signaling. Indirect support of a co-ligation model comes from the physical mechanisms involved in the NK cell lytic hit. Here, a finite portion of the effector NK cell's surface forms a tight connection with that of the target, which could result in the clustering and co-engagement of both the activating and inhibitory receptors at this site. Should the inhibitory ligands be present, the Src kinases activated by the as yet unidentified NK cell receptor, the engagement of integrins at the points of cell–cell contact, or both would facilitate the phosphorylation of Ly-49 ITIMs, resulting in the recruitment of SHP-1 and subsequent inhibition of the activation program. Activating receptors engaged on a different portion of the cell—one without inhibitory receptors or without access to inhibitory ligands—would transmit their signals intact and result in lysis of that unprotected target. Cold-target competition assays have confirmed that the presence of protected targets does not preclude the lysis of susceptible targets by a given population of NK cells (3).

Once an activating receptor complex has facilitated the phosphorylation of the ITIMs of a Ly-49 homodimer and led to the recruitment of SHP-1, what are the critical targets of the phosphatase? To date there are few data to address this question. As predicted by the model outlined above, there are reports of reductions in phosphorylation of several early tyrosine kinase substrates. They include the TCR zeta chains (TCRζ) phosphorylated in response to NK cell Fc receptor-mediated signaling, the Syk and Zap-70 tyrosine kinases, and phospholipase Cγ (88). One of the most intriguing reports of a specific target of ITIM-recruited SHP-1 is from Parham's laboratory (92). They reported that engagement of NK cells by targets protected by virtue of expression of inhibitory receptor ligands resulted in normal tyrosine phosphorylation of multiple substrates. However, a 36-kDa polypeptide, identified by its ability to form a complex with the adaptor protein Grb-2 and PLCγ1, demonstrated a marked reduction in tyrosine phosphorylation (92). These data suggest that pp36 is a critical mediator of the NK signaling pathway and imply that it may be the critical target of SHP-1. Recently a 36-kDa protein has been cloned from NK cells and T cells and termed the linker of activated T cells (LAT) (93,94). LAT forms signaling complexes with PLCγ1, Grb-2, and several other signal transduction molecules. Whether LAT is the pp36 regulated by inhibitory receptors in NK cells remains a mystery. Analysis of the role of LAT in NK cell signaling has only just begun, so a role for LAT in NK cell biology has not yet been established.

One report has suggested that the complex adaptor Slp-76 may be a critical target of SHP-1 recruited to ITIM-containing receptors (95). These data demonstrate phosphorylation of Slp-76 during effector target interactions. Co-ligation of KIRs prevents target-induced phosphorylation of Slp-76. Most convincing is the demonstration that the catalytic domain of SHP-1 specifically binds to tyrosine phosphorylated Slp-76 in far Western blots. These findings suggest that, even though receptor engagement may result in the tyrosine phosphorylation of several cellular substrates, SHP-1 may be highly specific in the selection of its substrates (95).

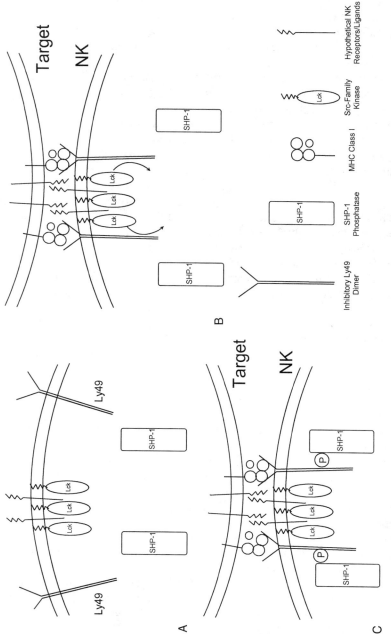

FIG. 4-1. Model for the induction of ITIM phosphorylation and recruitment of SHP-1 by co-crosslinking with activating receptors. **A:** Prior to engagement by target cells, Ly-49s and activating receptors are dispersed throughout the membrane. The ITIMs are unphosphorylated, and SHP-1 is free in the cytosol. **B:** Engagement by a target cell results in activation of protein tyrosine kinases functionally associated with activating receptors. Target cell MHC at the site of effector–target interaction results in the recruitment of Ly-49s into the proximity with the activating receptors. The activated kinases then can phosphorylate the ITIMs of the Ly-49s. **C:** Phosphorylated ITIMs serve to recruit and activate SHP-1.

Positive Receptors

In marked contrast to the inhibitory Ly-49 molecules, Ly-49D seems able to mediate the activation of murine NK cells; and a second Ly-49, Ly-49H, also appears to be a positively signaling receptor (30,96,97). Similarly, so-called noninhibitory KIRs have been described and their ability to activate NK cells documented (98–100). We have learned a great deal about the biochemical mechanisms involved in these activation pathways. These positive signaling receptors have two major features that distinguish them from their inhibitory counterparts: the total lack of ITIMs and the presence of charged residues within their transmembrane domains (2,60,101). In the case of Ly-49D, the canonical ITIM sequence is replaced with the sequence DxFxxV. In the KIRs the ITIM-containing carboxy-terminal tail of the receptors is truncated.

Perhaps the different approaches for neutralizing the inhibitory activity of these two classes of receptors is a result of their physical differences. Specifically, the fact that KIRs are type I receptors logistically simplifies their genetic truncation. In contrast, the Ly-49s are type II proteins, so truncation of the cytoplasmic tail would require an alternative translational start site downstream of the ITIM. Regardless, the results are Ly-49s with cytoplasmic tails of comparable length but lacking the ability to become tyrosine-phosphorylated. Notably, membrane proximal cytoplasmic tyrosine residues found in other Ly-49s are also absent in Ly-49D (60).

The presence of a charged amino acid residue in the putative transmembrane region of Ly-49D (Arg[54]) was recognized as a potential site of interaction with other receptor chains (63,102). Various receptors, including the TCR and the Fc receptors, utilize charged residues in their transmembrane domains to form salt bridges, with additional receptor chains containing oppositely charged residues. In support of this notion, we demonstrated that immunoprecipitation of Ly-49D from NK cells does not reveal tyrosine phosphorylation of the receptor itself but in the co-immunoprecipitation of low-molecular-weight tyrosine phosphoproteins, which we termed pp16 (63,103). Analysis of the components of this receptor complex using antiserum recognizing the TCRζ chain and the FcεRI gamma chain (FcεRIγ), both expressed by mouse NK cells, revealed that neither represented the Ly-49D co-immunoprecipitating bands. We took this analysis one step farther by demonstrating that mice with targeted disruptions in both the TCRζ (and therefore TCRδ) and FcεRIγ still express the Ly-49D-associated polypeptides (103). Similar observations were made with noninhibitory KIRs (104). These early studies allowed us to demonstrate the critical role of Arg[54] in the association of Ly-49D with these low-molecular-weight proteins. In fact, we were able to demonstrate not only that Arg[54] is required for association with pp16 but that mutation of Arg[54] in Ly-49D destroyed its ability to signal, suggesting an important role for pp16 in the signal transduction pathway of Ly-49D (103). Together with the reports of co-immunoprecipitating proteins with the noninhibitory KIRs in human NK cells, our data began to suggest a physical model of the Ly-49D receptor complex. The Ly-49s themselves are disulfied-linked homodimers, and so apparently was pp16 (103,104). Under nonreducing phosphotyrosine immunoblotting, this complex migrated as a ladder from 25 kDa to 32 kDa. Following reduction, a prominent 16-kDa band was seen with lesser phosphorylated species running below it at about 12 to 14 kDa. The interaction with Ly-49 was clearly mediated by Arg[54], implying that pp16 contains a transmembrane domain with one or more acidic residues. The potent tyrosine phosphorylation and laddered appearance of pp16 was reminiscent of the migration of phospho-TCRζ and phospho-FcεRIγ, suggesting that pp16 was similar to these chains biochemically. Lastly, the apparent ability of pp16 to mediate Ly-49D signal transduction suggested that it contained at least one ITAM

(103). Each of these characteristics was supported by studies of the noninhibitory KIRs (104,105). As for the expression patterns of pp16, we had detected it in NK cells and in the mastocytoma P815, suggesting expression in myeloid cells as well as NK cells (103). Others, however, concluded that it would be expressed only in NK cells (104).

The primary sequence of a low-molecular-weight polypeptide capable of physically associating with human noninhibitory KIRs was identified through a database search for the characteristics outlined above. The resulting cDNA was named DAP12 (106). The primary sequence confirmed the predictions made by several laboratories. DAP12 is a small type I transmembrane protein. It is comprised of a leader sequence followed by a 14-amino-acid extracellular domain, a putative transmembane domain containing a single aspartic acid residue, and a 48-amino-acid cytoplasmic domain that includes a single ITAM (106). The extracellular domain contains two cysteine residues that are likely involved in disulfide-mediated dimerization. Northern analysis confirmed the expression of DAP12 in the myeloid compartment and in NK cells. No expression is seen in T cells or in the B cell lines reported (106). Since the report of DAP12, we and others have confirmed that it is the Ly-49D-associated signal transduction chain (96,97). In addition, Ly-49H couples to DAP12 for its signal transduction (96,97). Subsequent studies in human NK cells have demonstrated that the activating heterodimer CD94/NKG2C also functionally couples to DAP12 (107).

As the story of noninhibitory KIRs has emerged, several other receptor families with homology to the KIRs have been identified (17,23–25,108,109). Like the noninhibitory KIRs, these new families have members that lack ITIMs and, instead, have charged residues in their putative transmembrane regions. Many of these receptors are expressed in monocytes and macrophages, prompting speculation that these activating receptors may also utilize DAP12. This does not appear to be the case. We and others have demonstrated that one such family, the paired Ig-like receptors (PIRs), do not couple to DAP12 but use FcεRIγ (110,111). Another family, the leukocyte immunoglobulin-like receptors (LIRs) also use FcεRIγ and not DAP12 (112). Close examination of the transmembrane domains of these receptors suggests a structural basis for these findings. In Ly-49D, Ly-49H, human KIRs, and CD94/NKG2C, the arginine residue involved in bridging to DAP12 is located almost exactly in the middle of putative transmembrane region. This fits well with the location of the aspartic acid residue of DAP12 near the middle of its transmembrane domain (106). In contrast, the newly described PIRs, LIRs, and Ig-like transcripts (ILT), like their homolog the Fcα receptor, carry their charge near the outer leaflet of the plasma membrane (17,23,109). In fact, these receptors all contain the motif LIRM with the arginine only four or five amino acids into the putative membrane span. This spacing likely prevents the association of these receptors with DAP12 and facilitates the association with FcεRIγ.

As mentioned above, tyrosine-based receptor systems are often initiated through the activation of tyrosine kinases that phosphorylate either the ITIMs or ITAMs. In the case of the DAP12-coupled Ly-49s, virtually nothing is known regarding the involvement of the Src family protein tyrosine kinases. What is known, however, is that unlike the inhibitory receptors crosslinking of Ly-49D alone results in prominent tyrosine phosphorylation of DAP12 (103), suggesting a physical association of DAP12 with tyrosine kinases. There are no data describing the co-immunoprecipitation of kinase activity with Ly-49D or Ly-49H. There are, however, data demonstrating co-immunoprecipitation of tyrosine kinase activity with noninhibitory KIRs and what we now know to be DAP12 (104). This report, unfortunately, does not address the identity of the kinase(s). One potential candidate is the Syk protein tyrosine kinase. Like its only other family member, Zap-70, Syk contains two amino-terminal SH2 domains and a carboxyterminal kinase catalytic domain. In characterized receptor systems that utilize FcεRIγ or TCRζ, Syk or Zap-70 bind the precisely spaced tyrosines of the phosphorylated ITAMs (113). These kinases are then activated through phosphorylation and are responsible for mediating many of the downstream events associated with receptor ligation. Evidence suggests that Syk may be the initiating kinase within the DAP12 pathway. It includes the fact that phosphopeptides derived from the DAP12 sequence readily bind both Syk and Zap-70 (106). Furthermore, there are multiple reports of Syk phosphorylation following crosslinking of Ly-49D, Ly-49H, CD94/NKG2C, or noninhibitory KIRs (96,97,106,107,114). Only one report, however, has documented activation of Syk catalytic activity following crosslinking (114). Although Syk and Zap-70 are similar in structure, their activation requirements appear to be different. *In vitro* experiments have shown that transfection of Syk along with an ITAM-containing receptor results in tyrosine phosphorylation of the ITAM and activation of Syk (115). In contrast, similar experiments using ZAP-70 demonstrated that co-transfection of an Src family kinase was required for efficient activation of Zap-70. Syk's apparent ability to phosphorylate ITAM-containing receptors readily and efficiently, together with its expression in all DAP12-expressing cells reported to date, suggest a model where prior to stimulation low amounts of Syk may be physically associated with the Ly-49D–receptor complex, perhaps even with DAP12 itself. Engagement of the receptor results in activation of the associated Syk, phosphorylation of DAP12, further recruitment and activation of Syk, and then phosphorylation of downstream targets (Fig. 4-2).

An alternative model for the initiation of Ly-49 and other DAP12-associated receptors is similar to the one outlined above for the inhibitory receptors. This model is built under the assumption that Ly-49s, whether positive or inhibitory, are designed solely as co-receptors. In fact, there are no data to suggest any biologic function of Ly-49s ligated by themselves; and the fact that they recognize cell-bound ligands, often on possible target cells, implies that multiple receptors including integrins and others are concurrently activated. Under this assumption, DAP12 ITAMs could become tyrosine-phosphorylated by Syk or Src family kinases activated as a consequence of effector-target conjugation. This initiation event would then facilitate the recruitment of additional Syk and the start of the downstream signaling events. Experiments underway should lead to clarification of these issues.

In addition to the phosphorylation of DAP12 and the activation of Syk, what other events are associated with Ly-49D crosslinking? Interestingly, activation of the second Syk family kinase, Zap-70, does not occur despite the expression of Zap-70 in murine NK cells (114). Several other cellular proteins are, however, phosphorylated following engagement of Ly-49D–DAP12 receptor complexes. These downstream substrates include PLCγ1, Cbl, and the mitogen-activated protein kinases (MAP kinases) Erk1 and Erk2 (105,114). Each of these substrates likely plays an important role in the biologic function of Ly-49D. PLCγ1, the enzyme responsible for the hydrolysis of phosphoinositol 4,5-bisphosphate into the second messengers diacylglycerol and inositol 1,4,5-trisphosphate, is most likely responsible for the vigorous mobilization of intracellular calcium demonstrated following crosslinking of Ly-49D or noninhibitory KIRs (105,114). In addition, the production of diacylglycerol suggests that Ly-49D–DAP12 might result in activation of protein kinase C (PKC). No one has yet directly demonstrated the activation of PKC by a DAP12-coupled receptor, but we and others have shown that the MAP kinase cascade, a downstream target of PKC, is activated following ligation of Ly-49D or noninhibitory KIRs (105,114). MAP kinases phosphorylate and activate transcription factors, suggesting stimulation of transcriptional activation by Ly-49D. To date, the

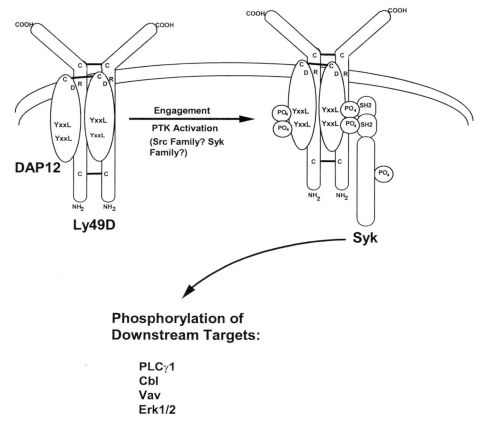

FIG. 4-2. Current model for NK activation by Ly-49D. Engagement of Ly-49D results in the tyrosine phosphorylation of Ly-49-associated DAP12 by an as yet unidentified tyrosine kinase. Tyrosine phosphorylated DAP12 mediates the recruitment and activation of the Syk protein tyrosine kinase. Following activation of Syk the additional substrates noted become tyrosine-phosphorylated and presumably mediate the events associated with Ly-49D activation. Amino acids involved in disulfide links, receptor–DAP12 interactions, or phosphorylation events are designated by a single letter.

most convincing demonstration of transcriptional activation by a DAP12-coupled receptor is the production of IFN-γ following crosslinking of Ly-49D on mouse NK cells (Mason et al., in preparation). One other report demonstrates IFN-γ production in response to crosslinking of noninhibitory KIRs in an NK cell clone (116). Are genes other than IFN-γ, induced by Ly-49D or other DAP12-coupled receptors, and if so by what transcription factors? This question is currently under study.

Although there are numerous reports of the induction of tyrosine phosphorylation by DAP12-coupled receptors, only one has identified Cbl as a target (114). Cbl, the product of the c-*cbl* proto-oncogene, functions as a multivalent adaptor molecule in a variety of immune receptor systems where it interacts with proteins such as Grb-2, the p85 regulatory subunit of phosphatidylinositol 3-kinase, and various protein tyrosine kinases including Syk (117–126). Recent work suggests that Cbl acts as an inhibitor by physically interacting with tyrosine kinases. In mast cells, Cbl reduces receptor-mediated activation of Syk (117). Overexpression of wild-type Cbl, but not the 70Z/3 transforming mutant, effectively reduces both receptor-mediated Syk tyrosine phosphorylation and catalytic activity, resulting in decreased FcεRI-mediated serotonin release. These observations suggest that Cbl functions in the Ly-49D pathway to attenuate DAP12-mediated Syk activation. It is worth noting that Syk activation by the Ly-49D–DAP12 complex is vigorous even in the presence of extensive phosphorylation of Cbl. Regardless, the possibility that Cbl negatively regulates the signal transduction cascade of DAP12-mediated receptors, and if so how, is currently under investigation.

FUTURE QUESTIONS

Many questions remain regarding the signal transduction of the inhibitory Ly-49 molecules. They include identification of the critical substrates of Ly-49 ITIM-mediated inhibition, dissection of the physical makeup of the heterologous complexes that result when positive and negative receptors are co-engaged, and clear delineation of the enzyme(s) responsible for the phosphorylation of Ly-49 ITIMs and therefore initiation of inhibitory signaling. Answers to these questions should help identify the receptor-mediated events regulated by Ly-49 inhibition and how these inhibitory pathways are insulated from the unaffected cellular processes.

Study of the signaling of the positive Ly-49s is still in its infancy. Several issues remain unresolved. The signaling events defined for Ly-49D thus far largely parallel those defined for other ITAM-containing receptor complexes, including receptors coupled to FcεRIγ. Why then have the Ly-49s evolved to use DAP12? Are there biochemical parameters that differ between the signaling of DAP12-coupled receptors and those that use other chains? If so, what are they? What are the signaling endpoints of a DAP12 pathway? Lastly, if monocytes express DAP12 but not Ly-49, what receptors are coupled to DAP12 in these cells? Might these receptors mediate NK-like functions in macrophages such as cellular cytotoxicity? These questions

and others will no doubt be addressed by the ongoing study of DAP12 signaling by us and in other laboratories.

REFERENCES

1. Lotzova E, Ades EW. Natural killer cells: definition, heterogeneity, lytic mechanism, functions and clinical application: highlights of the Fifth International Workshop on natural killer cells, Hilton Head Island, S.C., March 1988. *Nat Immun Cell Growth Regul* 1989;8:1–9.
2. Long EO, Burshtyn DN, Clark WP, et al. Killer cell inhibitory receptors: diversity, specificity, and function. *Immunol Rev* 1997;155:135–144.
3. Lanier LL. NK cell receptors. *Annu Rev Immunol* 1998;16:359–393.
4. Moretta L, Ciccone E, Mingari MC, Biassoni R, Moretta A. Human natural killer cells: origin, clonality, specificity, and receptors. *Adv Immunol* 1994;55:341–380.
5. Meyaard L, Adema GJ, Chang C, et al. LAIR-1, a novel inhibitory receptor expressed on human mononuclear leukocytes. *Immunity* 1997;7:283–290.
6. Yokoyama WM, Jacobs LB, Kanagawa O, Shevach EM, Cohen DI. A murine T lymphocyte antigen belongs to a supergene family of type II integral membrane proteins. *J Immunol* 1989;143:1379–1386.
7. Wong S, Freeman JD, Kelleher C, Mager D, Takei F. Ly-49 multigene family: new members of a superfamily of type II membrane proteins with lectin-like domains. *J Immunol* 1991;147:1417–1423.
8. Stoneman ER, Bennett M, An J, et al. Cloning and characterization of 5E6(Ly-49C), a receptor molecule expressed on a subset of murine natural killer cells. *J Exp Med* 1995;182:305–313.
9. Smith HR, Karlhofer FM, Yokoyama WM. Ly-49 multigene family expressed by IL-2-activated NK cells. *J Immunol* 1994;153:1068–1079.
10. Mason L, Giardina SL, Hecht T, Ortaldo J, Mathieson BJ. LGL-1: a nonpolymorphic antigen expressed on a major population of mouse natural killer cells. *J Immunol* 1988;140:4403–4412.
11. Lopez-Botet M, Perez-Villar JJ, Carretero M, Rodriguez A, Melero I. Functional resemblance between the Ig-related NK cell receptors specific for HLA class I molecules and the CD94 C-type lectin. *Chem Immunol* 1996;64:116–134.
12. Bottino C, Vitale M, Pende D, Bassoni R, Moretta A. Receptors for HLA class I molecules in human NK cells. *Semin Immunol* 1995;7:67–73.
13. Arm JP, Nwankwo C, Austen KF. Molecular identification of a novel family of human Ig superfamily members that possess immunoreceptor tyrosine-based inhibition motifs and homology to the mouse gp49B1 inhibitory receptor. *J Immunol* 1997;159:2342–2349.
14. Katz HR, Austen KF. A newly recognized pathway for the negative regulation of mast cell-dependent hypersensitivity and inflammation mediated by an

endogenous cell surface receptor of the gp49 family. *J Immunol* 1997;158:5065–5070.

15. Yabe T, McSherry C, Bach FH, et al. A multigene family on human chromosome 12 encodes natural killer-cell lectins. *Immunogenetics* 1993;37:455–460.

16. Houchins JP, Yabe T, McSherry C, Bach FH. DNA sequence analysis of NKG2, a family of related cDNA clones encoding type II integral membrane proteins on human natural killer cells. *J Exp Med* 1991;173:1017–1020.

17. Kubagawa H, Burrows PD, Cooper MD. A novel pair of immunoglobulin-like receptors expressed by B cells and myeloid cells. *Proc Natl Acad Sci USA* 1997;94:5261–5266.

18. Alley TL, Cooper MD, Chen M, Kubagawa H. Genomic structure of PIR-B, the inhibitory member of the paired immunoglobulin-like receptor genes in mice. *Tissue Antigens* 1998;51:224–231.

19. Ortega E, Schneider H, Pecht I. Possible interactions between the Fc epsilon receptor and a novel mast cell function-associated antigen. *Int Immunol* 1991;3:333–342.

20. Guthmann MD, Tal M, Pecht I. A secretion inhibitory signal transduction molecule on mast cells is another C-type lectin. *Proc Natl Acad Sci USA* 1995;92:9397–9401.

21. Cella M, Dohring C, Samaridis J, et al. A novel inhibitory receptor (ILT3) expressed on monocytes, macrophages, and dendritic cell involved in antigen processing. *J Exp Med* 1997;185:1743–1751.

22. Colonna M, Navarro F, Bellon T, et al. A common inhibitory receptor for major histocompatibility complex class I molecules on human lymphoid and myelomonocytic cells. *J Exp Med* 1997;186:1809–1818.

23. Borges L, Hsu ML, Fanger N, Kubin M, Cosman D. A family of human lymphoid and myeloid Ig-like receptors, some of which bind to MHC class I molecules. *J Immunol* 1997;159:5192–5196.

24. Cosman D, Fanger N, Borges L, et al. A novel immunoglobulin superfamily receptor for cellular and viral MHC class I molecules. *Immunity* 1997;7:273–282.

25. Blery M, Kubagawa H, Chen CC, Vely F, Cooper MD, Vivier E. The paired Ig-like receptor PIR-B is an inhibitory receptor that recruits the protein-tyrosine phosphatase SHP-1. *Proc Natl Acad Sci USA* 1998;95:2446–2451.

26. McQueen KL, Freeman DJ, Takei F, Mager DL. Localization of five new Ly49 genes, including three closely related to Ly49c. *Immunogenetics* 1998;48:174–183.

27. Daniels BF, Nakamura MC, Rosen SD, Yokoyama WM, Seaman WE. Ly-49A, a receptor for H-2Dd, has a functional carbohydrate recognition domain. *Immunity* 1994;1:785–792.

28. Brennan J, Mager D, Jefferies W, Takei F. Expression of different members of the Ly-49 gene family defines distinct natural killer cell subsets and cell adhesion properties. *J Exp Med* 1994;180:2287–2295.

29. Ortaldo JR, Mason AT, Winkler-Pickett RT, Raziuddin A, Murphy WJ, Mason LH. Ly-49 receptor expression and functional analysis in multiple mouse strains. *J Leukoc Biol* (1999, in press).

30. Mason LH, Anderson SK, Yokoyama WM, Smith HR, Winkler-Pickett R, Ortaldo JR. The Ly-49D receptor activates murine natural killer cells. *J Exp Med* 1996;184:2119–2128.

31. Uhrberg M, Valiante NM, Shum BP, et al. Human diversity in killer cell inhibitory receptor genes. *Immunity* 1997;7:753–763.

32. Valiante NM, Uhrberg M, Shilling HG, et al. Functionally and structurally distinct NK cell receptor repertoires in the peripheral blood of two human donors. *Immunity* 1997;7:739–751.

33. Ortaldo JR, Winkler-Pickett R, Mason AT, Mason LH. The Ly-49 family: regulation of cytotoxicity and cytokine production in murine CD3+ cells. *J Immunol* 1998;160:1158–1165.

34. Dorfman JR, Raulet DH. Acquisition of Ly49 receptor expression by developing natural killer cells. *J Exp Med* 1998;187:609–618.

35. Kaufman DS, Schoon RA, Leibson PJ. MHC class I expression on tumor targets inhibits natural killer cell-mediated cytotoxicity without interfering with target recognition. *J Immunol* 1993;150:1429–1436.

36. Mason LH, Ortaldo JR, Young HA, Kumar V, Bennett M, Anderson SK. Cloning and functional characteristics of murine large granular lymphocyte-1: a member of the Ly-49 gene family (Ly-49G2). *J Exp Med* 1995;182:293–303.

37. Brennan J, Lemieux S, Freeman JD, Mager DL, Takei F. Heterogeneity among Ly-49C natural killer (NK) cells: characterization of highly related receptors with differing functions and expression patterns. *J Exp Med* 1996;184:2085–2090.

38. Sentman CL, Hackett J Jr, Kumar V, Bennett M. Identification of a subset of murine natural killer cells that mediates rejection of Hh-1d but not Hh-1b bone marrow grafts. *J Exp Med* 1989;170:191–202.

39. Yu YY, George T, Dorfman JR, Roland J, Kumar V, Bennett M. The role of Ly49A and 5E6(Ly49C) molecules in hybrid resistance mediated by murine natural killer cells against normal T cell blasts. *Immunity* 1996;4:67–76.

40. Ortaldo JR, Mason LH, Gregorio TA, Stoll J, Winkler-Pickett RT. The Ly-49 family: regulation of cytokine production in murine NK cells. *J Leukoc Biol* 1997;62:381–388.

41. Orange JS, Biron CA. An absolute and restricted requirement for IL-12 in natural killer cell IFN-gamma production and antiviral defense: studies of natural killer and T cell responses in contrasting viral infections. *J Immunol* 1996;156:1138–1142.

42. Tay CH, Welsh RM. Distinct organ-dependent mechanisms for the control of murine cytomegalovirus infection by natural killer cells. *J Virol* 1997;71:267–275.

43. Baker MB, Podack ER, Levy RB. Perforin- and Fas-mediated cytotoxic pathways are not required for allogeneic resistance to bone marrow grafts in mice. *Biol Blood Marrow Transplant* 1995;1:69–73.

44. Gosselin P, Mason LH, Willette-Brown J, Ortaldo JR, McVicar DW, Anderson SK. Induction of DAP12 phosphorylation, calcium mobilization,

and cytokine secretion by Ly49H. *J Leukoc Biol* 1999;66:165–171.

45. Smith KM, Wu J, Bakker AB, Phillips JH, Lanier LL. Ly-49D and Ly-49H associate with mouse DAP12 and form activating receptors. *J Immunol* 1998;161:7–10.

46. Herberman RB. Multiple functions of natural killer cells, including immunoregulation as well as resistance to tumor growth. *Concepts Immunopathol* 1985;1:96–132.

47. Murphy WJ, Reynolds CW, Tiberghien P, Longo DL. Natural killer cells and bone marrow transplantation. *J Natl Cancer Inst* 1993;85:1475–1482.

48. Murphy WJ, Longo DL. The potential role of NK cells in the separation of graft-versus-tumor effects from graft-versus-host disease after allogeneic bone marrow transplantation. *Immunol Rev* 1997;157:167–176.

49. Raziuddin A, Longo DL, Mason L, Ortaldo JR, Murphy WJ. Ly-49 G2+ NK cells are responsible for mediating the rejection of H-2b bone marrow allografts in mice. *Int Immunol* 1996;8:1833–1839.

50. Raziuddin A, Longo DL, Mason L, Ortaldo JR, Bennett M, Murphy WJ. Differential effects of the rejection of bone marrow allografts by the depletion of activating versus inhibiting Ly-49 natural killer cell subsets. *J Immunol* 1998;160:87–94.

51. Murphy WJ, Raziuddin A, Mason L, Kumar V, Bennett M, Longo DL. NK cell subsets in the regulation of murine hematopoiesis. I. 5E6+ NK cells promote hematopoietic growth in H-2d strain mice. *J Immunol* 1995;155:2911–2917.

52. George T, Yu YY, Lui J, et al. Allorecognition by murine natural killer cells: lysis of T-lymphoblasts and rejection of bone-marrow grafts. *Immunol Rev* 1997;155:29–40.

53. Amigorena S, Bonnerot C, Drake JR, et al. Cytoplasmic domain heterogeneity and functions of IgG Fc receptors in B lymphocytes. *Science* 1992; 256:1808–1812.

54. Muta T, Kurosaki T, Misulovin Z, Sanchez M, Mussenzweig MC, Ravetch JV. A 13-amino acid motif in the cytoplasmic domain of Fc gamma RIIB modulates B-cell receptor signaling. *Nature* 1994; 368:70–73.

55. Isakov N. ITIMs and ITAMs: the yin and yang of antigen and Fc receptor-linked signaling machinery. *Immunol Res* 1997;16:85–100.

56. Gauen LK, Zhu Y, Letourneur F, et al. Interactions of p59fyn and ZAP-70 with T-cell receptor activation motifs: defining the nature of a signalling motif. *Mol Cell Biol* 1994;14:3729–3741.

57. Letourneur F, Klausner RD. T-cell and basophil activation through the cytoplasmic tail of T-cell-receptor zeta family proteins. *Proc Natl Acad Sci USA* 1991;88:8905–8909.

58. D'Ambrosio D, Hippen KL, Minskoff SA, et al. Recruitment and activation of PTP1C in negative regulation of antigen receptor signaling by Fc gamma RIIB1. *Science* 1995;268:293–297.

59. Burshtyn DN, Scharenberg AM, Wagtmann N, et al. Recruitment of tyrosine phosphatase HCP by the killer cell inhibitor receptor. *Immunity* 1996;4:77–85.

60. Takei F, Brennan J, Mager DL. The Ly-49 family:

genes, proteins, and recognition of class I MHC. *Immunol Rev* 1998;155:67–77.

61. Chan P-Y, Takei F. Molecular cloning and characterization of a novel murine T cell surface antigen, YE1/48. *J Immunol* 1989;142:1727–1736.

62. Olcese L, Lang P, Vely F, et al. Human and mouse killer-cell inhibitory receptors recruit PTP1C and PTP1D protein tyrosine phosphatases. *J Immunol* 1996;156:4531–4534.

63. Mason LH, Gosselin P, Anderson SK, Fogler WE, Ortaldo JR, McVicar DW. Differential tyrosine phosphorylation of inhibitory versus activating Ly-49 receptor proteins and their recruitment of SHP-1 phosphatase. *J Immunol* 1997;159: 4187–4196.

64. Nakamura MC, Niemi EC, Fisher MJ, Shultz LD, Seaman WE, Ryan JC. Mouse Ly-49A interrupts early signaling events in natural killer cell cytotoxicity and functionally associates with the SHP-1 tyrosine phosphatase. *J Exp Med* 1997;185: 673–684.

65. Neel BG. Structure and function of SH2-domain containing tyrosine phosphatases. *Semin Cell Biol* 1993;4:419–432.

66. Pawson T, Schlessinger J. SH2 and SH3 domains. *Curr Biol* 1993;3:434–442.

67. Songyang Z, Shoelson SE, Chaudhuri M, et al. SH2 domains recognize specific phosphopeptide sequences. *Cell* 1993;72:767–778.

68. Burshtyn DN, Yang W, Yi T, Long EO. A novel phosphotyrosine motif with a critical amino acid at position -2 for the SH2 domain-mediated activation of the tyrosine phosphatase SHP-1. *J Biol Chem* 1997;272:13066–13072.

69. Barford D, Neel BG. Revealing mechanisms for SH2 domain mediated regulation of the protein tyrosine phosphatase SHP-2. *Structure* 1998;6: 249–254.

70. Pei D, Lorenz U, Klingmüller U, Neel BG, Walsh CT. Intramolecular regulation of protein tyrosine phosphatase SH-PTP1: a new function for Src homology 2 domains. *Biochemistry* 1994;33:15483–15493.

71. Ono M, Bolland S, Tempst P, Ravetch JV. Role of the inositol phosphatase SHIP in negative regulation of the immune system by the receptor Fc-gamma RIIB. *Nature* 1996;383:263–266.

72. Gupta N, Scharenberg AM, Burshtyn DN, et al. Negative signaling pathways of the killer cell inhibitory receptor and Fc gamma RIIb1 require distinct phosphatases. *J Exp Med* 1997;186:473–478.

73. Ono M, Okada H, Bolland S, Yanagi S, Kurosaki T, Ravetch JV. Deletion of SHIP or SHP-1 reveals two distinct pathways for inhibitory signaling. *Cell* 1997;90:293–301.

74. Kaufman DS, Schoon RA, Robertson MJ, Leibson PJ. Inhibition of selective signaling events in natural killer cells recognizing major histocompatibility complex class I. *Proc Natl Acad Sci USA* 1995;92:6484–6488.

75. Scharenberg AM. PtdIns-3,4,5-P3: a regulatory nexus between tyrosine kinases and sustained calcium signals. *Cell* 1998;94:5–8.

76. Scharenberg AM, El-Hillal O, Fruman DA, et al. Phosphatidylinositol-3,4,5-trisphosphate (PtdIns-3,4,5-P3)/Tec kinase-dependent calcium signaling

pathway: a target for SHIP-mediated inhibitory signals. *EMBO J* 1998;17:1961–1972.

77. Ashman RF, Peckham D, Stunz LL. Fc receptor off-signal in the B cell involves apoptosis. *J Immunol* 1996;157:5–11.

78. McVicar DW, Blake TB, Burns CM, Conlon KC, Ortaldo JR, O'Shea JJ. Differential basal protein tyrosine phosphorylation in natural killer (NK) and T cells: a biochemical correlate of lymphoid functional activity. *Cell Immunol* 1996;169: 302–308.

79. Isakov N, Wang RL, Samelson LE. The role of tyrosine kinases and phosphotyrosine-containing recognition motifs in regulation of the T cell-antigen receptor-mediated signal transduction pathway. *J Leukoc Biol* 1994;55:265–271.

80. Brown MT, Cooper JA. Regulation, substrates and functions of src. *Biochim Biophys Acta* 1996; 1287:121–149.

81. Horejsi V. Association of leukocyte surface receptors with protein kinases. *Int Arch Allergy Immunol* 1996;110:1–6.

82. Timson Gauen LK, Kong AN, Samelson LE, Shaw AS. p59fyn tyrosine kinase associates with multiple T-cell receptor subunits through its unique amino-terminal domain. *Mol Cell Biol* 1992;12:5438–5446.

83. Samelson LE, Phillips AF, Luong ET, Klausner RD. Association of the fyn protein-tyrosine kinase with the T-cell antigen receptor. *Proc Natl Acad Sci USA* 1990;87:4358–4362.

84. Cone JC, Lu Y, Trevillyan JM, Bjorndahl JM, Phillips CA. Association of the p56lck protein tyrosine kinase with the Fc gamma RIIIA/CD16 complex in human natural killer cells. *Eur J Immunol* 1993;23:2488–2497.

85. Pignata C, Prasad KV, Robertson MJ, Levine H, Rudd CE, Ritz J. Fc gamma RIIIA-mediated signaling involves src-family lck in human natural killer cells. *J Immunol* 1993;151:6794–6800.

86. Salcedo TW, Kurosaki T, Kanakaraj P, Ravetch JV, Perussia B. Physical and functional association of p56lck with Fc gamma RIIIA (CD16) in natural killer cells. *J Exp Med* 1993;177:1475–1480.

87. Campbell MA, Sefton BM. Association between B-lymphocyte membrane immunoglobulin and multiple members of the Src family of protein tyrosine kinases. *Mol Cell Biol* 1992;12:2315–2321.

88. Binstadt BA, Brumbaugh KM, Dick CJ, et al. Sequential involvement of Lck and SHP-1 with MHC-recognizing receptors on NK cells inhibits FcR-initiated tyrosine kinase activation. *Immunity* 1996;5:629–638.

89. Daeron M. Regulation of high-affinity IgE receptor-mediated mast cell activation by murine low-affinity IgG receptors. *J Clin Invest* 1995;95: 577–585.

90. Malbec O, Fong DC, Turner M, et al. Fcε Receptor I-associated lyn-dependent phosphorylation of Fcγ receptor IIB during negative regulation of mast cell activation. *J Immunol* 1998;160:1647–1658.

91. Blery M, Delon J, Trautmann A, et al. Reconstituted killer cell inhibitory receptors for major histocompatibility complex class I molecules control mast cell activation induced via immunoreceptor tyrosine-based activation motifs. *J Biol Chem* 1997;272:8989–8996.

92. Valiante NM, Phillips JH, Lanier LL, Parham P. Killer cell inhibitory receptor recognition of human leukocyte antigen (HLA) class I blocks formation of a pp36/PLC-gamma signaling complex in human natural killer (NK) cells. *J Exp Med* 1996;184: 2243–2250.

93. Zhang W, Sloan-Lancaster J, Kitchen J, Trible RP, Samelson LE. LAT: the ZAP-70 tyrosine kinase substrate that links T cell receptor to cellular activation. *Cell* 1998;92:83–92.

94. Weber JR, Orstavik S, Torgersen KM, et al. Molecular cloning of the cDNA encoding pp36, a tyrosine-phosphorylated adaptor protein selectively expressed by T cells and natural killer cells. *J Exp Med* 1998;187:1157–1161.

95. Binstadt BA, Billadeau DD, Jevremovic D, et al. SLP-76 is a direct substrate of SHP-1 recruited to killer cell inhibitory receptors. *J Biol Chem* 1998;273:27518–27523.

96. Smith KA, Wu J, Bakker ABH, Phillips JH, Lanier LL. Ly49D and Ly49H associate with mouse DAP12 and form activating receptors. *J Immunol* 1998;161:7–10.

97. Gosselin P, Mason LH, Willette-Brown J, Ortaldo JR, McVicar DW, Anderson SK. Induction of DAP12 phosphorylation, calcium mobilization, and cytokine secretion by Ly49H. *J Leukoc Biol* 1999;165–171.

98. Bottino C, Vitale M, Olcese L, et al. The human natural killer cell receptor for major histocompatibility complex class I molecules: surface modulation of p58 molecules and their linkage to CD3 zeta chain, Fc epsilon RI gamma chain and the p56lck kinase. *Eur J Immunol* 1994;24:2527–2534.

99. Brumbaugh KM, Perez-Villar JJ, Dick CJ, Schoon RA, Lopez-Botet M, Leibson PJ. Clonotypic differences in signaling from CD94 (kp43) on NK cells lead to divergent cellular responses. *J Immunol* 1996;157:2804–2812.

100. Moretta A, Sivori S, Vitale M, et al. Existence of both inhibitory (p58) and activatory (p50) receptors for HLA-C molecules in human natural killer cells. *J Exp Med* 1995;182:875–884.

101. Moretta A, Biassoni R, Bottino C, et al. Major histocompatibility complex class I specific receptors on human natural killer and T lymphocytes. *Immunol Rev* 1997;155:105–117.

102. Vely F, Vivier E. Conservation of structural features reveals the existence of a large family of inhibitory cell surface receptors and noninhibitory/activatory counterparts. *J Immunol* 1997;159: 2075–2077.

103. Mason LH, Willette-Brown J, Anderson SK, et al. Cutting edge: characterization of an associated 16-kDa tyrosine phosphoprotein required for Ly-49D signal transduction. *J Immunol* 1998;160:4148–4152.

104. Olcese L, Cambiaggi A, Semenzato G, Bottino C, Moretta A, Vivier E. Human killer cell activatory receptors for MHC class I molecules are included in a multimeric complex expressed by natural killer cells. *J Immunol* 1997;158:5083–5086.

105. Campbell KS, Cella M, Carretero M, Lopez-Botet

M, Colonna M. Signaling through human killer cell activating receptors triggers tyrosine phosphorylation of an associated protein complex. *Eur J Immunol* 1997;28:599–609.

106. Lanier LL, Corliss BC, Wu J, Leong C, Phillips JH. Immunoreceptor DAP12 bearing a tyrosine-based activation motif is involved in activating NK cells. *Nature* 1998;391:703–707.

107. Lanier LL, Corliss BC, Wu J, Phillips JH. Association of DAP12 with activating CD94/NKG2C NK cell receptors. *Immunity* 1998;8:693–701.

108. Hayami K, Fukuta D, Nishikawa Y, et al. Molecular cloning of a novel murine cell-surface glycoprotein homologous to killer cell inhibitory receptors. *J Biol Chem* 1997;272:7320–7326.

109. Samaridis J, Colonna M. Cloning of novel immunoglobulin superfamily receptors expressed on human myeloid and lymphoid cells: structural evidence for new stimulatory and inhibitory pathways. *Eur J Immunol* 1997;27:660–665.

110. Maeda A, Kurosaki M, Kurosaki T. Paired immunoglobulin-like receptor (PIR)-A is involved in activating mast cells through its association with Fc receptor γ chain. *J Exp Med* 1998;188:991–995.

111. Taylor LS, McVicar DW. Functional association of FcεRIγ with arginine[632] of paired immunoglobulin receptor (PIR)-A3 in murine macrophages. *Blood* (1999, in press).

112. Nakajima H, Samaridis J, Angman L, Colonna M. Cutting edge: human myeloid cells express an activating ILT receptor (ILT1) that associates with Fc receptor gamma-chain. *J Immunol* 1999;162:5–8.

113. Geahlen RL, Burg DL. The role of Syk in cell signaling. *Adv Exp Med Biol* 1994;365:103–109.

114. McVicar DW, Taylor LS, Gosselin P, et al. DAP12 mediated signal transduction in NK cells: a dominant role for the Syk protein tyrosine kinase. *J Biol Chem* 1998;49:32934–32942.

115. Zoller KE, MacNeil IA, Brugge JS. Protein tyrosine kinases Syk and ZAP-70 display distinct requirements for Src family kinases in immune response receptor signal transduction. *J Immunol* 1997;158:1650–1659.

116. Mandelboim O, Kent S, Davis DM, et al. Natural killer activating receptors trigger interferon g secretion from T cells and natural killer cells. *Proc Natl Acad Sci USA* 1998;95:3798–3803.

117. Ota Y, Samelson LE. The product of the proto-oncogene c-cbl: a negative regulator of the Syk tyrosine kinase. *Science* 1997;276:418–420.

118. Cerboni C, Gismondi A, Palmieri G, Piccoli M, Frati L, Santoni A. CD16-mediated activation of phosphatidylinositol-3 kinase (PI-3K) in human NK cells involves tyrosine phosphorylation of Cbl and its association with Grb2, Shc, pp36 and p85 PI-3K subunit. *Eur J Immunol* 1998;28:1005–1015.

119. Fukazawa T, Reedquist KA, Trub T, et al. The SH3 domain-binding T cell tyrosyl phosphoprotein p120: demonstration of its identity with the c-cbl protooncogene product and in vivo complexes with Fyn, Grb2, and phosphatidylinositol 3-kinase. *J Biol Chem* 1995;270:19141–19150.

120. Fournel M, Davidson D, Weil R, Veillette A. Association of tyrosine protein kinase Zap-70 with the protooncogene product p120c-cbl in T lymphocytes. *J Exp Med* 1996;183:301–306.

121. Hartley D, Corvera S. Formation of c-Cbl.phosphatidylinositol 3-kinase complexes on lymphocyte membranes by a p56lck-independent mechanism. *J Biol Chem* 1996;271:21939–21943.

122. Gesbert F, Garbay C, Bertoglio J. Interleukin-2 stimulation induces tyrosine phosphorylation of p120-Cbl and CrkL and formation of multimolecular signaling complexes in T lymphocytes and natural killer cells. *J Biol Chem* 1998;273:3986–3993.

123. Panchamoorthy G, Fukazawa T, Miyake S, et al. p120cbl is a major substrate of tyrosine phosphorylation upon B cell antigen receptor stimulation and interacts in vivo with Fyn and Syk tyrosine kinases, Grb2 and Shc adaptors, and the p85 subunit of phosphatidylinositol 3-kinase. *J Biol Chem* 1996; 271:3187–3194.

124. Sasaki K, Odai H, Hanazono Y, et al. TPO/c-mpl ligand induces tyrosine phosphorylation of multiple cellular proteins including proto-oncogene products, Vav and c-Cbl, and Ras signaling molecules. *Biochem Biophys Res Commun* 1995;216: 338–347.

125. Tsygankov AY, Mahajan S, Fincke JE, Bolen JB. Specific association of tyrosine-phosphorylated c-cbl with Fyn tyrosine kinase in T cells. *J Biol Chem* 1996;271:27130–27137.

126. Smit L, Borst J. The Cbl family of signal transduction molecules. *Crit Rev Oncog* 1997;8:359–379.

Cytotoxic Cells: Basic Mechanisms and Medical Applications, edited by Michail V. Sitkovsky and Pierre A. Henkart. Lippincott Williams & Wilkins, Philadelphia © 2000.

Chapter 5

TCR-Initiated Adhesion and Signaling Cascades in CTL Activation

Matthew F. Mescher and Paige L. Jensen

Center for Immunology, University of Minnesota, Minneapolis, Minnesota 55455, USA

Mature, circulating CD8$^+$ T lymphocytes recognize foreign peptide antigens (Ags) bound to class I major histocompatibility complex (MHC-I) proteins (1) and, in the context of appropriate co-stimulation, are stimulated to proliferate and differentiate to become effector cytotoxic T lymphocytes (CTLs). These killer cells can then bind tightly to cells displaying the foreign peptide–class I complex on their surfaces and directly kill them by one of at least two mechanisms: granule exocytosis or fas-mediated induction of apoptosis (2). Because the foreign peptide can derive from a virus or bacterium infecting the cell or a protein that is mutated or overexpressed in a tumor, CTLs can provide protection against a broad range of potential threats. Direct killing of Ag-expressing cells is the most dramatic and apparent function of CTLs, but they also produce cytokines in response to Ag recognition and may produce different patterns of cytokines in a manner analogous to T-helper 1 lymphocytes (Th1) and Th2 CD4$^+$ T cells.

When a CTL encounters an Ag-bearing cell, it binds tightly to the target cell in an Ag-specific manner to form a strong cell–cell conjugate. Within minutes the CTL delivers the "lethal hit" to the target, at which point the CTL can dissociate from the still intact target. The target subsequently dies by apoptosis, and the CTL can go on to kill additional targets (3,4). T cell receptor (TCR) recognition of Ag is clearly central to these events, as evidenced by the Ag-specific nature of conjugate formation and cytolysis. However, as monoclonal antibodies (mAbs) specific for lymphocyte surface proteins became available, it was apparent from blocking studies that additional receptors on the surface of the CTLs were involved (5,6). In particular, CD8 and leukocyte function-associated antigen (LFA-1) appeared to be important for adhesion to form conjugates and for killing by many populations or cloned lines of CTLs. LFA-1 binds to intracellular adhesion molecules (ICAM-1), and CD8 binds to a conserved region of class I proteins, raising the question as to how receptors that bind ligands common to many cell types could contribute without the CTL simply adhering to every cell it contacts, irrespective of the presence of Ag, thereby being diverted from its function in immune surveillance. This question was answered when it was found that the TCR must recognize Ag and deliver a signal(s) to activate the adhesion function of CD8 (7) or integrins (8–11). Thus a CTL does not bind tightly to another cell even though it has class I protein, ICAM-1, and other integrin ligands on its surface unless Ag is also present to trigger upregulation of the adhesion functions of the receptors for these ligands.

In addition to mediating adhesion, CD8 and integrins can generate transmembrane signals upon binding to their ligands, and these signals can act in concert with signals from the TCR to activate the functional responses of the CTLs. Thus the various receptors expressed on the CTL surface act in a cascade of signaling and adhesion events that results in tight binding to the Ag-bearing target cell and activation of the lytic function of the CTL. Some of the signals generated downstream in this cascade may also provide feedback to deactivate adhesion and allow the CTL to release the target after the lethal hit has been delivered. These aspects of CD8+ effector T cell activation are reviewed here and are briefly contrasted with the adhesion and signaling events involved in activating naive CD8+ T cells to proliferate and differentiate.

TCR SIGNALING WITH CD4 OR CD8 AS CO-RECEPTORS

Ligation of the TCR initiates the formation of multimolecular signaling complexes and activation of numerous intracellular signaling pathways, which lead to functional responses. Extensive investigation has revealed a general scheme for the events critical for generating the signals and has provided a wealth of additional information that requires much more study before a fully integrated understanding of this complex signaling machinery can be developed. A detailed review of signaling by the TCRs is beyond the scope of this chapter. Instead, the current model of the general features is briefly summarized.

The TCR includes the Ag-binding α- and β-chain (or γ- and δ-chain) heterodimer together with the nonpolymorphic CD3 chains ε, γ, and δ and the TCRζ chain (12). Each of these nonpolymorphic chains includes immunoreceptor tyrosine-based activation motifs (ITAMs) that are necessary and sufficient to couple the TCR to signaling pathways (13,14). Tyrosine phosphorylation of the ITAMS by *src* kinase family members *lck* or *fyn* allows ZAP-70 to be recruited to the complex by binding to the TCRζ chain via

its SH2 domain. The bound ZAP-70, a member of another protein tyrosine kinase family that includes *Syk,* is then activated when it is in turn tyrosine-phosphorylated, also by *lck* or *fyn.* Formation of the multimolecular signaling complex then proceeds as additional proteins such as LAT, SLP-76, and p36 are recruited through SH2-SH3 domain interactions. This leads to activation of downstream signaling pathways including the phosphatidylinositol 3-kinase (PI3-k) pathway, pathways activated by p21^{ras}, and the pathway for polyphosphotidylinositol (PI) hydrolysis through activation of PLC-γ1, to result in protein kinase C (PKC) activation and a rise in $[Ca^{2+}]_{int}$ (15,16).

In many instances of T cell stimulation, and probably most involving TCR ligation by Ag (in contrast to crosslinking antibodies or superAgs), engagement of the TCR is not sufficient to fully activate the cells. Instead, the CD4 or CD8 co-receptors must bind class II or class I MHC proteins, respectively, and contribute to signal generation (17,18). It is likely that this occurs through the *lck* that is noncovalently associated with the co-receptors (19,20), and may involve *lck*-mediated phosphorylation of ZAP-70 that has been recruited to the TCR. The contribution of CD8 to signaling in CTLs is discussed in more detail below.

A variety of evidence has accumulated to make it clear that the TCR is not simply acting as an on/off switch. Instead, signaling through the receptor is a highly dynamic process with different outcomes possible. A single peptide–MHC complex can be serially engaged by multiple TCRs (21–23), which may be necessary for generating an activating signal and may account for how fewer than ten complexes per target can support CTL-mediated killing of the target (24). In addition, the TCR employs ''kinetic proofreading'' (25). The duration of engagement of ligand appears to be critical; TCR engagement with ligands that dissociate rapidly not only can fail to activate the cell but can prevent activation by an optimal ligand. Fast-dissociating ligands cause intracellular signaling events distinct from those caused by optimal ligands (26–28). These dynamic aspects of TCR-dependent signal generation have been realized only relatively recently, and much remains to be learned, particularly with respect to developing a quantitative understanding of these processes.

CD8 IS AN ADHESION MOLECULE ON EFFECTOR CTL

CD8 consists of α and β transmembrane polypeptide chains, both of which are glycosylated and are members of the immunoglobulin supergene family of proteins (17). It is expressed on the cell surface as both an $\alpha\beta$ heterodimer and an $\alpha\alpha$ homodimer. It was first suggested that CD8 might interact with class I protein based on the observations that CD8+ T cells were predominantly class I restricted (29) and that anti-CD8 antibodies (Abs) could block target cell lysis by at least some CTLs (30). Direct evidence for a CD8–class I protein binding interaction was provided by experiments demonstrating that CHO cells transfected with CD8 α-chain, so they expressed $\alpha\alpha$ homodimers, and could adhere to cells that expressed class I protein on their surfaces (31). This approach was used to map the interaction site to the $\alpha3$ domain of the class I heavy chain by mutational analysis (32), and it was subsequently confirmed by crystallographic analysis (33,34). The interaction site is a highly conserved region of the class I heavy chain, and CD8 thus binds any class I protein.

The binding of CD8 to class I protein that was detected in the experiments employing transfected CHO cells (31,32) was weak; the α-chain had to be expressed at high levels on the transfected cells, and the partner cell in the binding assay was an Ebstein-Barr virus (EBV) transformed B cell that expresses about tenfold higher levels of class I protein on its surface than do normal cells. Thus it was not surprising that when we examined cloned CTLs interacting with purified class I protein immobilized on a surface at a density comparable to that on normal cells we found

that the cells did not adhere if it was a class I protein not recognized by the TCR. We did find that adhesion to the immobilized protein was readily detectable when it included antigen recognized specifically by the CTL (35). Somewhat paradoxically, this adhesion appeared to depend on the CD8–class I protein interaction, as anti-CD8 Abs could block it. This suggested the possibility that CD8 is normally in an inactive state, unable to mediate adhesion to class I; but it becomes activated as a result of a signal from the TCR. That this was the case was demonstrated in experiments in which anti-TCR mAbs in solution were added to the CTL to ligate the TCR (7,36); cells treated in this way adhered to class I proteins irrespective of their specificity but did not adhere to irrelevant control proteins or class II MHC proteins (Fig. 5-1A,B).

These experiments demonstrated that signaling through the TCR could in fact upregulate CD8-mediated adhesion of the cells. It was important to show that this occurred when the TCR bound to Ag and was not an artifact of crosslinking the TCR with an Ab. This point was examined in experiments that employed low-density Ag together with a non-Ag class I protein immobilized on the same surface (37). When H-2D^b was immobilized at a low density and pulsed with Ag peptide, CTL clones specific for the D^b/peptide neither adhered to the surface (Fig. 5-1C) nor responded by undergoing degranulation. In contrast, when Ag complexes at this same surface density were co-immobilized with nonantigen class I protein the CTLs adhered to the surface (Fig. 5-1D) and were triggered to degranulate. In these experiments a total class I surface density comparable to that found on normal cells was sufficient to support adhesion and degranulation. Adhesion and response were both blocked by anti-CD8 Abs or by Abs directed against the immobilized class I protein. Thus TCR engagement of Ag at a level too low to mediate adhesion by itself or to trigger degranulation is nevertheless sufficient to

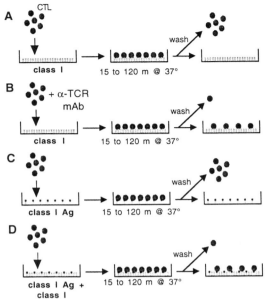

FIG. 5-1. CD8-dependent adhesion of cloned CTLs to class I protein requires TCR engagement. **A, B:** When labeled CTLs are incubated in mirotiter wells having immobilized class I protein that is not an antigen (Ag) for the TCR, adhesion of the cells to the wells is detected only if the cells are stimulated by addition of anti-TCR mAbs in solution (7). **C, D:** A low density of class I Ag complexes does not support adhesion but can provide the TCRs with a stimulus to activate adhesion if the total density of class I protein (Ag and non-Ag) is high (37).

signal the activation of CD8, which can then mediate adhesion provided the total class I protein is at a density comparable to that on cells. In contrast to CD8, CD4 does not undergo TCR-triggered upregulation to act as an adhesion molecule on CD4$^+$ T cells (38).

In the experiments examining binding of CD8 α-chain transfected CHO cells to class I expressing cells (31,32), high levels of expression were required, but there was no apparent requirement for signaling of CD8 activation. This, together with the results described above, suggests that there is basal binding of CD8 to class I protein and that it can be converted to high-avidity binding upon signaling through the TCR. The relation between low- and high-avidity binding by CD8 is further considered below when its co-receptor function is discussed.

SIGNALS FOR ACTIVATION OF CD8 ADHESION FUNCTION

The engagement of TCRs by antigen activates numerous signaling pathways, but only a subset of them are activated when CTLs are treated with anti-TCR mAbs in solution under the conditions that activate CD8-mediated adhesion. The PI hydrolysis pathway is not activated to any detectable extent, and intracellular free Ca^{2+} concentration does not increase (39,40). Thus although activation of these pathways is important for triggering degranulation, it does not appear to be important for activating CD8. Anti-TCR mAb does activate tyrosine phosphorylation, but it results in phosphorylation of only a subset of cellular substrates that are phosphorylated in response to stimulation with Ag (41). Inhibiting tyrosine phosphorylation with specific inhibitors completely inhibits TCR-triggered CD8-mediated adhesion to class I protein, indicating that it is critical for activating CD8 adhesion function (39).

Activation cannot simply result from direct phosphorylation of the receptor, however, as neither the α- nor β-chains of CD8 have a tyrosine in their cytoplasmic domains. Additional steps must be involved, and evidence suggests that activation of PI 3-kinase plays a role in enhancing the avidity of binding to class I protein. It has been shown that crosslinking of the TCR complex can result in an increase in PI3-k activity associated with p59^{fyn} tyrosine kinase (42). We found that this occurred upon treating cloned CTLs with anti-TCR mAbs under conditions that activate CD8-dependent adhesion, and that blocking the activity of PI3-k with specific inhibitors blocked adhesion to class I protein (Jensen and Mescher, manuscript in preparation). Furthermore, addition of genestein to inhibit tyrosine phosphorylation prevented the increase in *fyn*-associated PI3-k activity, indicating that upregulation of PI3-k occurs downstream of tyrosine kinase activation in the pathway leading to upregulation of CD8 adhesion function (Fig. 5-2).

The mechanism responsible for increasing the avidity of CD8-dependent adhesion to class I protein is not known. It may involve an alteration in CD8 to increase the binding affinity. Alternatively, it may involve changes in the distribution of CD8 on the cell surface or its association with other proteins, such as the cytoskeleton, so there is an increase in the binding avidity when numerous CD8 receptors on one cell engage class I proteins on the other cell. T cells undergo cytoskeletal reorganization when they are stimulated (43–46), and CD8-mediated adhesion of CTLs to class I protein is inhibited by agents that interfere with either microtubule or microfilament function (47). Thus an intact cytoskeleton is necessary for adhesion to occur. The cytoskeleton could be directly involved in increased adhesion through promoting the formation of CD8 microclusters on the cell surface. Treatment of polymorphonuclear leukocytes with phorbol myristic acetate (PMA) results in microclustering of C3bi receptors, and its extent correlates with the ability of the cells to bind to C3bi-coated particles (48). Clustering of CD8 receptors could potentially increase the avidity of binding to a class I protein-bearing surface by decreasing the apparent off-rate of the interaction.

Cytoskeletal-dependent deformation of the CTL to allow flattening and spreading onto the class I protein-bearing surface might also account for the importance of a functional cytoskeleton in CD8-mediated adhesion. CTLs interact with target cells over large regions of the cell surfaces (44), and CD8 binding to class I might act as a "zipper" to attach the surfaces as their contact region expands. Limiting the extent of spreading by interfering with the cytoskeleton could result in too few CD8–class I protein bonds forming to result in high-avidity attachment of the cells. This suggestion is consistent with the finding that class I protein must be presented on a large surface, approaching the dimensions of a cell, for CTLs to interact with it effectively (49).

Even if one or both of the above suggestions for a role for the cytoskeleton are correct, it does not rule out the possibility that additional changes may be critical to CD8 adhesion function, including a possible alteration of its affinity for class I protein. Clearly,

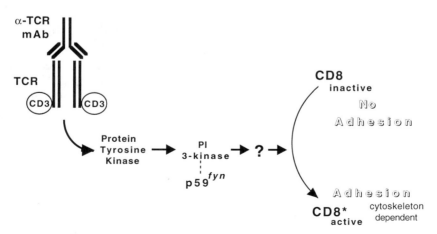

FIG. 5-2. Signals implicated in the activation of CD8 to mediate adhesion to class I protein. As discussed in the text, TCR-dependent activation of protein tyrosine kinase(s) is required upstream of *fyn*-associated PI3-k activation.

much remains to be learned regarding both the TCR-generated signals necessary to convert CD8 to its high-avidity state and the molecular basis for this conversion to high-avidity binding to class I protein.

CD8: A CO-RECEPTOR

The ability of anti-CD8 Abs to block Ag-specific CTL responses raised the possibility that CD8 might be involved in generating a transmembrane signal that contributes to activation of responses, although some evidence argued that crosslinking CD8 with Abs might generate a negative signal rather than interfering with generation of a positive signal (50). A signaling role received strong support when it was demonstrated that CD8 is noncovalently associated with p56^{lck} (19,20), which binds to the cytoplasmic region of the α-chain of CD8.

It became possible to demonstrate a co-signaling role of CD8 directly in the experiments employing anti-TCR mAbs in solution to trigger adhesion to class I protein. Treatment of CTLs with anti-TCR mAb in solution, which presumably results in bivalent crosslinking of the receptor, does not trigger detectable release of serine esterase activity into the medium (7). Release of serine esterase activity is a sensitive, quantitative measure of degranulation by the cells (51). Similarly, placing CTLs on non-Ag class I protein does not activate degranulation. However, when CTLs are treated with anti-TCR mAbs and then allowed to bind to class I protein via CD8, rapid and extensive degranulation occurs (7). This triggering is specific for class I protein and is blocked by anti-CD8 mAbs. Thus engagement of activated CD8 generates an additional signal that acts in cooperation with TCR-dependent signals to activate degranulation.

In the experiments described above using anti-TCR mAbs, the CD8 adhesion and co-receptor functions are supported by binding to class I protein that is not an Ag and thus is not bound by the TCRs. There is considerable evidence, however, that efficient co-re-ceptor function of CD8 requires that it bind to the same class I protein that is bound by the TCRs. When class I protein Ag is mutated in the region of the α3 domain that interacts with CD8, some CTLs can no longer lyse targets expressing the mutant Ag (32,52). This occurs despite the fact that the targets also express other nonantigen class I proteins on their surfaces that have the native α3 domain and can thus support CD8 interaction. This finding strongly supports the conclusion that CD8 and TCRs must bind the same class I protein for effective signaling—seemingly in contradiction to the fact that a nonantigen class I can support the co-stimulatory signaling role of CD8 when the CTL is stimulated with anti-TCR mAb (7).

A means of reconciling this apparent discrepancy is suggested by considering the likely possibility that co-signaling by CD8 involves its noncovalently associated *lck* tyrosine kinase phosphorylating components of the TCR complex to recruit and activate ZAP-70. If so, it would occur most efficiently when CD8 is held in close proximity to the ligated TCR by virtue of both receptors binding to the same class I protein. It is probably critical that this is accomplished in an efficient manner when a CTL is interacting with an Ag-bearing target, where the number of class I protein–Ag complexes is small (24,53–55). In contrast, when large numbers of TCRs are engaged by addition of anti-TCR mAbs in solution, inefficient transphosphorylation of TCR components by *lck* on an activated CD8 bound to class I protein is adequate to signal for functional responses. It may even yield as many fully activated TCR complexes as when class I protein–Ag complexes are present in low numbers.

Kane and colleagues demonstrated that the adhesion and co-receptor functions of CD8 can be dissociated (56). Class I protein with a Glu227 to Lys mutation in the acidic loop of the α3 domain could no longer provide co-stimulation for degranulation but could still support CTL adhesion by activated CD8. This does not rule out the high-avidity adhesion interaction being mediated by the acidic loop of the $\alpha3$ domain; it may simply be that the low-avidity interaction needed for co-receptor function is more dependent on Glu227. There is evidence, however, that CD8 can also interact with the $\alpha2$ domain of class I proteins (57–59). Binding at this distinct site(s) may be an important component of the high-avidity CD8-mediated adhesion.

Study of the Glu227 to Lys mutation in H-2K^b also indicated that efficient upregulation of the adhesion function of CD8 required its co-receptor function (56). Thus it may be that both TCR and CD8 need to interact with the class I protein–Ag complex and generate signals to upregulate CD8-mediated adhesion to the non-Ag class I proteins present on the target cell surface. Evidence for CD8 binding to the $\alpha3$ acidic loop prior to signaled activation was also obtained in independent studies by Luescher and coworkers (60), who employed photoaffinity labeling to examine binding of soluble class I protein–Ag complexes to TCRs on T cells. CD8 was shown to increase Ag binding by the TCRs substantially (i.e., to act as a coreceptor), and this effect was eliminated when Asp227 of the H-2K^d protein being examined was mutated to a Lys. Because binding of soluble monomeric class I protein–Ag complexes does not generate signals, this effect presumably involves CD8 binding to the acidic $\alpha3$ loop without needing to be activated to its high-avidity state. Garcia et al. (61) similarly found that CD8 could enhance binding of TCR to class I Ag in solution.

These results, obtained when examining the mutant class I proteins (56,60), suggest a model in which TCR and CD8 bind to the same class I protein–Ag complex while CD8 is still in the low-avidity state, with the interaction being critically dependent on residue 227 in the acidic loop of $\alpha3$. TCR binding of Ag is strengthened as a result of CD8 binding, and together the receptors generate the transmembrane signals that then convert CD8 to its high-avidity state. CD8 can then strengthen the cell–cell adhesion by binding

to any class I protein; this binding is less dependent on the residue in position 227 and may involve additional contacts with other sites on the class I protein.

SIGNALING EVENTS ACTIVATED BY TCR AND CD8 ENGAGEMENT

The experimental system employing anti-TCR mAbs in solution to activate CD8 provided an opportunity to distinguish the activation signals generated when the TCR was minimally ligated (by bivalent crosslinking or by Ag at low density) from those generated when CD8 was bound to class I protein. The earliest signaling events that can be detected upon stimulation with Ag are tyrosine phosphorylation of a variety of cellular substrates, including subunits of the TCR complex itself. As described above, stimulating CTLs with anti-TCR mAbs in solution causes phosphorylation of only a subset of the substrates that become phosphorylated in response to Ag. If these CTLs are then allowed to bind to class I protein via CD8, additional cellular substrates become phosphorylated (41). The combination of anti-TCR mAbs and nonantigen class I protein binding results in a tyrosine phosphorylation profile comparable to that obtained when the cells are stimulated with class I protein–Ag complexes.

The p59^{lck} tyrosine kinase associated with CD8 is the likely candidate for mediating at least some of this phosphorylation, and the activity of this enzyme increases upon CD8 binding to class I protein (41). In contrast to the phosphorylation of several cellular substrates seen when CD8 is bound to class I protein, Luo and Sefton (62) found that crosslinking CD8 with an mAb resulted in autophosphorylation of *lck,* but no phosphorylation of additional cellular substrates. It is likely that close juxtaposition of two *lck* molecules as a result of mAb crosslinking of CD8 results in transautophosphorylation. A similar juxtaposition does not occur when CD8 binds class I protein. These differing results raise an important cautionary note with respect to using crosslinking Abs to study signaling events that become activated upon receptor ligation; Ab crosslinking may not faithfully mimic the events that occur when a receptor engages its native ligand.

Treating CTLs with just anti-TCR mAbs does not activate polyphosphatidylinositol (PI) hydrolysis or cause a rise in $[Ca^{2+}]_{int}$, but both occur when the cells are then allowed to bind to class I protein via activated CD8 (39,40). Although activated *lck* might directly upregulate phospholipase C (PLC) to initiate PI hydrolysis, with a resulting inositol phosphate-mediated rise in $[Ca^{2+}]_{int}$, it is more likely that *lck* modifies the TCR complex (Fig. 5-3). *Lck* might mediate phosphorylation of zeta chain to allow recruitment of ZAP-70, phosphorylate ZAP-70 to activate it, or both, with ZAP-70 then initiating PLC activation for PI hydrolysis. As discussed above, these phosphorylation events might be expected to occur most efficiently when TCR and CD8 are bound to the same class I protein–Ag complex. Further work is

needed to determine the details of how CD8 binding to class I protein results in activation of these second messenger pathways that activate functional responses, including degranulation. Already, however, the results make it clear that qualitatively different signals are generated through the TCRs and CD8 receptors, rather than CD8 engagement simply causing a quantitative increase in the signals activated via the TCRs. Thus although CD8 can stabilize the binding to TCRs to class I Ag (60,61), it is not the only way in which it serves a co-receptor function.

IS DE-ADHESION A SIGNALED PROCESS?

A CTL forms a strong conjugate with an Ag-bearing target cell and delivers the "lethal hit" within minutes of initial contact. It can then release the target and proceed to bind and kill the next target while the initial target goes on to die by apoptosis over the next 15

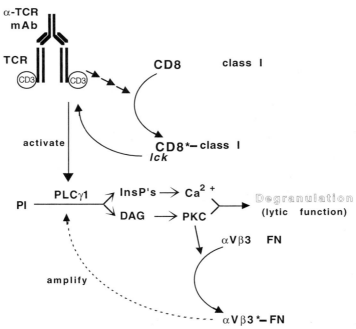

FIG. 5-3. Proposed model for the signaling events involved in co-stimulation by CD8 and $\alpha V\beta 3$ integrin.

to 30 minutes. This ability to recycle and kill multiple targets rapidly is presumably important to the efficient functioning of CTLs in eliminating infected or transformed cells. The ability of CTLs to release a still intact target following delivery of the lethal hit suggests that there may be signals that downregulate the activity of the adhesion receptors, such as CD8 and integrins, that mediate formation of the strong cell–cell conjugate. This was further suggested by the observation that CTLs binding to class I protein via TCR-activated CD8 had the properties of an equilibrium-binding process (63). Cells not only bind to the class I-bearing surface, they can also release and subsequently rebind.

Several observations suggest that activated protein kinase C (PKC) may provide an "off" signal for deactivating CD8 and allowing the CTLs to de-adhere from a class I-bearing surface. Treatment of the CTLs with PMA, which activates PKC, inhibits CD8-mediated binding to class I protein (40). Conversely, inhibiting PKC activity increases the equilibrium level of binding by decreasing the "off rate" of bound cells (Jensen and Mescher, in preparation). As discussed above, PI 3-kinase activation appears to be required to activate CD8 adhesion. PMA treatment can inhibit activation of PI 3-kinase in T cells (64), which seems also to be the case in CTLs (Jensen and Mescher, in preparation). Thus PKC might provide a signal for detachment by inactivating the PI 3-kinase required to upregulate CD8. Provision of an "off" signal via PKC is an attractive hypothesis in that one of the products of the CD8-dependent activation of the PI pathway would then feed back to deactivate the binding that initiated the pathway.

INTEGRINS: ADHESION AND SIGNALING

Signals delivered via TCRs can also upregulate the adhesion function of integrins expressed on T cells, including LFA-1 (8,9), and several of the $\beta 1$ (10) and $\beta 3$ (11) integrins. In addition, binding of the integrins to their ligands can provide co-stimulation for T cells (39,65–67), although it has been difficult to distinguish between adhesion effects that lead to increased TCR occupancy versus generation of transmembrane co-stimulatory signals by the integrin per se. Many long-term CTL lines express LFA-1 on their surface as well as the fibronectin (FN)-binding integrin $\alpha V\beta 3$, the vitronectin receptor (VNR). This provided the opportunity to compare the TCR signals for activating CD8 and integrins for adhesion and to compare the co-stimulatory signals generated when these receptors bind their ligands. We initially anticipated that activation of adhesion might involve a common pathway, and that co-stimulatory signaling by the different receptors would be redundant. In fact, the activation requirements are different for CD8 than for LFA-1 or $\alpha V\beta 3$, and all three receptors have distinct co-stimulatory functions.

The same treatment with anti-TCR mAbs in solution that activates CD8-mediated adhesion of CTLs to class I protein also activates LFA-1-dependent adhesion to ICAM-1 and $\alpha V\beta 3$-mediated adhesion to FN or vitronectin (VN) (11,39,68). However, the requirements for activating CD8 and integrin-mediated adhesions were distinguished in experiments examining the effects of pharmacologic agents. Treatment with PMA to activate PKC had been shown by others to activate integrin adhesion for other types of T cell (8,10), and it was also true for effector CTLs binding to either ICAM-1 or FN (11,68). In contrast, no increase in adhesion to class I protein could be detected upon PMA treatment (Fig. 5-4). In fact, when CD8-dependent adhesion to class I protein was triggered by anti-TCR mAbs, addition of PMA caused the adhesion to decrease, as discussed above.

Differences in TCR-activated CD8- and integrin-mediated adhesion were also found when a second Ab was added to further crosslink the TCRs. Binding to both ICAM-1 and FN were increased, but binding to class I protein was decreased (Fig. 5-4) (11,68).

Receptor	Stimulus			
	None	α-TCR Ab	α -TCR Ab + X-link	PMA
CD8	-	+	+/-	-
LFA-1	-	+	+ +	+ +
αVβ3	-	+	+ +	+ +

FIG. 5-4. Requirements for activating CD8 and integrin-dependent adhesions of CTL to the respective ligands differ. +, adhesion is activated; −, adhesion is not activated. Phorbol myristic acetate (PMA) activates protein kinase C.

The increase in integrin-mediated adhesion that occurs upon further crosslinking the TCR might simply result from a quantitative increase in the activating signals. Alternatively, more extensive crosslinking of the TCR might activate a new pathway(s) not activated upon bivalent crosslinking of the TCR, and the decreased binding to class I protein under these conditions suggested that this might in fact be the case. As described in a previous section, bivalent crosslinking of the TCR does not cause any detectable release of inositol phosphates or rise in $[Ca^{2+}]_{int}$, indicating that PLC and the PI hydrolysis pathway are not being activated. In contrast, PI hydrolysis is activated upon addition of a second Ab to further crosslink the TCR (40). PI hydrolysis leads to the production of diacylglycerol and activation of PKC. Thus the increased integrin adhesion and decreased class I adhesion that occur with either PMA treatment or further crosslinking of the TCR (Fig. 5-4) are consistent with activated PKC mediating these effects.

Further evidence for distinct signaling events becoming activated depending on the extent of TCR crosslinking comes from examining the effects of PI 3-kinase inhibitors on integrin-mediated adhesions. As is the case for CD8 binding to class I protein, VNR binding to FN triggered by anti-TCR mAb in solution can be completely inhibited by wortmannin at a concentration of 25 nM, where it is specific for PI 3-kinase (Jensen

and Mescher, in preparation). In contrast, when adhesion to FN is triggered by anti-TCR mAbs plus a second crosslinking Ab, wortmannin is an ineffective inhibitor, causing less than 20% decrease in adhesion even at 100 nM.

A variety of evidence demonstrates that the signals required for activating adhesion by CD8 are different from those for activation by the integrins. Furthermore, co-stimulatory signaling is distinct for the different receptors. CD8 initiates the PI hydrolysis pathway upon binding to class I protein (Fig. 5-3). In contrast, αVβ3 cannot initiate PI hydrolysis upon binding to FN. It can, however, substantially amplify the activity of this pathway (as measured by an increased rate of inositol phosphate release) once it has been initiated. Thus αVβ3 appears to act as a feedback amplifier for activation of functional responses (Fig. 5-3). Finally, LFA-1 binding to ICAM-1 has no effect on PI hydrolysis or degranulation that cannot be accounted for by its contribution to increased adhesion. This does not mean that LFA-1 cannot generate a signal; rather, if it does so in these cells, it is clearly distinct from signals generated by CD8 or αVβ3.

TCR INITIATES A CASCADE OF ADHESION AND SIGNALING

The findings summarized above suggest a model in which multiple receptors on CTLs contribute to binding and killing of the target cell by both increasing adhesion between the cell surfaces and generating transmembrane signals that contribute to activation of the lytic machinery. They do not do it in a concerted manner, however, and the signals they contribute are not redundant. Rather, they act in a cascade of adhesion and signal generation to form an Ag-specific conjugate with the target, activate the lytic machinery, and then release the target and recycle.

CD8 and the integrin receptors are normally in a low-avidity state, so the CTL does not simply bind to the first cell with which it comes into contact. Given the broad distribution of the ligands for these receptors, constitutive adhesion activity of the receptors would preclude the CTLs being able to circulate and carry out immune surveillance. However, if the TCR detects Ag on a cell the CTL contacts, signals are generated to upregulate the avidity of CD8 and allow it to begin to zip together the surfaces as it binds class I protein on the target. As CD8 binds class I protein, co-stimulatory signals are generated, probably via the associated *lck* kinase, that initiate PI hydrolysis and begin to generate the downstream second messengers that activate degranulation. The CD8 molecules bound to the same class I protein–Ag complex as the TCRs are probably the major contributors to co-stimulation, and CD8 molecules bound to any class I protein contribute to adhesion.

The PKC that is activated as a result of PI hydrolysis then signals for activation of the integrin receptors, and they then bind their ligands to the target with high avidity and contribute to tight binding of the target. At least in the case of $\alpha V\beta 3$, a new signal is generated that amplifies PI hydrolysis and degranulation. Finally, as second messengers reach high levels in the area of initial contact, they may provide "off" signals that begin to downregulate the adhesion activity of the receptors in that region.

This sequence of events can be envisioned as a wave of adhesion that begins at the site of initial contact and TCR engagement,

propagating outward in a circle as the adhesion receptors become activated. At somewhat longer times, de-adhesion begins in the central region of initial contact while new adhesion is still forming at the periphery of the wave. This sequence could potentially create a sealed space between the CTL and the target into which degranulation by the CTL could release the components of the lytic machinery, concentrating them at the surface of the Ag-bearing target and minimizing damage to bystander cells. Finally, as the spreading wave of adhesion reaches the limits of the cell contact region, it is overtaken by the central region of spreading de-adhesion, and the target is released to die while the CTL searches for another target.

ADHESION AND CO-STIMULATORY RECEPTORS ON RESTING CD8⁺ T CELLS

Many of the same receptors involved in effector CTL adhesion, signaling, and rapid functional response to Ag-bearing target cells are the same as those employed by resting CD8⁺ T cells to respond to Ag by proliferating and differentiating. Resting cells have additional receptors that can be critical, however, including cytokine receptors and the CD28 co-stimulatory receptor for B7 ligands (69–74). Although effector CTLs may express some of the latter receptors, they are not required for lytic function (73).

Even for the receptors employed by both effector CTLs and resting CD8 T cells, it is beginning to appear that they may not function in exactly the same ways. We have found that although CD8 appears to contribute to activation of resting T cells as a co-receptor, it cannot be upregulated via TCR signals to mediate adhesion of these cells to class I protein (Curtsinger et al., in preparation). This finding is consistent with the results of Kane's group, who demonstrated that the adhesion and co-receptor functions of CD8 can be dissociated (56). When resting CD8⁺ cells are stimulated *in vitro* with Ag over several days, the ability to undergo

TCR-triggered CD8-dependent adhesion to class I protein develops concomitantly with the development of lytic effector function. Thus the adhesion function of CD8 is developmentally regulated. This also appears to be the case for LFA-1 adhesion function, although the regulation is somewhat different than for CD8 (Curtsinger et al., in preparation). The importance of a co-stimulatory role for LFA-1 also appears to differ. As mentioned above, co-stimulation of degranulation by this integrin cannot be detected for effector CTLs. In contrast, LFA-1–ICAM-1 interactions make a clear co-stimulatory contribution to the TCR-dependent proliferation of resting CD8⁺ T cells (75).

CONCLUSIONS

The discovery that several of the receptors on T cells become activated to mediate high-avidity adhesion to their ligands only upon signaling through the TCR has revealed a novel means of regulating cell surface receptor function. In addition, it has clarified the long-standing puzzle of how effector CTLs can use receptors that recognize ligands common to numerous cell types without being diverted from immune surveillance as a result of binding tightly to every cell with which they come into contact. Some of the signaling pathways involved in activating these receptors and in mediating their co-stimulatory contributions have been defined, but much remains to be done to delineate these pathways and reveal the mechanisms responsible for mediating their high-avidity "activated" adhesion.

REFERENCES

1. Townsend A, Bodmer H. Antigen recognition by class I-restricted T lymphocytes. *Annu Rev Immunol* 1989;7:601–624.
2. Berke G. The binding and lysis of target cells by cytotoxic T lymphocytes: molecular and cellular aspects. *Annu Rev Immunol* 1994;12:735–773.
3. Martz E, Benacerraf B. Multiple target cell killing by the cytolytic T-lymphocyte and the mechanism of cytotoxicity. *Transplantation* 1976;21:5–11.
4. Zagury D, Bernard J, Thierness N, Feldman M, Berke G. Isolation and characterization of individual functionally reactive cytotoxic T lymphocytes: conjugation, killing and recycling at the single cell level. *Eur J Immunol* 1975;5:818–822.
5. Bierer B, Burakoff S. T cell adhesion molecules. *FASEB J* 1988;10:2584–2590.
6. Martz E, Heagy W, Gromkowski S. The mechanism of CTL-mediated killing: monoclonal antibody analysis of the roles of killer and target-cell membrane proteins. *Immunol Rev* 1983;72:73–96.
7. O'Rourke A, Rogers J, Mescher M. Activated CD8 binding to class 1 protein mediated by the T-cell receptor results in signalling. *Nature* 1990; 346:187–189.
8. Dustin M, Springer T. T-cell receptor cross-linking transiently stimulates adhesiveness through LFA-1. *Nature* 1989;341:619–624.
9. Van Kooyk Y, van de Wiel-van Kemenade P, Weder P, Kuijpers T, Figdor C. Enhancement of LFA-1-mediated cell adhesion by triggering through CD2 or CD3 on T lymphocytes. *Nature* 1989;342: 811–813.
10. Shimizu Y, Seventer G, Horgan K, Shaw S. Regulated expression and binding of three VLA (β1) integrin receptors on T cells. *Nature* 1990; 345:250–253.
11. Ybarrondo B, O'Rourke A, McCarthy J, Mescher M. Cytotoxic T lymphocyte interaction with fibronectin and vitronectin: activated adhesion and cosignalling. *Immunology* 1997;91:186–192.
12. Weissman AM. The T-cell antigen receptor: a multisubunit signaling complex. *Chem Immunol* 1994; 59:1–18.
13. Cambier JC. Antigen and Fc receptor signaling: the awesome power of the immunoreceptor tyrosine-based activation motif (ITAM). *J Immunol* 1995;155:3281–3285.
14. Wange RL, Samelson LE. Complex complexes: signaling at the TCR. *Immunity* 1996;5:197–205.
15. Weiss A, Littman DR. Signal transduction by lymphocyte antigen receptors. *Cell* 1994;76:263–274.
16. Cantrell D. T cell antigen receptor signal transduction pathways. *Annu Rev Immunol* 1996;14: 259–274.
17. Parnes J. Molecular biology and function of CD4 and CD8. *Adv Immunol* 1989;44:265–311.
18. Janeway C. The T cell receptor as a multicomponent signalling machine: CD4/CD8 coreceptors and CD45 in T cell activation. *Annu Rev Immunol* 1992;10:645–674.
19. Veillette A, Bookman M, Horak E, Bolen J. The CD4 and CD8 T cell surface antigens are associated with the internal membrane tyrosine-protein kinase p56lck. *Cell* 1988;55:301–308.
20. Rudd C. CD4, CD8 and the TCR-CD3 complex: a novel class of protein-tyrosine kinase receptor. *Immunol Today* 1990;11:400–406.
21. Valitutti S, Muller S, Cella M, Padovan E, Lanzavecchia A. Serial triggering of many T-cell receptors by a few peptide-MHC complexes. *Nature* 1995; 375:148–151.
22. Viola A, Lanzavecchia A. T cell activation determined by T cell receptor number and tunable thresholds. *Science* 1996;273:104–106.

23. Iezzi G, Karjalainen K, Lanzavecchia A. The duration of antigen stimulation determines the fate of naive and effector T cells. *Immunity* 1998;8:89–95.

24. Sykulev Y, Cohen RJ, Eisen HN. The law of mass action governs antigen-stimulated cytolytic activity of CD8$^+$ cytotoxic T lymphocytes. *Proc Natl Acad Sci USA* 1995;92:11990–11992.

25. McKeithan TW. Kinetic proofreading in T-cell receptor signal transduction. *Proc Natl Acad Sci USA* 1995;92:5042–5046.

26. Chau LA, Bluestone JA, Madrenas J. Dissociation of intracellular signaling pathways in response to partial agonist ligands and the T-cell receptor. *J Exp Med* 1998;187:1699–1709.

27. Malissen B. Translating affinity into response. *Science* 1998;281:528–529.

28. Neumeister Kersh E, Shaw AS, Allen PM. Fidelity of T cell activation through multistep cell receptor z phosphorylation. *Science* 1998;281:572–575.

29. Swain S. Significance of Lyt phenotypes: Lyt-2 antibodies block activities of T cells that recognize class I major histocompatibility complex antigens regardless of their function. *Proc Natl Acad Sci USA* 1981;78:7101.

30. Martz E, Davignon D, Kurzinger K, Springer T. The molecular basis for cytolytic T lymphocyte function: analysis with blocking monoclonal antibodies. *Adv Exp Med Biol* 1982;146:447–465.

31. Norment A, Salter R, Parham P, Engelhard V, Littman D. Cell-cell adhesion mediated by CD8 and MHC class I molecules. *Nature* 1988;336:79–81.

32. Salter R, Benjamin R, Wesley P, et al. A binding site for the T-cell co-receptor CD8 on the alpha 3 domain of HLA-A2. *Nature* 1990;345:41–46.

33. Gao GF, Tormo J, Gerth UC, et al. Crystal structure of the complex between human CD8αα and HLA-A2. *Nature* 1997;387:630–634.

34. Kern PS, Teng M-K, Smolyar A, et al. Structural basis of CD8 coreceptor function revealed by crystallographic analysis of murine CD8αα ectodomain fragment in complex with H-2K^b. *Immunity* 1998;9:519–530.

35. Kane K, Goldstein S, Mescher M. Class 1 alloantigen is sufficient for cytolytic T lymphocyte binding and transmembrane signalling. *Eur J Immunol* 1988;18:1925–1929.

36. O'Rourke A, Mescher M. T-cell receptor-activated adhesion systems. *Curr Opin Cell Biol* 1990; 2:888–893.

37. Kane K, Mescher M. Activation of CD8-dependent CTL adhesion and degranulation by peptide-class I complexes. *J Immunol* 1993;150:4788–4797.

38. O'Rourke A, Lasam M. Murine CD4$^+$ T cells undergo TCR-activated adhesion to extracellular matrix proteins but not to nonantigenic MHC class II proteins. *J Immunol* 1995;155:3839–3846.

39. O'Rourke A, Mescher M. Cytotoxic T-lymphocyte activation involves a cascade of signalling and adhesion events. *Nature* 1992;358:253–255.

40. O'Rourke A, Mescher M. Signals for activation of CD8-dependent adhesion and costimulation in cytotoxic T lymphocytes. *J Immunol* 1994;152:4358–4367.

41. Anel A, O'Rourke AM, Kleinfeld AM, Mescher MF. T cell receptor and CD8-dependent tyrosine phosphorylation events in cytotoxic T lymphocytes: activation of p56^{lck} by CD8 binding to class I protein. *Eur J Immunol* 1996;26:2310–2319.

42. Prasad KVS, Janssen O, Kapeller R, Raab M, Cantley LC, Rudd CE. Src-homology 3 domain of protein kinase p59fyn mediates binding to phosphatidylinositol 3-kinase. *Proc Natl Acad Sci USA* 1993;90:7366–7370.

43. Bykovskaja S, Rytenko A, Rauschenbach M, Bykovsky A. Ultrastructural alteration of cytolytic T lymphocytes following their interaction with target cells. II. Morphogenesis of secretory granules and intracellular vacuoles. *Cell Immunol* 1978;40:175–185.

44. Geiger G. Spatial relationships of microtubule organizing centers and the contact area of cytotoxic T lymphocytes and target cells. *J Cell Biol* 1982; 95:137–143.

45. Kupfer A, Dennert G. Reorientation of the microtubule-organizing center and the Golgi apparatus in cloned cytotoxic T lymphocytes triggered by binding to lysable target cells. *J Immunol* 1984;133:2762–2766.

46. Kupfer A, Singer S. Cell biology of cytotoxic and helper T-cell functions. *Annu Rev Immunol* 1989;7:309–338.

47. O'Rourke A, Apgar J, Kane K, Martz E, Mescher M. Cytoskeletal function in CD8- and T cell receptor-mediated interaction of cytotoxic T lymphocytes with class I protein. *J Exp Med* 1991;173:241–249.

48. Detmers P, Wright S, Olsen E, Kimball B, Cohn Z. Aggregation of complement receptors on human neutrophils in the absence of ligand. *J Cell Biol* 1987;105:1137–1145.

49. Mescher M. Surface contact requirements for activation of cytotoxic T lymphocytes. *J Immunol* 1992;149:2402–2405.

50. Hunig T. Monoclonal anti-Lyt-2.2 antibody blocks lectin-dependent cellular cytotoxicity of H-2-negative target cells. *J Exp Med* 1984;159:551–558.

51. Pasternak M, Eisen H. A novel serine esterase expressed by cytotoxic T lymphocytes. *Nature* 1985;314:743–745.

52. Potter T, Rajan T, Dick R, Bluestone J. Substitution at residue 227 of H-2 class I molecules abrogates recognition of CD8-dependent, but not CD8-independent, cytotoxic T lymphocytes. *Nature* 1989;337:73–75.

53. Vitiello A, Potter T, Sherman L. The role of β_2-microglobulin in peptide binding by class I molecules. *Science* 1990;250:1423–1426.

54. Christinck E, Luscher M, Barber B, Williams D. Peptide binding to class I MHC on living cells and quantitation of complexes required for CTL lysis. *Nature* 1991;352:67–70.

55. Falk K, Rotzschke O, Deres K, Metzger J, Jung G, Rammensee H-G. Identification of naturally processed viral nonapeptides allows their quantification in infected cells and suggests an allele-specific T cell epitope forecast. *J Exp Med* 1991;174:425–434.

56. Shen L, Potter TA, Kane KP. Glu227 → Lys substitution in the acidic loop of major histocompatibility complex class I a3 domain distinguishes low avidity CD8 coreceptor and avidity-enhanced CD8 accessory functions. *J Exp Med* 1996;184:1671–1683.

57. Sun J, Leahy DJ, Kavathas PB. Interaction between CD8 and major histocompatibility complex (MHC) class I mediated by multiple contact surfaces that include the α2 and α3 domains of MHC class I. *J Exp Med* 1995;182:1275–1280.
58. LaFace DM, Vestberg M, Yang Y, et al. Human CD8 transgene regulation of HLA recognition by murine T cells. *J Exp Med* 1995;182:1315–1325.
59. Newberg MH, Smith DH, Haertel SB, Vining DR, Lacy E, Engelhard VH. Importance of MHC class I α2 and α3 domains in the recognition of self and non-self MHC molecules. *J Immunol* 1996;156:2473–2480.
60. Luescher IF, Vivier E, Layer A, et al. CD8 modulation of T-cell antigen receptor-ligand interactions on living cytotoxic T lymphocytes. *Nature* 1995;373:353–356.
61. Garcia KC, Scott CA, Brunmark A, et al. CD8 enhances formation of stable T-cell receptor/MHC class I molecule complexes. *Nature* 1996;384:577–581.
62. Luo K, Sefton B. Cross-linking of T-cell surface molecules CD4 and CD8 stimulates phosphorylation of the *lck* tyrosine protein kinase at the autophosphorylation site. *Mol Cell Biol* 1990;10:5305–5313.
63. Mescher M, O'Rourke A, Champoux P, Kane K. Equilibrium binding of cytotoxic T lymphocytes to class I antigen. *J Immunol* 1991;147:36–41.
64. Hutchcroft JE, Franklin DP, Tsai B, Harrison-Findik D, Varticovski L, Bierer BE. Phorbol ester treatment inhibits phosphatidylinositol 3-kinase activation by, and association with, CD28, a T-lymphocyte surface receptor. *Proc Natl Acad Sci USA* 1995;92:8808–8812.
65. Van Seventer GA, Shimizu Y, Horgan KJ, Shaw S. The LFA-1 ligand ICAM-1 provides an important costimulatory signal for T cell receptor-mediated activation of resting T cells. *J Immunol* 1990;144:4579–4586.
66. Davis L, Oppenheimer-Marks N, Bednarczyk J, McIntyre B, Lipsky P. Fibronectin promotes proliferation of naive and memory T cells by signalling through both the VLA-4 and VLA-5 integrin molecules. *J Immunol* 1990;145:785–793.
67. Shimizu Y, Van Seventer A, Horgan KJ, Shaw S. Costimulation of proliferative responses of resting CD4+ T cells by the interaction of VLA-4 and VLA-5 with fibronectin or VLA-6 with laminin. *J Immunol* 1990;145:59–67.
68. Ybarrondo B, O'Rourke A, Brian A, Mescher M. Contribution of LFA-1/intercellular adhesion molecule-1 binding to the adhesion/signalling cascade of cytotoxic T lymphocyte activation. *J Exp Med* 1994;179:359–363.
69. Reiser H, Freeman G, Razi-wolf Z, Gimmi C, Benacerraf B, Nadler L. Murine B7 antigen provides an efficient costimulatory signal for activation of murine T lymphocytes via the T-cell receptor/CD3 complex. *Proc Natl Acad Sci USA* 1992;89:271–275.
70. Tan R, Teh S-J, Ledbetter J, Linsley P, Teh H-S. B7 costimulates proliferation of CD4⁻8⁺ T lymphocytes but is not required for the deletion of immature CD4⁺8⁺ thymocytes. *J Immunol* 1992;149:3217–3224.
71. Freeman G, Borriello F, Hodes R, et al. Murine B7-2, an alternative CTLA4 counter-receptor that costimulates T cell proliferation and interleukin 2 production. *J Exp Med* 1993;178:2185–2192.
72. Freeman G, Gribben J, Boussiotis V, et al. Cloning of B7-2: a CTLA-4 counter-receptor that costimulates human T cell proliferation. *Science* 1993;262:909–911.
73. Azuma M, Cayabyab M, Buck D, Phillips J, Lanier L. CD28 interaction with B7 costimulates primary allogeneic proliferative responses and cytotoxicity mediated by small, resting T lymphocytes. *J Exp Med* 1992;175:353–360.
74. Harding F, Allison J. CD28-B7 interactions allow the induction of CD8⁺ cytotoxic T lymphocytes in the absence of exogenous help. *J Exp Med* 1993;177:1791–1796.
75. Ni H-T, Deeths MJ, Li W, Mueller DL, Mescher MF. Signaling pathways activated by leukocyte function-associated Ag-1-dependent costimulation. *J Immunol* 1999;162:5183–5189.

Cytotoxic Cells: Basic Mechanisms and Medical Applications, edited by Michail V. Sitkovsky and Pierre A. Henkart. Lippincott Williams & Wilkins, Philadelphia © 2000.

Chapter 6

Lysis of Innocent Bystanders by Antigen-Specific Cytotoxic Lymphocytes

Hidefumi Kojima and Michail V. Sitkovsky

Laboratory of Immunology, National Institute of Allergy and Infectious Diseases, National Institutes of Health, Bethesda, Maryland 20892, USA

Exquisite specificity toward antigen-bearing cells (cognate targets) is considered to be one of the most important properties of the T-cell driven immune response, including target cell destruction by cytotoxic T cells (CTLs). It is believed that CTLs form contacts with all surrounding cells but that only the antigen-expressing (e.g., virus-infected or tumor) cells are recognized and destroyed after CTLs have formed appropriate conjugates and have been triggered to deliver the lethal hit. It is assumed that "innocent bystanders," a term that includes all antigen-nonexpressing cells, are not recognized and therefore are spared by CTLs.

The term "bystander" is applied to both CTLs and CTL targets. Indeed, CTLs themselves are called bystanders in studies of their activation in the absence of specifically recognized antigen. It was discussed, for example, that acute virus infection can cause expansion not only of virus-specific CTLs but also of bystander CTLs (1–4). According to published observations, activation by antigen A of CTLs with specificity to antigen A is accompanied by activation of bystander CTLs with specificity to antigen B. Bystander activation of CTLs was explained by "molecular mimicry" (1), that is, expansion or activation of bystander CTLs with T cell receptors (TCRs) that are able to recognize both antigens A and B. Studies of the mechanisms

of diabetes induced by coxsackie virus (5) were interpreted to suggest that the initiation of bystander damage, not molecular mimicry, best explains the experimental observations. It has been also suggested that cytokine-secreting, antigen-activated, antigen-specific T cells could activate surrounding bystander CTLs, and it was shown recently that type 1 interferon (IFN-α/β) can expand such bystander T cells (2); however, this explanation is not consistent with recent quantitative studies of bystander activation of CTLs by Ehl et al. (6) and Murali-Krishna et al. (7), who concluded that cytokine-driven accumulation of lytic CTLs does not have much biologic importance and that most of the accumulated CD8+ T cells during viral infection are accounted for by antigen-specific cells. The mechanisms of bystander activation of CTLs are far from being conclusively established, and studies in this area are of great interest. In this chapter we focus on the mechanisms of bystander target lysis by CTLs.

BYSTANDERS: SOME MORE VULNERABLE THAN OTHERS TO CTL-MEDIATED LYSIS

It could be expected from general considerations that bystander target lysis by CTLs either is not taking place or is not particularly damaging during the course of a normal immune response. Otherwise, every infection would be accompanied by severe immunopathologic reactions. Nevertheless, *in vitro* experiments have demonstrated the possibility of bystander lysis. It has been reported (8) that antigen-nonexpressing targets could be killed if they are bridged to antigen-activated CTLs by their own receptors (8). These experiments indicated that killing by CTLs is not exquisitely directional and requires cell–cell interactions.

Lysis of bystander targets was also reported by Duke in a more routine experimental setting. In his experiments, CTLs could lyse only syngeneic bystanders. This lysis was explained as being due to self-major histocompatibility complex (MHC) recognition by TCRs on activated CTLs (9). According to these observations, CTLs expressing TCRs with low affinity to self-MHC are most likely to become killers of bystanders.

The interest in studies of bystanders is par-

tially due to the potential application of bystander lysis for treatment of tumors. Indeed, it was demonstrated both *in vitro* and *in vivo* that melanoma cells could be lysed by MHC class II-restricted autoreactive T cells (10). The authors interpreted their data as supporting the hypothesis that autoreactive T cells destroy tumors by releasing lymphotoxin and IFN-γ after recognition of antigen at the injection site. Thus it is important in studies of bystander lysis to discriminate between mechanisms utilizing cell–cell contacts and cytokine-mediated bystander lysis.

Better understanding of the Fas-mediated death pathway in Fas-expressing cells (11, 12) and the conclusive demonstration of perforin- and Fas-mediated mechanisms of CTL cytotoxicity (13–16) have led to the expectation that bystander target lysis by CTLs should be more prevalent than is currently appreciated (17). Therefore, it was important to determine whether and to what extent CTLs killed antigen-free (noncognate) by-

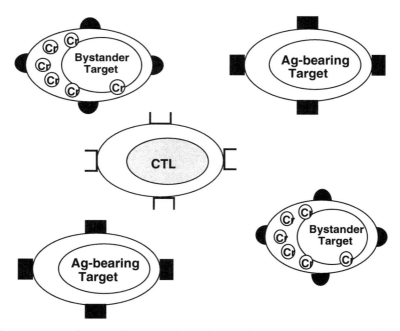

FIG. 6-1. The presence of non-antigen-bearing cells near interacting CTLs and antigen-expressing target cells could make them vulnerable to "bystander" lysis.

standers during lysis of specific antigen-bearing cells (cognate targets) (Fig. 6-1).

Advances in the field of CTL cytotoxicity have helped establish an experimental system to examine the mechanisms of bystander lysis by taking advantage of genetic tools and by using CTLs deficient in perforin or Fas ligand pathways of cytotoxicity. We used target cells that enabled us to discriminate between the Fas- and perforin-mediated death pathways. Both normal and functional Fas ligand (FasL)- deficient CTLs, as well as perforin-gene knockout FasL-expressing CTL clones, were used in these experiments. It was ascertained that the cytotoxic effects studied were mediated by CD8+ CTL clones and cell lines. Indeed, the treatment of CTL lines with anti-CD8 monoclonal antibody (mAb) and complement eliminated MHC class I (MHC-I)- restricted cytotoxic activity or strongly inhibited it if anti-CD8 mAbs were present during the assay, confirming that the cytotoxic effects of the CTLs studied are due to CD8+ CTLs.

The availability of anti-Fas mAb-resistant B-lymphoma cells and of Fas transfectants of the parental Fas-negative cell line L1210 (generously provided by Pierre Golstein) allowed us to use them as bystander targets in a well controlled assay to discriminate between Fas and perforin pathways of cytotoxicity.

The CTL cytotoxicity was measured using a routine chromium 51 (^{51}Cr) release assay. CTLs were mixed with ^{51}Cr-labeled bystanders and with unlabeled antigen-bearing stimulators and then were incubated for 4 hours at 37°C. When CD8+ CTLs, which kill antigen-bearing targets via the FasL-triggered pathway, were mixed with ^{51}Cr-labeled, Fas-expressing, antigen-free (nonspecific) targets, no lysis was usually observed (e.g., 13). We explained this by the fact that assays of CTL antigenic specificity were mostly done by mixing cells of only two types: ^{51}Cr-labeled targets and CTLs. It was reasoned that the better model of *in vivo* CTL activities required the simultaneous presence of three types of cell: (a) ^{51}Cr-labeled antigen-bearing

targets, which mimic *in vivo* activation of CTLs, surrounded by (b) antigen-free "innocent" bystanders and (c) CTLs (Fig. 6-1). Indeed, it was reported earlier that under such conditions a CD4+ ovalbumin-specific murine clone was able to lyse bystanders (18). At that time the authors explained this lysis as being due to nonspecific cytolytic activity induced by the clone's own interleukin-2 (IL-2), secreted in response to recognition of the specific target.

In our studies we observed the unexpectedly rapid and efficient lysis of bystanders by antigen-activated CTLs. Observations of such lysis of bystanders by antigen-specific CD8+ CTLs in short-term assays complement (but are different from) published observations of bystander lysis caused by CD4+ T-helper (Th1) cells in long-term assays (19) and by CD8+ CTL clones in short-term assays (9). The more detailed investigation of the molecular mechanisms of bystander lysis established that FasL/Fas cytotoxic mechanisms are primarily responsible for bystander lysis in short-term cytotoxicity assays. Even highly antigen-specific CTLs could efficiently kill antigen-free noncognate targets when the latter became bystanders during lysis of antigen-bearing cognate targets (Ag-TC) in a short-term 4-hour assay. For example, ^{51}Cr-labeled, antigen-free concanavalin A (Con A) blasts were not susceptible to lysis by CTLs in two cell-type assays; but the same ^{51}Cr-labeled, antigen-free Con A blasts were killed by CTLs as bystanders in the presence of antigen-bearing specific targets.

We determined that all vulnerable bystanders tested in our experiments expressed Fas, whereas resistant bystanders (e.g., P815 cells) did not, suggesting the importance of Fas antigen expression on bystander cells and the involvement of the FasL/Fas-mediated pathway of target cell death. Only the Fas-expressing transfected cells (not the Fas-negative parent cells) were killed as bystanders in these experiments.

Phorbol myristic acetate (PMA)/ionomycin pretreatment of CTLs mimicked TCR stimulation by antigen-bearing targets and was more powerful in triggering FasL/Fas mechanism-mediated bystander lysis. This experimental system has an advantage in facilitating the biochemical analysis of bystander lysis because of the absence of third-party antigen-bearing stimulator cells. It is important to note that even the powerful activation of CTLs by PMA/ionomycin treatment was not sufficient for lysis of bystanders in the absence of functional FasL expression.

Several lines of evidence point toward a major role of Fas ligand on CTLs in bystander lysis. These experiments include assays with a functional FasL-deficient C3H-*gld/gld*-origin GD1 CTL clone that was found not to kill Fas+ bystanders. In a parallel control, the same bystanders were killed by normal CTLs, whereas the same GD1 CTLs caused efficient lysis of specific antigen-bearing targets using the perforin-based mechanism of killing. Additional genetic evidence of the need for FasL–Fas interactions in bystander lysis was provided by use of a perforin gene-knockout CTL clone and by demonstrating that perforin deficiency did not eliminate the ability of CTLs to kill bystanders. Similar evidence on the predominant role of the Fas pathway in bystander lysis was obtained with Fas-expressing and Fas-resistant targets.

As discussed above, bystander lysis could be due to the effects of soluble factors. We addressed this possibility of bystander killing by soluble factors [including, for example, tumor necrosis factor (TNF) and soluble FasL] by testing the cytolytic potential of CTL supernatants and by using neutralizing anti-TNF antibody during the assay. It was shown that no supernatant had lytic activity toward Fas+ cells; in parallel controls, addition of anti-Fas antibody resulted in strong lysis of these cells, and the presence of neutralizing anti-TNF antibody did not block the lysis of Fas+ bystanders. Together with the short amount of time required to observe bystander lysis by CTLs, these observations suggest that solu-

ble FasL is not responsible for the effects of CTLs on bystanders.

VULNERABILITY OF BYSTANDERS TO CTL: TIME SENSITIVE AND LFA-1 -DEPENDENT

Time dependence studies showed that after 1 hour of preincubation bystander lysis was no longer dependent on CTL interactions with Ag-TC but that CTLs were able to kill bystanders no longer than 2 hours after their last interaction with Ag-TC. Indeed, we observed that after 2 hours of incubation with Ag-TC, CTLs lost the ability to kill bystanders; if fresh Ag-TC was added to the assay, however, bystander lysis by CTLs was resumed.

In experiments where ^{51}Cr-labeled Fas-expressing bystanders were added simultaneously with tested mAbs to cell surface proteins of preactivated CTLs, we compared the requirements for activation of CTLs by Ag-TC and for delivery of the lethal hit to bystanders by activated CTLs. The effects of anti-leukocyte function-associated antigen (anti-LFA-1) mAbs in these experiments revealed the need in LFA-1 for interactions between activated CTLs and bystanders, and the use of ^{51}Cr-labeled Con A blasts from intercellular adhesion molecule (ICAM-1)-gene-deficient mice as targets in a 4-hour assay confirmed the prediction that the LFA-1 partner, ICAM-1, is also required for CTL-mediated bystander lysis.

The relatively short "attention span" of activated CTLs toward bystanders can be explained by the relatively short-lived expression of antigen/TCR-upregulated FasL (13, 20) and by the limited time of expression of activated LFA-1 molecules on the surface of CTLs. It appears that only TCR-preactivated CTLs, in contrast to resting CTLs, enable their surface LFA-1 molecules to facilitate the strengthening of randomly formed nonspecific conjugates leading to bystander lysis.

The time course studies suggest that after activation CTLs no longer require the signals from Ag-TC to kill bystanders during CTL–

bystander interaction for at least 2 hours. Experiments using anti-CD8 mAbs have shown that the ability of anti-CD8 mAbs to inhibit bystander lysis was dramatically diminished if it was added 1 hour after the exposure of CTLs to antigen-bearing targets. Although the expression of FasL and LFA-1 on TCR-activated CTLs is necessary, expression of neither alone is sufficient for bystander lysis; both TCR-triggered FasL up-regulation and changes in LFA-1 are required for killing Fas$^+$ bystanders by CTLs. This may reflect the importance of changes in the affinity of adhesion proteins on the CTL surface (21), which may in turn facilitate CTL engagement and conjugation with the antigen-free target cell in nonspecific conjugates. These data led to the expectation that the requirements for lysis of the third-party bystander targets could differ from the requirements for lysis of antigen-bearing cells on the levels of recognition structures and of LFA-1–ICAM interactions.

REGULATION OF BYSTANDER LYSIS BY CTLs

Taken together, our observations are consistent with the following model of CTL activity (Fig. 6-2): (a) The first Fas-expressing bystander target cell encountered is spared by resting CTLs. (b) CTLs encounter and recognize the antigen-expressing target cell; and as the result of antigen/TCR-mediated signaling, they became activated CTLs with upregulated Fas ligand expression and more adhesive LFA-1 molecules. (c) The activated CTLs are able to form "productive" conjugates with randomly encountered bystanders due to the TCR-triggered activation of adhesion molecules LFA-1. (d) The randomly conjugated bystanders are then killed if they express sufficient levels of functional Fas (22) and ICAM-1 ligands for LFA-1. (e) The vulnerability of bystanders to CTL is transient and lasts only about 2 hours after the first encounter with Ag-TC. Bystanders encountered later than 2 hours are spared either because of downregulation of FasL or

deactivation of LFA-1 molecules. The time course of deactivation of LFA-1 and of downregulation of FasL, as yet undetermined, leads to better understanding of bystander lysis. (f) The encounter of the next Ag-TC can start this cycle of lysis of bystanders again (Fig. 6-2). The model described here is in agreement with the observations of Lancki et al. (23) and Smyth (24) and in partial agreement with those of Ando et al. (25), who demonstrated that lysis of susceptible bystanders by CTLs is mediated by FasL and TNF-α but not by perforin. In contrast, Kuwano and Arai (26) concluded that both perforin and FasL are involved in bystander lysis.

It was reasoned that if CTLs are able to kill bystanders there should be a mechanism to limit bystander lysis; otherwise, FasL-expressing CTLs may be able to inflict a lethal hit to any bystander targets, leading to indiscriminate lysis of all surrounding functional Fas-expressing cells during routine CTL surveillance. Indeed, the vulnerability of bystanders to activated CTL-mediated lysis could be controlled, minimized, or terminated by several mechanisms. The model described above clearly indicates that most cells are not vulnerable to CTLs when they lyse neighboring antigen-expressing targets. Several strict conditions must be satisfied before the antigen-nonexpressing bystanders become susceptible to the CTL lethal hit. First, the bystander must express functionally coupled molecules of Fas (22), and only a limited number of tissues do so. Second, bystanders must express molecules of ICAM-1 that are also not expressed on many cells. Finally, bystanders must be in the area of the CTL attack on Ag-TC, or relatively close, because CTLs are dangerous for no more than 2 hours after seeing the Ag-TC. In this respect, the termination of CTL stimulation by antigen due to disintegration of cognate targets could serve as the mechanism for limiting damage to bystanders. Thus there are several mechanisms for limiting, minimizing, and terminating bystander lysis by CTLs. Even if bystanders express ICAM-1, there is a pos-

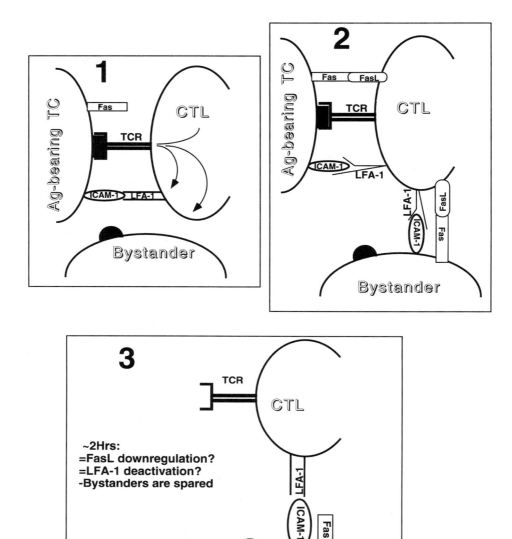

FIG. 6-2. Model of time-dependent, Fas-dependent, ICAM-1-dependent, antigen-expressing cell-dependent lysis of bystanders by antigen-specific CTL.

sibility that LFA-1–ICAM-1 interactions could be tightly regulated by a phosphorylation event(s), with PP2a phosphatase in CTLs playing the major role in downregulating the adhesive properties of CTLs (27). This view is based on our observations that inhibition of PP2a phosphatase resulted in enhancement of bystander lysis (Kojima and Sitkovsky, in preparation). The attractive and testable possibility is that the phosphorylation state of some yet unidentified LFA-1-associated intracellular protein X is important for maintaining LFA-1 molecules in an activated state.

Although the identity of a protein X is not yet known, PP2a phosphatase is currently being investigated as such a regulatory enzyme. PP2a phosphatase is implicated in this process due to our observations of enhanced lysis of Ag-TC and of bystanders (Kojima et al., manuscript in preparation) under conditions of inhibited PP2a phosphatase. It is important to note that PP2a phosphatase has been found to be associated with plasma membranes of lymphoid cells.

According to our working model, the recognition of antigen on the Ag-TC by the TCR–CD3 complex on the CTL surface results in signaling and Ser/Thr phosphorylation of protein X. The phosphorylated form of protein X is able to associate with LFA-1 molecules and cause changes in their affinity. That, in turn, allows efficient LFA-1–ICAM-1 interaction between CTLs and the T cell surface. As TCR signaling decreases in intensity, the membrane-associated PP2a phosphatase is constitutively dephosphorylating protein X, thereby determining the half-life of the activated state of LFA-1 and of LFA-1–ICAM-1-mediated contacts between CTLs and Ag-TC. It eventually leads to deactivation of LFA-1 and dissolution of CTL–Ag-TC conjugates. Thus the activity of this phosphatase may be part of the biochemical mechanism that terminates CTL–target cell conjugates.

Similarly, the same enzyme may control engagement of CTLs with bystanders because we have shown that LFA-1–ICAM-1 interactions are absolutely required for bystander lysis. Thus the activity of PP2a phosphatase is at least partially determining the time of engagement of CTLs with Ag-TC and with bystanders. Prolongation of contact may increase the probability of productive conjugates with the correct alignment of cell surface molecules on CTLs and target cells for the lethal hit delivery. This model is in agreement with our earlier observations of PP2a inhibitor (okadaic acid)-mediated enhancement of CTL–Ag-TC interactions (27)

and with observations of increased bystander lysis. These observations of cell–cell contact-dependent bystander lysis must be reconciled with the widely accepted notions of exquisite antigen specificity of the immune response in general and of CTL effector functions in particular.

The hypothesis that killing innocent bystanders represents an acceptable level of collateral damage during a normal CTL response is attractive. Such damage is likely limited owing to the above restrictions of Fas-mediated lysis and the relatively short duration of a normal immune response. The situation is expected to be more damaging during long-term, chronic infections accompanied by the persistent presence of antigen-expressing targets. This may cause immuno-pathologies involving Fas+ cells because of the cumulative effects of bystander killing by activated CTLs. Although many tissues do not express Fas, it is remarkable that among those that do are cells of the liver and heart. Cells in these vital tissues are among the most highly Fas-expressing cells (24,28).

Thus observations of Fas-mediated bystander lysis by CTLs leads to reevaluation of previous findings that antigen-specific CTLs from coxsackie virus B3-infected mice lyse both virus-infected and virus-uninfected myocytes (29,30). This finding suggests the possibility that Fas-mediated bystander lysis is one of the mechanisms of cardiomyocyte damage in the pathogenesis of myocarditis (31) and of liver damage during viral infections. If this is the case, one can expect the increased resistance of *lpr/lpr* mice compared with that of normal or *gld* mice to cardiomyocyte damage (31) by coxsackie virus-specific CTLs during experimental coxsackie virus infection and in other clinical situations (32). Future studies should address the relevance of bystander lysis *in vitro* observed here to CTL activities *in vivo*.

Acknowledgments

The authors thank Drs. Nobukata Shinohara (Mitsubishi-Kasei Life Sciences Institute, Japan) for valuable reagents and cell lines; Pierre Golstein (INSERM, France) for Fas-transfected cells; Jurg Tschopp (Lausanne, Switzerland) for anti-Fas ligand antibody; Y. Ito for advice in flow cytometry measurements; Ronald Germain for criticism and discussion; and Erastus Dudley (NIAID, NIH) for critical reading. We also thank Brenda Rae Marshall for editing and Ms. Shirley Starnes for manuscript preparation.

REFERENCES

1. Oldstone MBA. Molecular mimicry and autoimmune disease. Cell 1987;50:819–820.
2. Tough DF, Borrow P, Sprent J. Induction of bystander T cell proliferation by viruses and type I interferon in vivo. Science 1996;272:1947– 1950.
3. Butz EA, Bevan MJ. Massive expansion of antigen-specific CD8+ T cells during an acute virus infection. Immunity 1998;8:167–175.
4. Murali-Krishna K, Altman JD, Suresh M, et al. Counting antigen-specific CD8 T cells: a reevaluation of bystander activation during viral infection. Immunity 1998;8:177–187.
5. Horwitz MS, Bradley LM, Harbertson J, Krahl T, Lee J, Sarvetnick N. Diabetes induced by coxsackie virus: initiation by bystander damage and not molecular mimicry. Nat Med 1998;4:781–785.
6. Ehl S, Hombach J, Aichele P, Hengartner H, Zinkernagel RM. Bystander activation of cytotoxic T cells: studies on the mechanism and evaluation of in vivo significance in a transgenic mouse model. J Exp Med 1997;185:1241–1251.
7. Murali-Krishna K, Altman JD, Suresh M, et al. Counting antigen-specific CD8 T cells: a reevaluation of bystander activation during viral infection. Immunity 1998;8:177–187.
8. Lanzavecchia A. Is T-cell receptor involved in T-cell killing? Nature 1996;319:778–780.
9. Duke RC. Self-recognition by T-cells. I. Bystander killing of target cells bearing syngeneic MHC antigens. J Exp Med 1989;170:59–71.
10. Shiohara T, Ruddle NH, Horowitz M, Moellmann GE, Lerner AB. Anti-tumor activity of class II MHC antigen-restricted cloned autoreactive T cells. I. Destruction of B16 melanoma cells mediated by bystander cytolysis in vitro. J Immunol 1987;138:1971–1978.
11. Nagata S, Suda T. Fas and Fas ligand: lpr and gld mutations. Immunol Today 1995;16:39–43.
12. Schulze-Osthoff K, Walczak H, Drige W, Krammer PH. Cell nucleus and DNA fragmentation are not required for apoptosis. J Cell Biol 1994; 127:15–20.
13. Kojima H, Shinohara N, Hanaoka S, et al. Two distinct pathways of specific killing revealed by perforin mutant cytotoxic T lymphocytes. Immunity 1994;1:357–364.

14. Kagi D, Vignaux F, Ledermann B, et al. Fas and perforin pathways as major mechanisms of T cell-mediated cytotoxicity. Science 1994;265:528–530.
15. Lowin B, Hahne M, Mattmann C, Tschopp J. Cytolytic T-cell cytotoxicity is mediated through perforin and Fas lytic pathways. Nature 1994;370:650–652.
16. Walsh CM, Matloubian M, Liu CC, et al. Immune function in mice lacking the perforin gene. Proc Natl Acad Sci USA 1994;91:10854–10858.
17. Kojima H, Eshima K, Takayama H, Sitkovsky M. Leukocyte function-associated antigen-1-dependent lysis of Fas+ (CD95+/Apo-1+) innocent bystanders by antigen-specific CD8+ CTL. J Immunol 1997;159:2728–2734.
18. Gromkowsky SH, Hepler KM, Janeway CA Jr. Low doses of interleukin 2 induce bystander cell lysis by antigen-specific CD4+ inflammatory T cell clones in short-term assay. Eur J Immunol 1988;18:1385–1389.
19. Wang R, Rogers AM, Ratliff TL, Russel JH. CD95-dependent bystander lysis caused by CD4+ T helper 1 effectors. J Immunol 1996;157:2961–2968.
20. Vignaux F, Vivier E, Malissen B, Depraeter V, Nagata S, Golstein P. TCR/CD3 coupling to Fas based cytotoxicity. J Exp Med 1995;181:781–786.
21. Dustin ML, Springer TA. Role of lymphocyte adhesion receptors in transient interactions and cell locomotion. Annu Rev Immunol 1991;9:27–66.
22. Klas C, Debatin KM, Jonker RR, Krammer PH. Activation interferes with the APO-1 pathway in mature human T cells. Int Immunol 1993;5:625–630.
23. Lancki DW, Weiss A, Fitch FW. Requirements for triggering of lysis by cytolytic T lymphocyte clones. J Immunol 1987;138:3646–3653.
24. Smyth MJ. Fas ligand-mediated bystander lysis of syngeneic cells in response to an allogeneic stimulus. J Immunol 1997;158:5765–5772.
25. Ando K, Hiroishi K, Kaneko T, et al. Perforin, Fas/Fas ligand, and TNF-alpha pathways as specific and bystander killing mechanisms of hepatitis C virus-specific human CTL. J Immunol 1997;158:5283–5291.
26. Kuwano K, Arai S. Involvement of two distinct killing mechanisms in bystander target cell lysis induced by a cytotoxic T lymphocyte clone. Cell Immunol 1996;169:288–293.
27. Taffs RE, Redegeld FA, Sitkovsky MV. Modulation of cytolytic T lymphocyte functions by an inhibitor of serine/threonine phosphatase, okadaic acid: enhancement of cytolytic T lymphocyte-mediated cytotoxicity. J Immunol 1991;147:722–728.
28. Ogasawara J, Watanabe-Fukunaga R, Adachi M, et al. Lethal effect of the anti-Fas antibody in mice. Nature 1993;364:806–809.
29. Wong CY, Woodruff JF, Woodruf JJ. Generation of cytotoxic lymphocytes during coxsackie virus B3 infection: Model and viral specificity. J Immunol 1977;118:1159–1164.
30. Huber SA, Lodge PA. Coxsackie virus B-3 myocarditis in Balb/c mice. Am J Pathol 1984;116:21–29.
31. Rose NR. Myocarditis—from infection to autoimmunity. Immunologist 1996;4:67–75.
32. Wenig A, Irintchev A. A bystander damage of host muscle caused by implantation of MHC-compatible myogenic cells. J Neurol Sci 1995;130:190–196.

Cytotoxic Cells: Basic Mechanisms and Medical Applications, edited by Michail V. Sitkovsky and Pierre A. Henkart. Lippincott Williams & Wilkins, Philadelphia © 2000.

III / EFFECTOR CELL SIGNALING PATHWAYS

Chapter 7

Signaling for Cytotoxicity in LGLs

Dragan Jevremovic and Paul J. Leibson

Department of Immunology, Mayo Clinic and Foundation, Rochester, Minnesota 55905, USA

Natural killer (NK) cells and cytotoxic T lymphocytes (CTLs) act as data processors: Intracellular signals initiated from multiple cell surface receptors are integrated, and these signals ultimately regulate cytotoxic granule polarization and exocytosis. Various receptors on the surface of NK cells and T cells are responsible for initiating activation. In the case of NK cells, Fc receptor (FcR) recognition of antibody-coated targets generates second messengers that regulate the development of antibody-dependent cell-mediated cytotoxicity (ADCC) (1). Alternatively, separate receptors on NK cells can recognize specific ligands expressed on target cells, leading to "natural cytotoxicity" (2). For CTLs, heterodimeric, major histocompatibility complex (MHC)–peptide-recognizing receptors trigger cell-mediated killing. For each form of cytotoxicity, the triggering receptors initiate specific signaling cascades that positively regulate the delivery of the "lethal hit."

When NK cells or CTLs bind to potential target cells, a variety of other signal-generating receptors can be engaged. For example, MHC-recognizing receptors on NK cells can be ligated by specific MHC class I (MHC-I)-bearing targets (2–7). The signals generated by the MHC-recognizing receptors potently inhibit NK cell activation even in the presence of separate stimulatory ligands. Therefore, the capacity of cytotoxic lymphocytes to mediate killing appears to be determined by a balance between positive and negative regulatory events.

A diverse array of positive and negative signals are generated by protein tyrosine kinases (PTKs), protein tyrosine phosphatases, phospholipases, lipid kinases, and low-molecular-weight guanosine triphosphate (GTP)-binding (G) proteins (1). Despite this dramatic heterogeneity in generated second messengers, the fidelity of specific molecular interactions and the temporal sequence of events provide the order necessary for regulating specific functions (e.g., cell-mediated killing, cytokine secretion, proliferation). This review focuses on the transmembrane signaling events implicated in the regulation of NK cell-mediated cytotoxicity. Initial emphasis is placed on FcR-initiated signaling because the molecular identity of the triggering receptor is known, many of the signaling events have been characterized, and many of the same second messengers are utilized during the generation of natural cytotoxicity. We also highlight those signaling events that are differentially utilized during alternative modes of killing. Finally, recent data are described that provide new insights on the alteration in signaling induced by inhibitory MHC-recognizing receptors.

MULTICHAIN IMMUNE RECOGNITION RECEPTORS

The FcγRIIIA complex expressed on NK cells is a member of a broader family of multichain immune recognition receptors (MIRRs) (8). Other family members include the B cell antigen receptors (BCRs), the T cell antigen receptors (TCRs), and other FcRs. In each case the receptor complex is made up of separate ligand-binding and signal-transducing subunits. Although the signal-transducing subunits lack identifiable catalytic activity, they possess a conserved immunoreceptor tyrosine-based activation motif (ITAM) [consensus amino acid sequence $YxxL-(x)_{6-8}-YxxL$] in their cytoplasmic tails (9,10). Phosphorylation of the tyrosine residues in the ITAMs is among the earliest detectable events during receptor-initiated activation (11). The phosphorylated ITAMs then serve as high-affinity docking sites for nonreceptor PTK, and a subsequently generated multicomponent signaling complex translates the cell surface receptor stimulation into a cascade of intracellular second messengers.

The FcγRIIIA complex is specifically composed of a ligand binding α-subunit (CD16) and dimeric, ITAM-containing, signal-transducing subunits (1). The extracellular portion of CD16 has low affinity for the Fc portion of immunoglobulin G (IgG); but in the context of target cell bound IgG, this highly avid interaction activates NK cells. ITAM-containing zeta (ζ) and gamma (γ) subunits are found in FcγRIII complexes on the surface of human NK cells as either disulfide-linked homodimers or heterodimers (12–15). ζ Subunits are also part of the TCR–CD3 complex expressed on T cells and have three ITAMs (16). γ Subunits are also found in the high-affinity receptor for IgE (FcεRI) expressed on mast cells and basophils and have only one ITAM (17). Whereas both ζ and γ subunits can be found as part of the human FcγRIII complex, murine FcγRIII has only γ-γ homodimers coupled to the α-chain (18). The importance of the γ subunit in mouse NK cells is underscored by the observation that $\gamma^{-/-}$ mice lose their expression of CD16 and the ability of their NK cells to mediate ADCC (19). The relative importance of ζ versus γ subunits for human NK cells remains obscure.

One of the key features of the ITAM-containing ζ/γ subunits is their ability to facilitate CD16 expression on the cell surface. CD16 remains in the endoplasmic reticulum (ER) when expressed alone in COS-7 cells (20). Co-expression of CD16 with ζ or γ (or both) results in CD16 translocation from the ER to the cell surface. Surface expression of CD16 does not require interaction with the cytoplasmic portions of the ITAM-containing subunits, as truncated versions of ζ or γ lacking their cytoplasmic tails can facilitate CD16 expression. In contrast, interactions between the transmembrane portions of the receptor subunits appear to be critical (18,20) and may influence the affinity of the receptor for ligand (21).

The ITAM-containing subunits of the FcγRIII complex not only facilitate CD16 expression but form docking sites for proximal signaling elements. Phosphorylated tyrosine residues within the ITAM have high affinity for certain proteins containing Src-homology (SH)-2 domains. SH2 domains of multiple molecules, including Syk-family PTKs (i.e., ZAP-70 and Syk), phospholipase C (PLC)-γ, and phosphatidylinositol-3 kinase (PI-3K), can bind to phosphorylated ITAMs in vitro (22–25). Binding of these proteins to ITAMs leads to nucleation of the signaling complex and activation of multiple signaling pathways. The mutation of ITAM tyrosine residues to leucine or phenylalanine abrogates the FcγRIII-initiated signaling (26,27), underscoring the importance of ITAM tyrosine residues for cellular activation.

FcγRIIIA is not the only ITAM-containing activating receptor complex identified on NK cells. Specifically, receptors have been characterized whose extracellular domain bears homology with MHC-recognizing inhibitory receptors (28). However, their short cytoplasmic tails do not contain the immunoreceptor tyrosine-based inhibitory motifs (ITIMs) that are responsible for inhibitory function. Rather, their transmembrane regions have basic residues that facilitate their pairing with another ITAM-containing subunit, DAP12, which has an acidic aspartate residue in its membrane-spanning region

(29–31). Although ligation of these novel receptors *in vitro* with antibodies can initiate NK cell-mediated cytotoxicity (32–34), their role *in vivo* remains unclear. In addition, it is unknown whether DAP12 or other ITAM-containing subunits are involved in the cytotoxicity initiated by other NK cell receptors, such as NK-TR1, CD44, and LAG3.

EARLY ACTIVATION: PROTEIN TYROSINE KINASES

The tyrosine phosphorylation of multiple intracellular proteins is among the earliest detectable events following stimulation of multichain immune recognition receptors (10,11,35–37). Three families of tyrosine kinases have been implicated as mediators of these phosphorylations: Src-family, Syk-family, and Tec-family PTKs. Studies in various models of hematopoietic cell activation suggest the following paradigm for MIRR-initiated signaling: (a) membrane-associated, CD45-activated Src-family PTK phosphorylates tyrosine residues in the ITAMs of the signal-transducing subunits; (b) the SH2 domain of Syk-family PTK mediates their binding to the phosphorylated ITAMs; (c) recruited Syk-family PTKs are phosphorylated and activated by Src-family PTK, autophosphorylation, or both; (d) additional multidomain adaptor molecules (e.g., SLP-76, LAT) are recruited to the signaling complex; (e) PTK-activated PLC-γ cleaves membrane phosphoinositide to generate inositol-1,4,5-trisphosphate and *sn*-1,2-diacylglycerol, resulting in increased free calcium concentration ($[Ca^{2+}]_i$) and protein kinase C (PKC) activation, respectively; and (f) PI-3K-mediated recruitment of Tec-family PTK to the membrane also regulates PLC-dependent increases in $[Ca^{2+}]_i$.

Natural killer cell activation clearly involves some of the features of the above model (Fig. 7-1). Yet in some cases experimental data suggest certain unique features. NK cells do express Src-family PTK, including Lck, Lyn, Fyn, and Yes (38). FcR cross-linking on NK cells does induce Lck activation (39–41), and broad pharmacologic inhibition of Src-family PTK does abrogate

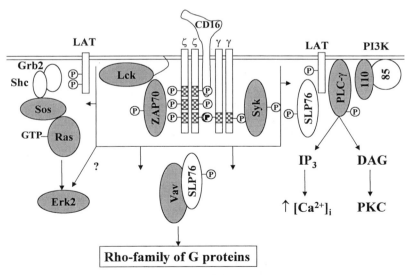

FIG. 7-1. Activation signaling. Receptor-mobilized protein tyrosine kinases activate downstream effectors resulting in the increased intracellular [Ca²⁺] and cytoskeletal rearrangements necessary for NK cell-mediated cytotoxicity. Proteins with known catalytic activity are represented by *shaded symbols.*

ADCC and natural cytotoxicity (37,42). Although T cell development and functions are severely compromised in mice lacking both Lck and Fyn, NK cell function remains intact (43). In addition, CD45-deficient mice, which should be unable to activate Lck fully, have normal NK cell development and cytotoxicity (44). It is possible that other Src-family PTK (e.g., Lyn, as in mast cells) (45) could provide redundant functions and can therefore substitute for each other in these genetic models. Alternatively, the presence of the ITAM-containing γ subunit and the Syk protein kinase may enable NK cells to become activated in a Src-family PTK-independent manner.

Unlike Src-family kinases, ZAP-70 and Syk (members of the Syk-family PTK) do not have a myristolation site. Their recruitment to the membrane signaling complex appears to be mediated by the binding of their tandem SH2 domains to phosphorylated tyrosines contained in the ITAMs (11). ZAP-70 clearly binds phosphorylated ITAMs in the ζ-chain (46–48). Although it has been difficult to detect Syk binding to the FcγRIIIA complex or NK cells, the SH2 domains of Syk can bind to the phosphorylated ITAM of the γ-chain following crosslinking of FcεRI, FcγRI, and FcγRIII on mast cells or macrophages (45,49–52).

As noted earlier, it is generally presumed that Src-family, not Syk-family, PTKs are responsible for the initial ITAM phosphorylation. This notion was challenged by experimental observations in well characterized genetic models in which Syk (but not ZAP-70) could phosphorylate the γ subunit ITAM in the absence of specific Src-family PTK (53). However, there remains a preponderance of evidence indicating that Syk is not acting alone to phosphorylate ITAMs in γ subunit-containing MIRRs. This includes the observations that FcεRI stimulation of cells lacking functional Syk leads to normal phosphorylation of the γ subunit (although downstream signaling is suppressed) (45,54). Similar results were obtained using piceatannol, a specific Syk-family PTK inhibitor (55). Thus, although Syk may have the potential to phosphorylate γ in NK cells, there are likely other kinases that share this function.

Both Syk and ZAP-70 are activated in NK cells upon FcR crosslinking (47,56,57), and both kinases are capable of phosphorylating similar sets of downstream signaling molecules. However, overexpressed Syk, but not ZAP-70, has the ability to enhance NK cell-mediated cytotoxicity (58). In addition, genetic transfer of kinase-inactive Syk, but not kinase-inactive ZAP-70, decreases the NK cell-mediated killing. Furthermore, ZAP-70 knockout mice (59) and ZAP-70-deficient patients (60,61) express normal NK cell functions. Therefore NK cells might preferentially use Syk PTK to mediate signals leading to cytotoxic responses. A potential model emerges in which two parallel modules may be employed in FcR-initiated activation of human NK cells. One pathway uses the ζ subunit, Lck, and ZAP-70 and is probably dispensable for generating ADCC. The other pathway couples the γ subunit to Syk and, depending on the intracellular context, may or may not be regulated by Src-family kinases.

Tec PTKs are a third family of tyrosine kinases involved in MIRR-initiated signaling. Members of the Tec-family have a pleckstrin homology (PH) domain at their N-terminus [mediates binding to membrane phosphatidylinositol-3,4,5 trisphosphate (PIP_3)], as well as SH2 (binds phosphotyrosine) and SH3 (binds proline-rich regions) domains (62). During B cell activation, BCR crosslinking leads to PI-3K recruitment to the receptor complex and a subsequent PI-3K-catalyzed increase in membrane PIP_3 (63,64). BTK, a Tec-family tyrosine kinase in B cells, is then recruited via the interaction of its PH domain with PIP_3 (65–68). Subsequent activation of BTK, perhaps by a Src-family PTK (69), phosphorylates and activates PLC-γ, leading to an increase in $[Ca^{2+}]_i$. In the absence of BTK, PLC-γ is not fully activated and the increase of $[Ca^{2+}]_i$ is only transient. A transient increase of $[Ca^{2+}]_i$ is insufficient for B cell activation, implying a crucial role for BTK in

BCR-initiated signaling. Much less is known about the roles of PI-3K and Tec-family PTK in FcR-initiated NK cell activation. PI-3K activation is necessary for the generation of ADCC (70), but the mechanism of its activation and its precise signaling role remain unclear. NK cells do express members of the Tec-family PTKs, and specifically Emt/Itk is phosphorylated upon FcR ligation (unpublished observations). It is conceivable that Emt or another Tec-family member has a role in the activation of PLC-γ in NK cells. However, to date no such data are available, and this issue awaits future investigation.

It must be emphasized that the PTK-dependent signaling pathways initiated by the FcγRIII on NK cells may or may not be similar to those employed during alternative modes of NK cell-mediated cytotoxicity. For example, NK cells stimulated through the activating forms of the MHC-recognizing receptors (which have the ITAM-containing DAP12 subunit in the complex) do activate Src-family and Syk-family PTK (33), which implies a conserved mechanism. However, separate forms of natural cytotoxicity can employ different second messenger pathways (70). As the heterogeneous group of "triggering" receptors on NK cells increases (e.g., NKR-P1, NK-TR, LAG3, integrins, CD44), the term "natural cytotoxicity" may soon become inappropriate. The challenge is to identify the signaling pathways utilized by the various receptors and to determine their specific relevance to antitumor and antimicrobial immunity.

ADAPTOR PROTEINS

Adaptor proteins are involved in scaffolding signaling complexes. Although adaptors do not have recognizable enzymatic activity, their structural features enable formation of docking sites for multiple downstream signaling effectors. Several proximal adaptor proteins have been identified to participate in NK cell activation. Shc and Grb2 have been described to couple MIRR-initiated PTK activation to the pathways involved in proliferation and differentiation. For NK cells, FcR crosslinking induces the tyrosine phosphorylation of Shc (71). The SH2 domain of Grb2 then directs its binding to Shc, and the proline-rich region of Grb2 binds to the SH3 domain of the guanine nucleotide exchange factor (GEF) Sos. When recruited to the membrane signaling complex, Sos promotes guanosine diphosphate (GDP) to GTP exchange on the low-molecular-weight G-protein Ras, placing it in the active state. Activated Ras promotes the activation of various transcription factors involved in the mitogenic pathway (72).

Another adaptor, originally identified as a Grb2-binding protein in T cells, is SLP-76 (73). SLP-76 contains three tyrosine residues that are targets for phosphorylation upon TCR-initiated activation of Syk-family kinases (74–76). In T cells, phosphorylated SLP-76 interacts with the SH2 domain of the GEF, Vav (77–79). Recruited Vav undergoes tyrosine phosphorylation and activation and has an increased ability to exchange GTP for GDP on specific Rho-family G-proteins (80,81). SLP-76 also binds to other adaptor proteins such as SLAP-130/Fyb (Fyn-binding protein) (82,83). SLP-76 deficiency in vivo blocks T cell development (84), and SLP-76 deficient T cell lines have impaired activation of both PLC-γ and Ras pathways (85). In NK cells, SLP-76 is phosphorylated upon crosslinking either FcγRIII (86) or activating forms of the CD94/NKG2 receptor (unpublished observations). NK cell binding to NK-sensitive targets also leads to SLP-76 phosphorylation. However, the functional significance of SLP-76 in NK-cell signaling and cytotoxicity remains unknown.

The recently cloned adaptor protein LAT (linker for the activation of T cells; p36) is expressed in T cells and NK cells (87). The presence of an N-terminal transmembrane domain makes LAT different from other known adaptors. Specifically, LAT may interact with the receptor complex and membrane-localized Src-family PTK not only directly but also by clustering in the same membrane subdomains (88,89). Upon TCR stimulation, phosphorylation of two C-terminal tyrosines on LAT facilitates its interaction with PLC-γ. In addition, LAT potentially interacts with Grb2, SLP-76, Vav, and the p85 regulatory subunit of PI-3K in T cells (87). NK cell recognition of sensitive tumor targets also induces LAT phosphorylation (unpublished observations). Like SLP-76, the functional significance of these biochemical modifications remain to be worked out.

DOWNSTREAM EFFECTORS

Multiple signaling pathways are activated downstream of receptor-associated PTKs. NK cells express two isoforms of PLC-γ, and they both become phosphorylated upon FcR ligation (90,91). PLC-γ activation appears to be influenced by Src-family PTK, Syk-family PTK, and (as discussed before) potentially Tec-family PTK (57,68,92–94). Current models propose that low-to-moderate levels of inositol trisphosphate in lymphocytes bind to their receptors on the ER, leading to transient elevations in $[Ca^{2+}]_i$ (68). In contrast, maximally activated PLC-γ may generate high levels of inositol trisphosphate, leading to additional calcium release from specialized stores that control "calcium release-activated calcium (CRAC) channels." The increased intracellular release of calcium stores facilitates the subsequent entry of extracellular Ca^{2+} from calcium-rich extracellular fluid. The resulting sustained increase in $[Ca^{2+}]_i$ is necessary for optimal activation of downstream effectors. PLC-γ-dependent cleavage of membrane phosphoinositides also results in the production of *sn*-1,2-diacylglycerol. In NK cells, diacylglycerol-mediated activation of PKC plays a critical role in some, but not all, forms of NK cell-mediated killing (70). Therefore, although potentially sharing early PTK-dependent signaling mechanisms, the various activating receptors may utilize different downstream signaling pathways.

Multiple G-proteins are involved in NK cell activation. Studies with neutralizing antibodies to specific heterotrimeric G-proteins suggest that G_o and G_z regulate cell-mediated killing (95). In addition, the low-molecular-weight Rho-family G-proteins RhoA and Rac-1 critically influence the generation of NK cell-mediated cytotoxicity. Inhibition of Rho A by the adenosine diphosphate (ADP)-ribosylating *Clostridium* C3 toxin inhibits NK killing (96). Also, overexpression of the Rac-1 GEF Vav enhances NK cell-mediated cytotoxicity, and expression of a dominant-negative mutant of Rac-1 blocks granule polarization and killing (97). Therefore Vav and Rac-1 in NK cells are pivotal regulators of granule exocytosis and cellular cytotoxicity.

Recent experiments also highlight an important downstream role in NK cells for the serine/threonine kinase ERK2 (98,99). ERK2 is a distal member of the mitogen-activated protein kinase (MAP kinase) cascade. This cascade of serine/threonine kinases, normally regulated by Ras, controls specific transcriptional events and influences proliferation and differentiation (72). Pharmacologic or molecular inhibition of ERK2 activity impairs granule polarization and NK cell-mediated killing (98,99). Because the delivery of the "lethal hit" by NK cells does not appear to require new gene transcription, these results suggest that ERK2 might function through a separate novel mechanism involving cytoskeletal or motor proteins.

ACTIVATION THROUGH OTHER RECEPTORS

A number of surface molecules are capable of activating NK cell effector mechanisms. Integrins are surface adhesion molecules involved in physical attachment and communication with other cells and extracellular matrix. They are composed of noncovalently associated α- and β-chains. Long considered passive connectors between cells, integrins are now recognized for their capacity to transfer signals from the cell surface (100). Signaling by integrins is mediated by the formation of multimolecular complexes at their cytoplasmic tails. These complexes include focal adhesion kinase (FAK), Src- and Syk-family kinases, and a tight interaction with cytoskeletal proteins (101–106). β_1 Integrins ($\alpha_4\beta_1$ and $\alpha_5\beta_1$ in NK cells) mediate binding to extracellular matrix protein fibronectin. In addition to activation of multiple PTK, crosslinking β_1 integrins enhance NK cell-mediated killing (107). Leukocyte function-associated antigen (LFA-1) heterotypic interactions with intercellular adhesion molecule (ICAM) 1, 2, or 3 can also critically affect NK cell responses to bound target cells. For example, ICAM-2, when localized in the cytoplasmic projections (uropods) of potential targets, can stimulate NK cell cytotoxicity (108). In fact, transfections of the cytoskeletal protein ezrin into otherwise resistant cell lines stimulates uropod formation and sensitivity to NK cell-mediated killing. Therefore these analyses suggest that integrins can regulate the *in vitro* capacity of NK cells to kill potential targets. The relative importance *in vivo* of integrins as activating receptors or as adhesion molecules required for killing remains to be determined.

Another potential triggering molecule is the C-type lectin NKR-P1 (109,110). Antibodies specific for this receptor can initiate NK cell-mediated killing (111). In addition, NKR-P1-deficient NK cells are unable to mediate natural killing against certain tumor targets (112). NKR-P1 associates with the ITAM-containing γ subunit, and cells from $\gamma^{-/-}$ mice cannot mediate NKR-P1-initiated killing (113). Although there are reports that heterotrimeric G proteins (114) and phospholipase A_2 (115) couple NKR-P1 to downstream effector functions, most studies have focused on how proximal PTK activation and PLC-dependent calcium signaling regulate granule release and killing (116–119). Therefore NKR-P1 activation appears to have clear similarities with signaling initiated by other multisubunit immune recognition receptors. Other "triggering" receptors have been identified on

NK cells, but for the most part the signaling pathways utilized and their functional roles remain to be determined.

INHIBITORY SIGNALING

When an NK cell encounters a potential target, there must be tight regulation as to whether the cytotoxic program is initiated. As discussed earlier in this chapter, one level of control involves NK cell triggering receptors recognizing stimulatory ligands on target cells. During the last several years abundant data have emerged that the capacity of NK cells to mediate killing is determined by a balance between positive and negative regulatory events. In particular, there has been broad interest in the observations that receptor-mediated recognition of MHC-I complexes on target cells can block NK cell function *in vitro* and *in vivo* (2–7,120,121). Therefore normal MHC-I-bearing cells are relatively resistant to NK cell-mediated killing because of their ability to engage the NK cell inhibitory receptors. In contrast, malignant or virus-infected cells with reduced MHC-I on their surface may fail to engage the NK cell inhibitory receptors and therefore can become more susceptible to NK cell-mediated killing.

The inhibitory MHC-recognizing receptors molecularly identified thus far include human killer cell inhibitory receptors (KIRs) (two or three immunoglobulin superfamily domains in their extracellular regions), human and rodent CD94/NKG2 (both subunits are members of the C-type lectin superfamily), and rodent Ly-49 (type II disulfide-linked dimeric integral membrane protein with homology to the C-type lectin superfamily). Despite heterogeneity in their extracellular domains, a major common characteristic of all of the MHC-recognizing inhibitory receptors is the presence of a specific immunoreceptor tyrosine-based inhibition motif (ITIM)—[I,V]xYxx[L,V])—in their cytoplasmic tail. Crosslinking of the MHC-recognizing inhibitory receptors induces phosphorylation of the tyrosine residue in the ITIM (122). Genetic analysis suggests that Src-family PTKs play a central role in this process (122,123). For example, no tyrosine phosphorylation is observed following the ligation of KIRs expressed in the Lck-deficient Jurkat line JCaM1 (123). The ITIM phosphorylation is efficiently restored by re-expression of wild-type Lck (but not Fyn, c-Src, or Lyn). In fibroblasts, Lyn can mediate the phosphorylation of KIRs transiently expressed in fibroblasts (122). Therefore although it remains to be determined which specific Src-family kinase or kinases mediate KIR phosphorylation in NK cells, members of this PTK family are likely candidates.

For all of the identified families of MHC-recognizing inhibitory receptors, phosphorylated ITIMs create a binding site for the cytoplasmic protein tyrosine phosphatase SHP-1 (122–128). This phosphatase is known to be involved in the down-modulation of signaling from several families of leukocyte receptors, including cytokine receptors, growth factor receptors, and lympho-cyte antigen receptors (129). SHP-1 contain two amino-terminal SH2 domains and a carboxy-terminal catalytic site (130,131). The N-terminal SH2 domain inhibits the catalytic activity of SHP-1 in the resting state presumably by intramolecular binding that compromises the active site (132,133). This inhibition can be overcome by the addition of specific phosphotyrosine-containing peptides that interact with the N-terminal or C-terminal SH2 domain (or both) and thus expose the catalytic domain. It is postulated that phosphorylated peptides mimic phosphorylated ITIMs of the inhibitory receptors. Based on this model, a sequence of events that occur *in vivo* upon engagement of KIRs on NK cells is proposed (4) (Fig. 7-2). An Src-family kinase phosphorylates ITIMs, generating a docking site for the SH2 domain-containing SHP-1 and resulting in two important characteristics: (a) SHP-1 is in an active conformation, capable of dephosphorylating its substrates; and (b) because activating and inhibitory receptors interact with the

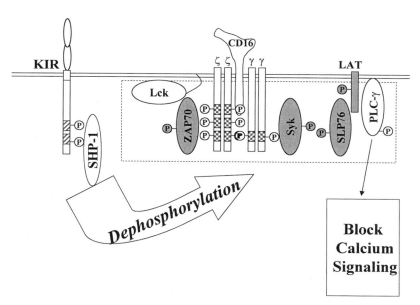

FIG. 7-2. Inhibitory signaling from MHC-recognizing receptors. Mobilization of the SHP-1 phosphatase to the cytoplasmic tail of KIR results in dephosphorylation of proximal signaling molecules and a subsequent block in calcium signaling. Potential direct targets of SHP-1 are represented by *shaded symbols.*

same target cell, SHP-1 is brought into close proximity with the activating signaling complex. Mobilizing activated SHP-1 to the site where triggering receptors are being engaged blocks NK cell activation. This inhibition occurs at a very proximal step in the activation pathway. Upon KIR co-engagement with FcγRIII, several key signaling molecules, including the ζ and γ subunits, ZAP-70, Syk, and PLC-γ, have inhibited tyrosine phosphorylation (33,123). As a result, FcγRIII-dependent increases in the intracellular content of inositol trisphosphate and calcium are blocked and NK cell-mediated cytotoxicity is suppressed (33,127,128,134). Overexpression in NK cells of a catalytically inactive version of SHP-1 reverses the normally inhibitory effects of the KIRs on protein tyrosine phosphorylation and restores NK cell-mediated killing of the target cells (122,123). Therefore the inhibitory effects of KIR-associated SHP-1 depends on its ability to catalyze the dephosphorylation of critical signaling elements.

A major unresolved issue is which molecules are direct targets for SHP-1-mediated dephosphorylation. Because the very proximal phosphorylation of ITAM-containing subunits is inhibited, the receptor or Src-family kinases are logical candidates. However, data showing these interactions have not been reported. On the other hand, two proximal signaling elements have been implicated as potential SHP-1 targets: LAT and SLP-76. Upon KIR interaction with MHC I-expressing cells, PLC-γ is phosphorylated but does not associate with tyrosine phosphorylated LAT (135). This observation would be consistent with a model in which the SHP-1 mediated dephosphorylation of LAT would uncouple PLC-γ from other proximal signaling events. In addition, recent analyses using a combination of direct binding and functional assays suggested that SLP-76 is a specific target for dephosphorylation by SHP-1 (86). Because tyrosine phosphorylation of SLP-76 appears to be required for optimal activation of cytotoxic lymphocytes, the targeted dephosphorylation of SLP-76 by

SHP-1 would be a potent negative regulator of NK cell function. Additional investigations are necessary to determine if the effects on LAT and SLP-76 are indirectly affecting ITAM or Syk-family PTK activation or if other SHP-1 targets serve this role.

CONCLUSIONS

This chapter summarizes selected key features of transmembrane signaling during NK cell activation. Recent progress has been fueled in part by the molecular characterization of specific activating and inhibitory receptors. The important role for the MHC-recognizing inhibitory receptors in NK cells have highlighted the need to determine the mechanisms regulating the balance between positive and negative signaling events for other hematopoietic cell types. As therapeutic approaches are designed to enhance NK cell activation (e.g., for antitumor or antiviral immunity) or to suppress NK cell function (e.g., to promote engraftment of hematopoietic cell progenitors), pharmacologic or molecular manipulations of the positive and signaling pathways are likely to be targeted. Future investigations of the signaling mechanisms regulating NK cell activation will likely be informative and challenging.

REFERENCES

1. Leibson PJ. Signal transduction during natural killer cell activation: inside the mind of a killer. *Immunity* 1997;6:655–661.
2. Lanier LL. NK cell receptors. *Annu Rev Immunol* 1998;16:359–393.
3. Colonna M. Natural killer cell receptors specific for MHC class I molecules. *Curr Opin Immunol* 1996;8:101–107.
4. Binstadt BA, Brumbaugh KM, Leibson PJ. Signal transduction by human NK cell MHC-recognizing receptors. *Immunol Rev* 1997;155:197–203.
5. Moretta A, Moretta L. HLA class I specific inhibitory receptors. *Curr Opin Immunol* 1997;9: 694–701.
6. Burshtyn DN, Long EO. Regulation through inhibitory receptors: lessons from natural killer cells. *Trends Cell Biol* 1997;7:473–479.
7. Yokoyama WM. HLA class I specificity for natural killer cell receptor CD94/NKG2A: two for one in more ways than one [comment]. *Proc Natl Acad Sci USA* 1998;95:4791–4794.

8. Keegan AD, Paul WE. Multichain immune recognition receptors: similarities in structure and signaling pathways. *Immunol Today* 1992;13:63–68.
9. Reth M. Antigen receptor tail clue. *Nature* 1989;338:383–384.
10. Cambier JC. Antigen and Fc receptor signaling: the awesome power of the immunoreceptor tyrosine-based activation motif (ITAM). *J Immunol* 1995;155:3281–3285.
11. Qian D, Weiss A. T cell antigen receptor signal transduction. *Curr Opin Cell Biol* 1997;9:205–212.
12. Anderson P, Caligiuri M, Ritz J, Schlossman SF. CD3-negative natural killer cells express ζTCR as part of a novel molecular complex. *Nature* 1989;341:159–162.
13. Lanier LL, Yu G, Phillips JH. Co-association of CD3ζ with a receptor (CD16) for IgG Fc on human natural killer cells. *Nature* 1989;342:803–805.
14. Orloff DG, Ra C, Frank SJ, Klausner RD, Kinet J-P. Family of disulphide-linked dimers containing the ζ and η chains of the T-cell receptor and the γ chain of Fc receptors. *Nature* 1990;347:189–191.
15. Kurosaki T, Gander I, Raveth JV. A subunit common to an IgG Fc receptor and the T-cell receptor mediates assembly through different interactions. *Proc Natl Acad Sci USA* 1991;88:3837–3841.
16. Weissman AM, Hou D, Orloff DG, et al. Molecular cloning and chromosomal localization of the human T-cell receptor ζ chain: distinction from the molecular CD3 complex. *Proc Natl Acad Sci USA* 1988;85:9709–9713.
17. Blank U, Ra C, Miller L, White K, Metzger H, Kinet J-P. Complete structure and expression in transfected cells of high affinity IgE receptor. *Nature* 1989;337:187–189.
18. Kurosaki T, Ravetch JV. A single amino acid in the glycosyl phosphatidylinositol attachment domain determines the membrane topology of FcγRIII. *Nature* 1989;342:805–807.
19. Taki T, Li M, Sylvester D, Clynes R, Ravetch JV. FcRγ chain deletion results in pleiotrophic effector cell defects. *Cell* 1994;76:519–529.
20. Lanier LL, Yu G, Phillips JH. Analysis of FcγRIII (CD16) membrane expression and association with CD3ζ and FcεRI-γ by site-directed mutation. *J Immunol* 1991;146:1571–1576.
21. Miller KL, Duchemin A-M, Anderson CL. A novel role for the Fc receptor γ subunit: enhancement of the FcγR ligand affinity. *J Exp Med* 1996; 183:2227–2233.
22. Songyang Z, Shoelson SE, Chaudhuri M, et al. SH2 domains recognize specific phosphopeptide sequences. *Cell* 1993;72:767–778.
23. Exley M, Varticovski L, Peter M, Sancho J, Terhorst C. Association of phosphatidylinositol 3-kinase with a specific sequence of the T cell receptor ζ chain is dependent on T cell activation. *J Biol Chem* 1994;269:15140–15146.
24. Cambier JC, Johnson SA. Differential binding activity of ARH1/TAM motifs. *Immunol Lett* 1995;44:77–80.
25. Isakov N, Wange RL, Burgess WH, Watts JD, Aebersold R, Samelson LE. ZAP-70 binding specificity to T cell receptor tyrosine-based activation motifs: the tandem SH2 domains of ZAP-70 bind

26. Bonnerot C, Amigorena S, Choquet D, Pavlovich R, Choukroun V, Fridman WH. Role of associated γ-chain in tyrosine kinase activation via murine FcγRIII. *EMBO J* 1992;11:2747–2757.
27. Paolini R, Renard V, Vivier E, et al. Different roles for the FcεRI γ chain as a function of the receptor context. *J Exp Med* 1995;181:247–255.
28. Vely F, Vivier E. Conservation of structural features reveals the existence of a large family of inhibitory cell surface receptors and noninhibitory/activatory counterparts. *J Immunol* 1997;159:2075–2077.
29. Lanier LL, Corliss BC, Wu J, Leong C, Phillips JH. Immunoreceptor DAP12 bearing a tyrosine-based activation motif is involved in activating NK cells. *Nature* 1998;391:703–707.
30. Lanier LL, Corliss B, Wu J, Phillips JH. Association of DAP12 with activating CD94/NKG2C NK cell receptors. *Immunity* 1998;8:693–701.
31. Smith KM, Wu J, Bakker AB, Phillips JH, Lanier LL. Ly-49D and Ly-49H associate with mouse DAP12 and form activating receptors. *J Immunol* 1998;161:7–10.
32. Perez-Villar JJ, Melero I, Rodriguez A, et al. Functional ambivalence of the Kp43 (CD94) NK cell-associated surface antigen. *J Immunol* 1995;154:5779–5788.
33. Brumbaugh KM, Perez-Villar JJ, Dick CJ, Schoon RA, Lopez-Botet M, Leibson PJ. Clonotypic differences in signaling from CD94 (kp43) on NK cells lead to divergent cellular responses. *J Immunol* 1996;157:2804–2812.
34. Mason LH, Anderson SK, Yokoyama WM, Smith HRC, Winkler-Pickett R, Ortaldo JR. The Ly-49D receptor activates murine natural killer cells. *J Exp Med* 1996;184:2119–2128.
35. Vivier E, Morin P, O'Brien C, Druker B, Schlossman SF, Anderson P. Tyrosine phosphorylation of the FcγRIII(CD16): ζ complex in human natural killer cells; induction by antibody-dependent cytotoxicity but not by natural killing. *J Immunol* 1991;146:206–210.
36. O'Shea JJ, Weissman AM, Kennedy ICS, Ortaldo JR. Engagement of the natural killer cell IgG Fc receptor results in tyrosine phosphorylation of the ζ chain. *Proc Natl Acad Sci USA* 1991;88:350–354.
37. Einspahr KJ, Abraham RT, Binstadt BA, Uehara Y, Leibson PJ. Tyrosine phosphorylation provides an early and requisite signal for the activation of natural killer cell cytotoxic function. *Proc Natl Acad Sci USA* 1991;88:6279–6283.
38. Eiseman E, Bolen JB. src-Related tyrosine protein kinases as signaling components in hematopoietic cells. *Cancer Cells* 1990;2:303–310.
39. Salcedo TW, Kurosaki T, Kanakaraj P, Ravetch JV, Perussia B. Physical and functional association of p56^lck with FcγRIIIA (CD16) in natural killer cells. *J Exp Med* 1993;277:1475–1480.
40. Pignata C, Prasad KVS, Robertson MK, Levine H, Rudd CE, Ritz J. FcγRIIIA-mediated signaling involves src family lck in human natural killer cells. *J Immunol* 1993;151:6794–6800.
41. Cone JC, Lu Y, Trevillyan JM, Bjorndahl JM, Phil-

lips CA. Association of the p56[lck] protein tyrosine kinase with the FcγRIIIA/CD16 complex in human natural killer cells. *Eur J Immunol* 1993; 23:2488–2497.

42. O'Shea JJ, McVicar DW, Kuhns DB, Ortaldo JR. A role for protein tyrosine kinase activity in natural cytotoxicity as well as antibody-dependent cellular cytotoxicity. *J Immunol* 1992;148:2497–2502.

43. Van Oers NSC, Lowin-Kropf B, Finlay D, Connolly K, Weiss A. αβT cell development is abolished in mice lacking both lck and fyn protein tyrosine kinases. *Immunity* 1996;5:429–436.

44. Yamada H, Kishihara K, Kong Y-Y, Nomoto K. Enhanced generation of NK cells with intact cytotoxic function in CD45 exon 6-deficient mice. *J Immunol* 1996;157:1523–1528.

45. Scharenberg AM, Lin S, Cuenod B, Yamamura H, Kinet J-P. Reconstitution of interactions between tyrosine kinases and the high affinity IgE receptor which are controlled by receptor clustering. *EMBO J* 1995;14:3385–3394.

46. Chan AC, Iwashima M, Turck CW, Weiss A. ZAP-70: A 70 kd protein-tyrosine kinase that associates with the TCR ζ chain. *Cell* 1992;71:649–662.

47. Vivier E, da Silva AJ, Ackerly M, Levine H, Rudd CE, Anderson P. Association of a 70-dKa tyrosine phosphoprotein with the CD16:ζ·γ complex expressed in human natural killer cells. *Eur J Immunol* 1993;23:1872–1876.

48. Hatada MH, Lu X, Laird ER, et al. Molecular basis for interaction of the protein tyrosine kinase ZAP-70 with the T-cell receptor. *Nature* 1995; 377:32–41.

49. Benhamou M, Ryba NJP, Kihara H, Nishikata H, Siraganian RP. Protein-tyrosine kinase p72[syk] in high affinity IgE receptor signaling. *J Biol Chem* 1993;268:23318–23324.

50. Kihara H, Siraganian RP. Src homology 2 domains of syk and lyn bind to tyrosine-phosphorylated subunits of the high affinity IgE receptor. *J Biol Chem* 1994;369:22427–22432.

51. Darby C, Geahlen RL, Schreiber AD. Stimulation of macrophage FcγRIIIA activates the receptor-associated protein tyrosine kinase syk and induces phosphorylation of multiple proteins including p95Vav and p62/GAP-associated protein. *J Immunol* 1994;152:5429–5437.

52. Durden DL, Liu YB. Protein-tyrosine kinase p72[syk] in Fcγ RI receptor signaling. *Blood* 1994;84:2102–2108.

53. Zoller KE, MacNeil IA, Brugge JS. Protein tyrosine kinases syk and ZAP-70 display distinct requirements for src family kinases in immune response receptor signal transduction. *J Immunol* 1997; 158:1650–1659.

54. Zhang J, Berenstein EH, Evans RL, Siraganian RP. Transfection of syk protein tyrosine kinase reconstitutes high affinity IgE receptor-mediated degranulation in a syk-negative variant of rat basophilic leukemia RBL-2H3 cells. *J Exp Med* 1996; 184:71–79.

55. Oliver JM, Burg DL, Wilson BS, McLaughlin JL, Geahlen RL. Inhibition of mast cell FcεR1-mediated signaling and effector function by the syk-

56. Stahls A, Liwszyc GE, Couture C, Mustelin T, Andersson LC. Triggering of human natural killer cells through CD16 induces tyrosine phosphorylation of the p72[syk] kinase. *Eur J Immunol* 1994;24:2491–2496.

57. Ting AT, Dick CJ, Schoon RA, Karnitz LM, Abraham RT, Leibson PJ. Interaction between lck and syk family tyrosine kinases in Fcγ receptor-initiated activation of natural killer cells. *J Biol Chem* 1995;270:16415–16421.

58. Brumbaugh KM, Binstadt BA, Billadeau DD, et al. Functional role for syk tyrosine kinase in natural killer cell-mediated natural cytotoxicity. *J Exp Med* 1997;186:1–9.

59. Negishi I, Motoyama N, Nakayama K-I, et al. Essential role for ZAP-70 in both positive and negative selection of thymocytes. *Nature* 1995;376: 435–438.

60. Elder ME, Lin D, Clever J, et al. Human severe combined immunodeficiency due to a defect in ZAP-70, a T cell tyrosine kinase. *Science* 1994;264:1596–1598.

61. Chan AC, Kadlecek TA, Elder ME, et al. ZAP-70 deficiency in an autosomal recessive form of severe combined immunodeficiency. *Science* 1994;264:1599–1601.

62. Rawlings DJ, Witte ON. The Btk subfamily of cytoplasmic tyrosine kinases: structure, regulation and function. *Semin Immunol* 1995;7:237–246.

63. Gold MR, Chan VW-F, Turck CW, DeFranco AL. Membrane Ig cross-linking regulates phosphatidylinositol 3-kinase in B lymphocytes. *J Immunol* 1992;148:2012–2022.

64. Tuveson DA, Carter RH, Soltoff SP, Fearon DT. CD19 of B cells as a surrogate kinase insert region to bind phosphatidylinositol 3-kinase. *Science* 1993;260:986–989.

65. Takata M, Kurosaki T. A role for bruton's tyrosine kinase in B cell antigen receptor-mediated activation of phospholipase C-γ2. *J Exp Med* 1996; 184:31–40.

66. Fluckiger A-C, Li Z, Kato RM, et al. Btk/Tec kinases regulate sustained increases in intracellular Ca²⁺ following B-cell receptor activation. *EMBO J* 1998;17:1973–1985.

67. Scharenberg AM, El-Hillal O, Fruman DA, et al. Phosphatidylinositol-3,4,5-trisphosphate (PtdIns-3,4,5-P₃)/Tec kinase-dependent calcium signaling pathway: a target for SHIP-mediated inhibitory signals. *EMBO J* 1998;17:1961–1972.

68. Scharenberg AM, Kinet J-P. PtdIns-3,4,5-P3: a regulatory nexus between tyrosine kinases and sustained calcium signals. *Cell* 1998;94:5–8.

69. Rawlings DJ, Scharenberg AM, Park H, et al. Activation of BTK by a phosphorylation mechanism initiated by src family kinases. *Science* 1996; 271:822–825.

70. Bonnema JD, Karnitz LM, Schoon RA, Abraham RT, Leibson PJ. Fc receptor stimulation of phosphatidylinositol 3-kinase in natural killer cells is associated with protein kinase C-independent granule release and cell-mediated cytotoxicity. *J Exp Med* 1994;180:1427–1435.

71. Ricciarda G, Palmieri G, Piccoli M, Frati L, Santoni A. CD16-mediated p21^{ras} activation is associated with Shc and p36 tyrosine phosphorylation and their binding with Grb2 in human natural killer cells. *J Exp Med* 1996;183:179–186.

72. McCormick F. Activators and effectors of *ras* p21 proteins. *Curr Opin Genet Dev* 1994;4:71–76.

73. Jackman JK, Motto DG, Sun Q, et al. Molecular cloning of SLP-76, a 76-kDa tyrosine phosphoprotein associated with Grb2 in T cells. *J Biol Chem* 1995;270:7029–7032.

74. Wardenburg JB, Fu C, Jackman JK, et al. Phosphorylation of SLP-76 by the ZAP-70 protein-tyrosine kinase is required for T-cell receptor function. *J Biol Chem* 1996;271:19641–19644.

75. Fang N, Motto DG, Ross SE, Koretzky GA. Tyrosines 113, 128, and 145 of SLP-76 are required for optimal augmentation of NFAT promoter activity. *J Immunol* 1996;157:3769–3773.

76. Musci MA, Motto DG, Ross SE, Fang N, Koretzky GA. Three domains of SLP-76 are required for its optimal function in a T cell line. *J Immunol* 1997;159:1639-1647.

77. Wu J, Motto DG, Koretzky GA, Weiss A. Vav and SLP-76 interact and functionally cooperate in IL-2 gene activation. *Immunity* 1996;4:593–602.

78. Tuosto L, Michel F, Acuto O. p95^{vav} associates with tyrosine-phosphorylated SLP-76 in antigen-stimulated T cells. *J Exp Med* 1996;184:1161–1166.

79. Raab M, da Silva AJ, Findell PR, Rudd CE. Regulation of Vav-SLP-76 binding by ZAP-70 and its relevance to TCRζ/CD3 induction of interleukin-2. *Immunity* 1997;6:155–164.

80. Bustelo XR. The VAV family of signal transduction molecules. *Crit Rev Oncog* 1996;7:65–66.

81. Crespo P, Schuebel KE, Ostrom AA, Gutkind JS, Bustelo XR. Phosphotyrosine-dependent activation of Rac-1 GDP/GTP exchange by the *vav* proto-oncogene product. *Nature* 1997;375:169–172.

82. Musci MA, Hendricks-Taylor LR. Motto DG, et al. Molecular cloning of SLAP-130, and SLP-76-associated substrate of the T cell antigen receptor-stimulated protein tyrosine kinases. *J Biol Chem* 1997;272:11674–11677.

83. Da Silva AJ, Li Z, De Vera C, Canto E, Findell P, Rudd CE. Cloning of a novel T-cell protein FYB that binds FYN and SH2-domain-containing leukocyte protein 76 and modulates interleukin 2 production. *Proc Natl Acad Sci USA* 94:7493–7498.

84. Clements JL, Yang B, Ross-Barta SE, et al. Requirement for the leukocyte-specific adapter protein SLP-76 for normal T cell development. *Science* 1998;281:416–419.

85. Yablonski D, Kuhne MR, Kadlecek T, Weiss A. Uncoupling of nonreceptor tyrosine kinases from PLC-γ1 in an SLP-76-deficient T cell. *Science* 1998;281:413–415.

86. Binstadt BA, Billadeau DD, Jevremovic D, et al. SLP-76 is a direct substrate of SHP-1 recruited to killer cell inhibitory receptors. *J Biol Chem* 1998;273:27518–27523.

87. Zhang W, Sloan-Lancaster J, Kitchen J, Trible RP, Samelson LE. LAT: the ZAP-70 tyrosine kinase substrate that links T cell receptor to cellular activation. *Cell* 1998;92:83–92.

88. Brdicka T, Cerny J, Horejsi V. T cell receptor signalling results in rapid tyrosine phosphorylation of the linker protein LAT present in detergent-resistant membrane microdomains. *Biochem Biophys Res Commun* 1998;248:356–360.

89. Zhang W, Trible RP, Samelson LE. LAT palmitoylation: its essential role in membrane microdomain targeting and tyrosine phosphorylation during T cell activation. *Immunity* 1998;9:239–246.

90. Ting AT, Karnitz LM, Schoon RA, Abraham RT, Leibson PJ. Fcγ receptor activation induces the tyrosine phosphorylation of both phospholipase C (PLC)-γ1 and PLC-γ2 in natural killer cells. *J Exp Med* 1992;176:1751–1755.

91. Azzoni L, Kamoun M, Salcedo TW, Kanakaraj P, Perussia B. Stimulation of Fc gamma RIIIA results in phospholipase C-gamma 1 tyrosine phosphorylation and p56^{lck} activation. *J Exp Med* 1992;176:1745–1750.

92. Ting AT, Einspahr KJ, Abraham RT, Leibson PJ. Fcγ receptor signal transduction in natural killer cells: coupling to phospholipase C via a G protein-independent, but tyrosine kinase-dependent pathway. *J Immunol* 1991;147:3122–3127.

93. Kolanus W, Romeo C, Seed B. T cell activation by clustered tyrosine kinases. *Cell* 1993;74:171–183.

94. Williams BL, Schreiber KL, Zhang W, et al. Genetic evidence for differential coupling of syk family kinases to the T-cell receptor: reconstitution studies in a ZAP-70-deficient Jurkat T cell line. *Mol Cell Biol* 1998;18:1388–1399.

95. Maghazachi AA, Al-Aoukaty A, Naper C, Torgersen KM, Rolstad B. Preferential involvement of G$_o$ and G$_z$ proteins in mediating rat natural killer cell lysis of allogeneic and tumor target cells. *J Immunol* 1997;157:5308–5314.

96. Lang P, Guizani L, Vitte-Mony I, et al. ADP-ribosylation of the *ras*-related, GTP-binding protein RhoA inhibits lymphocyte-mediated cytotoxicity. *J Biol Chem* 1992;267:11677–11680.

97. Billadeau DD, Brumbaugh KM, Dick CJ, Schoon RA, Bustelo XR, Leibson PJ. The Vav-Rac1 pathway in cytotoxic lymphocytes regulates the generation of cell-mediated killing. *J Exp Med* 1998;188:549–559.

98. Milella M, Gismondi A, Roncaioli P, et al. CD16 cross-linking induces both secretory and extracellular signal-regulated kinase (ERK)-dependent cytosolic phospholipase A$_2$ (PLA$_2$) activity in human natural killer cells: involvement of ERK, but not PLA$_2$, in CD16-triggered granule exocytosis. *J Immunol* 1997;158:3148–3154.

99. Wei S, Gamero AM, Liu JH, et al. Control of lytic function by mitogen-activated protein kinase/extracellular regulatory kinase 2 (ERK2) in a human natural killer cell line: identification of perforin and granzyme B mobilization by functional ERK2. *J Exp Med* 1998;187:1763–1765.

100. Newton RA, Thiel M, Hogg N. Signaling mechanisms and the activation of leukocyte integrins. *J Leukoc Biol* 1997;61:422–426.

101. Gismondi A, Milella M, Palmieri G, Piccoli M, Frati L, Santoni A. Stimulation of protein tyrosine

phosphorylation by interaction of NK cells with fibronectin via $\alpha_4\beta_1$ and $\alpha_5\beta_1$. *J Immunol* 1995;154:3128–3137.

102. Rabinowich H, Lin W-C, Manciulea M, Herberman RB, Whiteside TL. Induction of protein tyrosine phosphorylation in human natural killer cells by triggering via $\alpha_4\beta_1$ or $\alpha_5\beta_1$ integrins. *Blood* 1995;85:1858–1864.

103. Rabinowich H, Manciulea M, Herberman RB, Whiteside TL. β_1 Integrin-mediated activation of focal adhesion kinase and its association with Fyn and Zap-70 in human NK cells. *J Immunol* 1996;157:3860–3868.

104. Perez-Villar JJ, Melero I, Gismondi A, Santoni A, Lopez-Botet M. Functional analysis of $\alpha_1\beta_1$ integrin in human natural killer cells. *Eur J Immunol* 1996;26:2023–2029.

105. Gismondi A, Bisogno L, Mainiero F, et al. Proline-rich tyrosine kinase-2 activation by β_1 integrin fibronectin receptor cross-linking and association with paxillin in human natural killer cells. *J Immunol* 1997;159:4729–4736.

106. Hannigan GE, Dedhar S. Protein kinase mediators of integrin signal transduction. *J Mol Med* 1997; 75:35–44.

107. Palmieri G, Serra A, DeMaria R, et al. Cross-linking of $\alpha_4\beta_1$ and $\alpha_5\beta_1$ fibronectin receptors enhances natural killer cell cytotoxic activity. *J Immunol* 1995;155:5314–5322.

108. Helander TS, Carpen O, Turunen O, Kovanen PE, Vaheri A, Timonen T. ICAM-2 redistributed by ezrin as a target for killer cells. *Nature* 1996; 382:265–268.

109. Giorda R, Rudert WA, Vavassori C, Chambers WH, Hiserodt JC, Trucco M. NKR-P1, a signal transduction molecule on natural killer cells. *Science* 1990;249:1298–1300.

110. Lanier LL, Chang C, Phillips JH. Human NKR-P1A: a disulfide-linked homodimer of the C-type lectin superfamily expressed by a subset of NK and T lymphocytes. *J Immunol* 1994;153:2417–2428.

111. Chambers WH, Vujanovic NL, DeLeo AB, Olszowy MW, Herberman HB, Hiserodt JC. Monoclonal antibody to a triggering structure expressed on rat natural killer cells and adherent lymphokine-activated killer cells. *J Exp Med* 1989; 169:1373–1389.

112. Ryan JC, Niemi EC, Nakamura MC, Seaman WE. NKR-P1A is a target-specific receptor that activates natural killer cell cytotoxicity. *J Exp Med* 1995;181:1911–1915.

113. Arase N, Arase H, Park SY, Ohno H, Ra C, Saito T. Association with FcRγ is essential for activation signal through NKR-P1 (CD161) in natural killer (NK) cells and NK1.1$^+$ T cells. *J Exp Med* 1997;186:1957–1963.

114. Al-Aoukaty A, Rolstad B, Maghazachi AA. Functional coupling of NKR-P1 receptors to various heterotrimeric G proteins in rat interleukin-2-activated natural killer cells. *J Biol Chem* 1997; 272:31604–31608.

115. Cifone MG, Roncaioli P, Cironi L, et al. NKR-P1A stimulation of arachidonate-generating enzymes in rat NK cells is associated with granule release and cytotoxic activity. *J Immunol* 1997;159:309–317.

116. Ryan JC, Niemi EC, Goldfien RD, Hiserodt JC, Seaman WE. NKR-P1, an activating molecule on rat natural killer cells, stimulates phosphoinositide turnover and a rise in intracellular calcium. *J Immunol* 1991;147:3244-3250.

117. Josien R, Heslan M, Soulillou J-P, Cuturi M-C. Rat spleen dendritic cells express natural killer cell receptor protein 1 (NKR-P1) and have cytotoxic activity to select targets via a Ca^{2+}-dependent mechanism. *J Exp Med* 1997;186:467–472.

118. Campbell KS, Giorda R. The cytoplasmic domain of rat NKR-P1 receptor interacts with the N-terminal domain of p56^{lck} via cysteine residues. *Eur J Immunol* 1997;27:72–77.

119. Cerny J, Fiserova A, Horvath O, Bezouska K, Pospisil M, Hoejsi V. Association of human NK cell surface receptors NKR-P1 and CD94 with Src-family protein kinases. *Immunogenetics* 1997;46: 231–236.

120. Ljunggren H-G, Karre K. In search of the "missing self": MHC molecules and NK cell recognition. *Immunol Today* 1990;11:237–244.

121. Leibson PJ. MHC-recognizing receptors: they're not just for T cells anymore. *Immunity* 1995;3:5–8.

122. Burshtyn DN, Scharenberg AM, Wagtmann N, et al. Recruitment of tyrosine phosphatase HCP by the killer cell inhibitory receptor. *Immunity* 1996;4:77–85.

123. Binstadt BA, Brumbaugh KM, Dick CJ, et al. Sequential involvement of Lck and SHP-1 with MHC-recognizing receptors on NK cells inhibits FcR-initiated tyrosine kinase activation. *Immunity* 1996;5:629–638.

124. Olcese L, Lang P, Vely F, et al. Human and mouse killer-cell inhibitory receptors recruit PTP1C and PTP1D protein tyrosine phosphatases. *J Immunol* 1996;156:4531–4534.

125. Fry AM, Lanier LL, Weiss A. Phosphotyrosines in the killer cell inhibitory receptor motif of NKB1 are required for negative signaling and for association with protein tyrosine phosphatase 1C. *J Exp Med* 1996;184:295–300.

126. Campbell KS, Dessing M, Lopez-Botet M, Cella M, Colonna M. Tyrosine phosphorylation of a human killer inhibitory receptor recruits protein tyrosine phosphatase 1C. *J Exp Med* 1996;184:93–100.

127. Nakamura MC, Niemi EC, Fisher MJ, Shulz LD, Seaman WE, Ryan JC. Mouse Ly-49A interrupts early signaling events in natural killer cell cytotoxicity and functionally associates with the SHP-1 tyrosine phosphatase. *J Exp Med* 1997;185: 673–684.

128. Houchins JP, Lanier LL, Niemie EC, Phillips JH, Ryan JC. Natural killer cell cytolytic activity is inhibited by NKG2-A and activated by NKG2-C. *J Immunol* 1997;158:3603–3609.

129. Neel BH. Role of phosphatases in lymphocyte activation. *Curr Opin Immunol* 1997;9:405–420.

130. Plutzky J, Neel BG, Rosenberg RD. Isolation of a src homology 2-containing tyrosine phosphatase. *Proc Natl Acad Sci USA* 1992;89:1123–1127.

131. Yi T, Cleveland JL, Ihle JN. Protein tyrosine phosphatase containing SH2 domains: characterization, preferential expression in hematopoietic cells, and

localization to human chromosome 12p12-p13. *Mol Cell Biol* 1992;12:836–846.

132. Pei D, Lorezn U, Klingmuller U, Neel BG, Wlash CT. Intramolecular regulation of protein tyrosine phosphatase SH-PTP1: a new function for Src homology 2 domains. *Biochemistry* 1994;33:15483–15493.

133. Pei D, Wang J, Walsh CT. Differential functions of the two Src homology 2 domains in protein tyrosine phosphatase SH-PTP1. *Proc Natl Acad Sci USA* 1996;93:1141–1145.

134. Kaufman DS, Schoon RA, Robertson MJ, Leibson PJ. Inhibition of selective signaling events in natural killer cells recognizing major histocompatibility complex class I. *Proc Natl Acad Sci USA* 1995; 92:6484–6488.

135. Valiante NM, Phillips JH, Lanier LL, Parham P. Killer cell inhibitory receptor recognition of human leukocyte antigen (HLA) class I blocks formation of a pp36/PLC-γ signaling complex in human natural killer (NK) cells. *J Exp Med* 1996;184:2243–2250.

Cytotoxic Cells: Basic Mechanisms and Medical Applications, edited by Michail V. Sitkovsky and Pierre A. Henkart. Lippincott Williams & Wilkins, Philadelphia © 2000.

Chapter 8

Role of Nonimmune Extracellular Signaling Molecules in the Local Tissue Environment During CTL Differentiation and Effector Functions

Michail V. Sitkovsky and Sergey G. Apasov

Laboratory of Immunology, National Institute of Allergy and Infectious Diseases, National Institutes of Health, Bethesda, Maryland 20892, USA

It is proposed that T cell receptor (TCR)-driven differentiation and expansion of peripheral T cells, including cytotoxic T lymphocytes (CTLs), could be influenced by transmembrane signaling by nonimmune extracellular molecules in the local tissue environment. Many small molecules can signal through G-protein-coupled receptors including receptors to extracellular nucleotides (purinergic receptors) that have been found to be expressed on T lymphocytes and antigen-presenting cells (APCs). Such signaling could be TCR antagonizing or enhancing and thereby could affect positive and negative selection of thymocytes and effector functions of mature T cells. Similarly, signaling by nonimmune extracellular molecules in the local tissue environment could affect antigen presentation and initiation of the immune response and expansion of T cells by interfering with chemokine-mediated or other signaling on dendritic cells and macrophages. Both extracellular adenosine triphosphate (extATP) and extracellular adenosine (ext-Ado) have been demonstrated to act through specific purinergic receptors that are expressed on the surface of thymocytes, periph-

eral T cells, and macrophages. The pattern of expression of some purinergic receptors (e.g., P_{2y2}) is similar to that of immediate early response genes, suggesting the possibility of their involvement in feedback regulation. The other receptors (e.g., P_{2x7}, ATP-gated pores, and cation channels) have differentiation-related patterns of expression and may play a role in the regulation of T cell development. In addition to their possible role in normal processes of T cell differentiation, expansion, and CTL effector functions, experimental data point to a role of purinergic receptors under pathologic conditions upon accumulation of extracellular adenosine. Abnormal accumulation of adenosine may occur in a hypoxic environment, such as large solid tumors, or in the absence of adenosine deaminase (ADA) in ADA severe combined immunodeficiency (SCID) patients. An example of the critical effects of adenosine-triggered signaling is provided by studies of ADA deficiency *in vitro*. We propose a dual mechanism for ADA SCID in which the accumulation of adenosine causes the death of a large proportion of thymocytes by nonspecific intracellular toxicity, and adenosine-mediated signaling affects the threshold of TCR-dependent T cell selection. The inhibition of TCR-driven signaling may prevent the elimination of potentially autoreactive T cells in the process of negative selection and allow survival of potentially autoimmune CTLs. It is of note that adenosine in vitro blocked practically all stages of CTL–T cell interaction and of lethal hit delivery, including granule exocytosis and Fas ligand (FasL) upregulation. In addition to the conditions of adenosine deaminase deficiency, the accumulation of extracellular adenosine *in vivo* can be observed as the result of hypoxia or medical treatment with some pharmacologic agents. The issue of naturally occurring hypoxic conditions in various tissues requires special investigation, but the behavior of CTLs in the hypoxic areas of solid tumors is of special interest because accumulation of extAdo near solid tumors may serve to suppress antitumor immune responses.

INTRODUCTION

The processes of differentiation of immature thymocytes into mature CD8+ CTLs, and of CTL expansion and effector functions, take place in the thymus and various lymphoid and targeted tissues. The extracellular environment in different tissues is expected to contain a different number and "repertoire" of signaling molecules. We explore the hypothesis that the final outcome of the immune response (TCR-driven differentiation, expansion, and effector functions of peripheral T cells including CTLs) is at least partially determined by transmembrane signaling by nonimmune, physiologically abundant molecules in the local tissue extracellular environment (1–6) (Fig. 8-1). Such signaling could affect the differentiation of immature thymocytes into mature T cells during positive and negative selection of thymocytes, leading to survival of T cells with an inappropriate TCR repertoire. The effects of steroid hormones on thymocyte selection are examples of intracellular signaling that could be direct or in combination with TCR-mediated effects; a recent model (7) based on antagonism between TCR- and steroid-induced signals provides an attractive explanation for the effects of steroids in these processes.

The effector phase of the immune response involves recognition of antigen, expansion of CTLs and CTL-mediated lymphokine secretion, and lethal hit delivery. Each of these responses is driven by complex transmembrane signaling cascades and therefore is susceptible to modulation by ad-

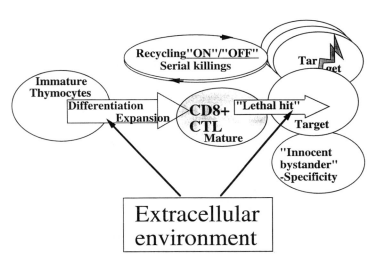

FIG. 8-1. Role of signaling molecules in a local tissue extracellular environment in the differentiation of thymocytes into effector T cells and lysis of antigen-bearing and bystander cells.

ditional extracellular signaling, resulting in the inhibition or enhancement of T cell functions. Thus signaling from the extracellular environment could affect the ability of CTLs both to recognize and to kill. Similarly, the extracellular environment of the local tissue could interfere with chemokine-mediated or other signaling in antigen-presenting dendritic cells and macrophages, thereby severely affecting the initiation of the immune response and the expansion of T cells. This TCR-independent signaling could be mediated by many small signaling molecules through G-protein-coupled receptors including, for example, receptors to extracellular

nucleotides (purinergic receptors), which have been found to be expressed on T lymphocytes and APCs (1–6).

Our most recent series of experiments have focused on the possible role of extAdo and extracellular ATP (extATP) and their receptors in the regulation of immune processes (Fig. 8-2). Both extAdo and extATP were shown to be able to signal through purinergic receptors, classified as P_1 and P_2 receptors, respectively. P_1 receptors for extAdo include A_1, A_{2a}, A_{2b}, and A_3 receptors; and P_2 for extATP receptors are divided into P_{2x} and P_{2y} subclasses (8,9). A_{2a} and A_3 adenosine receptors; and P_{2x7} ATP receptors are

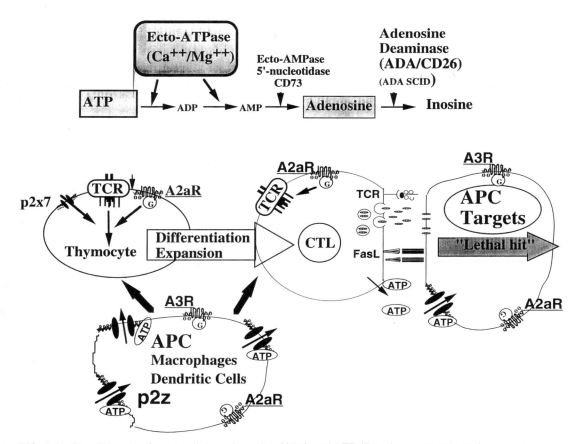

FIG. 8-2. Possible role of extracellular adenosine (A2a) and ATP (P2x7) receptors in antigen presentation and in differentiation of thymocytes into effector T cells and lysis of antigen-bearing and bystander cells. A well coordinated system of extracellular enzymes is involved in the regulation of concentrations of extracellular ATP and adenosine.

currently under the closest scrutiny in our studies (Fig. 8-2).

Purinergic receptor-mediated effects of extATP and extAdo are implicated in a variety of physiologic responses in various cellular systems (9–11). The functional role of purinergic receptors in lymphocytes has not yet been conclusively ascertained, whereas signaling, cell permeabilizing, and apoptotic effects of extATP on cells including thymocytes, T cells, and macrophages are well documented (1,12–15). The presence of extATP in biologic fluids has been demonstrated; notably, the activation of T cells with anti-TCR monoclonal anibody (mAb) led to the accumulation of extATP (16). The extATP could be degraded by ecto-ATPases on T cells (1) to form extAdo, which in turn could be degraded by adenosine deaminase (ADA) (Fig. 8-2). Studies of signal-transmitting properties of extATP and extAdo suggest that signaling through purinergic receptors may regulate the TCR-driven processes of T cell differentiation, expansion, and effector functions (1–6). A combination of purinergic receptor signaling with TCRs or steroid hormone-mediated signals (or both) can be critical at a particular stage of T cell development if purinergic receptors are differentially expressed to enable selective targeting of T cell subsets. Although the effects and possible role of purinergic receptors were the first we explored, other signaling molecules in the extracellular environment and G-protein-coupled receptors must also be investigated for their possible roles in regulation of the immune response.

EXPRESSION OF PURINERGIC RECEPTORS IN T LYMPHOCYTES

Extracellular adenosine and extATP receptors are expressed on the surface of thymocytes, peripheral T cells, and macrophages. Formal genetic evidence of the expression of purinergic receptors in T cells was provided by Northern blot and reverse transcriptase-polymerase chain reaction (RT-PCR) analysis of their mRNA expression

(2,4–6,17). The expression of functional P_2 purinergic receptors in T cells was evidenced by increases in intracellular Ca^{2+} after incubation of thymocytes and T cells with ATP and ATP analogs (17). We found that ATP [but not uridine triphosphate (UTP)] can trigger Ca^{2+} increases, whereas AMP and Ado are not efficient. The Ca^{2+} increases were detected during the first minutes of incubation with ATP but not with AMP or Ado. This finding complements pharmacologic observations identifying P_2 purinoreceptors as being responsible for these effects. The changes in $[Ca^{2+}]$ correlated with the cellular effects of extATP, as only ATP but not UTP was efficient in interfering with Dex-induced apoptosis (2). Virtually all thymocyte subsets responded to ATP by increases in $[Ca^{2+}]$, as is evident from inspection of the flow cytometry data (17); however, different thymocyte subsets are differentially susceptible to the effects of extATP and can be divided into at least two subpopulations: thymocytes that respond to ATP by low increases in $[Ca^{2+}]_i$ and thymocytes that have high $[Ca^{2+}]_i$ responses.

We found that exposure of thymocytes or cloned CTLs to extAdo or nonhydrolyzable Ado receptor agonists results in a rapid, sustained increase of intracellular cAMP levels. The selective A_{2a} receptor agonist was found to induce—whereas selective A_{2a} receptor antagonists decreased—cAMP accumulation in CTL clones. These observations virtually excluded cAMP level-decreasing A_1 and A_3 receptors as being responsible for the cAMP-increasing effects of extAdo in T cells. The predominant expression of A_{2a} receptors in T cells, which has been established in biochemical assays using selective A_{2a} receptor agonists and antagonists, is confirmed by Northern blot studies of A_1, A_{2a}, and A_3 mRNA expression in CTLs (5,6). Ongoing studies address the question of expression of A_1, A_{2a}, A_{2b}, and A_3 adenosine receptors in APCs, including dendritic cells.

Although we identified the A_{2a} receptor as the likely executor of effects of extAdo on purified T cells, we are also interested in the contribution of the A_3 class of these receptors in effects of adenosine on complex cell mixtures that include APCs. A_3 receptors were claimed to be involved in the proliferation of cytotoxic cells (18), but the authors based their conclusion on the observations that addition of ADA preparations in the culture inhibits proliferation of the interleukin-2 (IL-2)-dependent CTLs. We could not confirm these observations and subsequently demonstrated that the observed effects were due to the presence of ammonium sulfate in the ADA preparations, not to the enzymatic activity of ADA (19). Thus no data exist to date to implicate the A_3 receptor in any function of T lymphocytes. Despite our inability to detect expression of A_3 mRNA in T cells from spleen, lymph nodes (6), and *in vitro*-maintained T cell lines, it is still possible that low levels of A_3 receptors are expressed in T cells and could contribute to the effects described here. Another interesting possibility is that A_3 receptors are expressed in APCs, including dendritic cells and macrophages, and that their functioning in APCs could be important for CTL development. It is expected that the experiments with A_{2a} and A_3 receptor gene-deficient mice will provide important insights into the functioning of these receptors in the immune system.

Study of the expression of purinergic receptors was facilitated by their cDNA cloning. Experiments with the first available cDNA for the G-protein-coupled P_{2y2} receptors demonstrated that mRNA expression of this receptor is similar to the pattern of immediate early genes in murine T lymphocytes (4). The fact that expression of P_{2y2} mRNA could be rapidly induced by steroid hormones or anti-TCR mAbs in a protein synthesis-independent manner led to the proposal that purinergic receptors could serve in the feedback regulation of T cell responses (4). Accordingly, activated T cells may upregulate their purinergic receptor expression, which in turn makes these cells susceptible to the effects of extATP and extAdo and P_1/P_2 receptor-mediated transmembrane signaling. Such signaling could regulate the

expression of other genes in T cells and could be additive or counteract the effects of the original first signal, thereby providing a feedback mechanism of T lymphocyte responses.

Expression of P_{2x7} receptors in thymocytes and T cells follows a pattern in which expression of these receptors increases as thymocytes mature from $CD4^-CD8^-$ (double negative) to $CD4^+CD8^+$ (double positive) and $CD4^+$ (single positive) splenic T cells, reflecting the differentiation-related expression of these receptors (17). Such a pattern suggests the possibility that P_{2x7} receptor-mediated signaling may be involved in the regulation of differentiation and cell death in thymocytes and peripheral T cells (3,17); however, experimental evidence is still lacking about the role of these receptors in CTL differentiation. Thus the overall effects of extATP and extAdo and the possibility of feedback regulation will be determined by: (a) concentrations of extracellular nucleotides; (b) expression and activities of ecto-ATPases and ADA on individual cells; and (c) levels of expression and functional coupling of purinergic receptors.

EFFECTS OF extATP ON THYMOCYTES AND CTLs

The detectable *in vitro* effects of extracellular nucleotides support their possible role in normal processes of thymocyte differentiation, expansion, and CTL effector functions. The effects of extATP and extAdo on T cells in vitro (2,3,20) implied their possible physiologic role in T cell development and expansion, but conclusive evidence is yet to be provided. The most compelling data are related to the effects of extAdo. Detailed studies of the effects of extracellular nucleotides revealed that extAdo suppresses practically all stages of CTL–T cell interaction and of lethal hit delivery, including such short-term, TCR-triggered effector functions of T lymphocytes as granule exocytosis, perforin- and Fas-mediated cytotoxicity by T killer cells, and lymphokine secretion by T-helper cells.

The cytotoxicity mediated by CTLs involves several steps, including the early biochemical events of TCR-mediated signaling, conjugate formation, and lethal hit delivery. The two complementary mechanisms of CTL-mediated cytotoxicity—exocytosis of perforin- and granzyme-containing cytotoxic granules (see related chapters in this book) and FasL/Fas receptor interactions—share the requirement for TCR triggering. The experiments described below show that extAdo was able to block both types of cytotoxicity. To study the susceptibility of Fas-mediated versus perforin-mediated and FasL/Fas cytotoxicity pathways to inhibition by extAdo, we took advantage of the availability of Fas-expressing and Fas-mediated death pathway-sensitive targets to test the lysis of such targets by perforin-deficient CTLs. It was found that extAdo and Ado analogs were able to inhibit the cytotoxicity of these CTLs against the antigen-bearing target cells in a dose-dependent manner.

It was important to determine whether inhibition of Fas-mediated cytotoxicity could be due to (a) inhibition of adhesion protein-mediated CTL target conjugate formation, (b) interference of extAdo in the intracellular processes of cell death in targets, or (c) inhibition of TCR-triggered FasL upregulation. The ability of extAdo to inhibit FasL-mediated cytotoxicity of CTLs in a retargeting assay excluded the effect of extAdo on CTL–target conjugate formation. The Ado and Ado analogs had no effect on the Fas-mediated death pathway even at high concentrations (5 mM), thereby excluding interference in the processes of cell death.

The competitive RT-PCR procedure for FasL mRNA detection (5) was used to test the effect of extAdo on FasL expression in CTLs. We found that TCR triggering results in upregulation of FasL mRNA expression and that the addition of extAdo dramatically decreased FasL expression on CTLs. Of interest is that extAdo inhibited expression of FasL mRNA not only in activated CTLs but also in untreated control cells. This finding suggests that levels of FasL mRNA expression in control, nonactivated CTLs possibly

reflect the basal level of TCR signaling during culture of CTL clones, which are also antagonized by extAdo.

Perforin-based, CTL-mediated cytotoxicity requires completion of exocytosis of perforin-containing cytolytic granules. We found that Ado analogs significantly inhibit TCR-triggered granule enzyme secretion. As expected, the inhibition of granule exocytosis in CTLs by Ado resulted in inhibition of target cell lysis by CTLs. The fact that Ado and Ado analogs were inhibitory suggests that signaling, rather than Ado degradation (metabolism) products, is responsible for these effects. Both antigen receptor-triggered exocytosis of cytotoxic granules and specific antigen-triggered T cell lysis were inhibited by extAdo. Extracellular Ado does not inhibit only short-term protein synthesis-independent effector functions, as a decrease in IL-2 secretion was observed after incubation of T cells with anti-TCR mAbs. Thus practically all tested TCR-triggered effector functions—but not the Fas-triggered process of programmed cell death—were inhibited by extAdo. These results are in agreement with our hypothesis that Ado receptor signaling could be the underlying mechanism of the immunosuppressive effects of increased concentrations of Ado.

The extAdo concentration is tightly controlled by ADA, and it was necessary to establish a plausible mechanism for the prolongation of the effects of Ado beyond its presence in the T cell environment. Accordingly, experiments were designed to resolve these difficulties by extrapolating *in vitro* effects of extAdo on lymphocytes to *in vivo* effects.

T CELL MEMORY OF EXPOSURE TO extADO AND TO ADO RECEPTOR-MEDIATED SIGNALING

In our earlier studies we found that extAdo-induced cAMP accumulation in T cells persists long after the original exposure to extAdo. This finding suggested the possible existence of a memory of exposure to extAdo due to Ado receptor-induced increases in [cAMP]. To test whether short exposure to extAdo would affect the subsequent TCR-triggered T cell activation, CTLs were pretreated with Ado or Ado analogs (or both) followed by removal of Ado; assays of T cell granule exocytosis and lymphokine secretion were then performed. A 10-minute preincubation was sufficient to observe inhibition of CTLs, and statistically significant inhibition was observed after only a 1- or 5-minute exposure of CTLs to extAdo. Exposure to Ado as short as 20 minutes caused inhibition of TCR-triggered IL-2 secretion after 20 hours of T cell incubation.

Thus even short-term exposure to Ado was sufficient to observe inhibition of TCR-triggered effector functions of T killer cells. The fact that the presence of extAdo with cells during a 4-hour assay did not significantly alter the extent of inhibition suggested that the maximal effects of Ado/second messenger-mediated changes were inflicted during short-term preincubation of T cells with Ado. Together, these data suggested that inhibition of the TCR-triggered effector functions of T cells is likely to be due to Ado receptor-mediated signaling and to cAMP accumulation that persists longer than the original exposure to Ado. The inhibition of TCR-triggered effector functions could be due to the lymphotoxicity of Ado or its analogs, but this alternative interpretation is not compatible with the rescue of exposed T cells from TCR-triggered inhibition of proliferation that we observed (5). Indeed, extAdo was able to prevent TCR-induced apoptosis (20) and inhibition of T cell proliferation (6). This overall rescuing effect of extAdo, which results in maintenance of the T cell's ability to proliferate, is not consistent with the widely accepted intracellular lymphotoxicity model of Ado action (21). It is unlikely that extAdo can reverse TCR signaling and inhibition of proliferation by being toxic or by inhibiting DNA synthesis.

In addition to being "remembered," the extAdo-triggered cAMP-mediated pathway is able to cross-talk with TCR-triggered bio-chemical pathways, which was suggested by the results of experiments in which various T cells were pretreated with immobilized anti-TCR mAbs and then exposed to extAdo to detect changes in cAMP. We found that pretreatment of normal, untransformed T cells (including *ex vivo* splenocytes and thymocytes and CTL clones) with anti-TCR–CD3 complex mAbs decreased extAdo-triggered cAMP accumulation. These data reflect cross-talk between TCR-triggered and extAdo/A_{2a} receptor-triggered biochemical pathways because TCR-triggered processes are inhibited by the A_{2a}/cAMP pathway, whereas A_{2a}-triggered cAMP accumulation was affected by TCR triggering.

We were unable to determine whether pretreatment with anti-TCR mAbs causes downregulation of A_{2a} extAdo receptors or affects the coupling of A_{2a} receptors with transmembrane signaling pathways in T cells. These experiments require the availability of mAbs specific to Ado receptors.

POSSIBLE ROLE OF extADO-MEDIATED INHIBITION OF TCR-TRIGGERED T CELL FUNCTIONS IN THE PATHOGENESIS OF HUMAN DISEASES

The exact regulatory role of purinergic receptors in a normal immune response remains to be established, but strong experimental data point to the role of these receptors in CTL activity in pathologic conditions: accumulation of extAdo under the hypoxic conditions in large solid tumors and in the absence of ADA, as in ADA SCID patients.

The effects of extAdo described above provide an additional explanation of SCID, which is observed in the absence or with levels of ADA in humans. ADA SCID is characterized by a hypoplastic thymus, T lymphocyte depletion, and autoimmunity. Whereas ADA deficiency causes increased levels of both intracellular and extracellular Ado, only the intracellular lymphotoxicity of accumulated Ado was discussed to explain ADA

SCID. We proposed a dual mechanism of ADA SCID in which the intracellular toxicity of increased concentrations of Ado causes the death of a large proportion of thymocytes, and extAdo-mediated signaling causes changes in the TCR repertoire of surviving thymocytes (20). This signaling mechanism explains both autoimmunity and T cell deficiency in ADA SCID.

Our current working model is based on the assumption that, under the conditions of ADA deficiency, thymocytes and T cells are exposed to the effects of both intracellular and extracellular Ado, with excess intracellular Ado being toxic and eventually lethal to many but not all T cells. The extAdo may act on surviving thymocytes through Ado receptors directly or by counteracting the TCR signaling important for thymocyte selection. This, in turn, could lead to abnormal positive and negative selection of thymocytes and to changes in the TCR repertoire of surviving T cells. Thus CTLs among surviving T cells in ADA SCID patients could be autoimmune or have "holes" in their TCR repertoire. Even otherwise normal CTLs would have their effector functions inhibited owing to extAdo-mediated signaling under ADA-deficient conditions.

The inhibition of both perforin-based and Fas-mediated cytotoxicity may explain failures of immunotherapy for large solid tumors with tumor-specific CTL clones in the mouse model because high concentrations of Ado were observed in the areas of solid tumors and were considered important in the inhibition of killer cells (22). Indeed, both CTL activation and expansion could be inhibited under hypoxic conditions, which are known to cause accumulation of extAdo. Expansion of CTLs could be inhibited in hypoxic areas, as we recently showed that TCR-triggered upregulation of CD25 (IL-2 receptor chain) and the CD25-dependent proliferation of peripheral T cells are strongly inhibited by low concentrations of extAdo (6). If the hypoxic condition in solid tumors causes accumulation of Ado and subsequent inhibition of antitumor CTLs, the

simultaneous addition of CTLs and preparations of ADA (to degrade the extAdo) may improve the antitumor activity of injected CTLs.

Together these data demonstrate that extAdo affects T cells at all stages of their differentiation, expansion, and effector functions and suggest that the final outcome of the immune response is at least partially determined by the biochemical parameters of individual tissues. Accordingly, the organs with the highest concentrations of Ado (e.g., with hypoxic conditions) are the least susceptible to effective immunosurveillance by T cells. *In vivo* conditions with increased concentrations of extAdo include hypoxic conditions and some pharmacologic interventions. The issue of naturally occurring hypoxic conditions in various tissues is under investigation.

REFERENCES

1. Filippini A, Taffs RE, Agui T, Sitkovsky MV. Ecto–ATPase activity in cytolytic T lymphocytes: protection from the cytolytic effects of extracellular ATP. *J Biol Chem* 1990;265:334–340.
2. Apasov S, Koshiba M, Redegeld F, Sitkovsky M. Role of extracellular ATP and P₁ and P₂ classes of purinergic receptors in T cell development and cytotoxic T lymphocyte effector functions. *Immunol Rev* 1995;146:5–19.
3. Apasov SG, Koshiba M, Chused TM, Sitkovsky MV. Effects of extracellular ATP and adenosine on different thymocyte subsets: possible role of ATP-gated channels and G protein-coupled purinergic receptors. *J Immunol* 1997;158:5095–5105.
4. Koshiba M, Apasov S, Sverdlov V, et al. Transient up–regulation of P_{2Y2} nucleotide receptor mRNA expression is an immediate early gene response in activated thymocytes. *Proc Natl Acad Sci USA* 1997;94:831–836.
5. Koshiba M, Kojima H, Huang S, Apasov S, Sitkovsky MV. Memory of extracellular adenosine/A_{2a} purinergic receptor-mediated signaling in murine T cells. *J Biol Chem* 1997;272:25881–25889.
6. Huang S, Koshiba M, Apasov S, Sitkovsky M. Role of A_{2a} adenosine receptor mediated signaling in inhibition of T cell activation and expansion. *Blood* 1997;90:1600–1610.
7. Vacchio MS, Papadopoulos V, Ashwell JD. Steroid production in the thymus: implications for thymocyte selection. *J Exp Med* 1994;179:1835–1846.
8. Abbracchio MP, Cattabeni F, Fredholm BB, Williams M. Purinoceptor nomenclature: a status report. *Drug Dev Res* 1993;28:207–213.
9. Abbracchio MP, Burnstock G. Purinoceptors: are

there families of P_{2X} and P_{2Y} purinoceptors? *Pharmacol Ther* 1994;64:445–475.

10. Dubyak GR, El-Moatassim C. Signal transduction via P_2-purinergic receptors for extracellular ATP and other nucleotides. *Am J Physiol* 1993;265:c577–c606.

11. Weisman G, De BK, Friedberg I, Pritchard RS, Heppel LA. Cellular responses to external ATP which precede an increase in nucleotide permeability in transformed cells. *J Cell Physiol* 1984; 119:211–219.

12. Lin J, Krishnaraj R, Kemp RG. Exogenous ATP enhances calcium influx in intact thymocytes. *J Immunol* 1985;135:3403–3410.

13. Zheng LM, Zychlinsky A, Liu CC, Ojcius DM, Young JD. Extracellular ATP as a trigger for apoptosis or programmed cell death. *J Cell Biol* 1991;112:279–288.

14. Zanovello P, Bronte V, Rosato A, Pizzo P, DiVirgilio F. Responses of mouse lymphocytes to extracellular ATP. II. Extracellular ATP causes cell type-dependent lysis and DNA fragmentation. *J Immunol* 1990;145:1545–1550.

15. Steinberg T, Newman AS, Swanson JA, Silverstein SC. ATP^{4-} permeabilizes the plasma membrane of mouse macrophages to fluorescent dyes. *J Biol Chem* 1987;262:8884–8888.

16. Filippini A, Taffs RE, Sitkovsky MV. Extracellular ATP in T lymphocyte activation: possible role in effector functions. *Proc Natl Acad Sci USA* 1990;87:8267–8271.

17. Chused TM, Apasov S, Sitkovsky MV. Murine T lymphocytes modulate activity of an ATP-activated P2z-type purinoreceptor during differentiation. *J Immunol* 1996;157:1371–1380.

18. Antonysamy MA, Moticka EJ, Ramkumar V. Adenosine acts as an endogenous modulator of IL-2 dependent proliferation of cytotoxic T lymphocytes. *J Immunol* 1995;155:2813–2821.

19. Smith P, Armstrong J, Koshiba M, Apasov S, Sitkovsky M. Caveats and promises in evaluation of functional effects of purinergic receptors in immune response. *Drug Dev Res* 1998;45:229–244.

20. Apasov S, Sitkovsky M. The extracellular versus intracellular mechanisms of inhibition of TCR-triggered activation in thymocytes by adenosine under conditions of inhibited adenosine deaminase. *Int Immunol* 1999;11:179–189.

21. Hirschhorn R. Adenosine deaminase deficiency. *Immunodefic Rev* 1990;2:175–198.

22. Hoskin DW, Reynolds T, Blay J. Adenosine as a possible inhibitor of killer T cell activation in the microenvironment of solid tumours. *Int J Cancer* 1994;59:854–855.

Cytotoxic Cells: Basic Mechanisms and Medical Applications, edited by Michail V. Sitkovsky and Pierre A. Henkart. Lippincott Williams & Wilkins, Philadelphia © 2000.

IV / CYTOTOXIC EFFECTOR MOLECULES

Chapter 9

Overview of Cytotoxic Lymphocyte Effector Mechanisms

Pierre A. Henkart

Lymphocyte Cytotoxicity Section, Experimental Immunology Branch, National Cancer Institute, National Institutes of Health, Bethesda, Maryland 20892, USA

Studies on the molecular mechanisms of cell death have exploded over the last few years, but immunologists have studied cytotoxic T lymphocyte (CTL)-induced cell death *in vitro* for about 30 years. When compared to other agents capable of inducing cell death *in vitro,* CTLs show two distinct and interesting properties. First, they kill their target cells rapidly, requiring several hours or in some cases minutes, not many hours or days. Second, their cytotoxic effect is highly selective, which is seen most dramatically in experiments showing that "innocent bystander" cells are not killed; that is, cells lacking antigens to which the CTLs have been sensitized are generally spared lethal injury even when they are mixed in the same cell pellet with targets that were killed. (There are interesting exceptions where some bystander killing is observed—discussed elsewhere in this book.) Historically, these two features of cell death induced by CTLs have placed severe constraints on mechanistic proposals to explain target death, and hypotheses involving secretion of soluble mediators now seem implausible. For example, lymphotoxin was originally described as a soluble cytotoxic "factor" in the supernatants of antigen-stimulated T cells, and it was considered a candidate mediator of CTL-induced cytotoxicity. However, because lymphotoxin did not kill target cells nearly as rapidly as CTLs and its activity did not possess the requisite antigen

specificity, it was not considered a plausible mediator. In light of this history, it is interesting to note that we now recognize that Fas ligand (FasL) and tumor necrosis factor (TNF), molecules related to lymphotoxin, can be expressed in a surface-anchored form on T cells, and that it potentially allows them to kill target cells rapidly and with the required antigenic specificity.

The apoptotic character of cell death triggered by CTLs was recognized by morphologic studies during the 1970s (1) and with measurements of target DNA release and breakdown during the early 1980s (2). These studies were done before the concept of apoptosis was widely accepted but were interpreted as evidence that the lytic mechanism used by cytotoxic lymphocytes was distinct from the other major immunologic cell death mediator, complement. It has subsequently been found that some target cell deaths induced by CTLs are not characterized by the complete syndrome of apoptotic characteristics. Thus the amount of DNA breakdown and apoptotic nuclear morphology accompanying target lysis seems to vary with the target cells (3). If one assumes that cell death mechanisms can be meaningfully divided into two nonoverlapping categories of apoptotic and necrotic, such data imply that cytotoxic lymphocytes use at least two distinct mechanisms to induce target cell death. The significance of the apoptotic features of target cell death is currently open to debate, as is discussed elsewhere in this volume.

PERFORIN-DEPENDENT GRANULE EXOCYTOSIS AND FasL/Fas: MAJOR *in vitro* pathways of target cell damage used by CTLs

Figure 9-1 illustrates the two major pathways used by cytotoxic lymphocytes to kill target cells. In the *perforin-dependent pathway,* perforin and other preformed cytotoxic mediators are stored in secretory granules until cytoplasmic signaling from cell surface receptors triggers exocytosis, which is fusion of the granule membrane with the plasma membrane. As a result of this membrane fusion, the granule membrane becomes part of the plasma membrane, and the granule contents are delivered to the exterior. This secretory process is analogous to mast cell degranulation and the release of neurotransmitters into synapses, and it can occur rapidly after signaling as it does not require transcription or translation.

In contrast, the *FasL/Fas pathway* utilizes FasL expressed on the surface of the effector cell to crosslink Fas on the target cell. In principle, this pathway can also operate via a soluble form of FasL that is not attached to the membrane. The FasL/Fas pathway appears to be inherently slower than the perforin-dependent pathway, and this kinetic difference explains why the latter pathway normally predominates in short-term (4 hour) assays. As shown in Figure 9-1, FasL can be transported to the surface by the degranulation process or by newly synthesized FasL molecules transported directly to the surface membrane after translation.

Studies on CTLs from perforin knockout mice revealed that the most rapid *in vitro* cytotoxic activity from CTLs and natural killer (NK) cells was dependent on perforin (4) and hence occurred via the perforin-

dependent granule exocytosis pathway. For classic alloreactive CTL-mediated cytotoxicity *in vitro,* a variable but generally minor level of activity was seen in the absence of perforin, depending on the target cell and the length of the assay. This residual activity was shown to be accounted for by the FasL/Fas pathway, using target cells from the *lpr* mouse strain naturally defective in Fas in conjunction with CTLs from perforin-deficient mice (5,6). When both pathways were crippled, cytotoxicity was negligible. For normal NK cells, the FasL/Fas pathway seems to play a negligible role; but after interleukin-2 (IL-2) activation NK cells can express FasL, which can be a significant component of cytotoxicity if the target cell expresses Fas.

In addition to the FasL/Fas pathway, other members of this ligand family and receptor family may play a role in cytotoxicity, particularly *in vivo*. The receptor family includes those with a death domain (TNFR1, DR3, DR4, DR5) whose ligation may give rise to caspase activation and cell death. The ligands binding these receptors can be soluble cytokines or can be expressed as surface molecules on effector cells (similar to FasL), allowing a multivalent and potent crosslinking signal to be delivered to target cells. Experiments designed to evaluate the role of TNF in the cytotoxicity by CD8[+] CTLs suggested that it plays no role in standard 4-hour *in vitro* assays but can contribute to cytotoxicity measured in longer-term assays (7). Studies have provided evidence for the involvement of TRAIL receptor in this family in cytotoxicity by CD4[+] CTLs based largely on the ability of an anti-TRAIL monoclonal antibody (mAb) to block tumor target-cell killing (8).

Cloned CD4[+] T cells express some granule components in common with CD8[+] T cells and undergo T cell receptor (TCR)-triggered granule exocytosis (9). Some cytotoxic CD4[+] T cells kill target cells predominantly by the granule exocytosis pathway (10), whereas others appear predominantly to use the FasL/Fas pathway (11).

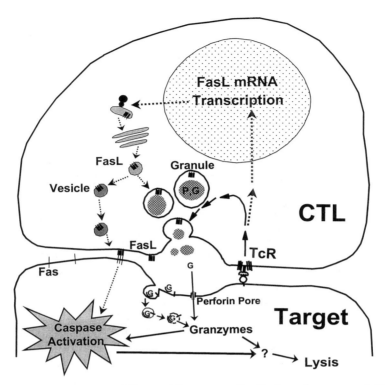

FIG. 9-1. Two pathways used by CTLs to kill target cells. Both pathways are initiated by TCR engagement of antigen on the target cell. Prior to the events shown here, TCR signaling induces cytoplasmic polarization, resulting in the secretory apparatus being oriented to face the bound target cell. The two cytotoxicity pathways share some immediate signaling steps after antigen recognition and then diverge. The granule exocytosis pathway (*solid arrows*) results in rapid release of the preformed proteins perforin and granzymes (*P, G*), initially bound to proteoglycan, into the synapse-like space between the effector and the target cell. There the ionic complex of perforin and granzymes dissolves, allowing perforin to undergo a calcium-induced conformational change and insert in the target membrane, oligomerize, and form pores. Granzymes may enter the target cell directly through the perforin pore or subsequent to endocytosis and endosome disruption. Once free in the cytoplasm, granzymes trigger both caspase-dependent and caspase-independent damage pathways. The FasL/Fas pathway, depicted with *dashed arrows,* is also initiated by the TCR. It results in FasL mRNA expression and de novo synthesis of the trimeric FasL membrane protein in the endoplasmic reticulum. This protein is processed by the Golgi apparatus, after which it is directed either directly to the plasma membrane via vesicles (*left side*) or to the granules where it can be released via a subsequent TCR stimulus. Trimeric surface FasL crosslinks Fas on the target cell, thereby triggering caspase activation via FADD and caspase-8, as shown in Figure 9-2. All target damage in the FasL/Fas pathway is blocked by caspase inhibitors.

PERFORIN-DEPENDENT PATHWAY

Lymphocyte Granules, Effector Polarization, Exocytosis

Rapid secretion of preformed mediators in response to stimuli occurs in many cell types and is associated with secretory granules, which release mediators via the process of exocytosis. Although lymphocytes are classically considered nongranular, it is now clear that CTLs contain a modest number of cytoplasmic granules that contain mediators associated with target cell death. Most cytokine secretion by T cells and NK cells has been thought to occur via the constitutive secretory pathway, which involves direct transport of newly synthesized proteins to the plasma membrane with no intracellular storage step. However, because chemokines can be secreted by a granule exocytosis pathway (see below), it is clear that lymphocyte granules can allow rapid, triggered secretion of diffusible mediators not directly involved in cytotoxicity.

The secretory granules of CTLs, though not numerous, can be seen by microscopy under favorable conditions. Naive CD8+ T cells do not contain granules, which develop during the differentiation process, leading to cytotoxic effector function. When NK effector cells were purified from blood, they were found to be larger than other resting lymphocytes with a moderate complement of cytoplasmic granules, giving rise to the term large granular lymphocyte (12). The existence of granules in CTLs was formerly contentious. Whereas cloned CTL lines cultured in IL-2 clearly possess cytoplasmic granules (13), the potently lytic CTLs found in vivo in the peritoneal cavity after rejection of allogeneic tumors appeared to be devoid of granules. Subsequent in vitro culture in IL-2 allowed the granules to be detected (14). However, earlier electron microscopy studies of such CTLs had revealed granules stained histochemically for lysosomal enzymes, with their activity being secreted by exocytosis after target cell engagement (15). This controversy emphasizes the difficulty of trying to detect low numbers of granules in lymphocytes where microscopic sections can easily miss the critical granule-containing region of cytoplasm. Evidence that these in vivo CTLs do have granules is inferred from their dramatic lack of functional activity against Fas-negative target cells in perforin knockout mice (4). Because perforin is released from the cell only by secretory pathways, and because CTL-mediated cytotoxicity occurs in the presence of inhibitors of RNA and protein synthesis, some preformed storage compartment must be present even if it is not recognized morphologically as granules.

The granules of CTLs are known largely from studies on in vitro cultured cells. They are typically 0.5 to 1.0 μm in diameter and have an internal structure consisting of two components. By electron microscopy the central core regions stain rather uniformly with moderate density and show some similarity to cores of mast cell granules. In some granules the cores are surrounded by a double membrane, whereas in others the cores are not bound by membranes (16). In addition to the cores, granules contain a typically cortical multivesicular region comprised of numerous membrane vesicles ranging from 30 to 150 nm in diameter. Some granules appear to contain no cores, whereas in others the cores appear to dominate the internal volume.

Studies using immunogold staining with electron microscopy have revealed that the granule cores contain perforin, granzymes, and proteoglycan; and the multivesicular regions contain soluble lysosomal enzymes and lysosomal membrane markers (16). By this approach the vesicles contain TCRs, CD8, and class I major histocompatibility complex (MHC-I) molecules. These membrane proteins are oriented with the normally extracellular domains facing the lumen of the granules, consistent with the hypothesis that they are derived from the plasma membrane by endocytosis. After an initial endocytic uptake event at the plasma membrane, endosomes fuse with granule membranes, followed by budding of the granule membranes to give rise to the observed intragranular vesicles.

As is typical for secretory granules, weak base pH probes show that CTL granules have an acidic interior, with an estimated internal pH of 5.4 (17). The proton pump maintaining this pH gradient can be blocked by concanamycin A, and the consequent neutralization of the granules selectively blocks cytotoxicity by the granule exocytosis pathway (18), a result of perforin inactivation and proteolytic degradation in the neutral pH granules (19).

As described above, secreted cytotoxic

mediators had for some years been regarded as implausible given the sparing of "innocent bystanders" lacking antigen. The granule exocytosis model accommodated these findings by proposing that the secretory process is highly polarized. Such polarization has been observed microscopically in both CTL and NK cells, as well as in helper-T cells, typically by using markers of granules or other cytoplasmic organelles, such as the microtubule organizing center. It has been found that target cell recognition induces rapid cellular polarization such that most of the cytoplasmic organelles in the CTLs are localized toward the bound target cell (20), a process dependent on extracellular calcium (21). Experiments indicate that it is regulated by cytoplasmic immunoreceptor tyrosine-based motifs (ITAMs) of the TCR complex (22), and there is a potential molecular linkage between adhesion receptors clustered near the TCR and the cytoskeleton (23).

Components of Cytotoxic Lymphocyte Granules

Cytotoxic lymphocyte granules have been purified from homogenates of cloned lymphocytes grown *in vitro*. When analyzed biochemically, such granules show a limited number of prominent protein bands. The most abundant proteins are perforin and the granzymes, components that have been studied for their functional role in target cell death. The biochemical properties of these components and their functional roles in cytotoxicity are discussed below.

One of the most appealing aspects of the granule exocytosis model is that the critical secretory process is in many respects highly analogous to that which occurs in mast cells and neutrophils. Thus studies of receptor-mediated signaling leading to degranulation in mast cells can be regarded as good models for the analogous process in CTLs, which themselves can be difficult to study because of the difficulty obtaining adequate numbers of purified cells.

Perforin

Perforin, also known as cytolysin or pore-forming protein, was originally believed to be solely responsible for target cell death via the granule exocytosis pathway, a view that has been modified with recognition of the importance of granzymes. Despite the currently different ideas about the details of how granule exocytosis leads to target death, there is agreement that perforin is necessary for target damage by this pathway.

A hallmark property of perforin is its ability to form pores in membranes; and because they are in many ways analogous to those formed by complement, it seemed plausible that target lysis would follow. The mechanism by which perforin forms membrane pores is still incompletely understood, but electron microscopy shows that the maximal pores appear large enough to allow passage of sizable proteins. Both purified perforin and complement are much more active in lysing red blood cells than nucleated cells, as was observed with effector cells secreting perforin without granzymes (24). As depicted in Figure 9-1, one explanation is that nucleated cells can rapidly endocytose patches of membrane containing inserted perforin, thereby avoiding diffusion of ions across the membrane and consequent osmotic lysis. Endocytosis by target cells can also result in the internal transport of surface-bound granzymes, and it has been proposed that this is the physiologic route of granzyme entry to the cytoplasm. In this case, perforin must mediate granzyme transport into the cytoplasm from endosomes, either by pore formation or by an uncharacterized endosome-disrupting activity of perforin.

Granzymes

The properties of granzymes have been previously reviewed (25–27), and studies of their role in target cell death are described elsewhere in this volume. Granzymes are a subfamily of serine proteases expressed in CTL granules. When several groups independently isolated genes selectively expressed in CTLs, about half of the discoveries turned out to be granzymes, showing that these proteases are among the major genes uniquely expressed by CTLs. The importance of granzymes for target cell death is inferred from experiments in which noncytotoxic rat basophilic leukemia cells were transfected to express various combinations of perforin, granzyme A, and granzyme B. Although perforin expression was adequate to allow potent cytotoxicity against red blood cell targets, both granzyme A and granzyme B were additionally required to confer strong cytotoxicity against tumor targets (28).

The various granzymes have several distinct proteolytic cleavage specificities: Granzyme A cleaves proteins after the basic amino acids arginine or lysine; granzyme B cleaves proteins after aspartic acid; and granzymes D, E, F, and G have a preference for cleavage at hydrophobic amino acids. Why such a variety of protease specificities is expressed in cytotoxic lymphocyte granules is still unexplained. Because mast cell granules also contain a variety of proteases implicated in inflammation (29), it is possible that at least some of the lymphocyte granule proteases have a parallel role and are not effector molecules for cytotoxicity.

Chemokines

In NK cells and CD8+ cloned CTLs, chemokines can be secreted via the "regulated secretory pathway" (i.e., by the same process of granule exocytosis used to deliver cytotoxic mediators) (30,31). Most chemokines are highly cationic, and it is likely that they are stored in granules as part of the insoluble core complexes held together by the electrostatic forces between the serglycin-linked glycosaminoglycans and the cationic proteins. Released chemokines, including the noncationic MIF-1α and MIF-1β, remain complexed to proteoglycans (31), but such complexes probably dissociate to yield free

chemokines, which can impair human immunodeficiency virus (HIV) replication by competing for viral co-receptors (32). Released chemokines rapidly amplify immune responses by recruiting other cells to the site where antigen is present and can themselves trigger further degranulation in the absence of antigen (33), suggesting a possible positive feedback loop. Chemokines enhance cytotoxicity and other lymphocyte activities, including proliferation and cytokine secretion (33,34).

Serglycin-Proteoglycans

As described above, granules contain an insoluble core that can be visualized by electron microscopy. This core is an electrostatic complex of cationic proteins with chrondroitin sulfate-containing proteoglycans covalently linked to the Ser-Gly repeat domain of the small protein termed serglycin (35). Electron microscopic immunolocalization studies showed that perforin and granzymes are in this core (36) along with a subset of mostly cationic granule components including the granzymes. Perforin is mildly cationic (pl is about 8), but there are several cationic peptide sequence motifs that could be involved in its interaction with proteoglycans; perforin binds to heparin affinity columns but is eluted before granzymes. After secretion the proteoglycan–protein core complex initially persists but then dissolves (presumably due to the change in pH and ionic environment); in mast cells, different proteases are solubilized from the analogous granule core at different rates, which has been proposed to be physiologically significant (37). Secreted serglycin-proteoglycans have the potential to crosslink CD44 and can function as activation co-stimulators (38).

Because proteoglycan binding to perforin inhibits its cytolytic activity, it may play a role in effector cell self-protection after degranulation. A satisfactory explanation for how this would selectively protect the effector cell has not been forthcoming, nor is there presently convincing experimental evidence in support of this hypothesis.

Lysosomal Enzymes

Lysosomal enzymes have been long known to be present in lymphocyte granules and to be secreted after antigen engagement (39). Lymphocyte activation is accompanied by an increase in lysosomal enzymes (40), attributable to upregulation of both transcription and translation (41). Electron microscopic histochemical studies showed that lysosomal enzymes are localized in the vesicular cortical region of granules. Because of their low pH optima, lysosomal enzymes may not be active in the extracellular environment after secretion. Lysosomal enzymes of other cells, such as fibroblasts, are also exocytosed in response to stimuli that increase intracellular Ca^{2+} (42). Although the physiologic role of this secretion is unclear, one could speculate that lysosome exocytosis is a means of eliminating undigestible material accumulated after intense endocytic activity.

Lysosomal cysteine proteases, including cathepsins B, H, and L, are unlikely to act as effector proteases in the manner of granzymes, as they have acidic pH optima and are unstable at neutral pH. These proteases seem designed to act within the granule, where (as described above) they may be involved in perforin processing. The dipeptidase DPPI (cathepsin C) removes hydrophobic dipeptides from the N-terminus of newly synthesized granzymes, a processing step required for expression of their enzymatic activity (43).

LAMP1 (CD107a) and LAMP2 (CD107b) are highly glycosylated lysosomal membrane proteins considered to be lysosomal membrane markers. Although they are not normally found on the cell surface, these markers are found to be surface-expressed on $CD56^+$ and $CD3^+$ human peripheral blood lymphocytes within 2 hours after *in vitro* phytohemagglutinin (PHA) activation (44). They are also found on peripheral blood mononuclear cells (PBMCs) from patients with

autoimmune diseases, where *in vivo* antigen activation may have occurred. In PHA-treated lymphocytes, significant expression is still seen in a subpopulation of cells 96 hours later. Cell surface LAMP2 mediates adhesion of activated PBMCs to vascular endothelial cells, possibly via endothelial selectins.

TNF Family Proteins

TNF family proteins can be secreted by the granule exocytosis pathway. They include FasL and are discussed below.

CTLA-4

CTLA-4 was originally identified as a gene selectively expressed in CTLs and has been recognized to function as a negative regulator of T lymphocyte activation (45). It is rapidly but transiently expressed on T cell surfaces after activation. As seen by fluorescent immunolocalization, CTLA-4 is primarily expressed as an intracellular membrane protein with a perinuclear expression pattern, and it co-localizes with perforin in vesicles polarized toward the direction of TCR engagement (46). After exposure on the surface membrane, CTLA-4 is rapidly reinternalized via clathrin-coated vesicles (47), which recycle the CTLA-4 to the granule-associated secretory compartment. This recycling activity is compatible with the dual secretory and endolysosomal nature of granules.

Granulysin

A relatively new type of granule mediator has been described in both NK cells and CTLs and has been suggested to play a role in target cell damage and the destruction of microorganisms (48). Two groups have studied this family for some time, starting in one case with porcine NK cells and isolating a small protein with antibacterial activity termed NK lysin (49), or starting with human CTLs and using a subtractive cDNA approach to isolate and characterize a protein termed granulysin with multiple mRNA species (50). This granule mediator is described in detail in Chapter 15.

FasL/Fas CYTOTOXICITY PATHWAY

The second major cytotoxicity pathway used by CTLs is the FasL/Fas pathway. This pathway critically depends on Fas expression on the target cell surface. Because studies have shown that Fas appears to be expressed in many tissues *in vivo* (51), it has the potential to play an important physiologic role. In contrast to Fas, FasL is expressed only under restricted circumstances. Early studies showed activated T lymphocytes to be unique in their high FasL expression, although in recent years FasL has been reported in other sites, particularly in tissues associated with "immune privilege," in tumors, and in sites of inflammation. In both $CD4^+$ and $CD8^+$ T cells, FasL mRNA appears to be transiently expressed after TCR engagement, and in some cells the newly transcribed protein is rapidly expressed on the plasma membrane to allow cytotoxic effector function by the FasL/Fas pathway. The TCR-triggered upregulation of FasL mRNA is described in Chapters 16 and 17.

The FasL is part of the TNF family of cytokines that signal cells via a family of specific receptors. One unusual property of the TNF lymphokine family is that the soluble proteins are secreted via a surface membrane intermediate, which is subsequently cleaved by a protease to release the soluble form of the protein. Although FasL and TNF have been generally thought to be expressed on the membrane via the constitutive secretory pathway after upregulation of their transcription, a granule-delivered pathway has been suggested by a study in which FasL was immunolocalized to granules of both NK and CTL cell lines (52). Domain-swapping experiments show that the FasL cytoplasmic domain contains a motif that can target the plasma membrane protein CD69 for localization in the secretory granules of transfected rat basophilic leukemia (RBL) cells, arguing that newly synthesized FasL goes directly to granules rather than arriving there after surface expression and subsequent endocytosis (52). Previous work showing that T cell FasL surface expression requires de novo mRNA and protein synthesis was largely derived from T hybridoma cells, which contain no granules. Despite the clear demonstration that FasL is found in granules in cloned lymphocytes, it is not yet clear whether such effector molecules are functional or are bound to Fas and hence functionally "neutralized." Fas expression in granules is not implausible given the demonstration that a variety of cell surface proteins are found there, apparently derived from endocytic activity consistent with the dual function of these secretory granules as endolysosomes (53).

Cytotoxic effector cells can express functional FasL in three distinct forms. The first and "classic" form is as an effector surface membrane protein. A second way the FasL membrane protein can be presented is on a membrane vesicle derived from granules. The release of such granule-derived vesicles by exocytosis has been described (16,54); and because TCR has been detected in such vesicles they could thus act as specific delivery vehicles for FasL to cells expressing TCR-recognized MHC–peptide complexes. The third form of FasL that effector cells may express is the soluble trimer, which is released from either of the above two membrane forms. Such a soluble FasL could be produced by the metalloprotease described (55), by lysosomal cathepsins in effector cell granules, or conceivably by granzymes from these granules. A precedent for FasL expression via granule exocytosis was found earlier in mast cells, where TNF-α is secreted after IgE crosslinking via both exocytosis of preformed TNF-α in granules and a more sustained constitutive secretory pathway route (56). It seems likely that both secretory pathways can operate for all the cytotoxic lymphocyte granule components (57).

FasL expression on effector cells may not be sufficient to deliver a functional death signal to any target cell it contacts. This issue arises in consideration of bystander lysis; and in some cases it appears that FasL expression is inadequate to mediate such lysis and that adhesion molecules must also be engaged (58).

Fas DEATH PATHWAY

Evidence that the Fas death pathway plays a physiologic role in the immune system comes from studies of natural and induced muta-tions in Fas and FasL. These mutations, in both the mouse and humans, give rise to lymphoproliferative and autoimmune syn-dromes, which argues strongly that this death pathway regulates immune responses (59,60). Further evidence suggesting that this pathway is important comes from findings that specific inhibitors blocking several steps of this pathway have evolved in a number of circumstances. The first level of blocking by these inhibitors is Fas crosslinking itself. A soluble "decoy receptor" termed DcR3 has been described that competes for FasL bind-ing and thus blocks effective crosslinking of functional Fas (61) (Fig. 9-2). DcR3 mRNA

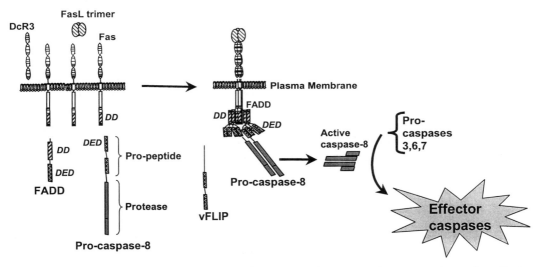

FIG. 9-2. FasL/Fas cytotoxicity pathway. FasL, expressed as a membrane protein on the effector cell or as the soluble form shown, spontaneously trimerizes. Upon binding to Fas, trimeric FasL triggers its oligomerization, which is the critical step in initiating signaling. One inhibitor of this system is the decoy receptor DcR3, a soluble member of the TNFR family that binds FasL, although it is not closely homologous to Fas in sequence. External crosslinking of membrane-bound Fas results in the close approximation of its cytoplasmic death domains (DDs). This fosters the binding of cytoplasmic DD-containing FADD adaptor molecules via like–like interactions, forming a complex on the internal portion of the membrane. The death effector domain (DED) of FADD now becomes oligomerized in this complex and binds to the DED on procaspase-8, again through like–like interac-tions. This step is potentially inhibited by DED-containing FLIP molecules, illustrated by vFLIP, which act as "dominant negative" competitors for the recruitment of procaspase-8. When multiple procaspase-8 molecules are recruited into the multiprotein complex, they autoactivate by proteolytic processing to form active caspase-8. This active caspase has lost its propeptide and is free to diffuse into the cytoplasm, where it can then process effector procaspases 3, 6, and 7. These effector caspases can cleave several cellular proteins important for maintenance of cell viability. This scheme omits a potential amplification step involving mitochondria and procaspase-9, which is required in some cells.

was found to be expressed in a variety of normal tissues and in several tumor cell lines. A remarkable finding was that the *DcR3* gene was found to be amplified in a sizable number of human cancer cell lines, suggesting that increased expression of *DcR3* may have been a selection factor that allows the tumor to escape *in vivo* Fas-based immune destruction.

The death pathway induced by crosslinking of surface Fas receptors has been elucidated more completely than other intracellular death pathways (62) and is a notable example of a well understood signal transduction process. As depicted in Figure 9-2, the initial event in this pathway is Fas crosslinking by the trimeric FasL, which oligomerizes the previously monomeric Fas molecules in the membrane. The cytoplasmic tail of Fas (as well as TNFR1 and several other TNFR family members) contains a protein domain known as a death domain (DD), which in its oligomerized form recruits soluble FADD adaptor molecules to form a complex at the cytoplasmic face of the membrane. FADD contains DD homologous to the DD of Fas, and these bind to the other DDs in the complex. The death effector domains (DEDs) in complexed FADD, in turn, recruit procaspase-8 by binding to the DED in the pro-region of this caspase. After oligomerization, procaspase-8 is able to autoactivate by self-processing to produce a freely soluble caspase-8, which in turn leads to a caspase activation cascade, including effector caspases 3, 6, and 7. It seems likely that cleavage of any one of several caspase substrates could lead to death. The importance of caspases in this pathway is shown by the blocking of all measurable target damage by caspase inhibitors (63).

Effective crosslinking of Fas by FasL does not ensure target cell death, as the downstream elements in the death pathway can be blocked by cytoplasmic inhibitors. In addition to more general inhibitors of apoptosis, such as the Bcl-2 family and IAPs, cell death via the DD-containing receptors can specifically be inhibited by naturally oc-curring "dominant negative" molecules that contain DEDs. The DEDs in these inhibitors (known by a variety of names including FLIPs) interacts with the DEDs in FADD molecules in the membrane complex (Fig. 9-2), blocking the recruitment of procaspase-8. FLIPs occur in two forms, cellular FLIPs (cFLIPs), expressed by T cells after activation, and viral FLIPs (vFLIPs), expressed by viruses during their intracellular infective cycle. Although FLIPs were originally described as inhibitors of this death pathway, in some cases FLIP expression can enhance death, perhaps by enhancing complex formation. In any case, FLIPs provide another mechanism that allows some target cells to become resistant to Fas-mediated death; and the functional status of this pathway, in particular Fas-bearing target cells, should be ascertained in cytotoxicity assays with highly multivalent Fas crosslinkers (FasL or anti-Fas).

Because of the importance of the FasL/Fas pathway in regulating immune responses, it is not easy to use the Fas or FasL natural mutations or knockout mice to assess the importance of this pathway as an effector mechanism for cytotoxic lymphocytes *in vivo*. However, the finding that both tumor cells and virally infected cells express inhibitors of this cytotoxicity pathway suggests that it plays an *in vivo* role in controlling these two abnormal cell systems classically ascribed to cytotoxic lymphocytes.

REFERENCES

1. Sanderson CJ, Glaueret AM. The mechanism of T cell mediated cytotoxicity. V. Morphological studies by electron microscopy. *Proc R Soc Lond* 1977; 198:315–323.
2. Russell JH. Internal disintegration model of cytotoxic lymphocyte-induced target damage. *Immunol Rev* 1983;72:97–118.
3. Sellins KS, Cohen JJ. Cytotoxic T lymphocytes induce different types of DNA damage in target cells of different origins. *J Immunol* 1991;147:795–803.
4. Kagi D, Ledermann B, Burki K, et al. Cytotoxicity mediated by T cells and natural killer cells is greatly impaired in perforin-deficient mice. *Nature* 1994; 369:31–37.

5. Kagi D, Vignaux F, Ledermann B, et al. Fas and perforin pathways as major mechanisms of T cell-mediated cytotoxicity. *Science* 1994;265:528–530.

6. Lowin B, Hahne M, Mattmann C, Tschopp J. Cytolytic T-cell cytotoxicity is mediated through perforin and Fas lytic pathways. *Nature* 1994;370:650–652.

7. Ratner A, Clark WR. Role of TNF-α in CD8$^+$ cytotoxic T lymphocyte-mediated lysis. *J Immunol* 1993;150:4303–4314.

8. Thomas WD, Hersey P. TNF-related apoptosis-inducing ligand (TRAIL) induces apoptosis in Fas ligand-resistant melanoma cells and mediates CD4 T cell killing of target cells. *J Immunol* 1998; 161:2195–2200.

9. Taplits MS, Henkart PA, Hodes RJ. T helper cell cytoplasmic granules: exocytosis in response to activation via the T cell receptor. *J Immunol* 1988; 141:1–9.

10. Williams NS, Engelhard VH. Identification of a population of CD4$^+$ CTL that utilizes a perforin-rather than a Fas ligand-dependent cytotoxic mechanism. *J Immunol* 1996;156:153–159.

11. Stalder T, Hahn S, Erb P. Fas antigen is the major target molecule for CD4$^+$ T cell-mediated cytotoxicity. *J Immunol* 1994;152:1127–1133.

12. Timonen T, Ortaldo JR, Herberman RB. Characteristics of human large granular lymphocytes and relationship to natural killer and K cells. *J Exp Med* 1981;153:569–582.

13. Griffiths G. The cell biology of CTL killing. *Curr Opin Immunol* 1995;7:343–348.

14. Berke G, Rosen D. Highly lytic in vivo primed cytolytic T lymphocytes devoid of lytic granules and BLT-esterase activity acquire these constituents in the presence of T cell growth factors upon blast transformation in vitro. *J Immunol* 1988;141:1429–1436.

15. David A, Bernard J, Thiernesse N, Nicolas G, Cerottini JC, Zagury D. Le processus d'exocytose lysosomale est-il responsable de l'action cytolytique des lymphocytes T tuers? *CR Acad Sci Paris* [D] 1979;288:441–444.

16. Peters PJ, Borst J, Oorschot V, et al. Cytotoxic T lymphocyte granules are secretory lysosomes, containing both perforin and granzymes. *J Exp Med* 1991;173:1099–1109.

17. Burkhardt JK, Hester S, Lapham CK, Argon Y. The lytic granules of natural killer cells are dual-function organelles combining secretory and pre-lysosomal compartments. *J Cell Biol* 1990;111:2327–2340.

18. Kataoka T, Shinohara N, Takayama H, et al. Concanamycin A, a powerful tool for characterization and estimation of contributed of perforin- and Fas-based lytic pathways in cell-mediated cytotoxicity. *J Immunol* 1996;156:3678–3686.

19. Kataoka T, Togashi K, Takayama H, Takaku K, Nagai K. Inactivation and proteolytic degradation of perforin within lytic granules upon neutralization of acidic pH. *Immunology* 1997;91:493–500.

20. Kupfer A, Singer SJ. Cell biology of cytotoxic and helper T cell functions: immunofluorescence microscopic studies of single cells and cell couples. *Annu Rev Immunol* 1989;7:309–337.

21. Kupfer A, Dennert G, Singer SJ. The reorientation of the Golgi apparatus and the microtubule-organizing center in the cytotoxic effector cell is a prerequisite in the lysis of bound target cells. *J Mol Cell Immunol* 1985;2:37–49.

22. Lowin-Kropf B, Shapiro VS, Weiss A. Cytoskeletal polarization of T cells is regulated by an immunoreceptor tyrosine-based activation motif-dependent mechanism. *J Cell Biol* 1998;140:861–871.

23. Dustin ML, Olszowy MW, Holdorf AD, et al. A novel adaptor protein orchestrates receptor patterning and cytoskeletal polarity in T-cell contacts. *Cell* 1998;94:667–677.

24. Shiver JW, Henkart PA. A noncytotoxic mast cell tumor line exhibits potent IgE-dependent cytotoxicity after transfection with the cytolysin/perforin gene. *Cell* 1991;62:1174–1181.

25. Pham CT, Ley TJ. The role of granzyme B cluster proteases in cell-mediated cytotoxicity. *Semin Immunol* 1997;9:127–133.

26. Darmon AJ, Bleackley RC. Proteases and cell-mediated cytotoxicity. *Crit Rev Immunol* 1998; 18:255–273.

27. Smyth MJ, O'Connor MD, Trapani JA. Granzymes: a variety of serine protease specificities encoded by genetically distinct subfamilies. *J Leukoc Biol* 1996;60:555–562.

28. Nakajima H, Park HL, Henkart PA. Synergistic roles of granzymes A and B in mediating target cell death by RBL mast cell tumors also expressing cytolysin/perforin. *J Exp Med* 1995;181:1037–1046.

29. Huang C, Sali A, Stevens RL. Regulation and function of mast cell proteases in inflammation. *J Clin Immunol* 1998;18:169–183.

30. Greenberg AH, Khalil N, Pohajdak B, Talgoy M, Henkart P, Orr FW. NK-leukocyte chemotactic factor (NK-LCF): a large granular lymphocyte (LGL) granule-associated chemotactic factor. *J Immunol* 1986;137:3224–3230.

31. Wagner L, Yang OO, Garcia-Zepeda EA, et al. Beta-chemokines are released from HIV-1 specific cytolytic T cell granules complexed to proteoglycans. *Nature* 1998;391:908–911.

32. Cocchi F, DeVico AL, Garzino-Demo A, Arya SK, Gallo RC, Lusso P. Identification of RANTES, MIP-1 alpha, and MIP-1 beta as the major HIV-suppressive factors produced by CD8$^+$ T cells. *Science* 1995;270:1811–1815.

33. Taub DD, Sayers TJ, Carter CRD, Ortaldo JR. Alpha and beta chemokines induce NK cell migration and enhance NK-mediated cytolysis. *J Immunol* 1995;155:3877–3888.

34. Taub DD, Ortaldo JR, Turcovski-Corrales SM, Key ML, Longo DL, Murphy WJ. Beta chemokines costimulate lymphocyte cytolysis, proliferation, and lymphokine production. *J Leukoc Biol* 1996; 59:81–89.

35. Stevens RL, Kamada MM, Serafin WE. Structure and function of the family of proteoglycans that reside in the secretory granules of natural killer cells and other effector cells of the immune response. *Curr Top Microbiol Immunol* 1989;140:93–108.

36. Masson D, Peters PJ, Geuze HJ, Borst J, Tschopp J. Interaction of chondroitin sulfate with perforin and granzymes of cytolytic T cells is dependent on pH. *Biochemistry* 1990;29:11229–11235.

37. Ghildyal N, Friend DS, Stevens RL, et al. Fate of two mast cell tryptases in V3 mastocytosis and normal BALB/c mice undergoing passive systemic anaphylaxis: prolonged retention of exocytosed mMCP-6 in connective tissues, and rapid accumulation of enzymatically active mMCP-7 in the blood. *J Exp Med* 1996;184:1061–1073.

38. Gullberg U, Andersson E, Garwicz D, Lindmark A, Olsson I. Biosynthesis, processing and sorting of neutrophil proteins: insight into neutrophil granule development. *Eur J Haematol* 1997;58:137–153.

39. Thiernesse N, David A, Bernard J, Jeanesson P, Zagury D. Activitie phosphatasique acide de la cellule T cytolytique au cours du processus de cytolyse. *CR Acad Sci Paris* [D] 1977;285:713–715.

40. Olsen I, Bou-Gharios G, Abraham D. The activation of resting lymphocytes is accompanied by the biogenesis of lysosomal organelles. *Eur J Immunol* 1990;20:2161–2170.

41. Olsen I, Adams G, Watson G, Chain B, Abraham D. Multi-level regulation of lysosomal gene expression in lymphocytes. *Biochem Biophys Res Commun* 1993;195:327–335.

42. Rodriguez A, Webster P, Ortego J, Andrews NW. Lysosomes behave as Ca^{+2}-regulated exocytic vesicles in fibroblasts and epithelial cells. *J Cell Biol* 1997;137:93–104.

43. McGuire MJ, Lipsky PE, Thiele DL. Generation of active myeloid and lymphoid granule serine proteases requires processing by the granule thiol protease dipeptidyl peptidase I. *J Biol Chem* 1993;268:2458–2467.

44. Kannan K, Stewart RM, Bounds W, et al. Lysosome-associated membrane proteins h-LAMP1 (CD107a) and h-LAMP2 (CD107b) are activation-dependent cell surface glycoproteins in human peripheral blood mononuclear cells which mediate cell adhesion to vascular endothelium. *Cell Immunol* 1996;171:10–19.

45. Greenfield EA, Nguyen KA, Kuchroo VK. CD28/B7 costimulation: a review. *Crit Rev Immunol* 1998;18:389–418.

46. Linsley PS, Bradshaw J, Greene J, Peach R, Bennett KL, Mittler RS. Intracellular trafficking of CTLA-4 and focal localization towards sites of TcR engagement. *Immunity* 1996;4:535–543.

47. Chuang E, Alegre ML, Duckett CS, Noel PJ, Vander Heiden MG, Thompson CB. Interaction of CTLA-4 with the clathrin-associated protein AP50 results in ligand-independent endocytosis that limits cell surface expression. *J Immunol* 1997;159:144–151.

48. Stenger S, Hanson DA, Teitelbaum R, et al. An antimicrobial activity of cytolytic T cells mediated by granulysin. *Science* 1998;282:121–125.

49. Andersson M, Gunne H, Agerberth B, et al. NK-lysin, a novel effector peptide of cytotoxic T and NK cells: structure and cDNA cloning of the porcine form, induction by interleukin 2, antibacterial and antitumor activity. *EMBO J* 1995;14:1615–1625.

50. Pena SV, Krensky AM. Granulysin, a new human cytolytic granule-associated protein with possible involvement in cell-mediated cytotoxicity. *Semin Immunol* 1997;9:117–125.

51. Leithauser F, Dhein J, Mechtersheimer G, et al. Constitutive and induced expression of APO-1, a new member of the nerve growth factor/tumor necrosis factor receptor superfamily, in normal and neoplastic cells. *Lab Invest* 1993;69:415–429.

52. Bossi G, Griffiths GM. Degranulation plays an essential part in regulating cell surface expression of Fas ligand in T cells and natural killer cells. *Nat Med* 1999;5:90–96.

53. Peters PJ, Geuze HJ, Donk HA, et al. Molecules relevant for T cell-target cell interaction are present in cytolytic granules of human T lymphocytes. *Eur J Immunol* 1989;19:1469–1475.

54. Henkart MP, Henkart PA. Lymphocyte mediated cytolysis as a secretory process. *Adv Exp Med Biol* 1982;146:227–242.

55. Kayagaki N, Kawasaki A, Ebata T, et al. Metalloproteinase-mediated release of human Fas ligand. *J Exp Med* 1995;182:1777–1783.

56. Gordon JR, Galli SJ. Release of both preformed and newly synthesized tumor necrosis factor α (TNF-α)/cachectin by mouse mast cells stimulated via the Fo$_g$RI: a mechanism for the sustained action of mast cell-derived TNF-α during IgE-dependent biological responses. *J Exp Med* 1991;174:103–107.

57. Isaaz S, Baetz K, Olsen K, Podack E, Griffiths GM. Serial killing by cytotoxic T lymphocytes: T cell receptor triggers degranulation, re-filling of the lytic granules and secretion of lytic proteins via a non-granule pathway. *Eur J Immunol* 1995;25:1071–1079.

58. Kojima H, Eshima K, Takayama H, Sitkovsky MV. Leukocyte function-associated antigen-1-dependent lysis of Fas$^+$ (CD95$^+$/Apo-1$^+$) innocent bystanders by antigen-specific CD8$^+$ CTL. *J Immunol* 1997;159:2728–2734.

59. Straus SE, Sneller M, Lenardo MJ, Puck JM, Strober W. An inherited disorder of lymphocyte apoptosis: the autoimmune lymphoproliferative syndrome. *Ann Intern Med* 1999;130:591–601.

60. Nagata S. Human autoimmune lymphoproliferative syndrome, a defect in the apoptosis-inducing Fas receptor: a lesson from the mouse model. *J Hum Genet* 1998;43:2–8.

61. Pitti RM, Marsters SA, Lawrence DA, et al. Genomic amplification of a decoy receptor for Fas ligand in lung and colon cancer. *Nature* 1998;396:699–703.

62. Ashkenazi A, Dixit VM. Death receptors: signaling and modulation. *Science* 1998;281:1305–1308.

63. Sarin A, Williams MS, Alexander-Miller MA, Berzofsky JA, Zacharchuk CM, Henkart PA. Target cell lysis by CTL granule exocytosis is independent of ICE/Ced-3 family proteases. *Immunity* 1997;6:209–215.

Cytotoxic Cells: Basic Mechanisms and Medical Applications, edited by Michail V. Sitkovsky and Pierre A. Henkart. Lippincott Williams & Wilkins, Philadelphia © 2000.

Chapter 10

Control of Perforin Gene Expression: A Paradigm for Understanding Cytotoxic Lymphocytes?

Mathias G. Lichtenheld

Department of Microbiology and Immunology, University of Miami, School of Medicine, Miami, Florida 33101, USA

Cytotoxic lymphocytes comprise crucial effector cells in both the first and second lines of defense against intracellular pathogens (1, 2). The first line of defense, or the innate cytotoxic reaction, is largely orchestrated by natural killer (NK) cells ready to kill various targets. The second line of defense, or the adaptive cytotoxic response, relies on activation of the immune system, which triggers conventional cytotoxic T lymphocytes (CTLs) [i.e., $CD8^+$ and TCR α/β^+ T cells that recognize antigen in the context of major histocompatibility complex class I (MHC-I)] to mature into antigen-specific killer cells. Common to both arms of the cytotoxic offensive is the expression of perforin, one of the molecules in the arsenal of weapons employed during lymphocyte-mediated cytotoxicity (3). The constitutively high expression of perforin by NK cells mirrors the innate component of cytotoxicity. The low but inducible expression of perforin in CTLs resembles the adaptive component of lymphocyte-mediated cytolysis. The development of armed NK cells and the activation of CTLs leading to their differentiation from impotent preeffector CTL into armed effector CTL may be coordinated by the activation of numerous gene products. Most of these products, such as molecules governing the cell cycle, are common to all cell types. On the other hand, a few gene products, such as perforin and certain granzymes, are involved in the acquisition of the specific immune function of NK cells and CTLs. They are expressed primarily by cytotoxic lymphocytes in contrast to other mediators of cytotoxicity, such as fas ligand. Therefore, understanding the control of the perforin gene is an excellent paradigm for elucidating which receptors, second messenger pathways, and nuclear events are involved in these processes. Knowledge is just emerging in these areas compared with what already has been learned about the regulation of other genes related to the activation of T-helper function. Eventually, the design of therapeutic strategies aimed at harnessing undesired responses of cytotoxic lymphocytes in transplant and autoimmunity settings or boosting responses against tumors and viral infections may integrate, and perhaps even evolve from, some of the available and forthcoming investigations.

Progress during the last decade since the isolation of the first molecular tools (4,5) required to decipher where, when, and how the perforin gene is expressed is summarized here in four parts. In support of the paradigm, "Perforin Expression in Disease and as a Diagnostic Marker," the first part highlights recent findings on the activation and local recruitment of cytotoxic lymphocytes as determined by the presence of perforin-expressing cells *in situ*. The diagnostic potential and limitations are discussed. The second part, "Cell-Type Specificity of Perforin Expression," emphasizes that the spectrum of perforin-expressing cells goes beyond NK cells and conventional CTLs. The third part, "Signals Regulating Perforin Gene Expression," stresses the importance of cytokine stimuli over T cell receptor (TCR) signals for activation of the perforin gene. The fourth part, "Transcriptional Control of the Perforin Gene," dissects the levels of regulation of perforin gene expression and highlights the *cis*- and *trans*-acting molecules, including ongoing work in our laboratory. All told, many aspects of cytotoxic lymphocytes can be learned by studying the control of perforin despite—and because of—its complexity.

PERFORIN EXPRESSION IN DISEASE AND AS A DIAGNOSTIC MARKER

The local expression of perforin in lymphocytic infiltrates *in situ* has been investigated in humans, mice, and rats in all general scenarios where lymphocyte-mediated cytotoxicity is known to occur (i.e., during virus infection, transplant rejection, and in some cases tumor rejection). Situations have been analyzed also where cytotoxicity could be suspected, namely autoimmune tissue destruction. The functional and historic hallmark of cytotoxic lymphocytes, their elimination of virus-infected cells (1), was one of the first scenarios to be investigated to validate the concept that the local expression of perforin *in situ*, either at the RNA or the protein level, can be a marker for the recruitment and activation of cytotoxic lymphocytes (6,7). These original observations beautifully represent the exponentially growing literature on the *in situ* expression of perforin in diverse clinical settings. The infection of mice with lymphotropic choriomeningitis virus (LCMV) is a well established and charac-

terized model for studying cytolytic immune responses *in vivo*. When mice are infected with a hepatotropic LCMV strain, perforin-expressing CD8[+] lymphocytes begin to infiltrate the liver. About 1 week later the organ is maximally filled with CTLs, at which point an LCMV-specific cytolytic response can be detected *in vitro*. Analogous findings are made when a different LCMV strain is inoculated intracerebrally, with the exception that the tropism of the infiltrate now becomes the meningi and the choroid plexus. At least in this instance, the appearance of perforin-expressing cells at the site of the antigen coincides with a cytotoxic response.

Other instances presumably reflecting events analogous to those described for LCMV are listed in Table 10-1, which incorporates investigations of the *in situ* expression of perforin in human diseases. The table is subdivided according to the assumed nature of the antigen (i.e., virus, transplant, tu-

TABLE 10-1. In situ *accumulation of perforin-expressing cells in human disease*

Virus
  Cytomegalovirus pneumonitis (8)
  Meningoencephalitis (9)
  Skin (10)
  Chronic hepatitis C (11)
Transplant
  Heart (12–15)
  Lung (16)
  Kidney (17–20)
  GVHD—skin (21,22)
Tumor
  Colorectal cancer (23)
  Follicular B cell lymphoma (24)
  EBV-associated gastric carcinoma (25)
Autoimmune or other
  Rheumatoid arthritis (26–28)
  Hashimoto's thyroiditis (29)
  Graves' disease (29)
  Sjögren syndrome (30)
  Takayasu's arteritis (31)
  Erythema multiforme (10)
  Ulcerative colitis (32)
  Crohn's disease (32)
  Polymyositis (33,34)
  Idiopathic cardiomyopathy (35)
  Alcoholic chronic pancreatitis (36)

Examples are given according to the nature of the antigen.
GVHD, graft-verus-host disease; EBV, Epstein-Barr virus.

mor, or, presumably, autoantigen). The variety of the diseases symbolizes that activation of the perforin gene during an immune response is a common theme rather than a unique event. Elevated numbers of perforin-positive cells can be found not only locally but also in peripheral blood mononuclear cells (PBMCs) of patients undergoing virus infections, transplant rejections, or autoimmune disease (9,37–44).

As intriguing as all these studies are, it is important to emphasize their limits of interpretation. Detection of a local accumulation of perforin-expressing cells is consistent with an immune response but does not necessarily imply that cytotoxic lymphocytes are an essential component of the disease process or that the expression of perforin is the essential mediator. Such conclusions should be reserved for experiments employing cells or animals that are deficient in perforin or other molecules (see Chapter 11). Many investigations have established the cell-surface phenotype of the perforin-expressing cells as a conventional CTL (i.e., CD8$^+$ T cell), but other cell types expressing perforin also were observed. Notably, a predominant CD4$^+$ and perforin-expressing T-cell infiltrate, or expansion in the blood, appears in several of the autoimmune diseases (29,32,44). This observation together with the possibility of perforin expression by other lymphoid lineages (see Cell-Type Specificity of Perforin Expression, below) emphasizes the relevance of establishing the phenotypes of the perforin-expressing cells, which may help us understand the immunologic component of a particular disease. Similarly, many of these analyses are snapshots and may not truly represent the entire dynamics of a cytotoxic response. Finally, in regard to the analysis of PBMCs, it is important to take into consideration that healthy individuals maintain a large and variable number of CTLs in the perforin-expressing effector stage (see Cell-Type Specificity of Perforin Expression, below). In light of these issues, it is interesting that only a few reports did not correlate the local expression of perforin to the disease or

the disease stage (45–47). On the other hand, particularly in transplant settings, the local increase of perforin-expressing lymphocytes generally appears to precede the acute rejection episode and presumably also the changes in peripheral blood. These observations suggest that the detection of perforin-expressing cells in transplant biopsies may serve as a diagnostic marker for an upcoming rejection and for monitoring the efficacy of immunosuppressive therapy (48). It is quite interesting that an immunosuppressive regimen of either cyclosporin A or donor-specific transfusion and anti-CD4 does not prevent infiltration of the transplant by CD8$^+$ T-cells. Instead, fewer cells of the infiltrate express perforin (49,50). This finding illustrates that perforin expression can be used to discriminate between unarmed and armed cytotoxic cells, and that the proliferation and arming of CTLs are under separate controls.

CELL-TYPE SPECIFICITY OF PERFORIN EXPRESSION

It is frequently assumed that perforin expression is restricted to conventional CTLs and NK cells, inducibly in the first and constitutively in the second. Based on numerous investigations during the last decade, this dogma requires several modifications. Also, another look must be taken at the common assumption that conventional CTLs in the peripheral blood of healthy individuals are comprised only of naive and memory CTLs that would require activation for their expression of cytotoxicity and perforin. The following sheds light on these and related issues.

CD4$^+$ T Cells

Perforin can be expressed not only by conventional CTLs but also by T cells with a conventional T-helper (Th) surface phenotype (i.e., CD4$^+$ and TCR α/β^+ cells) that recognize antigen in the context of MHC class II. This should not be surprising inasmuch as class II-restricted cytotoxic activity against alloantigens has been established for more than 20 years (51–54). Indeed, CD4+ T cells can employ a perforin-dependent pathway *in vivo* toward graft-versus-host disease in MHC-disparate recipients to the same degree as CD8+ T cells (55).

Much of the direct evidence for perforin gene expression by CD4+ T cells is based on the analysis of T cell clones. When a large number of cytotoxic human allospecific clones were investigated, perforin expression was documented in every clone irrespective of its expression of CD4 or CD8 (56) and in all analyzed cytotoxic CD4 clones (57). Class II-restricted, CD4+ CTL clones have been generated also against several viruses (58) including herpes simplex virus (HSV) and human immunodeficiency virus type 1 (HIV-1). In these instances perforin gene expression has been documented in every clone (59,60). Unlike conventional virus-specific CTLs, this MHC-II-restricted CD4+ CTL may be unable to attack *in vivo* the infected tissue expressing MHC-I (61). Instead, virus-specific CD4+ CTLs can be expected to recognize and lyse MHC-II-expressing cells *in vivo* that may have presented internalized and degraded viral protein (i.e., antigen-presenting cells). In this context their biologic function would entail a negative regulatory control of a viral immune response (58).

Of course, information gained from the analysis of long-term cultured T cell clones should be viewed with some skepticism and not be generalized. Also, unlike CD8+ CTL clones (see below), quite a number of CD4+ CTL clones—in particular murine clones—do not express perforin (62–64). The results of investigations of "normal" CD4+ T cells (i.e., primary lymphocytes obtained from blood or spleen) appear to contradict each other on first sight. Some investigations addressing the possibility of perforin gene expression by activated CD4+ T cells are negative (65–67). Other investigations clearly document perforin expression in this lineage at the RNA and protein levels as well as the single-cell level after *in vitro* or *in vivo* stimulation (29,32,37,44,68–70). These different results can be reconciled by the

more stringent activation requirements for the CD4+ lineage that probably were not met in the first set of investigations. Resting CD8+ T cells can be readily stimulated by the cytokine interleukin 2 (IL-2) on its own (see Signals Regulating Perforin Expression, below) because they, but not CD4+ T cells, constitutively express functional IL-2 receptors (IL-2R) (71). CD4+ T cells express the missing p75 IL-2R chain only upon TCR signaling. Second, perforin-dependent cytotoxicity may develop in CD4+ T-cells only in the absence of activated CD8+ T-cells (72), suggesting that activation of the perforin gene was forced toward the CD8+ lineage in experiments where both types of cells were stimulated simultaneously. Taken together, CD4+ T cells intrinsically may possess a potential for perforin gene expression similar to that of CD8+ T cells, but they have control mechanisms in place that refine this potential to fewer situations. Therefore, the number of perforin-expressing CD4+ peripheral T cells in healthy humans or mice is much lower (37,70,73) than that of CD8+ peripheral T cells (see below).

Naive, Effector, and Memory CD8+ T Cells

Unlike the situation with CD4+ T cells, perforin gene expression can be upregulated readily in conventional CTLs. This is also reflected in the analysis of CD8+ T cell clones where most if not all of them are found to express perforin (56,63). Regarding primary CD8+ peripheral T cells, many of us in the field have noticed significant amounts of perforin mRNA in cells freshly obtained from healthy individuals. Up to some time ago we took this as a sign of the presence of NK cells in the cell preparation, because NK cells express constitutively moderate levels of perforin mRNA (66,74). Studies at the single-cell level clearly show, however, that approximately 15% to 25% of conventional human peripheral CD8+ T cells express perforin and that this percentage increases upon stimulation with IL-2 (75–77). Several complementary investigations shed light on this issue, indicating that at least in humans a large number of conventional CTLs are maintained in a perforin-expressing effector CTL stage. In contrast, naive conventional CTLs (i.e., cells that never may have encountered their antigen) are discernible by their lack of detectable perforin protein expression. Finally, memory CTLs that allow a more rapid response to a second antigen encounter may retain the expression of perforin, albeit at lower levels.

Phenotypically, the perforin-expressing effector CTL subset can be identified most readily by the co-expression of CD8 and CD11b (37,78,79), but additional surface markers may be used also. This CTL subset is absent in cord blood T lymphocytes (80), and it increases with age (79,81). These cells, which do not express CD28, are cytolytically active *ex vivo* without stimulation (37,79, 81,82). They may play an essential role for protection against intracellular pathogens of the blood, particularly viral infections (83). The detection of perforin-expressing conventional CTLs in healthy mice suggests an analogous subset, but apparently as a smaller pool (73,84). It is possible that the effector-type CTLs of humans have a longer life-span. Equally as likely is that the persistence of antigen or cross-reactive antigens and non-specific stimulatory cytokines maintain this pool longer in a natural environment than in the animals housed under pathogen-free conditions. Most peripheral CD8+ T cells are perforin-negative naive CTLs in humans and mouse, and they co-express CD45RA and CD27 in humans (79). They are the only CD8+ T cells present in cord blood, consistent with their naive phenotype. The third CD8+ CTL population, which functionally and phenotypically resembles memory-type cells (CD45RA−CD27+), expresses perforin but less homogenously than the effector-cell type (79). Because effector CTLs may seed the memory CTL pool (85) it appears that expression of the perforin gene is maintained from the effector stage into the memory stage albeit at lower levels. Similar investigations of peripheral CD4+ T cells that exclu-

sively relied on surface markers suggested that a small fraction of these cells are maintained *in vivo* as perforin-expressing memory or effector cells (70).

Perforin and the Pattern of Cytokine Production

CD4+ T cells can be divided into two polarized groups, Th1 and Th2, based on their pattern of cytokine production correlating with the promotion of cell-mediated inflammatory reactions versus antibody and allergic responses (86). Analogous findings have been made recently for the cytokine profiles of CD8+ T cells but not necessarily their *in vivo* function (87). One may wonder whether a particular lymphokine profile secreted by a cell correlates with perforin expression by that cell. Regarding CD8+ T cells, functional experiments strongly suggest that perforin, but not fas ligand, is expressed by both subsets equally well (88), consistent with the notion that generally all CD8+ CTL clones can express perforin. Regarding CD4+ CTL clones, perforin appeared to be preferably expressed in cells secreting Th1 cytokines according to one report (58); but in another report it was associated with cells expressing Th2 lymphokines (63). Taken together, it appears unlikely that perforin expression by a T cell correlates with or is determined by the cytokine profile or vice versa. However, it is reasonable to assume that the levels of perforin could be modulated by a particular cytokine profile.

Constitutive Expression of Perforin by NK Cells, Granulated Metrial Gland Cells, and γ/δ T Cells

Unlike the conventional T cell subsets described above, NK cells, granulated metrial gland cells, and γ/δ T cells generally do not require prior activation for their abundant perforin gene expression or for their display of MHC-unrestricted cytolytic activity. In that sense, they represent an important component of innate immune reactions, albeit the functions of NK cells and γ/δ T cells are complex and entail more than cytotoxicity (2,89,90). Several investigations, including single-cell analyses, demonstrate that every NK cell in humans and mouse is expressing perforin protein and perforin mRNA without activation (37,66,73,74,77,84,91).

Morphologically and phenotypically, NK-like cells with high levels of perforin differentiate in the decidua during the first trimester of the human pregnancy, and they are found in the metrial gland in the uterus of pregnant mice (92–95). The function of these cells remains to be defined in light of the normal reproduction and pregnancy of perforin-deficient mice. However, the morphologic changes in the pregnant uterus of perforin-deficient mice (96) could indicate a functional compensation in consideration of the reported decrease in the prevalence of perforin-positive lymphoid cells during pregnancy failures in humans (97).

Lymphokine-activated killer (LAK) cells are generated *in vitro* by culturing lymphocytes with high doses of IL-2. They are functionally NK-like cells but are phenotypically heterogeneous cells of T and NK origin (98,99). The analysis of sublines and clones from such cultures suggests that most or all of the generated LAK cells express perforin (100,101).

Lastly, TCR γ/δ^+ lymphocytes, which prefer to accumulate in epithelial and mucosal tissues in rodents but preponderate in the blood and lymphoid organs in humans, may express perforin constitutively based on the analysis of the following tissues and cells: γ/δ T cell clones (102), so-called dendritic epidermal γ/δ T cells residing in the skin (103,104), intraepithelial γ/δ T cells residing in the gut (105), and γ/δ T cells residing in the blood (106).

Expression of Perforin by Immature Lymphocytes, Hematopoietic Progenitors, and Lymphoid Tumors

It is conceptually interesting to speculate about a developmentally common precursor for all cells that express perforin, assuming that the perforin gene locus becomes demarcated from its surrounding inactive chromatin at a particular stage of development prior to its transcription in analogy to other genes. Applied to the T cell- and NK cell-restricted expression of perforin described so far, this could suggest a bipotential progenitor cell for T and NK cells. Such cells may exist at least during fetal thymic ontogeny (107). It is therefore relevant to describe the developmental stages of progenitor cells in which perforin has been detected.

The earliest precursors investigated so far are cells already committed to becoming T cells or NK cells. Regarding the T cell lineage, perforin transcripts are detected by reverse transcriptase–polymerase chain reaction (RT-PCR) in CD3 low, double-positive fetal thymocytes (108). Interestingly, they continue to be present in single-positive cells of both the CD4 and CD8 phenotype but with prevalence in the CD8 phenotype, as noted above for the mature cells. Clearly, the small number of transcripts indicates only an accessibility of the perforin gene locus and not that perforin may be present in biologically significant amounts in thymocytes. Regarding phenotypically and functionally immature NK cells derived from cord blood cells, all of the stages investigated expressed perforin at probably biologically significant levels (109–111). As one might expect, normal CD34$^+$ marrow cells did not appear to express perforin (112,113), suggesting that the demarcation of the perforin gene locus occurs upon further differentiation. This finding is consistent with the observation that they, or an already committed derivative, can develop *in vitro* into perforin-positive NK-like cells after cytokine stimulation (113). After combined chemotherapy and granulocyte/macrophage colony-stimulating factor (GM-CSF) stimulation, CD34$^+$ cells accumulating in the peripheral blood also express perforin (112). Finally, after *in vitro* culture of mouse bone marrow in the presence of GM-CSF and IL-2, cells can be obtained that can differentiate further into either perforin-negative macrophage-like cells or perforin-positive NK-like cells (114). Although still sketchy, these results are consistent with demarcation of the perforin gene locus at an early progenitor stage during hematopoietic development that precedes the commitment to T cells and NK cells.

Tumors arising from hematopoietic cells can correspond to intermediate stages of the developing lineages. Therefore, they may also pinpoint the developmental point from which perforin can be expressed. As expected, perforin-expressing lymphomas and leukemias have been noted for all of the described mature cells of T cell or NK cell origin but not those of B cell origin (115–130). Based on the lack of commonly used T cell, B cell, or NK cell markers or the lack of rearranged TCR genes, perforin can be expressed also by less mature tumors (119,120,122), but their precise developmental stages remain to be defined.

Perforin Expression by Nonlymphoid Cells

Oddly enough, perforin expression has been observed in nonlymphoid cells in two instances. Keratinocytes freshly extracted from the human skin do not express perforin; but upon their *in vitro* culture, perforin expression can be detected (131). Perforin gene expression cannot be detected in the normal fetal or adult brain. However, perforin may be expressed by cultured astrocytes, some astrocytoma cell lines, and astrocytes reacting to certain degenerative diseases (132). These findings could suggest that keratinocytes, astrocytes, and perforin might play a role in inflammatory processes of the skin and brain; but further studies are required to strengthen this implication. The following focuses only on regulation of the perforin gene in lymphoid cells.

SIGNALS REGULATING PERFORIN GENE EXPRESSION

Discerning the signals that control the expression of perforin is of fundamental rele-vance if one maintains that activation of the perforin gene reflects a significant aspect of cytotoxic lymphocytes during an immune response. Appropriate interpretations of experiments addressing this issue involve several considerations, in particular when peripheral blood mononuclear cells (PBMCs) are investigated.

First, as already described, perforin can be expressed by all peripheral T cell lineages and by NK cells. Hence, documenting a rise in perforin mRNA or in the number of perforin-positive cells after stimulation of PBMCs on its own only implies that any of the conventional CTLs or Th cells or γ/δ T cells or NK cells may have been affected. Second, even when purified CD8$^+$ T cells are being used, the experiments alone cannot distinguish whether the signal activates the perforin gene in naive CTLs, or whether perforin expression is modulated or upregulated in a memory or effector CTL, or any combination of these possibilities. The requirements for perforin induction or upregulation may not be identical for these subsets considering that proliferative responses to various combinations of signals are quantitatively, and frequently qualitatively, distinct for each subset (79,133). Third, one cannot ignore the possibility of secondary events that in fact could comprise the essential primary event, in particular if activation requires longer periods of time. For example, CTL effectors can be induced in T cells by an optimal TCR signal alone, but their development is severely impaired by co-incubation with an anti-CD25 monoclonal antibody (mAb), indicating that the production of IL-2 and signals from the IL-2R are crucially involved (134). In heterogeneous populations, negative crosstalk upon activation also must be considered, including the already described block in the generation of perforin-dependent cytotoxicity in CD4$^+$ T cells by activated CD8$^+$ T cells (72). Within this review, it is impossible to discuss these important issues for each experimental setting reported. Instead, the literature is summarized with my conceptual view; I leave it to the reader to reconcile potential limitations. Observations of antigen- or cytokine-dependent CTL clones are not included. In our hands, the analysis of such CTLs is impeded by the following findings. Antigen- and cytokine-dependent CTL clones or lines generally appear to shut down more than 90% of their RNA and protein synthesis when they are deprived of stimuli for the time periods required to "downregulate" the perforin gene prior to its "activation." Furthermore, these starvation conditions induce apoptosis of the cells. In our hands, any signal required for the growth and survival of a particular clone affects perforin gene expression. Therefore, we believe that activation studies of such cells largely reflect unspecific events. Finally, the following is restricted to the activation or upregulation of the perforin gene in conventional CTLs and its modulation in NK cells and TCR γ/δ^+ lymphocytes because current information regarding other cell types is sketchy. Interestingly, there may be only one major direct pathway for perforin induction in CD8$^+$ T cells that can be extracted from the reported investigations. There are, however, several costimulatory-like pathways—costimulatory-like because either they are insufficient on their own or they result in much weaker responses over longer periods of time.

Perforin Gene Induction or Upregulation in Conventional CTLs by Cytokine

The direct response within hours of the perforin gene to IL-2 or IL-15, which was the first pathway to be identified, is experimentally the best characterized course of perforin gene activation (5,66,67,135–137). Both cytokines use identical receptor chains for the generation of their signals (138) and thus comprise an interchangeable pathway to the perforin gene. As alluded to already, resting CD4$^+$ T cells cannot respond to these cytokines (66) by virtue of their lack of functional receptors (71), but they may respond concomitantly with their induction of one of the signaling subunits of the receptor (68). In

CD8$^+$ T cells this pathway of perforin mRNA induction does not require newly synthesized proteins (67) and is not inhibited by rapamycin (139; unpublished observations), an immunosuppressive drug known to inhibit selectively certain signaling pathways of the IL-2R, including some required for the IL-2-induced progression of the cell cycle (140). In contrast, the IL-2/IL-15 pathway of perforin induction or upregulation is completely blocked if the cells are exposed to transforming growth factor-β (TGF-β) at or before their stimulation but not at later times (141).

Based on elegant *in vitro* investigations at the mRNA and single-cell levels, the IL-2 response of conventional CTLs is primarily accompanied by an increase in the number of cells expressing perforin mRNA (about fivefold), while the increase of mRNA per individual cell is less (about 2.5-fold) (142). Qualitatively similar data have been reported for perforin protein expression at the single-cell level using flow cytometry (37,76). The frequency of perforin-positive cells increases also *in vivo* upon administration of IL-2 (143). An increase in the frequency of perforin-expressing cells suggests that the IL-2R signals affect not only the effector or memory CTLs already expressing perforin but also naive CTLs. The physiologic source of IL-2 during an immune response *in vivo* may be autocrine or paracrine from another T cell activated by the same antigen-presenting cell (APC) or one nearby. The important role for IL-2 or IL-15 for the generation of effector CTLs *in vivo* is emphasized by the failure of IL-2R β-deficient animals to generate virus-specific effector CTLs, although this phenotype is unlikely to be exclusively linked to perforin gene expression because of additional abnormalities in these animals (144).

Interleukin-12 is another cytokine that may directly upregulate perforin in conventional CTLs (145). The kinetics of its induction, but not the magnitude, are reminiscent of that observed for IL-2. The two cytokines together exert an additive effect, suggesting that their signals act independently of each other. The smaller response to IL-12 could be determined by the very low expression of the receptor by resting peripheral blood T cells (146). Somewhat more potent effects can be observed if IL-12 is included during MHC-I allospecific mixed lymphocyte cultures (147). The primary source of IL-12 during an adaptive immune response may be the APCs (146). In tumor models, systemic administration of IL-12 has been associated with an increased number of perforin-expressing effector CTLs infiltrating the tumor (148,149).

The cytokines described next are less potent or entirely ineffective on their own. Under suboptimal stimulations of the IL-2R, they act additively and in one case synergistically. IL-6 alone does not affect the levels of perforin expression. In the presence of low doses of IL-2, however, IL-6R signals act in synergy to upregulate the levels of perforin mRNA to at least the levels seen after optimal IL-2R stimulation (150). The observed synergy may entail upregulation of the IL-2R chains by IL-6R signals and may occur in naive, effector, and memory CTLs (150–152). Because the two potential biologic sources for IL-6 during the activation of CTLs may entail T cells and APCs, it is interesting to note that the presence of monocytes also enhances perforin expression in IL-2-stimulated CD8$^+$ T cells (153). Other monokines, such as IL-1, may play a similar role (154). IL-7 alone is able to weakly increase perforin mRNA levels after longer periods of incubation. Once again under suboptimal IL-2R signals, however, perforin mRNA levels are augmented by IL-7 but not as potently as by IL-6 (155). IL-4, tumor necrosis factor-α (TNF-α), interferon-α (IFN-α), and IFN-γ on their own do not affect perforin expression (155). Under particular culture conditions, however, IL-4 prevents upregulation of perforin and primes the cells to produce Th-2 cytokines (156). This negative effect is likely to be mediated indirectly because it takes place over several days and is depen-

dent on the presence of second-messenger pathway activating agents and cytokines.

Direct Versus Indirect Roles of TCR Signals for Perforin Gene Induction or Upregulation in Conventional CTLs

It is well established that conventional CTLs can be activated by TCR signals via pharmacologic agents or by crosslinking of the TCRs to produce cytokine and to proliferate. In contrast, there is little evidence for a direct signal from the TCR to the perforin gene. Notably, phorbol ester and Ca ionophore alone or in combination have little or no effect under conditions that lead to robust cytokine induction and proliferation (66, 67,135). Moreover, experiments using pharmacologic agents in the presence of lectins or accompanied by crosslinking of the TCR are consistent with indirect effects due to cytokine production and upregulation of cytokine receptors. Unlike the rapid response of the perforin gene to cytokine (within 6 hours), all of the conditions tested result in significant increases only after 1 to 2 days (135,142). At this time cytokines, including IL-2, can be readily detected in the cultures (66), making a strong argument for an indirect effect. Second, this CTL generation, which is TCR-initiated but cytokine-dependent, can be blocked by anti-IL-2R or anti-IL-2 antibodies (157).

Two experimental settings are consistent with, albeit not proof for, a direct link of a TCR signal to the perforin gene. Both circumstances require an additional signal derived from monocytes. Under these conditions crosslinking of the TCRs can increase perforin mRNA within 9 hours, before IL-2 protein can be detected (66). This pathway is blocked by TGF-β (141), as was described above for the IL-2R pathway of perforin gene activation. Also dependent on a signal derived from monocytes, the elevation of intracellular Ca^{2+} results in profound and transient induction of perforin mRNA that is faster and stronger than that controlled by IL-2R signals (67). In the latter scenario perforin induction occurs independently of de novo protein synthesis and thus independently of IL-2. This pathway is blocked by cyclosporin A. The requirement for monocytes begs the question whether any of the soluble cytokines described above could be involved. It also raises the issue of receptor-mediated costimulation involving B7–CD28, LFA3–CD2, ICAM–LFA1, or other interactions. No reports are available regarding perforin and costimulation via B7–CD28 interactions. In our hands, the increases are small and correlate well with the potent increases in IL-2 production. However, we never addressed to our satisfaction whether they are exclusively due to IL-2. In fact, an IL-2-independent component of this costimulus appears to be important for granzyme B induction (158). On the other hand, CTL responses against LCMV infection require perforin-dependent CTLs (159), but they are not impaired in CD28-deficient mice (160). Regarding CD2 and LFA-1, little and, respectively, no effect at all was observed for perforin under the experimental conditions analyzed (161,162).

All told, TCR signals and costimulatory receptor signals directly involved in perforin gene regulation in conventional CTLs are open for speculation and remain to be established experimentally. Along a similar vein is the question of whether the TCR signal that is absolutely necessary for conventional Th cells to express perforin is merely required for the expression of a functional IL-2R by these cells. On the other hand, the role of cytokine-dependent perforin gene regulation is well established, leading to the suggestion that the cytokine environment and responsiveness of a naive CTL may in fact be the primary determinant for this cell to express perforin. Antigen encounter may simply lower the threshold of activation and is of relevance for the clonal expansion of cells primed to express perforin. Both aspects are important, of course, for generating a biologically effective CTL response. This point is highlighted by the observation that *in vivo* administration of anti-CD3 mAbs plus IL-2 to tumor-bearing animals results in significant perforin mRNA expression at the site of certain tumors only in the presence of both stimuli (163,164).

Signals Modulating Perforin Expression in NK Cells, γ/δ T Cells, and Granulated Metrial Gland Cells

NK cells, $\gamma\delta$ T cells, and granulated metrial gland cells express constitutively moderate levels of perforin mRNA (66,155,165) and protein (37,92,106). Therefore, it is not surprising that the studied cytokine effects generally appear to be small. The only exception concerns *in situ* investigations of developing granulated metrial gland cells because here cytokine may also be required for their *in situ* expansion.

Perforin levels show little or no modulation in NK cells (66). Approximately twofold increases have been reported in response to IL-2R signals (i.e., IL-2 and IL-15), particularly when the cells have undergone short-term *in vitro* culture. These cytokines increase the levels of perforin per individual cell (74,76,166–168). This modulation is abolished in the presence of TGF-β (169) and IL-4 (166,168). Modulations similar to those seen with IL-2 or IL-15 occur also in the presence of IL-12 (167,168,170), but they may not be inhibited by IL-4 (168). Regarding granulated metrial gland cells, investigations of the expression of several cytokines and their receptors in the pregnant uterus along with *in vitro* stimulation indicate that these NK-like cells develop *in situ* and express perforin under the control of IL-15 rather than IL-2 (165). Regarding TCR γ/δ^+ lymphocytes, modulations of perforin mRNA by cytokines appear unremarkable in freshly isolated cells (155), although IL-12 was reported to increase perforin mRNA in a transformed line (171).

TRANSCRIPTIONAL CONTROL OF THE PERFORIN GENE

Perforin gene expression is tightly controlled *in vivo* (see Perforin Expression in

Disease and as a Diagnostic Marker, above). During lymphoid development it becomes restricted to mature cells of T and NK origin (see Cell-Type Specificity of Perforin Expression, above). Within these lineages, perforin is largely expressed constitutively by NK cells, TCR γ/δ^+ lymphocytes, and conventional effector CTLs. In contrast, it is inducible by cytokine in conventional naive CTLs and by more stringent conditions in conventional Th cells (see Signals Regulating Perforin Expression, above). Understanding the respective regulatory events in molecular terms may shed light on nuclear events that are of relevance not only for perforin but also for other genes involved in the development and maturation of cells expressing perforin (i.e., cytotoxic lymphocytes). The progress made despite the difficulty of addressing these events experimentally and despite their emerging complexities is summarized here in four parts. The first describes the structure of the perforin gene. The second establishes that the regulatory events taking place during perforin gene activation involve, largely or exclusively, changes at the level of transcription initiation, while a posttranscriptional regulatory event is confined to a unique and unrelated event. The third part describes the function of the perforin promoter in the context of its known *cis*-acting elements and their respective transcription factors. Finally, some of the ongoing work by our laboratory toward the indentification and function of two new enhancers that add the level of cytokine regulation to the cytokine-unresponsive promoter is briefly summarized.

Structure of the Perforin Gene Locus and Its Transcript

The original assignments of the first exon and promoter of the perforin gene and its chromosomal localization can be reconciled as follows for the mouse and human genes. Both genes, which are quite compact, are comprised of three exons embedded within approximately 6 kb (human) and 7 kb (mouse) of DNA (172–174). Both genes are localized in a syntenic region on chromosome 10, and the human gene maps to 10q22 (175,176). Distinct sequences were reported for DNA upstream of the murine perforin promoter (approximately 1,200 bp upstream of the transcription initiation sites) (173,174). The authenticity of these murine upstream sequences has been confirmed in only one case (173). The presently known neighboring genes are at least 2 Mbp away, based on a recent survey of the mouse and human genome projects on the Internet. The most proximal genes are expressed in the inner ear and, respectively, in the central nervous system (CNS) and the reproductive system. Obviously, perforin is not part of a huge and coordinately regulated gene cluster encompassing these genes. It remains interesting to identify potentially closer genes.

The first exon of the perforin gene, which exclusively contains 5′ untranslated sequences, is alternatively spliced to the second exon in both the human (unpublished observation) and the mouse gene (174), albeit the localization of the acceptor sites is not conserved between humans and mouse. The second exon contains the remainder of the 5′ untranslated sequence and coding sequences. The alternative splicing of the 5′ untranslated sequence appears to be without functional relevance because it does not affect the coding sequences of the perforin gene, nor does it alter the translation efficiencies of the two mRNA species (177). The third exon contains the remaining coding sequences and the 3′ untranslated sequences. Two distinct sequences were reported for the 3′ untranslated region of the murine perforin mRNA (175,178), but only one of them (175) may be authentic (unpublished observation), suggesting that no additional exons are present. After transcription and processing of the primary transcripts, the polyadenylated perforin mRNAs comprise approximately 2,900 bp, almost twice as much as the actual coding sequence.

```
CCCggGtGAgATG  TGaC CATGTGGcCTGGgGtCTGttggCtACTTaTTCCCATCATgTACTcACTTAgGgGtttgtgAGaacTaccccCa      murine
CCCatGaGAcATGaTGtCaCATGTGGtCTGGacCTG  cccCACTtCTTCCCATCATaTACaCagTTALGAg  aacaAGttgtHgagaaCc         human
                                                                        AP-1        Ets? (NP3)
cCCTgCaTggtTTACCCACCT  CataacCagCAcCAAttTtTTtTtTTaagCCCCCagtAGtatCcaTGAGTCAcTCtgCCATGGAAA           murine
aCCT CcT cccTTACCCAgCTgCcccaCcccCAgAAgccgTgTgaTTtgCCCCC  cAGtgcccTgAGTCAcTCcaCCCATGGAAA            human

CCT  CCCACagTaACCTCAgGACgCAgaaCAGAGTGgccAActgtctTCCaCaCGTaCTAgCCtGctCAa                            murine
CCTcacCCCCAaCCcTgACCTCAaGCAaggCAGAGTGcagAAgacatgTcTccGTgCTA CCaGacCActtcaccagcacccacgacct            human

cagcagggctggagccagcgtggagccaactggctgtcctcacaaagcgaggagcgaggagccccctgttcgaggaacatgcttggagtt          human
                             Ets-like (NF-P2)
    AcCtgaGGtTcaGcTGGGATGTAGGTaTGgaCAGGAAGTGGgT  aCCAGcTTtGAG  tATCTCTC  CcCaCtCcCAGGGAGGAG       murine
    cggAgCCctgGGcTaggGtTGGGATGTAGGT  TGaCAGGAAGTGGaTgGatgCAaGaTTaGAGcaacATCTCTCTtCtCcCaCTCAGGGAGGAG   human

GGAacagTcCACAtgtatTGAgAaTGgAgtAAaGatCgtGtctAGTtcctAAGCACTgCA      CCaT    GTCTtCATG   TcCccTC     murine
GGAAtggCcCACAgGctcTGAcACTcAagAAgGgcCagGacaGTtccAAGCACTtCAcaacaacCCCTaggGTCTaCATGaccTaCaaTC          human

tC ATgGaCAcTG tGA  TtAGCACAcTtttGaatgAGgAGcTgAgatGT gAagCgGCTGaaaccCCTtgCCcAGCcaCtCAAGC            murine
cCAATtGttCAgTGaaGAAacTGaGGcCACAgTgagGctgaaGaAcCCtAccaGTccAcaCtGCTG  gtgCaTaaCCgaGCtgCcCAAGC        human

CCaGGC    cactct  TcAGCaaCtcttcCTGacaGCgcaTccCATCCCAaACA      CTcaaC  TCAGAAG                      murine
CCCGGCggtctggcgtgtaggcccatgctc  TgAGCcgCcgcctCTGcctcTGcCtctaCATCCCACACAtgcgatgCTgtgCATCAGAAG        human

CAgGGAGcaG  tCAgtTGGCCTGcCTggTCcACACCA                                                             murine
CAaGGAGatGgccCTgCTGGCCTGtCtcaTcaACACCAggccgagtctcaaagtcctcaaagtcctcagcgcccgccctcctccgcctgtgccct     human

GAGTCCCgcAcCCCaacTgCtCtGCTCTtgCTtGGCAGATGAGCC  cCTTGGCCTTcacaGCTgaCTTCCTGaaGGCTGTCA    caAGCCGG   murine
GAGTCCCgcAgCCC  CaGcaGCTCTaCTcGGCAGATGAGCC  tCTGGCCCT  gctcGCTcgcTTCCTGAgGGCTGTCAgtggggAGCCGG     human
                                                               Sp-1        Ets
ATGAGGAGgTGAcaACAGGGTGGGTGCTGgGTGGGA          ACCTGTGACCACActCTGGGGGCaGGGCAGGAAGTAG              murine
ATGAGG GcTGAggACAGGgTGGGTGCTcGTGGGA  ggggagagcacaaagg ACCTGTGACCACA gCTGGGGGCgGGGCAGGAAGTAG      human
                               Sp-1-like                    multiple initiation sites
ATGAGGAGgTGAcaACAGGGTGGGTGCTGgGTGGGA                                                             
     multiple initiation sites

tAaTGATaTGA  cGTtGG      CCAgGGTGGGCcTGCCT GGGGataGATcgCAgCATTtTaAaAGCCTcCATTGACAacG             murine
aaGTGATgTGAgtGGtTGGCtggtgcaaggagagCCAcaGTGGGC TGCCTgTGGGGgctGATgCCACaTTccAggAGCCT CggTGA AgaG      human

caGgTgTCCcccCTGGcttCaGtggCgTCTtggtGGGAcTtCAG   murine
agGaTaTCCatcCTGtagCCcGcttC TCTatacGGGAtTcCAG   human
                                            intron
```

Transcriptional Versus Posttranscriptional Regulatory Events

Control of a cell-type specific expression pattern, such as that of perforin, is usually exerted by developmentally active transcription factors and therefore is at the transcriptional level. Indeed, the perforin promoter mediates this function (see below). Regarding regulation of perforin mRNA levels within the various lineages, several but not all of the signals described have been experimentally addressed. The stimulation of conventional CTLs by IL-2 or by the elevation of intracellular Ca^{2+} in the presence of a signal derived from monocytes requires de novo transcription for perforin mRNA upregulation and does not affect mRNA stability (67), which is consistent with a transcriptional control. Direct measurements of the levels of transcription in a CTL/tumor hybrid, in which perforin can be induced by IL-1, show in this case that perforin mRNA induction is controlled at the transcriptional level (177). Our own analogous experiments in a similar system in which perforin is inducible by IL-2 show that this induction occurs at the level of transcription initiation (manuscript submitted). The modulation of perforin mRNA levels in NK cells by IL-2 or IL-12 is mirrored by a pronounced effect by the intrinsically insensitive nuclear run-on analyses, albeit an increase in the stability of the mRNA after IL-2 stimulation of NK cells was reported at the same time (74). The half-life of perforin mRNA in NK cells and in activated conventional CTLs is of similar intermediate length (90–100 minutes) (67,74). The longer half-life reported for a CTL/tumor hybrid is most likely related to the use of a different internal control standard (177). The cumulative evidence described indicates that cell-type specificity and the upregulation of perforin upon CTL or NK activation is largely, if not exclusively, determined at the level of transcription initiation.

Recently, a rapid loss of perforin mRNA (and granzymes and TNF-α) was observed when certain CTLs and NK-like clones, as well as LAK cells, engaged target cells with and without triggering cytotoxicity (179–182). In molecular terms, this process occurs at the posttranscriptional level and appears to require destabilizing sequences spread over the coding sequences but not the 3' untranslated sequences, as well as a preexisting nuclease (183). The biologic significance of this phenomenon remains to be established.

Function of the Perforin Promoter

So far all investigations have focused on the functional analysis of the mouse perforin promoter. The alignment of the mouse and human sequences shown in Figure 10-1 strongly suggests that analogous regulatory events occur for the human gene. Notably, the depicted sequences are likely to contain all functionally relevant sequences of the proximal and distal promoter region and all the neighboring upstream regulatory elements because the human and mouse sequences diverge upstream of the shown alignment. However, this is not to say, or exclude, that additional enhancers or silencers could reside further upstream in the functionally analyzed DNAs because the position

FIG. 10-1. Alignment of the murine and human perforin promoter sequences and identified *cis*-acting elements. Sequences of the promoters along with upstream regulatory DNA were aligned until no further homology could be found. Included are the 5' untranslated sequences of the first exon up to the splice site. Only the farthest upstream and farthest downstream transcription initiation sites are indicated. Boxed areas represent the presently best characterized *cis*-acting elements. The respective transcription factors, indicated on the top of the boxes, are described in more detail in the text.

of these potential regulatory domains in relation to the promoter may not be conserved between the two species.

Regarding transcription initiation, neither gene contains classic TATA-box sequences (Fig. 10-1) known to direct the RNA polymerase II to initiate transcription from a single start site. Instead, there are multiple initiation sites in both genes that can be detected using RNAse protection assays or S1 nuclease assays but may not be apparent in primer extension analyses (173; unpublished observation for the human gene). Figure 10-1 depicts only the farthest upstream site, for which we have also identified 5′ RACE cDNA clones derived from spliced mRNA species, as well as the farthest downstream mapped site (173). The presence of multiple initiation sites has resulted in the dilemma that each investigator, including ourselves, refers to a different site as +1. Therefore, no numbering has been included in Figure 10-1. Regardless, the perforin promoters do not contain initiator-like sequences (184), which also could direct the RNA polymerase II. Instead, the indicated Sp-1 and Sp-1-like binding sites and the additional G-rich stretches in the proximal promoter area that comprise potential Sp-1 binding sequence stretches (185) may direct transcription initiation of the perforin gene. They are known to perform this function in TATA- and initiater-deficient promoters (186–188). This interpretation is consistent with *in vitro* footprints of the G-rich sequences (189), the binding of Sp-1 and Sp-1-like proteins to the indicated elements in Figure 10-1, and their requirement for full promoter activity (190).

The functions of the remaining sequences within the homology area (shown in Fig. 10-1) have been investigated by several laboratories using different approaches and different T cell clones or tumor cell lines. Therefore, it is not surprising that some of the findings are similar, whereas others appear to be distinct. Rather than being mutually exclusive, they are likely to complement each other *in vivo* in normal cells to account for the phenotype of several independent

transgenic lines in which the function of the entire murine promoter and upstream DNA has been analyzed in tissues, at the single-cell level, and upon lymphocyte activation (191). On the other hand, results from the *in vitro* investigations are unlikely to relate to functions that could not be documented in these animals. At integration sites permissive for transgene expression, every lymphocyte that can express perforin (i.e., conventional CTLs, conventional Th cells, γ/δ T cells, and NK cells), but not, for example, B cells or monocytes, express the transgene. The transgene is also expressed by thymocytes but not by immature cells of the lymphoid or myeloid lineage. Thus, the most appropriate description of the transgenic phenotype is that the perforin promoter confers developmentally accurate expression, resulting in the appropriate cell type-specific expression by terminally differentiated lymphoid cells. (The peculiar expression of perforin by keratinocytes and astrocytes was unknown at the time and was not analyzed.) Interestingly, conventional CTLs and conventional Th cells express identical levels of the transgene, consistent with the already developed idea that conventional CTLs and conventional Th cells have intrinsically the same probability of expressing perforin. The term probability is particularly descriptive in view of the observation that at the single-cell level each cell expresses the transgenic surface-tag with identical frequencies of expression turned on and expression turned off (unpublished observation). Unexpectedly, however, the probability of NK cells or γ/δ T cells (high levels of endogenous perforin expression) and the probability of naive T cells (low levels of endogenous perforin gene expression) to express the transgene, as well as the steady-state levels of transgene expression by these populations, are identical. Similarly, the probability of appropriately activated T cells to express the transgene do not differ from that of unactivated T cells. These findings, together with the observation that the expression levels on a per-transgene copy basis are lower than those derived from the two endogenous perforin genes, indicate that *cis*-acting DNAs in addition to the promoter and upstream regulatory DNA are required for the high probability of an NK cell, and for the increased probability of an activated conventional CTL, to transcribe the perforin gene (see below). Regardless, most or all of the qualitative information required for the developmentally determined, lineage-restricted expression of perforin must be found in the depicted homology area of the promoter and upstream DNA, emphasizing the relevance of the regulatory mechanisms described next.

The *in vitro* dissection of the promoter DNA indicates that two mechanisms are in place to restrict perforin gene expression: gene repression in cells of noncytolytic lineages and gene activation in lineages that can express perforin (173,189,190,192,193). Best characterized at the molecular level are those elements and transcription factors that are included in Figure 10-1.

Regarding positive regulators, an Ets or Ets-like transcription factor acts in direct proximity to Sp-1 within the proximal promoter region (190). Strikingly, an identical sequence (CAGGAAGT), which is also functionally relevant (193), occurs in the distal promoter region. Both elements are completely conserved between human and mouse. Transcriptional activation via the distal binding site may involve two novel Ets-related proteins, one of which is ubiquitously expressed (NF-P1). The second one (NF-P2) may be expressed only by perforin-expressing cells (193). Because NF-P2 is a derivative of NF-P1, it was suggested that a cell-type specific dissociation of a subunit component, an alteration in the conformation of NF-P1, or both result in the formation of a functionally competent NF-P2 transcription factor (194). At present, it is not clear whether this protein is also involved in the transcriptional activation via the proximal Ets consensus. The identity of NF-P1 and NF-P2 should provide interesting clues because Ets transcription factors are of fundamental relevance for lymphoid development and activation (195).

A situation similar to NF-P1 and NF-P2

but with an opposite expression pattern and opposite function (i.e., gene repression in non-perforin-expressing lineages) involves a third and weak Ets-like consensus farther upstream (189). Here, a ubiquitously expressed protein called NP2 binds to the DNA with an affinity and fine specificity that is distinct from a second protein called NP3, which is present only in perforin-negative lineages. This element is in close proximity to a second element that binds the AP-1 family of transcription factors, which can be activated ubiquitously. Therefore, NP3 not only may repress transcription in resting perforin-negative cells but may be even more important during their activation (189).

Additional transcriptional events of activation and repression by sequences within the perforin promoter area have been described, but so far they have not been narrowed down to *cis*-acting elements (173,189,190,192,193). They are likely to be represented by some of the highly homologous or even identical sequence stretches in Figure 10-1.

Other Regulatory Domains in the Perforin Gene Locus

Expression of perforin is readily upregulated when conventional CTLs are activated by IL-2R signals. As described above, this induction occurs at the level of transcription initiation but not via regulatory elements within the perforin promoter region (191). Instead, this event involves two separate enhancers (manuscript submitted). They were localized by analyzing the expression of a transgenic human perforin gene locus (extending the structural gene by more than 25 kb on each end) in a murine CTL tumor model for perforin gene activation by IL-2R signals. DNA containing both regulatable enhancers also allows activation of a reporter gene construct in T cells of transgenic mice. The core enhancer functions are contained within approximately 150 bp and, respectively, 120 bp, shown in Figure 10-2 along with similarities to or identities with known

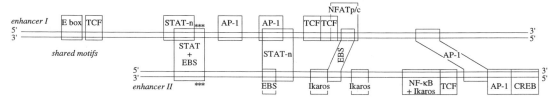

FIG. 10-2. Alignment of structural motifs of two novel IL-2 responsive enhancers in the human perforin gene locus. Similarities to or identities with consensus to known transcription factor binding sites are indicated in boxes labeled with the name of the respective motifs or transcription factors that are described in more detail in the text. Asterisks denote point mutations that result in a loss of enhancer function.

transcription factor-binding sites. The most striking structural feature of both enhancers entails a consensus for signal transducers and activators of transcription proteins (STATs) (196,197) that overlaps with an Ets binding site core (EBS). This consensus is followed by an imperfect consensus for STAT proteins (STAT-n) at identical spacings in both enhancers. Based on the introductions of point mutations, the enhancer functions are dependent on the STAT binding site among other binding sites. Another interesting finding for one of the enhancers is a potential NFATp/c consensus. It is located, however, within a stretch of sequences that could comprise other binding sites (Fig. 10-2). In lymphocytes, NF-AT proteins mediate responses from the TCR (198), thereby reopening the question of a direct versus an indirect link between TCR signals and perforin gene expression. Regardless, our experiments are consistent with lineage-specific activation of the enhancer function that involves a direct signal from the IL-2R via STAT proteins to the perforin gene. Notably, this pathway of perforin gene activation is consistent with its described independence of de novo protein synthesis and its insensitivity to rapamycin.

Thus, the transcriptional regulation of the perforin gene is controlled by at least three regulatory regions with overlapping and distinct functional properties. The promoter region confers appropriate but low constitutive activity during lymphoid development, resulting in a low probability of transcribing

the gene in all of the perforin-expressing lineages. In contrast, the two enhancers, whose individual function is also cell-type specific, can be activated by STAT proteins when conventional CTLs receive IL-2R signals. It will be interesting for us to determine whether these enhancers are constitutively active in NK cells and γ/δ T cells and, if so, which molecules are involved in this scenario.

PERSPECTIVE

Perforin gene expression is tightly controlled during lymphoid development and during an immune response consistent with its biologic function (see Chapters 9 and 11). Several mechanisms guarantee perforin expression in cytotoxic lymphocytes, and other mechanisms prevent expression in noncytotoxic lymphocytes. These controls involve receptors, in particular cytokine receptors (e.g., the IL-2R), signaling molecules such as STATs, and ultimately a combination of transcription factors, including STATs and unique Ets-like proteins. The dissection of all these control levels for each of the numerous crucial events in the life of a cytotoxic lymphocyte is still in progress, leaving much more to be revealed than has been emphasized here.

Acknowledgment

This work was supported by grant RO1 CA55811 from the National Institutes of Health to M.G.L.

REFERENCES

1. Doherty PC, Allan W, Eichelberger M, Carding SR. Roles of alpha beta and gamma delta T cell subsets in viral immunity. *Annu Rev Immunol* 1992;10:123–151.

2. Whiteside TL, Herberman RB. Role of human natural killer cells in health and disease. *Clin Diagn Lab Immunol* 1994;1:125–133.

3. Henkart PA. Lymphocyte-mediated cytotoxicity: two pathways and multiple effector molecules. *Immunity* 1994;1:343–346.

4. Shinkai Y, Takio K, Okumura K. Homology of perforin to the ninth component of complement (C9). *Nature* 1988;334:525–527.

5. Lichtenheld MG, Olsen KJ, Lu P, et al. Structure and function of human perforin. *Nature* 1988; 335:448–451.

6. Muller C, Kagi D, Aebischer T, et al. Detection of perforin and granzyme A mRNA in infiltrating cells during infection of mice with lymphocytic choriomeningitis virus. *Eur J Immunol* 1989;19: 1253–1259.

7. Young LH, Klavinskis LS, Oldstone MB, Young JD. In vivo expression of perforin by CD8+ lymphocytes during an acute viral infection. *J Exp Med* 1989;169:2159–2171.

8. Humbert M, Magnan A, Ladurie FL, et al. Perforin and granzyme B gene-expressing cells in bronchoalveolar lavage fluids from lung allograft recipients displaying cytomegalovirus pneumonitis. *Transplantation* 1994;57:1289–1292.

9. Navikas V, Haglund M, Link J, et al. Cytokine mRNA profiles in mononuclear cells in acute aseptic meningoencephalitis. *Infect Immun* 1995;63: 1581–1586.

10. Sayama K, Watanabe Y, Tohyama M, Miki Y. Localization of perforin in viral vesicles and erythema multiforme. *Dermatology* 1994;188:305–309.

11. Fukuda R, Ishimura N, Nguyen XT, et al. Gene expression of perforin and granzyme A in the liver in chronic hepatitis C: comparison with peripheral blood mononuclear cells. *Microbiol Immunol* 1995;39:873–877.

12. Clement MV, Haddad P, Soulie A, et al. Perforin and granzyme B as markers for acute rejection in heart transplantation. *Int Immunol* 1991;3:1175–1181.

13. Griffiths GM, Namikawa R, Mueller C, et al. Granzyme A and perforin as markers for rejection in cardiac transplantation. *Eur J Immunol* 1991; 21:687–693.

14. Fox WMD, Hameed A, Hutchins GM, et al. Perforin expression localizing cytotoxic lymphocytes in the intimas of coronary arteries with transplant-related accelerated arteriosclerosis. *Hum Pathol* 1993;24:477–482.

15. Legros-Maida S, Soulie A, Benvenuti C, et al. Granzyme B and perforin can be used as predictive markers of acute rejection in heart transplantation. *Eur J Immunol* 1994;24:229–233.

16. Clement MV, Legros-Maida S, Israel-Biet D, et al. Perforin and granzyme B expression is associated with severe acute rejection: evidence for in situ

localization in alveolar lymphocytes of lung-transplanted patients. *Transplantation* 1994;57:322–326.

17. Matsuno T, Sakagami K, Saito S, et al. Expression of intercellular adhesion molecule-1 and perforin on kidney allograft rejection. *Transplant Proc* 1992;24:1306–1307.

18. Lipman ML, Stevens AC, Strom TB. Heightened intragraft CTL gene expression in acutely rejecting renal allografts. *J Immunol* 1994;152:5120–5127.

19. Sharma VK, Bologa RM, Li B, et al. Molecular executors of cell death—differential intrarenal expression of Fas ligand, Fas, granzyme B, and perforin during acute and/or chronic rejection of human renal allografts. *Transplantation* 1996;62: 1860–1866.

20. Strehlau J, Pavlakis M, Lipman M, Maslinski W, Shapiro M, Strom TB. The intragraft gene activation of markers reflecting T-cell-activation and cytotoxicity analyzed by quantitative RT-PCR in renal transplantation. *Clin Nephrol* 1996;46:30–33.

21. Clement MV, Soulie A, Legros-Maida S, et al. Perforin and granzyme B: predictive markers for acute GVHD or cardiac rejection after bone marrow or heart transplantation. *Nouv Rev Fr Hematol* 1991;33:465–470.

22. Takata M. Immunohistochemical identification of perforin-positive cytotoxic lymphocytes in graft-versus-host disease. *Am J Clin Pathol* 1995; 103:324–329.

23. Nakanishi H, Monden T, Morimoto H, Kobayashi T, Shimano T, Mori T. Perforin expression in lymphocytes infiltrated to human colorectal cancer. *Br J Cancer* 1991;64:239–242.

24. Leger-Ravet MB, Devergne O, Peuchmaur M, et al. In situ detection of activated cytotoxic cells in follicular lymphomas. *Am J Pathol* 1994;144: 492–499.

25. Saiki Y, Ohtani H, Naito Y, Miyazawa M, Nagura H. Immunophenotypic characterization of Epstein-Barr virus-associated gastric carcinoma: massive infiltration by proliferating CD8+ T-lymphocytes. *Lab Invest* 1996;75:67–76.

26. Young LH, Joag SV, Lin PY, et al. Expression of cytolytic mediators by synovial fluid lymphocytes in rheumatoid arthritis. *Am J Pathol* 1992; 140:1261–1268.

27. Griffiths GM, Alpert S, Lambert E, McGuire J, Weissman IL. Perforin and granzyme A expression identifying cytolytic lymphocytes in rheumatoid arthritis. *Proc Natl Acad Sci USA* 1992;89:549–553.

28. Muller-Ladner U, Kriegsmann J, Tschopp J, Gay RE, Gay S. Demonstration of granzyme A and perforin messenger RNA in the synovium of patients with rheumatoid arthritis. *Arthritis Rheum* 1995;38:477–484.

29. Wu Z, Podack ER, McKenzie JM, Olsen KJ, Zakarija M. Perforin expression by thyroid-infiltrating T cells in autoimmune thyroid disease. *Clin Exp Immunol* 1994;98:470–477.

30. Tsubota K, Saito I, Miyasaka N. Expression of granzyme A and perforin in lacrimal gland of Sjögren's syndrome. *Adv Exp Med Biol* 1994; 350:637–640.

31. Seko Y, Minota S, Kawasaki A, et al. Perforin-secreting killer cell infiltration and expression of

a 65-kD heat-shock protein in aortic tissue of patients with Takayasu's arteritis. *J Clin Invest* 1994;93:750–758.

32. Muller S, Lory J, Corazza N, et al. Activated CD4+ and CD8+ cytotoxic cells are present in increased numbers in the intestinal mucosa from patients with active inflammatory bowel disease. *Am J Pathol* 1998;152:261–268.

33. Andreetta F, Bernasconi P, Torchiana E, Baggi F, Cornelio F, Mantegazza R. T-cell infiltration in polymyositis is characterized by coexpression of cytotoxic and T-cell-activating cytokine transcripts. *Ann NY Acad Sci* 1995;756:418–420.

34. Cherin P, Herson S, Crevon MC, et al. Mechanisms of lysis by activated cytotoxic cells expressing perforin and granzyme-B genes and the protein TIA-1 in muscle biopsies of myositis. *J Rheumatol* 1996;23:1135–1142.

35. Badorff C, Noutsias M, Kuhl U, Schultheiss HP. Cell-mediated cytotoxicity in hearts with dilated cardiomyopathy: correlation with interstitial fibrosis and foci of activated T lymphocytes. *J Am Coll Cardiol* 1997;29:429–434.

36. Hunger RE, Mueller C, Z'Graggen K, Friess H, Buchler MW. Cytotoxic cells are activated in cellular infiltrates of alcoholic chronic pancreatitis [see comments]. *Gastroenterology* 1997;112:1656–1663.

37. Nakata M, Kawasaki A, Azuma M, et al. Expression of perforin and cytolytic potential of human peripheral blood lymphocyte subpopulations. *Int Immunol* 1992;4:1049–1054.

38. Navikas V, Link J, Persson C, et al. Increased mRNA expression of IL-6, IL-10, TNF-alpha, and perforin in blood mononuclear cells in human HIV infection. *J Acquir Immune Defic Syndr Hum Retrovirol* 1995;9:484–489.

39. Rukavina D, Balen-Marunic S, Rubesa G, Orlic P, Vujaklija K, Podack ER. Perforin expression in peripheral blood lymphocytes in rejecting and tolerant kidney transplant recipients. *Transplantation* 1996;61:285–291.

40. Portales P, Djamali A, Tinland O, Clot J, Mourad G. Perforin intracytoplasmic expression by peripheral blood lymphocytes in renal transplantation. *Transplant Proc* 1997;29:2315–2317.

41. Nakamura T, Ebihara I, Osada S, Okumura K, Tomino Y, Koide H. Perforin gene expression in T lymphocytes correlates with disease activity in immunoglobulin A nephropathy. *Clin Sci* 1992; 82:461–468.

42. Matusevicius D, Navikas V, Palasik W, Pirskanen R, Fredrikson S, Link H. Tumor necrosis factor-alpha, lymphotoxin, interleukin (IL)-6, IL-10, IL-12 and perforin mRNA expression in mononuclear cells in response to acetylcholine receptor is augmented in myasthenia gravis. *J Neuroimmunol* 1996;71:191–198.

43. Matusevicius D, Kivisakk P, Navikas V, Soderstrom M, Fredrikson S, Link H. Interleukin-12 and perforin mRNA expression is augmented in blood mononuclear cells in multiple sclerosis. *Scand J Immunol* 1998;47:582–590.

44. Rubesa G, Podack ER, Sepcic J, Rukavina D. Increased perforin expression in multiple sclerosis patients during exacerbation of disease in peripheral blood lymphocytes. *J Neuroimmunol* 1997; 74:198–204.

45. Bugeon L, Cuturi MC, Paineau J, Anegon I, Soulillou JP. Similar levels of granzyme A and perforin mRNA expression in rejected and tolerated heart allografts in donor-specific tolerance in rats. *Transplantation* 1993;56:405–408.

46. Bugeon L, Cuturi MC, Paineau J, Chabannes D, Soulillou JP. Decreased IFN-gamma and IL-2 mRNA expression in peripheral tolerance to heart allografts with conserved granzyme A, perforin, and MHC antigens mRNA expression. *Transplant Proc* 1993;25:314–316.

47. Suthanthiran M. Molecular analyses of human renal allografts: differential intragraft gene expression during rejection. *Kidney Int Suppl* 1997;15–21.

48. Griffiths GM, Mueller C. Expression of perforin and granzymes in vivo: potential diagnostic markers for activated cytotoxic cells. *Immunol Today* 1991;12:415–419.

49. Mueller C, Shao Y, Altermatt HJ, Hess MW, Shelby J. The effect of cyclosporine treatment on the expression of genes encoding granzyme A and perforin in the infiltrate of mouse heart transplants. *Transplantation* 1993;55:139–145.

50. Chen RH, Bushell A, Fuggle SV, Wood KJ, Morris PJ. Expression of granzyme A and perforin in mouse heart transplants immunosuppressed with donor-specific transfusion and anti-CD4 monoclonal antibody. *Transplantation* 1996;61:625–629.

51. Wagner H, Gotze D, Ptschelinzew L, Rollinghoff M. Induction of cytotoxic T lymphocytes against I-region-coded determinants: in vitro evidence for a third histocompatibility locus in the mouse. *J Exp Med* 1975;142:1477–1487.

52. Swain SL, Dennert G, Wormsley S, Dutton RW. The Lyt phenotype of a long-term allospecific T cell line: both helper and killer activities to IA are mediated by Ly-1 cells. *Eur J Immunol* 1981;11: 175–180.

53. Meuer SC, Schlossman SF, Reinherz EL. Clonal analysis of human cytotoxic T lymphocytes: T4+ and T8+ effector T cells recognize products of different major histocompatibility complex regions. *Proc Natl Acad Sci USA* 1982;79:4395–4399.

54. Krensky AM, Reiss CS, Mier JW, Strominger JL, Burakoff SJ. Long-term human cytolytic T-cell lines allospecific for HLA-DR6 antigen are OKT4+. *Proc Natl Acad Sci USA* 1982;79:2365–2369.

55. Blazar BR, Taylor PA, Vallera DA. CD4+ and CD8+ T cells each can utilize a perforin-dependent pathway to mediate lethal graft-versus-host disease in major histocompatibility complex-disparate recipients. *Transplantation* 1997;64:571–576.

56. Geisberg M, Terry LA, Flomenberg N, Dupont B. Cytotoxic and proliferative allospecific T-cell clones contain perforin and mediate anti-CD3-induced cytotoxicity. *Hum Immunol* 1992;35: 239–245.

57. Susskind B, Shornick MD, Iannotti MR, et al. Cytolytic effector mechanisms of human CD4+ cytotoxic T lymphocytes. *Hum Immunol* 1996;45: 64–75.

58. Hahn S, Gehri R, Erb P. Mechanism and biological

significance of CD4-mediated cytotoxicity. *Immunol Rev* 1995;146:57–79.

59. Yasukawa M, Yakushijin Y, Hasegawa H, et al. Expression of perforin and membrane-bound lymphotoxin (tumor necrosis factor-beta) in virus-specific CD4+ human cytotoxic T-cell clones. *Blood* 1993;81:1527–1534.

60. Miskovsky EP, Liu AY, Pavlat W, et al. Studies of the mechanism of cytolysis by HIV-1-specific CD4+ human CTL clones induced by candidate AIDS vaccines. *J Immunol* 1994;153:2787–2799.

61. Oxenius A, Bachmann MF, Zinkernagel RM, Hengartner H. Virus-specific MHC-class II-restricted TCR-transgenic mice: effects on humoral and cellular immune responses after viral infection. *Eur J Immunol* 1998;28:390–400.

62. Strack P, Martin C, Saito S, Dekruyff RH, Ju ST. Metabolic inhibitors distinguish cytolytic activity of CD4 and CD8 clones. *Eur J Immunol* 1990;20:179–184.

63. Lancki DW, Hsieh CS, Fitch FW. Mechanisms of lysis by cytotoxic T lymphocyte clones: lytic activity and gene expression in cloned antigen-specific CD4+ and CD8+ T lymphocytes. *J Immunol* 1991;146:3242–3249.

64. Takayama H, Shinohara N, Kawasaki A, et al. Antigen-specific directional target cell lysis by perforin-negative T lymphocyte clones. *Int Immunol* 1991;3:1149–1156.

65. Garcia-Sanz JA, Plaetinck G, Velotti F, et al. Perforin is present only in normal activated Lyt2+ T lymphocytes and not in L3T4+ cells, but the serine protease granzyme A is made by both subsets. *EMBO J* 1987;6:933–938.

66. Smyth MJ, Ortaldo JR, Shinkai Y, et al. Interleukin 2 induction of pore-forming protein gene expression in human peripheral blood CD8+ T cells. *J Exp Med* 1990;171:1269–1281.

67. Lu P, Garcia-Sanz JA, Lichtenheld MG, Podack ER. Perforin expression in human peripheral blood mononuclear cells: definition of an IL-2-independent pathway of perforin induction in CD8+ T cells. *J Immunol* 1992;148:3354–3360.

68. Smyth MJ, Norihisa Y, Ortaldo JR. Multiple cytolytic mechanisms displayed by activated human peripheral blood T cell subsets. *J Immunol* 1992;148:55–62.

69. Nishimura T, Nakamura Y, Takeuchi Y, et al. Generation propagation, and targeting of human CD4+ helper/killer T cells induced by anti-CD3 monoclonal antibody plus recombinant IL-2: an efficient strategy for adoptive tumor immunotherapy. *J Immunol* 1992;148:285–291.

70. Rutella S, Rumi C, Lucia MB, Etuk B, Cauda R, Leone G. Flow cytometric detection of perforin in normal human lymphocyte subpopulations defined by expression of activation/differentiation antigens. *Immunol Lett* 1998;60:51–55.

71. Theze J, Alzari PM, Bertoglio J. Interleukin 2 and its receptors: recent advances and new immunological functions [see comments]. *Immunol Today* 1996;17:481–486.

72. Williams NS, Engelhard VH. Perforin-dependent cytotoxic activity and lymphokine secretion by CD4+ T cells are regulated by CD8+ T cells. *J Immunol* 1997;159:2091–2099.

73. Kawasaki A, Shinkai Y, Kuwana Y, et al. Perforin, a pore-forming protein detectable by monoclonal antibodies, is a functional marker for killer cells. *Int Immunol* 1990;2:677–684.

74. Salcedo TW, Azzoni L, Wolf SF, Perussia B. Modulation of perforin and granzyme messenger RNA expression in human natural killer cells. *J Immunol* 1993;151:2511–2520.

75. Kataoka K, Naomoto Y, Orita K. In vitro induction of perforin mRNA and cytotoxic activities in human splenocytes by the streptococcal preparation, OK-432. *Jpn J Clin Oncol* 1991;21:330–333.

76. Kataoka K, Naomoto Y, Kojima K, et al. Flow cytometric analysis on perforin induction in peripheral blood mononuclear cells with interleukin-2 or OK-432. *J Immunother* 1992;11:249–256.

77. Konjevic G, Schlesinger B, Cheng L, Olsen KJ, Podack ER, Spuzic I. Analysis of perforin expression in human peripheral blood lymphocytes, CD56+ natural killer cell subsets and its induction by interleukin-2. *Immunol Invest* 1995;24:499–507.

78. McFarland HI, Nahill SR, Maciaszek JW, Welsh RM. CD11b (Mac-1): a marker for CD8+ cytotoxic T cell activation and memory in virus infection. *J Immunol* 1992;149:1326–1333.

79. Hamann D, Baars PA, Rep MH, et al. Phenotypic and functional separation of memory and effector human CD8+ T cells. *J Exp Med* 1997;186:1407–1418.

80. Berthou C, Legros-Maida S, Soulie A, et al. Cord blood T lymphocytes lack constitutive perforin expression in contrast to adult peripheral blood T lymphocytes. *Blood* 1995;85:1540–1546.

81. Fagnoni FF, Vescovini R, Mazzola M, et al. Expansion of cytotoxic CD8+ CD28− T cells in healthy ageing people, including centenarians. *Immunology* 1996;88:501–507.

82. Azuma M, Phillips JH, Lanier LL. CD28− T lymphocytes: antigenic and functional properties. *J Immunol* 1993;150:1147–1159.

83. Bachmann MF, Kundig TM, Hengartner H, Zinkernagel RM. Protection against immunopathological consequences of a viral infection by activated but not resting cytotoxic T cells: T cell memory without "memory T cells"? *Proc Natl Acad Sci USA* 1997;94:640–645.

84. Kawasaki A, Shinkai Y, Yagita H, Okumura K. Expression of perforin in murine natural killer cells and cytotoxic T lymphocytes in vivo. *Eur J Immunol* 1992;22:1215–1219.

85. Zimmerman C, Brduscha-Riem K, Blaser C, Zinkernagel RM, Pircher H. Visualization, characterization, and turnover of CD8+ memory T cells in virus-infected hosts. *J Exp Med* 1996;183:1367–1375.

86. Mosmann TR, Sad S. The expanding universe of T-cell subsets: Th1, Th2 and more. *Immunol Today* 1996;17:138–146.

87. Mosmann TR, Li L, Sad S. Functions of CD8 T-cell subsets secreting different cytokine patterns. *Semin Immunol* 1997;9:87–92.

88. Carter LL, Dutton RW. Relative perforin- and

Fas-mediated lysis in T1 and T2 CD8 effector populations. *J Immunol* 1995;155:1028–1031.

89. Reyburn H, Mandelboim O, Vales-Gomez M, et al. Human NK cells: their ligands, receptors and functions. *Immunol Rev* 1997;155:119–125.

90. Kaufmann SH. Gamma/delta and other unconventional T lymphocytes: what do they see and what do they do? *Proc Natl Acad Sci USA* 1996;93:2272–2279.

91. Ortaldo JR, Winkler-Pickett R, Kopp W, et al. Relationship of large and small CD3⁻ CD56⁺ lymphocytes mediating NK-associated activities. *J Leukoc Biol* 1992;52:287–295.

92. Parr EL, Young LH, Parr MB, Young JD. Granulated metrial gland cells of pregnant mouse uterus are natural killer-like cells that contain perforin and serine esterases. *J Immunol* 1990;145:2365–2372.

93. Lin PY, Joag SV, Young JD, Chang YS, Soong YK, Kuo TT. Expression of perforin by natural killer cells within first trimester endometrium in humans. *Biol Reprod* 1991;45:698–703.

94. Zheng LM, Joag SV, Parr MB, Parr EL, Young JD. Perforin-expressing granulated metrial gland cells in murine deciduoma. *J Exp Med* 1991;174:1221–1226.

95. Gudelj L, Christmas SE, Laskarin G, Johnson PM, Podack ER, Rukavina D. Membrane phenotype and expression of perforin and serine esterases by CD3⁻ peripheral blood and decidual granular lymphocyte-derived clones. *Am J Reprod Immunol* 1997;38:162–167.

96. Stallmach T, Ehrenstein T, Isenmann S, Muller C, Hengartner H, Kagi D. The role of perforin-expression by granular metrial gland cells in pregnancy. *Eur J Immunol* 1995;25:3342–3348.

97. Gulan G, Podack ER, Rukavina D, et al. Perforin-expressing lymphocytes in peripheral blood and decidua of human first-trimester pathological pregnancies. *Am J Reprod Immunol* 1997;38:9–18.

98. Ortaldo JR, Mason A, Overton R. Lymphokine-activated killer cells: analysis of progenitors and effectors. *J Exp Med* 1986;164:1193–1205.

99. Phillips JH, Lanier LL. Dissection of the lymphokine-activated killer phenomenon: relative contribution of peripheral blood natural killer cells and T lymphocytes to cytolysis. *J Exp Med* 1986;164:814–825.

100. Testa U, Care A, Montesoro E, et al. Interleukin-2-dependent long-term cultures of low-density lymphocytes allow the proliferation of lymphokine-activated killer cells with natural killer, Ti gamma/delta or TNK phenotype. *Cancer Immunol Immunother* 1990;31:11–18.

101. Kato K, Sato N, Tanabe T, Yagita H, Agatsuma T, Hashimoto Y. Establishment of mouse lymphokine-activated killer cell clones and their properties. *Jpn J Cancer Res* 1991;82:456–463.

102. Koizumi H, Liu CC, Zheng LM, et al. Expression of perforin and serine esterases by human gamma/delta T cells. *J Exp Med* 1991;173:499–502.

103. Kobata T, Shinkai Y, Iigo Y, et al. Thy-1-positive dendritic epidermal cells contain a killer protein perforin. *Int Immunol* 1990;2:1113–1116.

104. Krahenbuhl O, Gattesco S, Tschopp J. Murine

Thy-1⁺ dendritic epidermal T cell lines express granule-associated perforin and a family of granzyme molecules. *Immunobiology* 1992;184:392–401.

105. Guy-Grand D, Malassis-Seris M, Briottet C, Vassalli P. Cytotoxic differentiation of mouse gut thymodependent and independent intraepithelial T lymphocytes is induced locally: correlation between functional assays, presence of perforin and granzyme transcripts, and cytoplasmic granules. *J Exp Med* 1991;173:1549–1552.

106. Nakata M, Smyth MJ, Norihisa Y, et al. Constitutive expression of pore-forming protein in peripheral blood gamma/delta T cells: implication for their cytotoxic role in vivo. *J Exp Med* 1990;172:1877–1880.

107. Carlyle JR, Michie AM, Furlonger C, et al. Identification of a novel developmental stage marking lineage commitment of progenitor thymocytes. *J Exp Med* 1997;186:173–182.

108. Vandekerckhove BA, Barcena A, Schols D, Mohan-Peterson S, Spits H, Roncarolo MG. In vivo cytokine expression in the thymus: CD3 high human thymocytes are activated and already functionally differentiated in helper and cytotoxic cells. *J Immunol* 1994;152:1738–1743.

109. Bennett IM, Zatsepina O, Zamai L, Azzoni L, Mikheeva T, Perussia B. Definition of a natural killer NKR-P1A⁺/CD56⁻/CD16⁻ functionally immature human NK cell subset that differentiates in vitro in the presence of interleukin 12. *J Exp Med* 1996;184:1845–1856.

110. Gaddy J, Broxmeyer HE. Cord blood CD16⁺56⁻ cells with low lytic activity are possible precursors of mature natural killer cells. *Cell Immunol* 1997;180:132–142.

111. Nakazawa T, Agematsu K, Yabuhara A. Later development of Fas ligand-mediated cytotoxicity as compared with granule-mediated cytotoxicity during the maturation of natural killer cells. *Immunology* 1997;92:180–187.

112. Berthou C, Marolleau JP, Lafaurie C, et al. Granzyme B and perforin lytic proteins are expressed in CD34⁺ peripheral blood progenitor cells mobilized by chemotherapy and granulocyte colony-stimulating factor. *Blood* 1995;86:3500–3506.

113. Vaz F, Hoffman R, Almeida-Porada G, Ascensao JL. Definition of early progenitors and functional maturation of human natural killer cells: requirements for cytocidal activity. *Pathobiology* 1998;66:41–48.

114. Li H, Pohler U, Strehlow I, et al. Macrophage precursor cells produce perforin and perform Yac-1 lytic activity in response to stimulation with interleukin-2. *J Leukoc Biol* 1994;56:117–123.

115. Boulland ML, Kanavaros P, Wechsler J, Casiraghi O, Gaulard P. Cytotoxic protein expression in natural killer cell lymphomas and in alpha beta and gamma delta peripheral T-cell lymphomas. *J Pathol* 1997;183:432–439.

116. Chiang AK, Chan AC, Srivastava G, Ho FC. Nasal T/natural killer (NK)-cell lymphomas are derived from Epstein-Barr virus-infected cytotoxic lymphocytes of both NK- and T-cell lineage. *Int J Cancer* 1997;73:332–338.

117. Cooke CB, Krenacs L, Stetler-Stevenson M, et al. Hepatosplenic T-cell lymphoma: a distinct clinicopathologic entity of cytotoxic gamma delta T-cell origin. *Blood* 1996;88:4265–4274.

118. Daum S, Foss HD, Anagnostopoulos I, et al. Expression of cytotoxic molecules in intestinal T-cell lymphomas: the German Study Group on Intestinal Non-Hodgkin Lymphoma. *J Pathol* 1997; 182:311–317.

119. Foss HD, Anagnostopoulos I, Araujo I, et al. Anaplastic large-cell lymphomas of T-cell and null-cell phenotype express cytotoxic molecules. *Blood* 1996;88:4005–4011.

120. Foss HD, Demel G, Anagnostopoulos I, Araujo I, Hummel M, Stein H. Uniform expression of cytotoxic molecules in anaplastic large cell lymphoma of null/T cell phenotype and in cell lines derived from anaplastic large cell lymphoma. *Pathobiology* 1997;65:83–90.

121. Horiuchi T, Yasukawa M, Yanagisawa K, Hato T, Fujita S. Immunological analysis of T cells bearing T cell receptor alpha/beta or gamma/delta in patients with granular lymphocyte proliferative disorder. *Acta Haematol* 1993;89:174–179.

122. Krenacs L, Wellmann A, Sorbara L, et al. Cytotoxic cell antigen expression in anaplastic large cell lymphomas of T- and null-cell type and Hodgkin's disease: evidence for distinct cellular origin. *Blood* 1997;89:980–989.

123. Martin AR, Chan WC, Perry DA, Greiner TC, Weisenburger DD. Aggressive natural killer cell lymphoma of the small intestine. *Mod Pathol* 1995;8:467–472.

124. Mori N, Yatabe Y, Oka K, et al. Expression of perforin in nasal lymphoma: additional evidence of its natural killer cell derivation. *Am J Pathol* 1996;149:699–705.

125. Ng CS, Lo ST, Chan JK, Chan WC. CD56$^+$ putative natural killer cell lymphomas: production of cytolytic effectors and related proteins mediating tumor cell apoptosis? *Hum Pathol* 1997;28:1276–1282.

126. Ohshima K, Suzumiya J, Shimazaki K, et al. Nasal T/NK cell lymphomas commonly express perforin and Fas ligand: important mediators of tissue damage. *Histopathology* 1997;31:444–450.

127. Oshimi K, Shinkai Y, Okumura K, Oshimi Y, Mizoguchi H. Perforin gene expression in granular lymphocyte proliferative disorders. *Blood* 1990; 75:704–708.

128. Salhany KE, Feldman M, Kahn MJ, et al. Hepatosplenic gammadelta T-cell lymphoma: ultrastructural, immunophenotypic, and functional evidence for cytotoxic T lymphocyte differentiation. *Hum Pathol* 1997;28:674–685.

129. Seko Y, Azuma M, Yagita H, et al. Perforin-positive leukemic cell infiltration in the heart of a patient with T-cell prolymphocytic leukemia. *Intern Med* 1995;34:782–784.

130. Yamashita Y, Yatabe Y, Tsuzuki T, et al. Perforin and granzyme expression in cytotoxic T-cell lymphomas. *Mod Pathol* 1998;11:313–323.

131. Berthou C, Michel L, Soulie A, et al. Acquisition of granzyme B and Fas ligand proteins by human keratinocytes contributes to epidermal cell defense. *J Immunol* 1997;159:5293–5300.

132. Gasque P, Jones J, Singhrao SK, Morgan B. Identification of an astrocyte cell population from human brain that expresses perforin, a cytotoxic protein implicated in immune defense. *J Exp Med* 1998;187:451–460.

133. De Jong R, Brouwer M, Miedema F, van Lier RA. Human CD8$^+$ T lymphocytes can be divided into CD45RA$^+$ and CD45RO$^+$ cells with different requirements for activation and differentiation. *J Immunol* 1991;146:2088–2094.

134. De Jong R, Brouwer M, Rebel VI, Van Seventer GA, Miedema F, Van Lier RA. Generation of alloreactive cytolytic T lymphocytes by immobilized anti-CD3 monoclonal antibodies: analysis of requirements for human cytolytic T-lymphocyte differentiation. *Immunology* 1990;70:357–364.

135. Liu CC, Rafii S, Granelli-Piperno A, Trapani JA, Young JD. Perforin and serine esterase gene expression in stimulated human T cells: kinetics, mitogen requirements, and effects of cyclosporin A. *J Exp Med* 1989;170:2105–2118.

136. Gamero AM, Ussery D, Reintgen DS, Puleo CA, Djeu JY. Interleukin 15 induction of lymphokine-activated killer cell function against autologous tumor cells in melanoma patient lymphocytes by a CD18-dependent, perforin-related mechanism. *Cancer Res* 1995;55:4988–4994.

137. Ye W, Young JD, Liu CC. Interleukin-15 induces the expression of mRNAs of cytolytic mediators and augments cytotoxic activities in primary murine lymphocytes. *Cell Immunol* 1996;174:54–62.

138. Waldmann T, Tagaya Y, Bamford R. Interleukin-2, interleukin-15, and their receptors. *Int Rev Immunol* 1998;16:205–226.

139. Makrigiannis AP, Hoskin DW. Inhibition of CTL induction by rapamycin: IL-2 rescues granzyme B and perforin expression but only partially restores cytotoxic activity. *J Immunol* 1997;159:4700–4707.

140. Miyazaki T, Liu ZJ, Kawahara A, et al. Three distinct IL-2 signaling pathways mediated by bcl-2, c-myc, and lck cooperate in hematopoietic cell proliferation. *Cell* 1995;81:223–231.

141. Smyth MJ, Strobl SL, Young HA, Ortaldo JR, Ochoa AC. Regulation of lymphokine-activated killer activity and pore-forming protein gene expression in human peripheral blood CD8$^+$ T lymphocytes: inhibition by transforming growth factor-beta. *J Immunol* 1991;146:3289–3297.

142. Liu CC, Rafii S, Koizumi H, Granelli-Piperno A, Young JD. Perforin gene expression in stimulated human peripheral blood T cells studied by in situ hybridization and northern blotting analysis. *Immunol Lett* 1992;33:79–85.

143. Leger-Ravet MB, Mathiot C, Portier A, et al. Increased expression of perforin and granzyme B genes in patients with metastatic melanoma treated with recombinant interleukin-2. *Cancer Immunol Immunother* 1994;39:53–58.

144. Suzuki H, Kundig TM, Furlonger C, et al. Deregulated T cell activation and autoimmunity in mice lacking interleukin-2 receptor beta. *Science* 1995;268:1472–1476.

145. Cesano A, Visonneau S, Clark SC, Santoli D. Cel-

lular and molecular mechanisms of activation of MHC nonrestricted cytotoxic cells by IL-12. *J Immunol* 1993;151:2943–2957.

146. Trinchieri G. Proinflammatory and immunoregulatory functions of interleukin-12. *Int Rev Immunol* 1998;16:365–396.

147. Chouaib S, Chehimi J, Bani L, et al. Interleukin 12 induces the differentiation of major histocompatibility complex class I-primed cytotoxic T-lymphocyte precursors into allospecific cytotoxic effectors. *Proc Natl Acad Sci USA* 1994;91:12659–12663.

148. Tannenbaum CS, Wicker N, Armstrong D, et al. Cytokine and chemokine expression in tumors of mice receiving systemic therapy with IL-12. *J Immunol* 1996;156:693–699.

149. Dias S, Thomas H, Balkwill F. Multiple molecular and cellular changes associated with tumour stasis and regression during IL-12 therapy of a murine breast cancer model. *Int J Cancer* 1998;75:151–157.

150. Smyth MJ, Ortaldo JR, Bere W, Yagita H, Okumura K, Young HA. IL-2 and IL-6 synergize to augment the pore-forming protein gene expression and cytotoxic potential of human peripheral blood T cells. *J Immunol* 1990;145:1159–1166.

151. Bass HZ, Yamashita N, Clement LT. Heterogeneous mechanisms of human cytotoxic T lymphocyte generation. II. Differential effects of IL-6 on the helper cell- independent generation of CTL from CD8$^+$ precursor subpopulations. *J Immunol* 1993;151:2895–2903.

152. Greene AL, Makrigiannis AP, Fitzpatrick L, Hoskin DW. Anti-CD3-activated killer T cells: interleukin-6 modulates the induction of major histocompatibility complex-unrestricted cytotoxicity and the expression of genes coding for cytotoxic effector molecules. *J Interferon Cytokine Res* 1997;17:727–737.

153. Sugihara K, Sone S, Shono M, et al. Enhancement by monocytes of perforin production and its gene expression by human CD8$^+$ T cells stimulated with interleukin-2. *Jpn J Cancer Res* 1992;83:1223–1230.

154. Fujiwara T, Grimm EA. Specific inhibition of interleukin 1 beta gene expression by an antisense oligonucleotide: obligatory role of interleukin 1 in the generation of lymphokine-activated killer cells. *Cancer Res* 1992;52:4954–4959.

155. Smyth MJ, Norihisa Y, Gerard JR, Young HA, Ortaldo JR. IL-7 regulation of cytotoxic lymphocytes: pore-forming protein gene expression, interferon-gamma production, and cytotoxicity of human peripheral blood lymphocytes subsets. *Cell Immunol* 1991;138:390–403.

156. Erard F, Wild MT, Garcia-Sanz JA, Le Gros G. Switch of CD8 T cells to noncytolytic CD8$^-$CD4$^-$ cells that make TH2 cytokines and help B cells. *Science* 1993;260:1802–1805.

157. Bass HZ, Yamashita N, Clement LT. Heterogeneous mechanisms of human cytotoxic T lymphocyte generation. I. Differential helper cell requirement for the generation of cytotoxic effector cells from CD8$^+$ precursor subpopulations. *J Immunol* 1992;149:2489–2495.

158. Guerder S, Carding SR, Flavell RA. B7 costimulation is necessary for the activation of the lytic function in cytotoxic T lymphocyte precursors. *J Immunol* 1995;155:5167–5174.

159. Kagi D, Ledermann B, Burki K, et al. Cytotoxicity mediated by T cells and natural killer cells is greatly impaired in perforin-deficient mice. *Nature* 1994;369:31–37.

160. Shahinian A, Pfeffer K, Lee KP, et al. Differential T cell costimulatory requirements in CD28-deficient mice. *Science* 1993;261:609–612.

161. Nelson PJ, Geller RL, Podack E, Bach FH. Molecular events in late stages of T-cell functional maturation. *Scand J Immunol* 1992;35:311–320.

162. Hommel-Berrey G, Bochan M, Brahmi Z. Increase in tumor necrosis factor-alpha mRNA but not perforin mRNA expression in response to two newly characterized anti-LFA-1 monoclonal antibodies. *Nat Immun* 1994;13:301–314.

163. Nakajima F, Khanna A, Xu G, et al. Immunotherapy with anti-CD3 monoclonal antibodies and recombinant interleukin 2: stimulation of molecular programs of cytotoxic killer cells and induction of tumor regression. *Proc Natl Acad Sci USA* 1994;91:7889–7893.

164. Asano T, Khanna A, Lagman M, Li B, Suthanthiran M. Immunostimulatory therapy with anti-CD3 monoclonal antibodies and recombinant interleukin-2: heightened in vivo expression of mRNA encoding cytotoxic attack molecules and immunoregulatory cytokines and regression of murine renal cell carcinoma. *J Urol* 1997;157:2396–2401.

165. Ye W, Zheng LM, Young JD, Liu CC. The involvement of interleukin (IL)-15 in regulating the differentiation of granulated metrial gland cells in mouse pregnant uterus. *J Exp Med* 1996;184:2405–2410.

166. Clement MV, Haddad P, Soulie A, et al. Involvement of granzyme B and perforin gene expression in the lytic potential of human natural killer cells. *Res Immunol* 1990;141:477–489.

167. Aste-Amezaga M, D'Andrea A, Kubin M, Trinchieri G. Cooperation of natural killer cell stimulatory factor/interleukin-12 with other stimuli in the induction of cytokines and cytotoxic cell-associated molecules in human T and NK cells. *Cell Immunol* 1994;156:480–492.

168. Salvucci O, Mami-Chouaib F, Moreau JL, Theze J, Chehimi J, Chouaib S. Differential regulation of interleukin-12- and interleukin-15-induced natural killer cell activation by interleukin-4. *Eur J Immunol* 1996;26:2736–2741.

169. Malygin AM, Meri S, Timonen T. Regulation of natural killer cell activity by transforming growth factor-beta and prostaglandin E2. *Scand J Immunol* 1993;37:71–76.

170. DeBlaker-Hohe DF, Yamauchi A, Yu CR, Horvath-Arcidiacono JA, Bloom ET. IL-12 synergizes with IL-2 to induce lymphokine-activated cytoxicity and perforin and granzyme gene expression in fresh human NK cells. *Cell Immunol* 1995;165:33–43.

171. Klein JL, Fickenscher H, Holliday JE, Biesinger B, Fleckenstein B. Herpesvirus saimiri immortalized gamma delta T cell line activated by IL-12. *J Immunol* 1996;156:2754–2760.

172. Lichtenheld MG, Podack ER. Structure of the human perforin gene: a simple gene organization with

interesting potential regulatory sequences. *J Immunol* 1989;143:4267–4274.

173. Lichtenheld MG, Podack ER. Structure and function of the murine perforin promoter and upstream region: reciprocal gene activation or silencing in perforin positive and negative cells. *J Immunol* 1992;149:2619–2626.

174. Youn BS, Liu CC, Kim KK, Young JD, Kwon MH, Kwon BS. Structure of the mouse pore-forming protein (perforin) gene: analysis of transcription initiation site, 5′ flanking sequence, and alternative splicing of 5′ untranslated regions. *J Exp Med* 1991;173:813–822.

175. Trapani JA, Kwon BS, Kozak CA, Chintamaneni C, Young JD, Dupont B. Genomic organization of the mouse pore-forming protein (perforin) gene and localization to chromosome 10: similarities to and differences from C9. *J Exp Med* 1990; 171:545–557.

176. Fink TM, Zimmer M, Weitz S, Tschopp J, Jenne DE, Lichter P. Human perforin (PRF1) maps to 10q22, a region that is syntenic with mouse chromosome 10. *Genomics* 1992;13:1300–1302.

177. Garcia-Sanz JA, Podack ER. Regulation of perforin gene expression in a T cell hybrid with inducible cytolytic activity. *Eur J Immunol* 1993; 23:1877–1883.

178. Lowrey DM, Aebischer T, Olsen K, et al. Cloning, analysis, and expression of murine perforin 1 cDNA, a component of cytolytic T-cell granules with homology to complement component C9. *Proc Natl Acad Sci USA* 1989;86:247–251.

179. Bajpai A, Kwon BS, Brahmi Z. Rapid loss of perforin and serine protease RNA in cytotoxic lymphocytes exposed to sensitive targets. *Immunology* 1991;74:258–263.

180. Kim KK, Blakely A, Zhou Z, Davis J, Clark W, Kwon BS. Changes in the level of perforin and its transcript during effector and target cell interactions. *Immunol Lett* 1993;36:161–169.

181. Bochan MR, Brahmi Z. Target cell-directed rapid degradation of TNF-alpha messenger RNA in human cytotoxic T cells. *Immunol Lett* 1994;40:37–42.

182. Bochan M, Hommel-Berrey G, Brahmi Z. Target cell-directed degradation of perforin mRNA in CTL: lack of correlation with loss of protein and lytic ability. *Mol Immunol* 1994;31:401–410.

183. Goebel WS, Schloemer RH, Brahmi Z. Target cell-induced perforin mRNA turnover in NK3.3 cells is mediated by multiple elements within the mRNA coding region. *Mol Immunol* 1996;33:341–349.

184. Garraway IP, Semple K, Smale ST. Transcription of the lymphocyte-specific terminal deoxynucleotidyltransferase gene requires a specific core promoter structure. *Proc Natl Acad Sci USA* 1996;93:4336–4341.

185. Berg JM. Sp1 and the subfamily of zinc finger proteins with guanine-rich binding sites. *Proc Natl Acad Sci USA* 1992;89:11109–11110.

186. Blake MC, Jambou RC, Swick AG, Kahn JW, Azizkhan JC. Transcriptional initiation is controlled by upstream GC-box interactions in a TATAA-less promoter. *Mol Cell Biol* 1990;10: 6632–6641.

187. Azizkhan JC, Jensen DE, Pierce AJ, Wade M. Transcription from TATA-less promoters: dihydrofolate reductase as a model. *Crit Rev Eukaryot Gene Expr* 1993;3:229–254.

188. Smale ST. Transcription initiation from TATA-less promoters within eukaryotic protein-coding genes. *Biochim Biophys Acta* 1997;1351:73–88.

189. Zhang Y, Lichtenheld MG. Non-killer cell-specific transcription factors silence the perforin promoter. *J Immunol* 1997;158:1734–1741.

190. Youn BS, Kim KK, Kwon BS. A critical role of Sp1- and Ets-related transcription factors in maintaining CTL-specific expression of the mouse perforin gene. *J Immunol* 1996;157:3499–3509.

191. Lichtenheld MG, Podack ER, Levy RB. Transgenic control of perforin gene expression: functional evidence for two separate control regions. *J Immunol* 1995;154:2153–2163.

192. Smyth MJ, Kershaw MH, Hulett MD, McKenzie IF, Trapani JA. Use of the 5′-flanking region of the mouse perforin gene to express human Fc gamma receptor I in cytotoxic T lymphocytes. *J Leukoc Biol* 1994;55:514–522.

193. Koizumi H, Horta MF, Youn BS, et al. Identification of a killer cell-specific regulatory element of the mouse perforin gene: an Ets-binding site-homologous motif that interacts with Ets-related proteins. *Mol Cell Biol* 1993;13:6690–6701.

194. Horta MF, Fu KC, Koizumi H, Young JD, Liu CC. Cell-free conversion of a ubiquitous nuclear protein into a killer-cell- specific form that binds to the NF-P enhancer element of the mouse perforin gene. *Eur J Biochem* 1996;238:639–646.

195. Bassuk AG, Leiden JM. The role of Ets transcription factors in the development and function of the mammalian immune system. *Adv Immunol* 1997;64:65–104.

196. Horvath CM, Darnell JE. The state of the STATs: recent developments in the study of signal transduction to the nucleus. *Curr Opin Cell Biol* 1997;9:233–239.

197. Ihle JN, Nosaka T, Thierfelder W, Quelle FW, Shimoda K. Jaks and Stats in cytokine signaling. *Stem Cells* 1997;15:105–111.

198. Rao A, Luo C, Hogan PG. Transcription factors of the NFAT family: regulation and function. *Annu Rev Immunol* 1997;15:707–747.

Cytotoxic Cells: Basic Mechanisms and Medical Applications, edited by Michail V. Sitkovsky and Pierre A. Henkart. Lippincott Williams & Wilkins, Philadelphia © 2000.

Chapter 11

Perforin: Structure, Biosynthesis, and Immune Regulatory Functions

Eckhard R. Podack

Department of Microbiology and Immunology, University of Miami School of Medicine, Miami, Florida 33101, USA

Perforin derived its name from its ability to perforate membranes as deduced by electron microscopy (1,2). Other names for perforin, coined at about the same time, are cytolysin (3), C9-related protein (4), and pore-forming protein (PFP) (5). Earlier electron microscopy studies (6) and functional studies (7) had suggested that lymphocyte-mediated cytolysis and complement-mediated lysis may be related mechanistically. At the time of the initial perforin description, research in the field of the membrane attack complex of complement had progressed to the point that it was clear that a single protein, complement component C9, was able, under appropriate conditions, to form a transmembrane pore through membrane insertion and polymerization (8,9). This discovery allowed the conceptual hypothesis that a single lymphocyte protein may be able to induce membrane pores and cell lysis.

Following the unambiguous demonstration of perforin-induced membrane lesions by cloned natural killer (NK) cells and cytotoxic T lymphocytes (CLTs), an intense search for the intracellular localization of perforin began. The groups of Henkart (10) and Podack (11) succeeded at about the same time to demonstrate that perforin is contained in cytoplasmic granules of CTLs and NK cells, that isolated granules are cytotoxic in the presence of Ca, lysing most cells with high efficiency, and that isolated granules were able to form polyperforin complexes. This demonstration was followed by the purification of perforin (12–14) and subsequent cloning of the cDNA (15–17).

STRUCTURE OF PERFORIN

Homology comparison of perforin (Fig. 11-1) confirmed the predicted homology of perforin with C9. However, only two domains of about 50 amino acids each (P-domains in Fig. 11-1) showed significant homology to the terminal complement proteins, whereas the complement proteins C6, C7, C8α, C8β, and C9 show significantly more homology to each other over the entire length of the molecule. The complement proteins contain domains shared with the low density lipoprotein (LDL) receptor (18) and with thrombospondin, which are not present in perforin. Perforin, in contrast, contains a C2 domain that is homologous to similar domains in Ca-dependent phospholipid-binding proteins such as protein kinase C and phospholipase.

The C2 domain, uncovered after intracellular proteolytic cleavage of the C-terminal perforin peptide (19), is likely to be responsible for the Ca-dependent binding of perforin to phospholipid head groups (20,21); and the P domains may be responsible for concerted membrane insertion and polymerization.

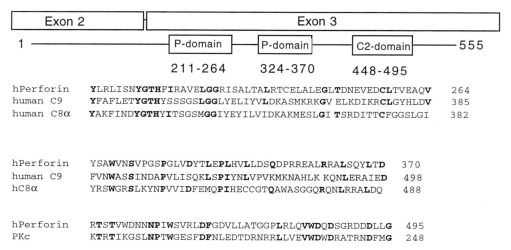

FIG. 11-1. Domain structure of perforin and homology alignment with complement component C9, C8α, and protein kinase C (PKC). The two P-domains have been found only in perforin and the complement proteins C6, C7, C8α, C8β, and C9; they are believed to be important for membrane insertion, polymerization, and channel formation. The C2 domain is not contained in the complement proteins but is found in a number of Ca-dependent phospholipid-binding proteins such as PKC.

The membrane insertion process of pore-forming proteins has been best characterized for C9 by electron microscopy and electrophysiology (8,9,22,23); and it is assumed that perforin membrane insertion works analogously (3). According to this model, phospholipid molecules are the receptors for perforin, which binds in a Ca-dependent process. Close apposition of two or more perforin molecules results in their Ca-dependent unfolding, polymerization, and membrane insertion, with perforin simultaneously undergoing a hydrophilic to amphiphilic transition. Membrane pores are generated if this process leads to membrane insertion of the polyperforin complex, the pore size depending on the number of perforin protomers per complex. The minimum number is likely to be a perforin dimer, and the maximum number of about 16 to 20 is reached upon circularization of the polymeric complex (Fig. 11-2). Transmembrane channel sizes therefore may vary from about 1 to 16 nm. Membrane pores are detectable by electron microscopy only if the complex is almost fully assembled, whereas functional and biologic effects are detectable for any of the smaller complexes.

If perforin polymerizes in the absence of membranes, it assumes the same structural conformation as membrane-bound perforin. This indicates that the structural transition from monomeric perforin to the polymeric form is driven by the protein–protein interacting forces during polymerization. These forces may provide also the energy for membrane insertion of perforin, displacement of lipids, and creation of an aqueous internal channel across the hydrophobic phase of the membrane. Perforin polymerized in solution is unable to insert itself into membranes and is inactive in membrane lysis. The inability of polyperforin to insert into membranes explains the short half-life of active perforin in the presence of Ca ions. Ca-induced polymerization results in the generation of inactive complexes unless polymerization is coupled with membrane insertion. Because extracellular Ca is ubiquitous, perforin cannot act at a distance. The biochemistry of perforin thus requires close killer target cell

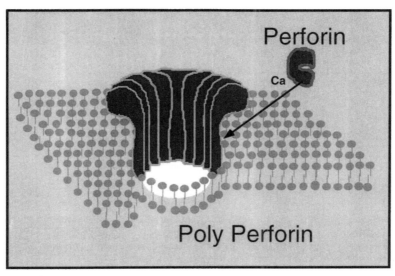

FIG. 11-2. Calcium-dependent perforin polymerization in phospholipid bilayers.

contact and direct secretion of perforin onto the target membrane.

FUNCTIONAL EFFECTS OF POLYPERFORIN ON TARGET MEMBRANES

Membrane insertion of perforin causes transmembrane pore formation, which has been observed directly through step conductance increases across lipid bilayers perforated by perforin (14). Step conductance increases vary more than tenfold from 400pS to 6nS in 0.1 M NaCl, indicating different pore sizes due to formation of perforin complexes of varying oligomeric number. The membrane pores are not ion-specific or voltage-independent. Perforin polymers assembled on phospholipid vesicles result in the efflux of vesicle-entrapped solutes limited by the Stoke's radius of the solute relative to the polyperforin pore size. Polyperforin inserted into nucleated cells causes rapid and sustained membrane depolarization. The effect on cell viability is perforin dose-dependent; at high doses of perforin, cells do not recover

their membrane polarization and die owing to the membrane damage caused by perforin. At lower perforin doses, cells may survive through active membrane repair if the perforin dose does not exceed the repair capacity. We have measured that tumor cells (Raji) can repair pores caused by 2×10^5 C9 molecules within 2 minutes (unpublished). Repair is dependent on Ca and is usually effected by endocytosis of the perforated membrane (24) or, in polymorphonuclear granulocytes, by pinching off and sloughing of the membrane (25). Exclusion of Ca, which blocks membrane repair, results in increased sensitivity of target cells to membrane pore formers (26); in the absence of intracellular Ca, nucleated target cells do not undergo DNA degradation, which is normally associated with cell death upon CTL or NK attack.

Calcium-dependent repair of perforin pores by endocytosis results in the pinocytosis of extracellular fluid containing granzymes (27) if perforin is secreted by the granule exocytosis mechanism (Fig. 11-3). As described in other chapters in this book, granzymes are responsible for triggering

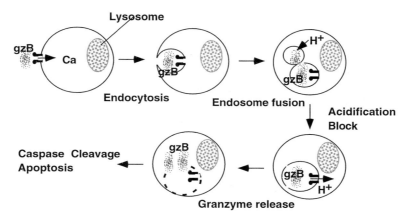

FIG. 11-3. Perforin-induced repair endocytosis is triggered by Ca influx, followed by removal of the membrane pore and uptake of granzymes. Polyperforin-containing endosome resistant to proteolytic removal is generated. Polyperforin pore prevents acidification and fusion with lysosome. The sequence ends by release of granzymes and triggering of apoptosis.

apoptosis in the target cell. Polyperforin, similar to poly-C9 (28), is exceedingly resistant to proteolysis. Endosomes containing polyperforin complexes therefore cannot be acidified and do not undergo the usual fusion with acidic lysosomes. It is likely that the stability of polyperforin and its resistance to proteolytic degradation is a prerequisite for its delivery function of granzymes and other granule components to the cytoplasm of the target cell. The stability of polyperforin and its pore-forming capacity prevents endosome–lysosome fusion and destruction of granzymes in the lysosomal furnace.

The combination of perforin with granzymes in the cytolytic granules of CTLs and NK cells confronts the target cell upon attack with an unenviable choice: repair perforin membrane lesions and take up granzymes causing apoptosis or do not repair and die of membrane depolarization and loss of ionic equilibrium. This deadly combination therefore does not require compliance of the target cell and distinguishes perforin mediated killing from apoptotic processes such as those mediated by Fas and Fas ligand (FasL), which can be modulated by genes of the tar-

get cell, by viral genes upon infection, and by oncogenic transformation.

BIOSYNTHESIS OF PERFORIN

Perforin is encoded by a single gene on chromosome 10q22 in humans (29) and 10 in mouse (30). Three exons comprise the mature transcript (31): Exon 1 codes for most of the 5' untranslated region; exon 2 encodes the start signal, signal peptide, and the protein coding sequence up to but not including the first P-domain, which is encoded by exon 3 together with the second P-domain, the C2 domain, and the 3' untranslated sequence. Perforin expression is regulated by transcriptional control. Several cytokines, including IL-2 (16), IL-2 plus IL-6 (32), IL-1 plus IL-2 (33), IL-12 (34), and Ca signals (35) are strong signals for perforin transcription, whereas TGF-β suppresses (36) the induction of perforin transcription. Only activated T cells and NK cells express perforin; recently it was reported that activated keratinocytes also express perforin, granzyme B, and FasL (37).

The cell specificity of perforin expression is determined by the 1800 basepair (bp) long promoter region, upstream of the transcription start site (38). This sequence contains elements for the binding of transcriptional repressors, preventing perforin expression in non-T and non-NK cells (39,40). Although the 1,800-bp promoter of perforin accounts for the cell specificity of perforin expression *in vitro* and *in vivo* in transgenic mice (31), it does not contain the elements responsible for perforin induction by IL-2. This inducibility by cytokines appears to be controlled by two novel STAT-dependent enhancer elements approximately 15 kb upstream of the perforin promoter (M. G. Lichtenheld, unpublished observations).

TRANSPORT OF PERFORIN TO CYTOPLASMIC GRANULES

Granules are storage organelles for secretory products that are released by a Ca-dependent stimulus through the TCR or are bypassed by phorbol esters (41). Cytotoxic granules of T cells and NK cells have properties of both storage granules and lysosomes (42) and have been termed granulosomes (43). Proteins targeted to granulosomes come from the cell surface (44) and from the endoplasmic reticulum (45). Whereas most granzymes use the lysosomal–endosomal sorting system of the mannose-6-phosphate receptor pathway, perforin does not use this targeting system and is glycosylated with complex carbohydrates when it leaves the trans-Golgi. The targeting signals for perforin to traffic to granules so far have not been defined. Although the largest portion of perforin and granzymes is directed to and stored in granules, a substantial proportion of both molecules enters the constitutive secretory pathway (46) and may be responsible for bystander lysis.

Posttranslational proteolytic processing of intracellular perforin, recently observed by Griffiths' group (19), suggested that proteolytic removal of the C-terminus of perforin next to the C2 domain may be necessary for the acquisition of functional activity. Removal of the C-terminal amino acid along with the associated glycan may uncover the C2 domain and enable it, upon secretion, to undergo Ca-dependent phospholipid binding, initiating membrane insertion and polymerization.

WHY DOES PERFORIN NOT KILL THE KILLER CELL?

It has long been recognized that cytotoxic T cells can go through several rounds of target killing without getting killed themselves in the process. This has been interpreted to indicate that killer cells are not susceptible to perforin and may be endowed with specific protective molecules preventing perforin attack ("protection") (47,48). The homologous restriction factor CD59, which restricts binding and polymerization of C8 and C9, does not restrict perforin lysis (16,49). DAF (CD55) and CD59 inhibit complement lysis at the level of C3 and C8/C9, respectively. Complement is specialized to lyse extracellular pathogens through antibody or alternative pathway recognition, and cells must be protected from accidental bystander lysis. Absence of CD59 or DAF through acquired defects in hematopoietic progenitor cells leads to the life-threatening syndrome of paroxysmal nocturnal hemoglobinuria, caused by complement lysis of unprotected blood cells. In contrast to complement, cytotoxic T cells and NK cells are mandated to lyse homologous cells to clear intracellular pathogens. To protect cells, even T cells and CTLs, from perforin lysis would result in the inability of removing virus-infected cells by perforin, one of the principal antiviral weapons of the immune system. It would also lead to the possibility that viruses acquire a similar gene and paralyze the cytotoxic response similar to what is observed in perforin deficiency (50).

How, then, are killer cells protected from lysis by perforin? We favor the hypothesis that the local delivery mechanism of perforin and granules is responsible for the ability of CTLs to unidirectionally kill targets without damaging themselves. The contact zone between killer and target cell at the site of granule exocytosis is shown in Figure 11-4. Several factors are postulated to guarantee the unidirectionality of the lytic attack.

1. Once exposed to extracellular Ca the half-life of perforin is extremely short (milliseconds), allowing only very short distances for diffusion in the active form.
2. Diffusion is further restricted by membrane apposition and a high density of adherence receptors (51) surrounding the exocytotic locus (Fig. 11-4).
3. Because perforin is secreted in a large supramolecular complex of proteoglycan associated also with granzymes, diffusion is further restricted by the high molecular mass and Stoke's radius of the complex (Fig. 11-4).
4. These physical constraints limit diffusion and access of perforin. Only the target membrane opposite the granule exocytosis and the granule membrane itself

are exposed to perforin. The latter may be coated with proteoglycan, blocking perforin access.

In this model restriction of perforin killing to target cells is dictated by the physical constraints of granule release to the target. The only part of the killer cell potentially coming into contact with perforin is the specialized granule membrane.

PERFORIN FUNCTION IN THE INDUCTION OF THE IMMUNE RESPONSE

Allogeneic bone marrow transplantation is becoming a routine procedure for many medical conditions. Although beneficial and life-saving, bone marrow transplantation is associated with significant risk of graft-versus-host disease (GVHD) characterized by donor T cells attacking recipient tissues. Primary target tissues in the recipient are skin (responding with dermatitis, alopecia, and depigmentation), liver, and small intestines, responding with hepatitis and enteritis, respectively. Target tissues are infiltrated with cytotoxic lymphocytes expressing granule proteins including perforin (52). GVHD is accompanied by progressive weight loss, cachexia, and death.

Using perforin-deficient or FasL-deficient T cells as grafts for bone marrow transplantation revealed the involvement of the two major cytotoxic pathways in different aspects of GVHD in allogeneic recipients disparate at major or minor MHC loci. The absence of FasL on grafted T cells eliminated skin and hepatic disease and ameliorated gastrointestinal disorders, but it had no effect on weight loss and survival (53). FasL therefore is responsible for many of the pathognomonic symptoms of GVHD but not for mortality and weight loss. The data are also useful for the prediction of tissue Fas expression and susceptibility *in vivo,* which appear to be high in the skin and liver and moderate in the intestinal organs. GVHD also is accompanied by immune suppression, particularly in

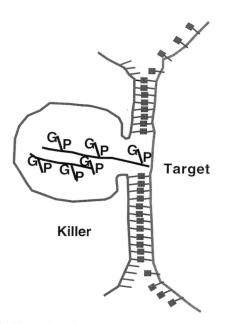

FIG. 11-4. Restriction of perforin to target lysis and killer cell self-protection by physical constraints. The locus of granule exocytosis is shown. Perforin diffusion is restricted by adhesion molecules via binding to proteoglycan complexes and rapid inactivation through Ca (see text).

the B cell compartment. FasL deficiency of grafted T cells allows recovery of B cells, indicating that immune suppression is mediated by the Fas/FasL pathway (54).

Bone marrow transplantation requires ablation of stem cells and T cells of the recipient to prevent graft rejection and allow engraftment. It is usually achieved in mice by sublethal irradiation. When wild-type bone marrow is transplanted using this regimen, the recipient is reconstituted with the donor-type hematopoietic system with little or no chimerism. In contrast, using FasL-deficient T cells in donor grafts, a substantial chimerism in the reconstituted recipient is seen (54), indicating that some stem cells that survive irradiation of the recipient are killed by wild-type T cells in the graft but not by FasL-deficient T cells. The creation of chimerism in this way may open new avenues for tolerance induction for organ transplantation.

Bone marrow allografts containing perforin-deficient T cells were significantly delayed in causing the onset of GVHD, and more perforin-deficient T cells were needed for disease induction (53,55). The acceleration of GVHD by perforin probably is due to tissue destruction by this cytolytic pathway and increased antigen presentation of liberated alloantigens, causing in turn accelerated expansion of alloantigen-specific T cells and more tissue destruction.

These studies indicate that both perforin and FasL contribute to GVHD but that neither is essential. An additional component of GVHD is mediated by TNF-R1 (56), and other factors and death receptors may play a role in this complex disease.

Braun et al. (57) reported that T cells with combined perforin/FasL deficiency had lost their ability to induce GVHD. This finding suggests that TNF receptor and other death receptors are not contributors to this disease. On the other hand, it is possible that perforin/FasL-deficient T cells are more easily rejected by the recipient of the graft and therefore do not cause disease. The latter possibility has not been excluded.

PERFORIN FUNCTION IN THE DOWNREGULATION OF THE IMMUNE RESPONSE

Perforin/FasL double-deficient mice develop severe pancreatitis, and female mice also have hysterosalpingitis and die within 10 to 12 weeks of birth. Female mice are infertile. The severe pancreatitis is characterized by the loss of exocrine cells and by survival of the islets of Langerhans. The pancreas is infiltrated with Mac1 (CD11b)-positive CD8 T cells and macrophages. Treatment of mice with intraperitoneal injection of carrageenan, a macrophage toxic agent, once per week from the age of 4 weeks significantly delays disease onset and restores the fertility of female mice. Perforin/FasL-deficient CD8$^+$ and CD4$^+$ T cells are unable to kill cognate syngeneic macrophages despite the fact that they produce quantities of TNF that are able to kill TNF-sensitive targets (58).

Generation of cytotoxic T cells by APCs requires a 3-day induction period during which the T cells begin to express FasL and perforin and differentiate into CTLs. The original APC is the ideal target for the newly formed CTLs and is lysed by the FasL or perforin pathway (Fig. 11-5). In this model the original stimulus of cytotoxicity also contains the signal for negative feedback regulation by lysis through the CTLs just gener-

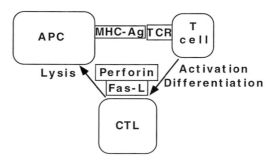

FIG. 11-5. Perforin and FASL-mediated lysis of antigen-presenting cells (*APC*). This mechanism may result in acceleration of early immune responses and dampening of immune responses after differentiation of CTLs.

ated. If both lytic effector molecules (FasL and perforin) are missing, the original stimulus cannot be turned off by lysis and continues to activate T cells, leading to disease. The effector molecules causing disease have not yet been identified, but they cannot be perforin or FasL. We propose that TNF, Tweak, or Trail are candidate effector molecules in this autoimmune disease and in GVHD.

PERFORIN EXPRESSION DURING PREGNANCY

The decidua of the pregnant uterus is the site of the highest concentration of perforin expression under physiologic conditions (59–61). The cell type expressing perforin may be classified as a subpopulation of NK cells based on the expression of CD56 and the absence of CD16. Human decidua-associated granular cells do not express CD16 and do not mediate antibody-dependent cytotoxicity. In addition they are only weakly cytotoxic for the typical NK target K562 despite their high perforin content. The function of these cells and their normal target are not understood at this time, but they are believed to provide a protective function for the fetus. Perforin deficiency in mice has no deleterious effect on fertility and pregnancy, suggesting that redundant pathways may serve the same function.

Perforin/FasL double-deficient female mice are infertile presumably owing to inflammatory infiltrates in the uterus. This condition can be corrected by weekly injections of carrageenan, restoring fertility. Perforin/FasL-deficient female mice treated with carrageenan have normal litters, indicating that the combined absence of perforin and FasL is not detrimental to an established pregnancy.

CONCLUSIONS

Perforin has been clearly established as the primary effector molecule against intracellular pathogens. Its cooperation with gran-

zymes make it a powerful mechanism for lysing cells through membrane damage and triggering apoptosis.

In addition to this primary function, perforin contributes to immune regulation and homeostasis. As revealed in GVHD, perforin accelerates the allogeneic immune response, most likely through the lysis of target cells, release of antigens, and representation by APCs. FasL-mediated apoptosis may not have the same effect because death by this pathway may downregulate antigen presentation.

Perforin in addition has a downregulatory function in the immune response through the killing of APCs. This function normally is performed by FasL-inducing apoptosis of APCs following T cell activation. However, in the absence of FasL, perforin can substitute for this function to some extent. In the absence of both effectors, severe autoimmunity ensues and causes early death.

REFERENCES

1. Dennert G, Podack ER. Cytolysis by H-2-specific T killer cells: assembly of tubular complexes on target membranes. *J Exp Med* 1983;157:1483–1495.
2. Podack ER, Dennert G. Assembly of two types of tubules with putative cytolytic function by cloned natural killer cells. *Nature* 1983;302:442–445.
3. Blumenthal R, Millard PJ, Henkart MP, Reynolds CW, Henkart PA. Liposomes as targets for granule cytolysin from cytotoxic large granular lymphocyte tumors. *Proc Natl Acad Sci USA* 1984;81:5551–5.
4. Zalman LS, Brothers MA, Muller-Eberhard HJ. A C9 related channel forming protein in the cytoplasmic granules of human large granular lymphocytes. *Biosci Rep* 1985;5:1093–1100.
5. Young JD, Damiano A, DiNome MA, Leong LG, Cohn ZA. Dissociation of membrane binding and lytic activities of the lymphocyte pore-forming protein (perforin). *J Exp Med* 1987;165:1371–1382.
6. Dourmashkin RR, Deteix P, Simone CB, Henkart P. Electron microscopic demonstration of lesions in target cell membranes associated with antibody-dependent cellular cytotoxicity. *Clin Exp Immunol* 1980;42:554–560.
7. Mayer MM, Hammer CH, Michaels DW, Shin ML. Immunologically mediated membrane damage: the mechanism of complement action and the similarity of lymphocyte-mediated cytotoxicity. *Transplant Proc* 1978;10:707–714.
8. Podack ER, Tschopp J. Polymerization of the ninth component of complement (C9): formation of poly(C9) with a tubular ultrastructure resembling

the membrane attack complex of complement. *Proc Natl Acad Sci USA* 1982;79:574–578.

9. Tschopp J, Muller-Eberhard HJ, Podack ER. Formation of transmembrane tubules by spontaneous polymerization of the hydrophilic complement protein C9. *Nature* 1982;298:534–538.

10. Millard PJ, Henkart MP, Reynolds CW, Henkart PA. Purification and properties of cytoplasmic granules from cytotoxic rat LGL tumors. *J Immunol* 1984;132:3197–204.

11. Podack ER, Konigsberg PJ. Cytolytic T cell granules: isolation, structural, biochemical, and functional characterization. *J Exp Med* 1984;160:695–710.

12. Podack ER, Young JD, Cohn ZA. Isolation and biochemical and functional characterization of perforin 1 from cytolytic T-cell granules. *Proc Natl Acad Sci USA* 1985;82:8629–8633.

13. Masson D, Tschopp J. Isolation of a lytic, pore-forming protein (perforin) from cytolytic T-lymphocytes. *J Biol Chem* 1985;260:9069–9072.

14. Young JD, Hengartner H, Podack ER, Cohn ZA. Purification and characterization of a cytolytic pore-forming protein from granules of cloned lymphocytes with natural killer activity. *Cell* 1986;44:849–859.

15. Shinkai Y, Takio K, Okumura K. Homology of perforin to the ninth component of complement (C9). *Nature* 1988;334:525–527.

16. Lichtenheld MG, Olsen KJ, Lu P, et al. Structure and function of human perforin. *Nature* 1988;335:448–451.

17. Kwon BS, Wakulchik M, Liu CC, et al. The structure of the mouse lymphocyte pore-forming protein perforin. *Biochem Biophys Res Commun* 1989;158:1–10.

18. Tschopp J, Masson D, Stanley KK. Structural/functional similarity between proteins involved in complement- and cytotoxic T-lymphocyte-mediated cytolysis. *Nature* 1986;322:831–834.

19. Uellner R, Zvelebil MJ, Hopkins J, et al. Perforin is activated by a proteolytic cleavage during biosynthesis which reveals a phospholipid-binding C2 domain. *EMBO J* 1997;16:7287–7296.

20. Yue CC, Reynolds CW, Henkart PA. Inhibition of cytolysin activity in large granular lymphocyte granules by lipids: evidence for a membrane insertion mechanism of lysis. *Mol Immunol* 1987;24:647–653.

21. Tschopp J, Schafer S, Masson D, Peitsch MC, Heusser C. Phosphorylcholine acts as a Ca^{2+}-dependent receptor molecule for lymphocyte perforin. *Nature* 1989;337:272–274.

22. Young JD, Cohn ZA, Podack ER. The ninth component of complement and the pore-forming protein (perforin 1) from cytotoxic T cells: structural, immunological, and functional similarities. *Science* 1986;233:184–190.

23. Podack ER. Molecular composition of the tubular structure of the membrane attack complex of complement. *J Biol Chem* 1984;259:8641–8647.

24. Carney DF, Hammer CH, Shin ML. Elimination of terminal complement complexes in the plasma membrane of nucleated cells: influence of extracellular Ca^{2+} and association with cellular Ca^{2+}. *J Immunol* 1986;137:263–270.

25. Morgan BP, Dankert JR, Esser AF. Recovery of human neutrophils from complement attack: removal of the membrane attack complex by endocytosis and exocytosis. *J Immunol* 1987;138:246–253.

26. Hameed A, Olsen KJ, Lee MK, Lichtenheld MG, Podack ER. Cytolysis by Ca-permeable transmembrane channels: pore formation causes extensive DNA degradation and cell lysis. *J Exp Med* 1989;169:765–777.

27. Podack ER, Lowrey DM, Lichtenheld MG, Hameed A. Function of granule perforin and esterases in T-cell mediated reactions: components required for delivery of molecules to target cells. *Ann NY Acad Sci* 1988;532:292–302.

28. Podack ER, Tschopp J. Circular polymerization of the ninth component of complement: ring closure of the tubular complex confers resistance to detergent dissociation and to proteolytic degradation. *J Biol Chem* 1982;257:15204–15212.

29. Fink TM, Zimmer M, Weitz S, Tschopp J, Jenne DE, Lichter P. Human perforin (PRF1) maps to 10q22, a region that is syntonic with mouse chromosome 10. *Genomics* 1992;13:1300–1302.

30. Trapani JA, Kwon BS, Kozak CA, Chintamaneni C, Young JD, Dupont B. Genomic organization of the mouse pore-forming protein (perforin) gene and localization to chromosome 10: similarities to and differences from C9. *J Exp Med* 1990;171:545–557.

31. Lichtenheld MG, Podack ER, Levy RB. Transgenic control of perforin gene expression: functional evidence for two separate control regions. *J Immunol* 1995;154:2153–2163.

32. Smyth MJ, Ortaldo JR, Bere W, Yagita H, Okumura K, Young HA. IL-2 and IL-6 synergize to augment the pore-forming protein gene expression and cytotoxic potential of human peripheral blood T cells. *J Immunol* 1990;145:1159–1166.

33. Garcia-Sanz JA, Podack ER. Regulation of perforin gene expression in a T cell hybrid with inducible cytolytic activity. *Eur J Immunol* 1993;23:1877–1883.

34. Aste-Amezaga M, D'Andrea A, Kubin M, Trinchieri G. Cooperation of natural killer cell stimulatory factor/interleukin-12 with other stimuli in the induction of cytokines and cytotoxic cell-associated molecules in human T and NK cells. *Cell Immunol* 1994;156:480–492.

35. Lu P, Garcia-Sanz JA, Lichtenheld MG, Podack ER. Perforin expression in human peripheral blood mononuclear cells: definition of an IL-2-independent pathway of perforin induction in $CD8^+$ T cells. *J Immunol* 1992;148:3354–3360.

36. Smyth MJ, Strobl SL, Young HA, Ortaldo JR, Ochoa AC. Regulation of lymphokine-activated killer activity and pore-forming protein gene expression in human peripheral blood $CD8^+$ T lymphocytes: inhibition by transforming growth factor-beta. *J Immunol* 1991;146:3289–97.

37. Berthou C, Michel L, Soulie A, et al. Acquisition of granzyme B and Fas ligand proteins by human keratinocytes contributes to epidermal cell defense. *J Immunol* 1997;159:5293–5300.

38. Lichtenheld MG, Podack ER. Structure of the hu-

man perforin gene: a simple gene organization with interesting potential regulatory sequences. *J Immunol* 1989;143:4267–4274.

39. Lichtenheld MG, Podack ER. Structure and function of the murine perforin promoter and upstream region: reciprocal gene activation or silencing in perforin positive and negative cells. *J Immunol* 1992;149:2619–2626.

40. Zhang Y, Lichtenheld MG. Non-killer cell-specific transcription factors silence the perforin promoter. *J Immunol* 1997;158:1734–1741.

41. Takayama H, Sitkovsky MV. Antigen receptor-regulated exocytosis in cytotoxic T lymphocytes. *J Exp Med* 1987;166:725–743.

42. Burkhardt JK, Hester S, Lapham CK, Argon Y. The lytic granules of natural killer cells are dual-function organelles combining secretory and pre-lysosomal compartments. *J Cell Biol* 1990;111:2327–2340.

43. Podack ER, Hengartner H, Lichtenheld MG. A central role of perforin in cytolysis? *Ann Rev Immunol* 1991;9:129–157.

44. Peters PJ, Geuze HJ, van der Donk HA, Borst J. A new model for lethal hit delivery by cytotoxic T lymphocytes. *Immunol Today* 1990;11:28–32.

45. Burkhardt JK, Hester S, Argon Y. Two proteins targeted to the same lytic granule compartment undergo very different posttranslational processing. *Proc Natl Acad Sci USA* 1989;86:7128–7132.

46. Isaaz S, Baetz K, Olsen K, Podack E, Griffiths GM. Serial killing by cytotoxic T lymphocytes: T cell receptor triggers degranulation, re-filling of the lytic granules and secretion of lytic proteins via a non-granule pathway. *Eur J Immunol* 1995;25:1071–1079.

47. Muller C, Tschopp J. Resistance of CTL to perforin-mediated lysis: evidence for a lymphocyte membrane protein interacting with perforin. *J Immunol* 1994;153:2470–2478.

48. Ojcius DM, Jiang SB, Persechini PM, Detmers PA, Young JD. Cytoplasts from cytotoxic T lymphocytes are resistant to perforin-mediated lysis. *Mol Immunol* 1991;28:1011–1018.

49. Meri S, Morgan BP, Wing M, et al. Human protectin (CD59), an 18–20-kD homologous complement restriction factor, does not restrict perforin-mediated lysis. *J Exp Med* 1990;172:367–370.

50. Kagi D, Ledermann B, Burki K, et al. Cytotoxicity mediated by T cells and natural killer cells is greatly impaired in perforin-deficient mice [see comments]. *Nature* 1994;369:31–37.

51. Podack ER, Kupfer A. T-cell effector functions: mechanisms for delivery of cytotoxicity and help. *Ann Rev Cell Biol* 1991;7:479–504.

52. Sale GE, Anderson P, Browne M, Myerson D. Evidence of cytotoxic T-cell destruction of epidermal cells in human graft-vs-host disease: immunohistology with monoclonal antibody TIA-1. *Arch Pathol Lab Med* 1992;116:622–625.

53. Baker MB, Altman NH, Podack ER, Levy RB. The role of cell-mediated cytotoxicity in acute GVHD after MHC-matched allogeneic bone marrow transplantation in mice. *J Exp Med* 1986;183:2645–2656.

54. Baker MB, Riley RL, Podack ER, Levy RB. Graft-versus-host-disease-associated lymphoid hypoplasia and B cell dysfunction is dependent upon donor T cell-mediated Fas-ligand function, but not perforin function. *Proc Natl Acad Sci USA* 1997;94:1366–1371.

55. Blazar BR, Taylor PA, Vallera DA. CD4[+] and CD8[+] T cells each can utilize a perforin-dependent pathway to mediate lethal graft-versus-host disease in major histocompatibility complex-disparate recipients. *Transplantation* 1997;64:571–576.

56. Speiser DE, Bachmann MF, Frick TW, et al. TNF receptor p55 controls early acute graft-versus-host disease. *J Immunol* 1997;158:5185–5190.

57. Braun MY, Lowin B, French L, Acha-Orbea H, Tschopp J. Cytotoxic T cells deficient in both functional fas ligand and perforin show residual cytolytic activity yet lose their capacity to induce lethal acute graft-versus-host disease. *J Exp Med* 1996;183:657–661.

58. Lee RK, Spielman J, Zhao DY, Olsen KJ, Podack ER. Perforin, Fas ligand, and tumor necrosis factor are the major cytotoxic molecules used by lymphokine-activated killer cells. *J Immunol* 1996;157:1919–1925.

59. Rukavina D, Rubesa G, Gudelj L, Haller H, Podack ER. Characteristics of perforin expressing lymphocytes within the first trimester decidua of human pregnancy. *Am J Reprod Immunol* 1995;33:394–404.

60. Ye W, Zheng LM, Young JD, Liu CC. The involvement of interleukin (IL)-15 in regulating the differentiation of granulated metrial gland cells in mouse pregnant uterus. *J Exp Med* 1996;184:2405–2410.

61. Parr EL, Parr MB, Young JD. Localization of a pore-forming protein (perforin) in granulated metrial gland cells. *Biol Reprod* 1987;37:1327–1335.

Cytotoxic Cells: Basic Mechanisms and Medical Applications, edited by Michail V. Sitkovsky and Pierre A. Henkart. Lippincott Williams & Wilkins, Philadelphia © 2000.

Chapter 12

Granule-Mediated Apoptosis: Delivering Death

Christopher J. Froelich

Evanston Northwestern Healthcare Research Institute, Evanston, Illinois 60201, USA

Both innate [natural killer (NK) cells] and adaptive defenses [cytotoxic T cells-(CTLs)] against intracellular pathogens, tumors, and non-self cells depend on granule-mediated apoptosis (1). The granules of cytotoxic cells contain the pore-forming protein [perforin (PFN)] chaperoned by the Ca-binding protein calreticulin, a serine carboxypeptidase (2), acid hydrolases, the antibacterial protein, granulysin (3), and granzymes bound to serglycin, a species of chondroitin A sulfate proteoglycan. The granzymes are granule-associated serine proteases with counterparts in the mouse, rat, and humans (4,5). Enzymatically, the various granzymes express trypsin-like, aspase, metase, or chymase activities.

Human: Granzyme A (GrA, trypsin-like activity) and granzyme B (GrB, aspase activity) have counterparts in the mouse and rat. Granzyme K (trypsin-like activity) and granzyme M (metase) have homologs in the rat (4)

Murine: Granzymes A to G (1,6)

Rat: Granzymes A, B, and K (7) plus M (8) and the recently described chymase (9). The latter lacks homologs in humans.

Among the many granule constituents, PFN and the granzymes appear to contribute directly to the phenomenon of cellular cytotoxicity. Two forms may exist: (a) PFN-mediated *necrosis* and (b) PFN/granzyme-induced *apoptosis.* Although it is unclear whether PFN-mediated lysis of target cells

occurs *in vivo* to a significant degree (10), the accumulated data from PFN and granzyme knockout mice indicate both are required for an effective defense against virus-infected and tumor cells (11–13). Furthermore, gene-deletion studies in mice have provided compelling evidence that GrB is most crucial for rapid induction of apoptosis (13,14), whereas other members elicit a delayed response (7,15).

Operationally, granule-mediated apoptosis is divisible into three steps: (a) signal-dependent exocytosis of the granule components; (b) intracellular delivery of the granzymes by PFN; and (c) induction of apoptotic pathways by the granzymes. Although substantial progress has been made in understanding the signals that initiate granule exocytosis, we have not firmly established how PFN facilitates delivery of the granzymes or, until recently, how the granzymes then induce cell death. The experimental systems described below by our laboratory and collaborators have provided some insights to the mechanism of granule-mediated apoptosis, particularly for GrB.

EXPERIMENTAL MODELS FOR GRANZYME/PFN-MEDIATED APOPTOSIS

Perforin

Perforin is synthesized as a 70-kDa inactive precursor (16) that is cleaved at the C-terminus to yield a more potent 60-kDa form. Cleavage occurs at the boundary of a C2 domain, exposing a calcium-dependent binding site that interacts with phospholipid membranes (17). Following exocytosis, pore formation is divisible into three steps: (a) Ca-dependent binding of the monomers to the membrane; (b) insertion into the bilayer, and (c) aggregation in the plane of the membrane to form a functional pore. Because PFN is primarily hydrophilic, the monomers must undergo conformational change to expose amphiphilic and hydrophobic domains to interact with the acyl chains of the lipid bilayer and hydrophilic residues to line the interior of the pore. Hence the barrel stave model has been proposed where the pore size is then proportional to the number of the monomers that aggregate. Based on conductance studies and osmotic protection assays, PFN is reported to form pores of 5 to 20 nM, allowing diffusion of fluorescent markers up to 17 kDa. An ion channel requires three or four monomers, but a greater number are required to form pores that allow diffusion of the fluorescent marker. Interestingly, the N-terminus (AA 1-34) of the PFN protein appears to have pore-forming activity but only small-diameter pores are generated. The pores formed by the peptide allow the influx of Ca killing tumor cells, but erythrocytes are not lysed (18,19). This suggests that other domains of the PFN protein may be necessary to facilitate formation of the larger pores that cause hemolysis (20). Nevertheless, depending on the pore size, PFN may have different biologic effects: Prior to removal from the membrane, small pores may transiently act as ion channels killing susceptible tumor cells, whereas large pores may be responsible for lytic necrosis. It is not clear, however, how the pores' size would influence the capacity of PFN to deliver the granzymes intracellularly.

Granzyme Gene Reconstitution Studies

Reconstitution-style experiments were the first to support a role for GrA and GrB in granule-mediated apoptosis. In this elegant model system, Henkart and colleagues transfected basophils with PFN plus either or both granzyme A and B expression constructs (21–23). Immunoglobulin E (IgE) anti-TNP antibodies bound to the target stimulated the Fc-IgE receptor of the basophil, inducing granule exocytosis and apoptotic cell death in the target. The results provided the first evidence that the apoptotic process was due to the combination of PFN and granzymes and tended to corroborate the model that PFN forms a conduit allowing the soluble granzymes to flow to the cytosol of the target cell ("granule injection" model) (24).

Granzyme Gene Ablation Studies

Complementing the reconstitutive experiments described above, cellular and animal gene ablation studies confirmed the crucial role played by GrB in granule-mediated apoptosis. We studied a human NK cell line (YT) that contained GrB and PFN but lacked GrA and GrK. Despite the absence of the two tryptases, YT cells retain potent cytotoxic activity toward a number of murine and human targets (25). After transfection with an anti-sense GrB construct, the level of GrB protein in the cell line was reduced by 80%, and apoptotic activity (DNA fragmentation) was decreased by more than 95% (26). Although these results suggested an important role for GrB in granule-mediated apoptosis, the function of this granzyme was unequivocally established by the development of GrB knockout mouse. CTLs and NK cells from these mice were unable to induce rapid apoptosis, but target cells would die after prolonged incubation (13,27). GrB clearly has an essential role in granule-mediated apoptosis, mediating rapid cell death. Subsequent work suggested that granule-mediated apoptosis was normal in GrA knockouts. However, distinguishing rapid and delayed apoptosis, the Ley laboratory showed that GrA-defective CTLs manifested a modest defect in delayed killing that was attributed to the loss of the GrA gene and the maintenance of GrK activity (28). Taken together, GrB appears to play a dominant role in granule-mediated apoptosis, overshadowing the activity of the tryptases GrA and GrK, which have ancillary roles in the production of cell death (29).

Reconstitution of Granule-Mediated Apoptosis *In Vitro*: Lessons from Purified Granzymes and PFN

The aforementioned descriptive studies, although instrumental in delineating the crucial role of the granzymes in granule-mediated apoptosis, failed to provide mechanistic insights to the function of PFN and the granzymes. Greenberg and colleagues took the first step toward unraveling how the granzymes and PFN induce target cell apoptosis by showing that the simultaneous addition of purified rat PFN and a granzyme resulted in cell death (30,31). In these landmark studies a "sublytic" concentration of PFN was found to be sufficient for apoptosis; and cytochalasin B, a microfilament inhibitor, partially inhibited the response. Because "sublytic" concentrations of PFN were sufficient to induce apoptosis, the "granule injection" model was modified by stating that soluble granzymes entered the target cell during pinocytotic repair of the PFN pores.

Summary

On the basis of these studies, the accepted model is summarized as follows: After effector–target interaction, the granule contents are discharged into the intercellular cleft. PFN polymerizes into pores of varying diameter in the target cell membrane. If large pores (20 nm) are generated, necrosis may ensue. The genesis of smaller sublytic pores allows the soluble granzymes to be taken up during pinocytotic repair of the damaged membrane. The soluble granzymes then somehow reach cytosolic and nuclear substrates causing apoptosis (1). It remained unclear how PFN might deliver the granzymes from the pinocytotic vesicles or what substrates, either plasma membrane-associated or intracellular, might be cleaved by the various granzymes to induce apoptosis.

GRANZYME ENTRY INTO CELLS

Binding of GrB to the Cell Surface—Prerequisite for Entry

Although granzyme delivery by transmembrane PFN pores or by pinocytotic uptake provides compelling models for granzyme delivery, we were intrigued that investigators failed to consider the possibility that granule-mediated apoptosis might adhere to established cell biologic tenets such as receptor-dependent endocytosis. Elaborating on the model originally described by Podack and Kupfer (32) and stimulated by the observation that cytochalasin B partially abrogated apoptosis in targets treated with PFN and GrB (30), we asked whether targets pulsed with GrB undergo apoptosis when subsequently treated with PFN. The previous design had co-incubated PFN and GrB, so it was impossible to distinguish fluid- from receptor-dependent internalization of the granzyme. Jurkat cells (human T cell lymphoma) were simply exposed to GrB (30 nM), washed free of soluble granzyme, and then treated with sublytic concentrations of human PFN. This sequential treatment indeed produced apoptosis (33). Because soluble GrB is removed, the protease could not enter the cytoplasm through channels formed by PFN or by pinocytosis. On the basis of these results, we tentatively postulated that GrB binds to cell membrane proteins and undergoes endocytosis. Importantly, internalization of GrB alone did not kill the target. As determined by assays that measure rates of proliferation and mitochondrial function (MTT assay), GrB was entirely nontoxic (C. Froelich, unpublished data). Two possibilities were considered: (a) GrB and PFN both provide a transmembrane signal or (b) PFN somehow delivers the internalized granzyme to the cytosol where the latter causes apoptosis.

Because GrB appeared to bind to the Jur-kat cells, this interaction might result in sig-nal transduction. Despite significant effort, we have not observed evidence of transmem-brane signaling in targets treated with GrB. As measured by the calcium-sensitive dye Fluo-3 and ultraviolet (UV) spectrophotom-etry, no change in the intracellular calcium levels could be detected (C. Froelich, un-published data). Studies designed to detect variations in the phosphorylation of various cytosolic and nuclear proteins also were neg-ative. Although more subtle activation of secondary messenger pathways (e.g., specific kinases) could occur, the data suggested that GrB does not contribute to the apoptotic response by initiating a robust transmem-brane signal. With these negative data in hand, we postulated that the GrB binding sites may serve to internalize the granzyme to a vesicular compartment, where the prote-ase is then released by PFN.

Taking the first step to critically evaluate this hypothesis, experiments were designed to characterize the binding of free GrB to Jurkat cells. The presence of binding sites were detected with proteolytically active io-dine 125 (^{125}I)-GrB in the presence and ab-sence of a 150-fold excess of unlabeled prote-ase (33). GrB binding and internalization were time- and concentration-dependent as well as specific and saturable (K_d about 10 nM). The calculated number of binding sites were relatively few (1×10^4 to 3×10^4 per cell). Unlabeled active protease blocked up-take of ^{125}I-GrB, indicating that the identified binding sites participated in granzyme inter-nalization. GrB that was inactivated with DCI also inhibited binding and internaliza-tion of the radioligand, suggesting that the active site was not crucial for interaction with the cells. In a related study, the binding re-quirement for apoptosis was addressed by incubating cells at 4°C (a temperature that minimizes internalization) and removing cell-associated granzyme by an acid wash. Target cells treated at 4°C and washed at neutral pH exhibited a level of apoptosis similar to cells treated at 37°C, whereas target cells

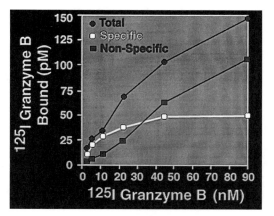

FIG. 12-1. Specific binding of radiolabeled gran-zyme B (GrB) to Jurkat cells. Specific binding of GrB to Jurkat cells was determined by measuring the membrane-associated CPM in the presence and absence of 150-fold excess of unlabeled GrB. After adding either medium or unlabeled GrB for 30 minutes at 4°C, cells were incubated at room temperature with radiolabeled GrB for 1 hour. CPM released by trypsin treatment repre-sents bound or membrane-associated GrB. CPM of pelleted cells, obtained by cutting the tip of the microfuge tubes, represents endocytosed gran-zyme. Nonspecific binding was in presence of 150-fold excess GrB.

washed with an acidic buffer did not undergo apoptosis (34). The latter studies further em-phasize that GrB probably is internalized by the target cell and that a second "process" facilitates release of the granzyme from vesi-cles to the cytosol where the protease then initiates the apoptotic response (Fig. 12-1).

Nature of the Vesicular Pathway Traversed by Internalized GrB

Because GrB appeared to undergo endocy-tosis by targets cells via a receptor-depen-dent process, studies were performed to de-lineate vesicular trafficking. Small Ras-like proteins of the Rab family are known to or-chestrate the interaction of numerous vesicu-lar compartments (35). Rab5 is found in vesi-cles near the plasma membrane and in newly formed early endosomes and perinuclear re-cycling endosomes, and Rab4 has been identified in early endosomes and endocytic vesicles that recycle plasma membrane-constituents from early endosomes. To determine whether GrB was internalized to these compartments, co-localization studies were performed with antibodies to the granzyme and respective endosomal markers followed by imaging with confocal laser scanning microscopy (CLSM) and immunogold electron microscopy techniques (34). To evaluate the early trafficking events, HeLa cells adherent to glass coverslips were incubated with fluoresceinated-GrB at 20°C, a temperature that minimizes membrane fusion of trafficking vesicles. Cells were fixed, permeabilized, and immunolabeled with anti-Rab4 or anti-Rab5 antibody and a corresponding Texas Red-conjugated antiserum. GrB was observed to accumulate in early endosomes and perinuclear recycling vesicles characterized by Rab5 staining; and a lesser amount co-localized with Rab4$^+$ vesicles. Because it had been reported that GrB appeared to translocate across the plasma membrane autonomously (36), a more detailed view of the early trafficking events then was performed by immunoelectron microscopy. HeLa cells were allowed to bind GrB at 4°C for 60 minutes; they were then washed and shifted to 20°C for 45 minutes to allow uptake of the granzyme. After processing, GrB was again found to co-localize with Rab4$^+$ endosomes. Together, these observations further validated the radioligand binding and CLSM studies, indicating that GrB was taken up by target cells via receptor-dependent endocytosis.

To characterize the vesicular pathway traversed by GrB, double-label studies were performed with the following markers: Rab4, Rab5, mannose 6-phosphate receptor (late endosomes and Golgi apparatus), cathepsin D (lysosomes), lgp120 (lysosomes), and cytochrome c (mitochondria). When target cells were incubated with fluoresceinated GrB at 37°C for 60 minutes, the granzyme no longer predominantly co-localized with Rab5 or Rab4. GrB, however, did not associate with the other markers described above. These

data suggest that GrB is indeed transported through the Rab5/Rab4 endosomal compartment. The granzyme then either accumulates in a cellular compartment that remains unidentified or might recycle to the cell surface (34). Consistent with the latter possibility, when target cells are pulsed with radiolabeled GrB, incubated for progressively longer periods of time, and then rinsed again, the amount of cell-associated label declines, suggesting that the granzyme is not targeted to the lysosomes but, rather, follows a recycling vesicular pathway back to the plasma membrane where molecules may be released extracellularly (33).

Delivery of GrB to the Cytosol by Microinjection is Sufficient for Apoptosis

If we presume that PFN facilitates the induction of apoptosis by releasing GrB from a vesicular compartment to the cytosol, microinjection of the granzyme into target cells should be sufficient to induce cell death. Working with Kevin Tomaselli and Feng Li (IDUN Pharmaceuticals), our laboratory learned that the microinjection of GrB into MCF-7 cells (breast carcinoma line) produces an apoptotic morphology (34). Because microinjection of GrB into the cytoplasm of a target cell resulted in apoptosis and internalization to an endocytic pathway fails to cause cell death, the data confirm the hypothesis that a key step in the process of GrB-mediated apoptosis is release of GrB to the cytosol.

Our results, however, must be contrasted with another study where microinjection of rat GrB into B16 melanoma cells and rat fibroblasts failed to produce any morphologic abnormalities except transient membrane blebbing (36). These conflicting data are easily reconciled by differences in the amount and activity of the GrB microinjected. In our experiments microinjection resulted in delivery of 54 fg/cell, whereas the value in the negative study was approximately 4 fg/cell. This issue notwithstanding, the biologic significance of the results is more difficult to interpret. First, a cell undergoes apoptosis when "injected" with a variety of proteases (37). Second, because the amount of GrB delivered by a CTL to a target cell is unknown, it is not clear whether the quantity of GrB that produces apoptosis by this technique is physiologic. Therefore the microinjection technique does not exclude important ancillary roles for PFN (e.g., Ca^{2+} influx, K^+ efflux) that might synergize with GrB to induce cell death. A more physiologic approach would be helpful to ascertain whether PFN functions solely to deliver the internalized granzyme to the cytosol.

Discovery of a Substitute for PFN in GrB-Mediated Apoptosis

A number of laboratories have attempted to identify agents that could act as a substitute for PFN during granule-mediated apoptosis. Complement terminal attack complex, a bacterial pore-forming protein (staphylococcal toxin), calcium ionophores, phorbol esters, and detergents (Triton X-100, saponin, digitonin, NP-40) have failed to replace PFN (33,36,38). If the primary function of PFN is to transfer GrB to the cytosol of the target cell, a substitute that mediates intracellular delivery of vesicle-bound granzyme should produce apoptosis. The replication-deficient type 2 adenovirus (AD), employed extensively to deliver genetic constructs, also transfers protein ligands intracellularly (39). Following interaction with their respective binding sites, the protein ligand and AD are co-internalized to a coated vesicle that fuses with an early endosome. In the acidic vesicle, the AD cysteine protease cleaves the capsid-stabilizing protein, disassembling the penton coat (penton base and fiber). These proteins disrupt the endosomal membrane by a poorly understood process, releasing the virus and internalized protein to the cytosol.

When the endocytosis of labeled AD virions are imaged, AD internalizes with a $t_{1/2}$ of 2.5 minutes, breaking out of endosomes early, likely prior to further endosome–endosome fusion. The virus then exhibits cytosolic velocities averaging 0.58 μm/s and translocates to the nucleus where more than 80% of internalized virus localizes 60 minutes after infection (40). Because Jurkat cells appeared to bind and internalize GrB, we speculated that AD might serve to deliver the granzyme and thereby replace PFN. Fulfilling numerous criteria for apoptosis, the sequential or co-administration of GrB and AD to Jurkat cells caused this form of cell death, whereas GrB or AD alone had no effect (33). The biologic relevance of this system was supported by showing that similar results could be obtained by treating Jurkat cells with GrB and sublytic PFN (41). Complementing the microinjection studies, these data provide proof of the principle that PFN only need deliver the granzyme. Once targeted to the cytosol, GrB is sufficient to initiate the biochemical events that culminate in apoptosis. Furthermore, based on the radioligand binding data, we estimate that under steady-state conditions a target contains approximately 0.04 fg/cell, a value that is 1,350-fold less than the amount required to cause cell death by microinjection. Although the amount of GrB delivered to the cytosol by AD (or sublytic PFN) might still greatly exceed the value provided by a CTL, the fact that it is markedly less than the quantities used in the microinjection experiments suggests delivery by AD should provide a more physiologic strategy for intracytoplasmic targeting of the granzyme.

At this point the data indicate that GrB must reach the cytosol to initiate apoptosis and that two distinct membranolytic agents (PFN and AD) have the capacity to deliver the granzyme. To further establish the "transporter" function for PFN (and AD) a series of CLSM studies were performed to visualize the shift in the intracellular distribution of GrB. Because GrB may contribute to apoptosis by cleaving nuclear as well as cytosolic substrates (38,41,42), the detection of GrB in nuclei would imply that the protease was released from the endosomal compartment to the cytosol, where it subsequently translocates through membrane pores to the nucleus. Tumor cells were preincubated with GrB, washed, and then exposed to sublytic PFN or AD. Although treatment with GrB alone showed the predicted vesicular pattern, the addition of PFN or AD resulted in significant translocation of GrB from vesicles to the nucleus. Importantly, such translocation was associated with apoptotic changes in the nucleus as measured by the TUNEL method (34,43). To ensure that this observation was not due to the apoptotic process per se, GrB-treated cells were exposed to anti-Fas antibody, a potent death stimulus, and the distribution of GrB was imaged. Although the cells showed nuclear fragmentation, GrB remained in a cytoplasmic distribution (34). The imaging data therefore confirm that PFN (or AD) releases GrB from a vesicular pathway to the cytosol where the protease then may act on preferred substrates initiating the apoptotic process.

Induction of Apoptosis Occurs Primarily Via Release of GrB from a Vesicular Compartment and Not by Entry at the Plasma Membrane

We emphasize that the data reported for our experimental models do not exclude the possibility that a portion of the GrB delivered by PFN occurs at the plasma membrane. When mixed with a cell suspension rich in Ca^{2+}, PFN molecules are instantly inactivated in the aqueous phase, or a highly variable number of molecules bind each target cell where the monomers insert, forming pores of diameters ranging from 5 to 20 nm. As a consequence, both the number and size of PFN pores on each cell varies considerably, yielding a heterogeneous population where the outcome ranges from undamaged cells without PFN deposition to cells that experience transient ionic flux or undergo immediate lysis owing to the insertion of numerous large pores. A sublytic quantity of PFN merely indicates that a few cells are lysed over time, and the survivors somehow dispose of the potentially le-thal pores. Prior to their removal, PFN pores could permeabilize the plasma membrane, allowing minute quantities of membrane-dissociated GrB to enter the cell.

Together with various collaborators, five studies have been performed to address the question: Does PFN function primarily as an endosomolytic factor? First, after exposure of target cells to sublytic PFN and GrB, membrane pore size was estimated by determining the exclusion limit of proteins of increasing relative molecular mass (M_r). Due to the heterogeneity of PFN binding and attendant variation in pore diameter, only cells that died by apoptosis and thereby had GrB delivered to the cytosol were analyzed. In the presence of sublytic PFN, cells excluded proteins larger than yeast cdk (13 kDa) but an 8-kDa bacterial azurin was able to enter cells. Therefore transmembrane pores large enough to allow passive diffusion of GrB (32 kDa) were not likely to contribute to the cytoplasmic delivery of the granzyme (43). Nevertheless, it should be emphasized that these studies may not detect transiently expressed, larger pores that might allow entry of plasma membrane-dissociated GrB.

We have found that target cells remain susceptible to apoptosis when PFN is added as long as 3 hours after a pulse of GrB (33). This result suggested that GrB and PFN may not have to be co-internalized to the same vesicle as might occur during CTL-mediated apoptosis. Therefore it was asked whether fusion of vesicles that contained PFN and GrB could induce cell death. To address this question, COS cells transfected with the murine GrB construct were exposed to PFN. These cells do not secrete the granzyme and lack detectable plasma membrane-associated protease. Despite the absence of membrane-bound GrB, the COS cells underwent apoptosis when incubated with PFN (or AD), and the granzyme was identified in the nucleus of the dying cells (34). Mock-transfectants exposed to exogenous GrB and PFN did not die, suggesting that GrB released from dying COS cells was unlikely to bind neighboring cells in amounts sufficient for cell death after addition of PFN. Although these remarkable data suggest that PFN- and GrB-filled vesicles could fuse resulting in the release of the granzyme, to our knowledge the results provide the first evidence that PFN must be internalized to deliver the granzyme effectively. Consistent with these results, when cells were first pulsed with PFN, washed, and then treated with GrB, the cells once again died further, suggesting that PFN is internalized by the target cell (34).

Manipulating targets with sublytic activities of PFN may not recapitulate the membrane-associated events that occur when PFN is delivered by a CTL. With this issue in mind, Kawasaki et al. have studied membrane trafficking after CTL contact using FM1-43 (44). This is a hydrophilic styryl dye that has been used extensively to visualize exocytic and endocytic activity of secretory vesicles and to monitor the level and rate of fluid-phase and receptor-dependent endocytic activity (45–47). When cells are incubated in media containing the dye, a minor portion partitions at the aqueous–lipid interface of the membrane and becomes fluorescent. Because FM1-43 readily diffuses from the cell surface, after the cells are washed only vesicles formed by endocytosis in the presence of FM1-43 are visible by fluorescence. When such vesicles are exocytosed to the medium that does not contain the dye, the fluorescence vanishes immediately as the dye rapidly diffuses into the medium.

A perforin-positive murine CTL clone was incubated with antigen-specific targets in media containing FM1-43, and changes in the membrane distribution of the dye were visualized by confocal microscopy in target cells. Three minutes after CTL–target contact, FM1-43 fluorescence became visible in the target cell. The dye appeared to form an overlapping pattern of punctate stains and to associate with intracellular membrane structures such as the nuclear envelope. To learn whether the dye entered

the target through transmembrane pores, the experiments were repeated using the membrane impermeant dye HPTS to monitor permeabilization. The CTLs induced the expected translocation of FM1-43, but there was no apparent influx of HPTS into the target cytosol. Importantly, application of sublytic doses of purified perforin to target cells resulted in a similar translocation of FM1-43 without influx of HPTS. The subsequent addition of digitonin, however, induced a striking influx of both dyes. Thus when the plasma membrane was damaged, HPTS was able to diffuse to the cytosol. During the attack of the CTL, the translocation of the FM-143 into the target cell may occur through association with the plasma membrane remnant of the endocytic vesicle, through influx of soluble dye past transmembrane pores, or through uptake of soluble dye by fluid-phase endocytosis. In most reports, internalization of FM1-43 is associated with the development of a pattern of punctate stains consistent with a vesicular distribution (48). In the images generated after CTL contact, there was an unanticipated dramatic increase in staining of the nuclear membrane and mitochondria. Because generalized permeabilization of the target cell plasma membrane could not be detected, what process could explain this massive transfer of the dye to these intracellular structures? The dye may be released from perforin-damaged vesicles and diffuse to intracellular structures. Alternately, the fusogenic potential of the vesicles may be enhanced by PFN, facilitating fusion with intracellular organelles. Subsequently, through lateral diffusion, FM1-43 associates with the membranous components of the organelles. Regardless of the precise mechanism, these data suggest that during a CTL attack perforin polymerizes in the plasma membrane and delivers the FM1-43 intracellularly without overt membrane permeabilization. Comparable results were obtained when target cells were exposed to purified PFN, so exposure of targets to isolated PFN and GrB may indeed be a reasonable *in vitro* model for CTL-mediated apoptosis.

If PFN should function as an endosomolytic agent, the activity might be mimicked by other pore-forming proteins after application to cells at sublytic concentrations. Studies performed with Trapani et al. (43) were undertaken to assess the capacity of the following bacterial porins to deliver GrB and cause cell death in the absence of plasma membrane permeabilization: staphylococcal alpha toxin (SAT), streptolysin O (SLO), pneumolysin (PLO), and listeriolysin (LLO). The diameter of SLO and PLO pores are apparently concentration-dependent, resulting in internal diameters ranging up to 40 nM, whereas SAT consistently polymerizes into pores of 2 to 5 nM. Unlike these toxins, LLO optimally forms pores at acidic pH; therefore although the toxin may produce pores at the plasma membrane it is also predicted to be most active within acidic vesicles (49). The toxins were titrated for intracellular delivery of GrB (i.e., cell death), and the integrity of the plasma membrane was monitored by exclusion of fluoresceinated dextran species (4–20 kDa). SAT, regardless of concentration, failed to deliver GrB, whereas SLO, PLO, and LLO induced apoptosis at concentrations that did not permeabilize the plasma membrane to the fluorescent markers (Trapani and Froelich, unpublished observations). These data suggest that sublytic concentrations of SLO, PLO, and LLO also deliver GrB to the cytosol through a process that occurs within the cell and not the plasma membrane. LLO, similar to AD, is an established endosomolytic; therefore the capacity to deliver GrB is not unexpected. SLO and PLO, on the other hand, are reported to form pores at the plasma membrane and thereby more closely approximate the function proposed for PFN. Unfortunately, we are unaware of data that describe whether the toxins are subjected to endocytic clearance from the plasma membrane. Furthermore, it is unclear why SAT failed to deliver the granzyme. Because this toxin forms a stable 5-nM pore perhaps endocytosis of a pore larger than 5 nm in diameter may be necessary for permeabilization and release of the granzyme from a vesicle. Nevertheless, the fact that three distinct bacterial toxins have the capacity to deliver GrB to the cytosol without obvious permeabilization of the plasma membrane indirectly supports the hypothesis that PFN also may function as an endosomolytic agent.

In comparison to transmembrane delivery systems (liposomes, electroporation), which directly transfer proteins through the plasma membrane by fusion or generation of large, nonspecific pores, AD-mediated protein delivery is exceedingly efficient (50). Therefore we have speculated that PFN-mediated granzyme delivery recapitulates this process. Viruses [e.g., human immunodeficiency virus (HIV)], however, also enter a cell by fusion at the plasma membrane. This process is equivalent to translocation of a single fusogenic protein across the membrane. In the case of granule delivery, PFN, the "fusogenic protein," is responsible for the delivery of an entirely separate protein that is also bound to the membrane. GrB might dissociate from the binding site and diffuse through transiently generated pores generated by PFN. We contend, however, that delivery of the GrB by internalization and subsequent PFN-mediated endosomolysis offers a more efficient delivery system.

Although the data provided here indirectly support the concept that PFN functions as an endosomolytic agent, experiments must be undertaken to directly establish the biologic effects of this fascinating protein. The first step would be to characterize the disposition of cell-associated PFN. The pore-forming protein might be cleared by budding from the membrane or, as we have postulated, by endocytosis. If the latter is a dominant mechanism, it should be possible using cell fraction techniques to characterize the vesicular trafficking of the internalized PFN. Thereafter, using endosome fusion techniques, the capacity of PFN to permeabilize endocytic vesicles could be evaluated.

INDUCTION OF APOPTOSIS BY INTRACELLULAR GrB

Physiologic Substrates Identified

Apoptosis is essential for ontogenetic development and remodeling of normal adult tissues. Operationally, apoptosis is initiated by death receptors (TNF, Fas, DR3, DR4, and DR5), by p53 dependent and independent cellular stress (genotoxic) pathways, and by the secretion of PFN and granzymes from cytotoxic cells. As a consequence, a family of phylogenetically conserved cysteine proteases (caspases) are activated (51). The caspases are divided into apical (caspases 2, 8, 9, and 10) and executioner subsets (caspases 3, 6, and 7). Ligation of a death receptor or cellular stress results in activation of specific apical members. Regardless of the stimulus, we have suggested that all apical caspases converge at caspase-3, after which caspase-6 and caspase-7 become activated (52,53). These executioner caspases then cleave regulatory and structural proteins that produce the apoptotic phenotype.

Although the substrates for the tryptases, GrA and GrK, remain elusive, an important clue that has served to clarify the function of GrB is a preference for cleavage of peptide bonds after the Asp residue. Caspase zymogens are processed by cleavage at specific Asp residues to form active heterodimeric enzymes. Thus GrB may have evolved to process and activate the caspases. Except for caspase-1 and caspase-2 (54,55), all members tested as GrB substrates are processed *in vitro,* including caspase-3 (56–58), caspase-6 (59,60), caspase-7 (61–63), caspase-8 (64–66), caspase-9 (67), and caspase-10a/b (68,69). Studies that examine processing of the caspases during granule-mediated apoptosis *in vivo* are more limited. Caspase-2 and caspase-3 undergo proteolysis in targets treated with CTLs (55,56), and targets where GrB is delivered internally contain processed

TABLE 12-1. *Nomenclature for caspases*

Designation	Alternative names	References
Caspase 1	Ice	73
Caspase 2	Ich-1	74
Caspase 3	Apopain, CPP32, Yama	75–77
Caspase 4	ICE$_{(rel)}$II, TX, Ich-2	78–80
Caspase 5	ICE$_{(rel)}$III, TY	78, 81
Caspase 6	Mch2	60
Caspase 7	Mch3, Ice-LAP3, Cmh-1	63, 82, 83
Caspase 8	FLICE 1, MACH, Mch5	64–66
Caspase 9	Ice-LAP6, Mch6	67, 84
Caspase 10a/b	Mch4, Flice2	68, 69

caspase-1 (70), caspase-3, caspase-7, caspase-6 (33,61,70,71), and caspase-8 (72). Nevertheless, these studies neither clarified which caspase is first cleaved by GrB to trigger the cascade nor provide insights to the sequence in which the caspases are activated during GrB-induced apoptosis (Table 12-1).

Caspase Processing by GrB in Whole Cells: Dependence on Preferred Substrates and Their Accessibility to Proteolysis

Subsite mapping through a combinatorial oligopeptide library approach showed that GrB prefers to cleave the caspases at the IXXD sequence, which lay at the juncture of the large and small subunits (85). Therefore one might postulate that GrB would initiate the caspase cascade *in vivo* by cleaving one of those members that contain this sequence (caspases 3, 7, or 10). The caspase then would undergo automaturation and proceed downstream to activate other members (Fig. 12-2).

To identify the caspase that GrB might first activate to trigger the death cascade, we assessed systematically the ability of the granzyme to process the human caspases. Among the 10 family members, GrB was indeed found to strongly prefer caspase-7 followed by caspase-10 and then caspase-3, cleaving at the IXXD sequence (71,86). Consequently, on the basis of rates of proteolysis, GrB would be predicted to first activate cas-

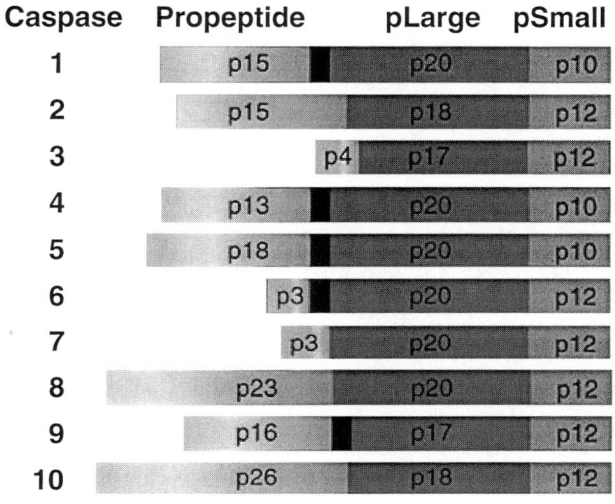

				CLEAVAGE SITES		
Caspase	Propeptide	pLarge	pSmall	*C-pro*	*NH-pL*	*C-pS*
1	p15	p20	p10	AVQD	WFKD	FEDD
2	p15	p18	p12	EHSD	????	DQQD
3	p4	p17	p12	ESMD	--------	IETD
4	p13	p20	p10	ESTD	WVRD	LEED
5	p18	p20	p10	LNMD	WVRD	LEAD
6	p3	p20	p12	TETD	DVVD	TEVD
7	p3	p20	p12	DSVD	-------	IQAD
8	p23	p20	p12	T I SD	????	VETD
9	p16	p17	p12	????	PEPD	DQLD
10	p26	p18	p12	NLKD	-------	IEAD

FIG. 12-2. Caspases: putative maturation sites. Predicted cleavage sites required to mature human caspases. *C-pro, NH-pL,* and *C-pS* represent, respectively, sites of cleavage to remove the propeptide, the spacer segment between the propeptide, and the pLarge subunit, and the cut between the pLarge and pSmall subunits (interdomain linker site).

pase-7, after delivery into whole cells. However, it was learned that caspase-7 cannot not be directly processed by GrB because the site preferred by the granzyme, IQAD, is cleaved after a cut is made that removes the propeptide segment (33). GrB therefore was postulated to cleave either or both caspase-3 and caspase-10, the remaining preferred substrates, to activate the cascade (71).

Although attempts had been made to dissect the pathway with oligopeptide inhibitors, this approach has failed to provide definitive results (87). To identify the caspase activated by GrB unequivocally required the identification of cells deficient in caspases-3 and -10. Fortunately, we found that MCF-7 cells lacked these caspases (71). After generating stable transfectants expressing either caspase-3 or caspase-10, a series of experiments were performed to delineate the steps of the pathway activated by GrB.

Foremost, GrB was found to function as an apical caspase in an undescribed two-step process where accessibility and susceptibility

to proteolysis contribute to the sequence in which the two executioner caspases are matured by the granzyme. GrB first activates caspase-3 even though this substrate is not the most preferred member of the death protease family. Caspase-3 then cleaves the N-peptide of procaspase-7, making it accessible to maturation by the granzyme. Unlike active caspase-3 and caspase-7, GrB has a marked preference for the IXXD sequence of caspase-7; therefore our results strongly suggested that GrB is responsible for maturation of the released caspase-7. Because GrB processes many different caspases *in vitro*, the granzyme has been regarded as a polyspecific activator of the caspase cascade *in vivo*. The inability of the granzyme to directly process caspases 7, 8, 9, and 10 as well as caspase-6 in the absence of caspase-3 was an unexpected finding, indicating that only a single GrB-induced pathway may exist for CTL-mediated activation of this death pathway (94).

Delineating the sequence in which the caspases are activated following ligation of death receptors or after genotoxic stress has been hampered by the notion that apical caspases mediate ubiquitous transactivation of executioner and other apical caspases. However, caspase-8, activated by ligation of the TNF receptor, also does not process other caspases in the absence of caspase-3 (88). Therefore not only does GrB function like an apical caspase, the granzyme appears to share the inability of apical caspases to activate other family members in the absence of caspase-3. Our observations raise two fascinating questions: How does caspase-3 access caspase-7 and presumably caspase-6, and where are these executioners compartmentalized to prevent their activation by GrB and the apical caspases? From this perspective it is intriguing to note that procaspase-3 is located in the cytosol as well as mitochondria in certain cell lines (89). The compartmentalization of caspase-3 to mitochondria suggests that the caspase localized there might be activated through caspase-9, whereas the cytosolic caspase-3 is processed by apical members activated through death receptors and by GrB, providing different avenues for the efficient activation of this important death protease. Because procaspase-7 is processed by GrB only after detergent extraction of the MCF-7null cells, the zymogen appears to be located in an inaccessible vesicular compartment. Others have observed, based on cell fractionation studies, that procaspase-7 is compartmentalized to the endoplasmic reticulum (ER) and mitochondia (90), further supporting a compartmentalization of apical and executioner caspases.

The sequestration of the executioner caspase-7 provides a previously undefined level of regulation in this enzymatic cascade. As a consequence of this sequestration, two distinct proteases are required for proper maturation of caspase-7: caspase-3 to remove the propeptide and GrB to cleave the interdomain linker site. Using the MCF-7 sublines treated with TNF, caspase-8 appears to function similarly to the granzyme (91). These results may define a common mechanism shared by the granzyme and apical caspases (2, 8, 9, and 10) to process the executioner caspases (Fig. 12-3). Subsequently, uninvolved apical caspases may be activated in a process that serves to amplify the portion of the cascade that converges at caspase-3, underscoring the central role of this protease in producing cell death. Therefore further studies of the proteolytic signal delivered from the apical to executioner caspases must take into account the different locations and intracellular trafficking patterns of the various family members in the cell and the efficiency that a particular caspase trans-activates another.

GrB: Killing Independently of the Caspase Cascade

To delay or prevent cell death, viruses have evolved proteins that inactivate the caspases. The cytokine response modifier A of the cowpox virus (92) and the description of a new family of viral inhibitors (93) exemplify this tactic. Although we have delineated the dominant death pathway GrB is likely to use when delivered intracellularly, the granzyme may not be able to cleave other caspases if caspase-3 is blocked (e.g., by a viral inhibitor). However, because GrB appears to function as an apical caspase, the granzyme should be able to kill cells by cleaving substrates recognized by caspases. This hypothesis was tested by showing that GrB was able to kill targets despite the presence of caspase inhibitors that blocked activation of caspase-3 (71). Furthermore, the delivery of GrB by AD or microinjection into caspase-3-deficient cells also causes apoptosis (34,94). Together, the results indicate that GrB should be able to access and cleave cellular substrates independently of the caspase cascade. In this regard, DNA-PKcs and NuMA have been recently found to be directly and efficiently cleaved by GrB *in vitro* and *in vivo,* generating unique substrate fragments not observed during other forms of apoptosis (95).

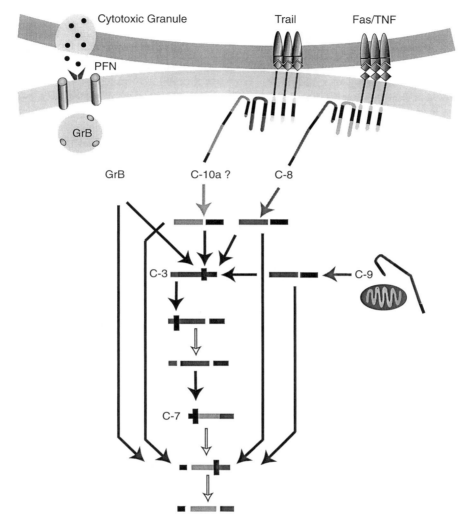

FIG. 12-3. Proposed pathway for activation of caspase death pathway. The death pathway of cell may be activated by a transmembrane signal transmitted through death receptors, by activation of the "genotoxic" pathway, or by delivery of granzyme B (GrB) to the cytosol. Ligation of death receptors results in activation of the linked apical caspases Fas/TNF [caspase-8 (C-8)] and Trail [caspase-10a (C-10a) (proposed)], whereas genotoxic stress leads to activation of apical caspase-9 (C-9). As described in the text, GrB also functions as an apical caspase after delivery to the cytosol. All apical caspases (and GrB) then converge at caspase-3 to activate this family member. Thereafter, caspase-3 (C-3) and the respective apical caspase act, in concert, to mature caspase-7 (C-7). GrB, granzyme B; Fas/TNF, Fas/tumor necrosis factor receptors; Trail, trail receptor.

Is GrB Able to Kill Targets Independently of PFN?

The biologic function of the granzymes is considered inextricably dependent on the pore-forming action of PFN. The observa- tion, however, that GrB induces apoptosis in AD-infected targets suggests an alternate mechanism for the intracellular delivery of GrB. In this instance, GrB is endocytosed by a cell previously infected by a pathogen that has disrupted vesicular trafficking (96); after entering the cell the granzyme is inadvertently discharged to the cytosol, causing apoptosis. Consistent with this possibility, GrB causes apoptosis in vesicular stomatitis virus (VSV)-infected U937 cells (97). A member of the rhabdovirus family, VSV enters the cell by receptor-dependent endocytosis and escapes to the cytosol when the hydrophobic domains of the M or G protein (or both) fuse with the endosomal membrane (98). Being a lytic virus, targets normally start to undergo apoptosis by 8 hours. Therefore it was asked if internalized GrB could accelerate the rate of apoptosis and inhibit viral replication in the VSV-infected cells. As determined by the TUNEL assay, 75% of the cells infected with VSV for 4 hours became apoptotic 2 hours after exposure to GrB. Importantly, Northern analysis confirmed that viral transcripts are degraded, a finding associated with 80% reduction in plaque formation.

What is the likelihood that a target cell encounters GrB in the absence of PFN *in vivo*? Activated CTLs are reported to secrete the granzymes constitutively (99); therefore GrB could diffuse to infected targets adjacent to the site where the killer cell is eliminating its foe. The possibility that GrB mediates a biologic effect independently of PFN is further strengthened by the observation that elevated levels of active GrB are detectable by capture immunoassay in the plasma of patients experiencing acute viral infection (e.g., Epstein-Bar virus, HIV-1) (100). Together the evidence supports a PFN-independent role for the granzymes in host defense. These findings should stimulate studies to learn whether cells infected with other intracellular pathogens (e.g., *Listeria monocytogenes*) also succumb to GrB-induced apoptosis *in vitro* and in animals rendered PFN-deficient.

providing an overview of granule-mediated apoptosis, may not accurately recapitulate events *in vivo*. The biologically relevant form of the granzyme may be a macromolecular complex where the various family members are bound to a granule-associated proteoglycan (PG), namely serglycin (SG). SG is distinct from other proteoglycans owing to a high degree of glycosylation and resistance to proteolysis. Various serglycins have been characterized in distinct cell types, differing primarily on the basis of the glycosaminoglycan side chains: serosal mast cells—heparin sulfate; bone marrow mast cells—chondroitin-4,6-sulfate; NK cells, eosinophils, and HL-60 promyelocytes—chondroitin-4-sulfate; and megakaryocytes—chondroitin-6-sulfate. Serglycins function to ensure the proper packaging of granule constituents and act as a carrier for granule proteins after granule secretion (101). All mast cell proteases except mast cell tryptase (murine mast cell protease 7) (102) are secreted as a macromolecular complex into the extracellular space.

The highly cationic granzymes are packaged with chondroitin-4-sulfate SG in an electrochemically neutral form within cytotoxic granules. Similar to mast cell proteases and chemokines secreted by mast cells and CTLs, respectively (103), the granzymes have been reported to be exocytosed as a macromolecular complex (104,105). The ligand–receptor studies suggest that free GrB specifically interacts with target cells. GrB, however, is highly cationic, suggesting that the specific interaction may be artifactual. On the basis of this information, a series of experiments was performed to determine if GrB formed stable complexes with chondroitin-4-sulfate glycosaminoglycans (GAGs) and if the complexes could induce apoptosis when delivered by AD or PFN.

NATURE OF EXOCYTOSED GRANZYMES

Our studies and data reported by others have examined the effect of purified GrB on target cells. These *in vitro* models, though useful for

GrB: Forming a Stable Complex with Anionic Glycosaminoglycan, Chondroitin Sulfate

We have reported that GrB binds tightly to a cation exchange column eluting at ionic strength of 590 mM NaCl (106). In a model system that consisted of desalted chondroitin A-4-sulfate and isolated human GrB, the strength of ionic interaction was examined by increasing the NaCl concentration (M), separating the free and bound granzyme by cation-exchange chromatography, and measuring the amount of GrB that dissociated from chondroitin-4-sulfate by the capture immunoassay. GrB did not begin to dissociate until the salt concentration exceeded 550 mM, indicating maintenance of a stable complex under physiologic conditions. Furthermore, the ionic interaction was stable at neutral pH and the acidic pH encountered in cytotoxic granules (pH 5.5). Together with studies showing that GrA is secreted complexed to PGs (104), the data suggest that GrB is likely to exist as a macromolecular complex following exocytosis. Consequently, the target cell is predicted to interact with complexed GrB after CTL attack.

GrB–Chondroitin A Complexes and Apoptosis

The question was then addressed whether equivalent amounts of active free GrB and GrB in chondroitin-4-sulfate complexes (CS–GrB) produce similar levels of apoptosis after delivery by AD. Because the average CS was approximately 50 kDa, and if it was presumed GrB bound CS in equimolar quantities, the molecular weights of the free CS versus CS–GrB delivered to the cells would be 32 and 82 kDa, respectively. For this comparison we quantitatively measured the levels of caspase-3-like activity in Jurkat cells using the fluorogenic substrate DEVD-AMC. Although we have not yet measured the amount of complexed GrB that might be internalized by the target cells, both forms produced comparable time-dependent increases in DEVD-AMC activity. To mimic conditions *in vivo*, PFN was used to deliver CS–GrB to target cells. Jurkat cells were first pulsed with the complexes and treated with a sublytic concentration of PFN as previously

described (33). In comparison to the free GrB, the CS–GrB delivered by PFN induced a similar percentage of target cells for death.

GrB is Secreted as a Macromolecular Complex and Retains Apoptotic Activity

If the biologically relevant form of GrB is a complex of the granzyme and granule-associated proteoglycan, the serine protease should be detected as a high-molecular-weight complex following exocytosis. When supernatant from anti-CD2-stimulated LAK cells were fractionated using a 100-kDa membrane filter, active GrB was completely retained in the high-molecular-weight fraction (107). Comparable to CS–GrB, this high-molecular-weight form of the granzyme also induced apoptosis following delivery into target cells with AD.

MODELS FOR A NEW FORM OF INTERCELLULAR SIGNALING

Consistent with data reported for most of the mast cell proteases, preliminary evidence suggests that the granzymes are exocytosed as a neutral high-molecular-weight complex. Studies designed to examine either the proteolytic or apoptotic activity of GrB *in vitro* have been confined to the free enzyme. The highly cationic nature of the granzyme would not only favor nonspecific interaction with the negatively charged plasma membrane but could also lead to artifactual vesicular trafficking and anomalous interaction with intracellular membranes and cytosolic proteins after intracytoplasmic delivery. Overall, intracellular proteins could act as a nonspecific "sink" for free GrB, modifying the correct localization of the granzyme in the cell. For example, after delivery by PFN, GrB is reported to readily bind and enter the nucleus of the target cell (43). This pattern of trafficking, which is apparently dependent on cytosolic factors, may not occur when complexed GrB is delivered to target cells. Furthermore, the proteolytic activity of GrB may be influenced by nonspecific interactions with cytosolic and intracellular membrane-associated proteins. When the rates of proteolysis of CS–GrB and free GrB were compared against caspase-3 and caspase-7, the cationic form manifested greater proteolytic activity. However, when the two forms of granzyme were added to cell lysates containing these caspases, a marked reduction in the rate of proteolysis was observed only for free-GrB (107). Reports exist where cells overexpressing Bcl-2 have been found to inhibit GrB/PFN but not cytotoxic cell-mediated apoptosis. As described above, free-GrB appears to initiate the caspase cascade by activating the less preferred but more accessible caspase-3. Then caspase-3 and GrB work in tandem to activate caspase-7. It will be interesting to learn whether this pathway is also activated by the complexed form of GrB. Nevertheless, we suggest that *in vitro* studies of granule-mediated apoptosis should be performed not with cationic GrB but, at a minimum, with CS–GrB complexes to recapitulate events enacted by CTLs.

A new paradigm is offered for granule-mediated apoptosis that focuses on the cytosolic delivery of granzymes. Contrary to the accepted view, GrB and other granzymes enter target cells by receptor dependent endocytosis in a process that is entirely independent of PFN. The pore-forming protein is crucial, however, for proper targeting of the granzyme to the cytosol being functionally equivalent to pore-forming or fusogenic proteins created by the pathogens (108). Therefore we speculate that granule-mediated apoptosis recapitulates the tactics that pathogens have devised to enter the cytosol. Although stoichiometric studies have not been performed, binding to the plasma membrane may occur through the multiple granzymes residing on a single molecule of SG. If SG has a relatively linear topology similar to other PGs (101) and each SG proteoglycan is covered by multiple granzyme molecules in a radial distribution to ensure electrochemical neutrality, the proteoglycan may serve to focus the interaction of granzyme molecules with membrane binding sites, encouraging "receptor" multimerization and internalization. Equally plausible, a contiguous array of GrB molecules could act as a template that facilitates the processing of the caspase-3. Because PFN delivers this macromolecular signaling complex consisting of an array of granzymes ionically linked to the scaffold of SG, we have named the paradigm the "multimeric granzyme complex model" of granule-mediated apoptosis. Thus the pore-forming protein not only delivers GrB but other members of the deadly granzyme family, ensuring the death of the target cell.

Although the granzyme–SG complexes and PFN are probably internalized coincidentally by the target cell during CTL-mediated killing, more than one model is necessary to fully explain our data. During the attack by the cytotoxic effector, granzymes are endocytosed into the target cell with plasma membrane containing sublytic PFN pores. The disrupted integrity of the vesicle could allow immediate release of the internalized GrB near the plasma membrane (Fig. 12-4a), or the granzyme escapes when the vesicle fuses with an early endosome (Fig. 12-4b). Alternately, PFN and the granzyme are internalized separately to vesicles that subsequently fuse, releasing the protease. A caveat of the latter model implies that secreted GrB alone could play a role in host defense against pathogen-mediated diseases that disrupt vesicular trafficking (Fig. 12-4).

Acknowledgments

We thank the many individuals who have participated in the described studies and specifically acknowledge the following: R. Christopher Bleackley, Vishva Dixit, William Hanna, Kim Orth, Robert Talanian, and Joseph Trapani. The work reported here was funded by the Rice Foundation, the Retirement Foundation, and the GCC and National Arthritis Foundations

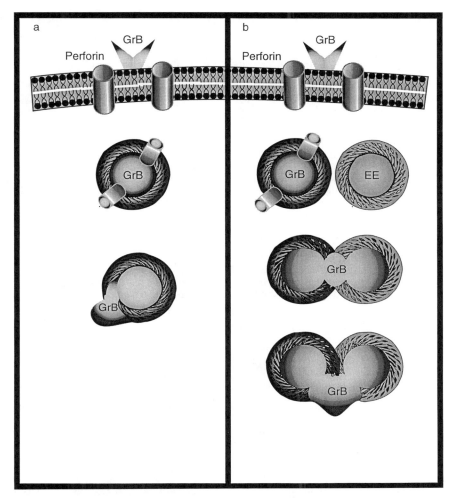

FIG. 12-4. Postulated mechanisms for the intracellular delivery of GrB. **a:** After interaction with specific binding sites, GrB is endocytosed with adjacent sublytic PFN pores. The compromised integrity of the vesicle then results in the escape of granzyme to the cytosol. **b:** GrB is endocytosed with PFN, and the granzyme is released when the vesicle fuses with an early endosome (*EE*). A third possibility (not shown) may occur in pathogen-infected cells. In this instance, GrB alone is internalized and released to the cytosol by an intracellular pathogen that disrupts the newly formed vesicle.

REFERENCES

1. Tschopp J, Nabholz M. Perforin-mediated target cell lysis by cytolytic lymphocytes. *Annu Rev Immunol* 1990;8:279–302.
2. Hanna WL, Turbov J, Jackman HL, Tan F, Froelich CJ. The dominant chymotrypsin-like esterase activity in human lymphocyte granules is mediated by the serine carboxypeptidase called cathepsin A-like protective protein (CAPP). *J Immunol* 1994;153:4663–4672.
3. Pena SV, Hanson DA, Carr BA, Goralski TJ, Krensky AM. Processing, subcellular localization and function of 519 (granulysin), a human late T cell activation molecule with homology to small lytic granule proteins. *J Immunol* 1997;158:2680–2688.
4. Hudig D, Ewoldt GR, Woodard SL. Proteases and lymphocyte cytotoxic killing mechanisms. *Curr Opin Immunol* 1993;5:90–96.
5. Greenberg AH, Lichtfield DW. Granzymes and apoptosis: targeting the cell cycle. *Curr Top Microbiol Immunol* 1995;198:95–118.

6. Jenne D, Tschopp J. Granzymes: a family of serine proteases of cytolytic T cells. *Curr Top Microbiol Immunol* 1988;140:268–271.

7. Shi L, Kam C-M, Powers JC, Aebersold R, Greenberg AH. Purification of three cytotoxic lymphocyte granule serine proteases that induce apoptosis through distinct substrate and target cell interactions. *J Exp Med* 1992;176:1521–1529.

8. Smyth MJ, Wiltrout T, Trapani JA, et al. Purification and cloning of a novel serine protease, RNK-Met-1, from the granules of a rat natural killer cell leukemia. *J Biol Chem* 1992;267:24418–24425.

9. Woodard SL, Fraser SA, Winkler U, et al. Purification and characterization of lymphocyte chymase I, a granzyme implicated in perforin-mediated lysis. *J Immunol* 1998;160:4988–4993.

10. Kyburz D, Speiser DE, Battegay M, Hengartner H, Zinkernagel RM. Lysis of infected cells in vivo by antiviral cytolytic T cells demonstrated by release of cell internal viral proteins. *Eur J Immunol* 1993;23:1540–1545.

11. Kägi D, Ledermann B, Bürki K, Zinkernagel RM, Hengartner H. Molecular mechanisms of lymphocyte-mediated cytotoxicity and their role in immunological protection and pathogenesis in vivo. *Annu Rev Immunol* 1996;14:207–232.

12. Van den Broek MF, Kägi D, Ossendorp F, et al. Decreased tumor surveillance in perforin-deficient mice. *J Exp Med* 1996;184:1781–1790.

13. Heusel JW, Wesselschmidt RL, Shresta S, Russell JH, Ley TJ. Cytotoxic lymphocytes require granzyme B for the rapid induction of DNA fragmentation and apoptosis in allogeneic target cells. *Cell* 1994;76:977–987.

14. Ebnet K, Hausmann M, Lehmann-Grube F, et al. Granzyme A-deficient mice retain potent cell-mediated cytotoxicity. *EMBO J* 1995;14:4230–4239.

15. Shresta S, Russell JH, Ley TJ. Mechanisms responsible for granzyme B-independent cytotoxicity. *Blood* 1997;89:4085–4091.

16. Lichtenheld MG, Olsen KJ, Lu P, et al. Structure and function of human perforin. *Nature* 1988; 335:448–451.

17. Uellner R, Zvelebil MJ, Hopkins J, et al. Perforin is activated by a proteolytic cleavage during biosynthesis which reveals a phospholipid-binding C2 domain. *EMBO J* 1997;16:7287–7296.

18. Ojcius DM, Persechini PM, Zheng L-M, Notaroberto PC, Adeodato SC, Young JD-E. Cytolytic and ion channel-forming properties of the N terminus of lymphocyte perforin. *Proc Natl Acad Sci USA* 1991;88:4621–4625.

19. Binah O, Liu CC, Young JDE, Berke G. Channel formation and $[Ca^{2+}]_i$ accumulation induced by perforin N-terminus peptides: comparison with purified perforin and whole lytic granules. *Biochem Biophys Res Commun* 1997;240:647–650.

20. Podack ER. Execution and suicide: cytotoxic lymphocytes enforce draconian laws through separate molecular pathways. *Curr Opin Immunol* 1995; 7:11–16.

21. Shiver JW, Su L, Henkart PA. Cytotoxicity with target DNA breakdown by rat basophilic leukemia cells expressing both cytolysin and granzyme A. *Cell* 1992;71:315–322.

22. Nakajima H, Henkart PA. Cytotoxic lymphocyte granzymes trigger a target cell internal disintegration pathway leading to cytolysis and DNA breakdown. *J Immunol* 1994;152:1057–1063.

23. Williams MS, Henkart PA. Intracellular proteolysis triggers cell death generally accompanied by apoptotic morphology and DNA breakdown. *J Immunol* 1993;150:208A.

24. Henkart MP, Henkart PA. Lymphocyte mediated cytolysis as a secretory phenomenon. *Adv Exp Med Biol* 1982;146:227–242.

25. Su B, Bochan MR, Hanna WL, Froelich CJ, Brahmi Z. Human granzyme B is essential for DNA fragmentation of susceptible target cells. *Eur J Immunol* 1994;24:2073–2080.

26. Bochan MR, Goebel WS, Brahmi Z. Stably transfected antisense granzyme B and perforin constructs inhibit human granule-mediated lytic ability. *Cell Immunol* 1995;164:234–239.

27. Shresta S, MacIvor DM, Heusel JW, Russell JH, Ley TJ. Natural killer and lymphokine-activated killer cells require granzyme B for the rapid induction of apoptosis in susceptible target cells. *Proc Natl Acad Sci USA* 1995;92:5679–5683.

28. Shresta S, Goda P, Wesselschmidt R, Ley TJ. Residual cytotoxicity and granzyme K expression in granzyme A-deficient cytotoxic lymphocytes. *J Biol Chem* 1997;272:20236–20244.

29. Simon MM, Hausmann M, Tran T, et al. In vitro- and ex vivo-derived cytolytic leukocytes from granzyme A × B double knockout mice are defective in granule-mediated apoptosis but not lysis of target cells. *J Exp Med* 1997;186:1781–1786.

30. Shi L, Kraut RP, Aebersold R, Greenberg AH. A natural killer cell granule protein that induces DNA fragmentation and apoptosis. *J Exp Med* 1992;175:553–566.

31. Cesano A, Santoli D. Two unique human leukemic T-cell lines endowed with a stable cytotoxic function and a different spectrum of target reactivity analysis and modulation of their lytic mechanisms. *In Vitro Cell Dev Biol* 1992;28A:648–656.

32. Podack ER, Kupfer A. T-cell effector functions: mechanisms for delivery of cytotoxicity and help. *Annu Rev Cell Biol* 1991;7:479–504.

33. Froelich CJ, Orth K, Turbov J, et al. New paradigm for lymphocyte granule-mediated cytotoxicity: targets bind and internalize granzyme B but a endosomolytic agent is necessary for cytosolic delivery and apoptosis. *J Biol Chem* 1996;271:29073–29081.

34. Pinkoski MJ, Hobman M, Heiben JA, et al. Cytosolic granzyme B is necessary and sufficient to induce apoptotic cell death. *Blood* 1998;92:1044–1054.

35. Novick P, Zerial M. The diversity of Rab proteins in vesicle transport. *Curr Opin Cell Biol* 1997;9: 496–504.

36. Shi L, Mai S, Israels S, Browne KA, Trapani JA, Greenberg AH. Granzyme B (GraB) autonomously crosses the cell membrane and perforin initiates apoptosis and GraB nuclear localization. *J Exp Med* 1997;185:855–866.

37. Williams MS, Henkart PA. Apoptotic cell death induced by intracellular proteolysis. *J Immunol* 1994;153:4247–4257.

38. Jans DA, Jans P, Briggs LJ, Sutton V, Trapani JA. Nuclear transport of granzyme B (fragmentin-2): dependence on perforin in vivo and cytosolic factors in vitro. *J Biol Chem* 1996;271:30781–30789.

39. Seth P. A simple and efficient method of protein delivery into cells using adenovirus. *Biochem Biophys Res Commun* 1994;203:582–587.

40. Leopold PL, Ferris B, Grinberg I, Worgall S, Hackett NR, Crystal RG. Fluorescent virions: dynamic tracking of the pathway of adenoviral genetransfer vectors in living cells. *Hum Gene Ther* 1998;10:367–378.

41. Froelich CJ, Hanna WL, Poirier GG, et al. Poly-(ADP-ribose) polymerase is cleaved by two different pathways during granzyme B mediated apoptosis of Jurkat cells. *Biochem Biophys Res Commun* 1996;227:658–665.

42. Pinkoski MJ, Winkler U, Hudig D, Bleackley RC. Binding of granzyme B in the nucleus of target cells: recognition of an 80-kilodalton protein. *J Biol Chem* 1996;271:10225–10229.

43. Trapani JA, Jans P, Smyth MJ, et al. Perforin-dependent nuclear entry of granzyme B precedes apoptosis, and is not a consequence of nuclear membrane dysfunction. *Cell Death Differ* 1998;5:488–496.

44. Kawasaki Y, Saito T, Shirota-Someya Y, et al. Cell death associated translocation of plasma membrane components to intracellular membrane structures induced by cytotoxic T lymphocytes. (1999; submitted)

45. Smith CB, Betz WJ. Simultaneous independent measurement of endocytosis and exocytosis. *Nature* 1996;380:531–534.

46. Ryan TA, Smith SJ, Reuter H. The timing of synaptic vesicle endocytosis. *Proc Natl Acad Sci USA* 1996;93:5567–5571.

47. Ribeiro F, Coelho PM, Vieira LQ, Powell K, Kusel JR. Membrane internalization processes in different stages of Schistosoma mansoni as shown by a styryl dye (FM 1-43). *Parasitology* 1998;6:51–59.

48. Henkel AW, Lübke J, Betz WJ. FM1-43 dye ultrastructural localization in and release from frog motor nerve terminals. *Proc Natl Acad Sci USA* 1996;93:1918–1923.

49. Beauregard KE, Lee KD, Collier RJ, Swanson JA. pH-dependent perforation of macrophage phagosomes by listeriolysin O from Listeria monocytogenes. *J Exp Med* 1997;186:1159–1163.

50. Novoa I, Benavente J, Cotten M, Carrasco L. Permeabilization of mammalian cells to proteins: poliovirus 2A^pro as a probe to analyze entry of proteins into cells. *Exp Cell Res* 1997;232:186–190.

51. Chinnaiyan AM, Dixit VM. The cell-death machine. *Curr Biol* 1996;6:555–562.

52. Froelich CJ, Dixit VM, Yang X. Granule mediated apoptosis: a matter of viral mimicry. *Immunol Today* 1998;19:30–36.

53. Li P, Nijhawan D, Budihardjo I, et al. Cytochrome c and dATP-dependent formation of Apaf-1/caspase-9 complex initiates an apoptotic protease cascade. *Cell* 1997;91:479–489.

54. Darmon AJ, Ehrman N, Caputo A, Fujinaga J, Bleackley RC. The cytotoxic T cell proteinase granzyme B does not activate interleukin-1b-con-

verting enzyme. *J Biol Chem* 1994;269:32043–32046.

55. Li H, Bergeron L, Cryns VL, et al. Activation of caspase-2 in Apoptosis. *J Biol Chem* 1997;272:21010–21017.

56. Darmon AJ, Nicholson DW, Bleackley RC. Activation of the apoptotic protease CPP32 by cytotoxic T-cell-derived granzyme B. *Nature* 1995;377:446–448.

57. Quan LT, Tewari M, O'Rourke K, et al. Proteolytic activation of the cell death protease Yama/CPP32 by granzyme B. *Proc Natl Acad Sci USA* 1996;93:1972–1976.

58. Martin SJ, Amarante-Mendes GP, Shi LF, et al. The cytotoxic cell protease granzyme B initiates apoptosis in a cell-free system by proteolytic processing and activation of the ICE/CED-3 family protease, CPP32, via a novel two-step mechanism. *EMBO J* 1996;15:2407–2416.

59. Orth K, Chinnaiyan AM, Garg M, Froelich CJ, Dixit VM. The CED-3/ICE-like protease Mch2 is activated during apoptosis and cleaves the death substrate lamin A. *J Biol Chem* 1996;271:16443–16446.

60. Fernandes-Alnemri T, Litwack G, Alnemri ES. Mch2, a new member of the apoptotic Ced-3/Ice cysteine protease gene family. *Cancer Res* 1995;55:2737–2742.

61. Chinnaiyan AM, Orth K, Hanna WL, et al. Cytotoxic T cell-derived granzyme B activates the apoptotic protease ICE-LAP3. *Curr Biol* 1996;6:897–899.

62. Gu Y, Sarnecki C, Fleming MA, Lippke JA, Bleackley RC, Su MSS. Processing and activation of CMH-1 by granzyme B. *J Biol Chem* 1996;271:10816–10820.

63. Fernandes-Alnemri T, Takahashi A, Armstrong R, et al. Mch3, a novel human apoptotic cysteine protease highly related to CPP32. *Cancer Res* 1995;55:6045–6052.

64. Boldin MP, Goncharov TM, Goltsev YV, Wallach D. Involvement of MACH, a novel MORT1/FADD-interacting protease, in Fas/APO-1- and TNF receptor-induced cell death. *Cell* 1996;85:803–815.

65. Muzio M, Chinnaiyan AM, Kischkel FC, et al. FLICE, a novel FADD-homologous ICE/CED-3-like protease, is recruited to the CD-95 (FAS/Apo-1) death-inducing signaling complex (DISC). *Cell* 1996;86:817–821.

66. Srinivasula SM, Ahmad M, Fernandes-Alnemri T, Litwack G, Alnemri ES. Molecular ordering of the Fas-apoptotic pathway: the Fas/APO-1 protease Mch5 is a CrmA-inhibitable protease that activates multiple Ced-3/ICE-like cysteine proteases. *Proc Natl Acad Sci USA* 1996;93:14486–14491.

67. Duan HJ, Orth K, Chinnaiyan AM, et al. ICE-LAP6, a novel member of the ICE/Ced-3 gene family, is activated by the cytotoxic T cell protease granzyme B. *J Biol Chem* 1996;171:16720–16724.

68. Fernandes-Alnemri T, Armstrong RC, Krebs J, et al. In vitro activation of CPP32 and Mch3 by Mch4, a novel human apoptotic cysteine protease containing two FADD-like domains. *Proc Natl Acad Sci USA* 1996;93:7464–7469.

69. Vincenz C, Dixit VM. Fas-associated-death domain protein interleukin-1b-converting enzyme 2 (FLICE2), an ICE/Ced-3 homologue, is proximally involved in CD95- and p55-mediated death signaling. *J Biol Chem* 1997;272:6578–6583.

70. Shi LF, Chen G, MacDonald G, et al. Activation of an interleukin 1 converting enzyme-dependent apoptosis pathway by granzyme B. *Proc Natl Acad Sci USA* 1996;93:11002–11007.

71. Talanian RV, Yang X, Turbov J, et al. Granule-mediated cell killing: mechanisms of granzyme B initiated apoptosis. *J Exp Med* 1997;186:1323–1331.

72. Medema JP, Toes REM, Scaffidi C, et al. Cleavage of FLICE (caspase-8) by granzyme B during cytotoxic T lymphocyte-induced apoptosis. *Eur J Immunol* 1997;27:3492–3498.

73. Cerretti DP, Kozlosky CJ, Mosley B, et al. Molecular cloning of the interleukin-1beta converting enzyme. *Science* 1992;256:97–100.

74. Wang L, Miura M, Bergeron L, Zhu H, Yuan JY. Ich-1, an Ice/ced-3-related gene, encodes both positive and negative regulators of programmed cell death. *Cell* 1994;78:739–750.

75. Fernandes-Alnemri T, Litwack G, Alnemri ES: CPP32, a novel human apoptotic protein with homology to Caenorhabditis elegans cell death protein Ced-3 and mammalian interleukin-1b-converting enzyme. *J Biol Chem* 1994;269:30761–30764.

76. Nicholson DW, Ali A, Thornberry NA, et al. Identification and inhibition of the ICE/CED-3 protease necessary for mammalian apoptosis. *Nature* 1995;376:37–43.

77. Tewari M, Quan LT, O'Rourke K, et al. Yama/CPP32b, a mammalian homolog of CED-3, is a CrmA-inhibitable protease that cleaves the death substrate poly(ADP-ribose) polymerase. *Cell* 1995;81:801–809.

78. Munday NA, Vaillancourt JP, Ali A, et al. Molecular cloning and pro-apoptotic activity of $ICE_{rel}II$ and $ICE_{rel}III$, members of the ICE/CED-3 family of cysteine proteases. *J Biol Chem* 1995;270:15870–15876.

79. Faucheu C, Diu A, Chan AWE, et al. A novel human protease similar to the interleukin-1b converting enzyme induces apoptosis in transfected cells. *EMBO J* 1995;14:1914–1922.

80. Kamens J, Paskind M, Hugunin M, et al. Identification and characterization of ICH-2, a novel member of the interleukin-1b-converting enzyme family of cysteine proteases. *J Biol Chem* 1995;270:15250–15256.

81. Kumar S, Harvey NL. Role of multiple cellular proteases in the execution of programmed cell death. *FEBS Lett* 1995;375:169–173.

82. Duan HJ, Chinnaiyan AM, Hudson PL, Wing JP, He WW, Dixit VM. ICE-LAP3, a novel mammalian homologue of the Caenorhabditis elegans cell death protein ced-3 is activated during fas- and tumor necrosis factor-induced apoptosis. *J Biol Chem* 1996;271:1621–1625.

83. Lippke JA, Gu Y, Sarnecki C, Caron PR, Su MSS. Identification and characterization of CPP32/2Mch2 homolog 1, a novel cysteine protease similar to CPP32. *J Biol Chem* 1996;271:1825–1828.

84. Srinivasula SM, Fernandes-Alnemri T, Zangrillia J, et al. The Ced-3/interleukin 1b converting enzyme-like homolog Mch6 and the lamin-cleaving enzyme Mch2a are substrates for the apoptotic mediator CPP32. *J Biol Chem* 1996;271:27099–27106.

85. Thornberry NA, Rano TA, Peterson EP, et al. Combinatorial approach defines specificities of members of the caspase and granzyme B family. *J Biol Chem* 1997;272:17907–17911.

86. Zhou Q, Salvesen GS. Activation of pro-caspase-7 by serine proteases includes a non-canonical specificity. *Biochem J* 1997;324:361–364.

87. Darmon AJ, Ley TJ, Nicholson DW, Bleackley RC. Cleavage of CPP32 by granzyme B represents a critical role for granzyme B in the induction of target cell DNA fragmentation. *J Biol Chem* 1996;271:21709–21712.

88. Jänicke RU, Sprengart ML, Wati MR, Porter AG. Caspase-3 is required for DNA fragmentation and morphological changes associated with apoptosis. *J Biol Chem* 1998;273:9357–9360.

89. Mancini M, Nicholson DW, Roy S, et al. The caspase-3 precursor has a cytosolic and mitochondrial distribution: implications for apoptotic signaling. *J Cell Biol* 1998;140:1485–1495.

90. Chandler JM, Cohen GM, MacFarlane M. Different subcellular distribution of caspase-3 and caspase-7 following Fas-induced apoptosis in mouse liver. *J Biol Chem* 1998;273:10815–10818.

91. Stennicke HR, Jurngensmeier JM, Shin H, et al. Pro-caspase-3 is a major physiologic target of caspase-8. *J Biol Chem* 1998;273:27084–27090.

92. Komiyama T, Ray CA, Pickup DJ, et al. Inhibition of interleukin-1b converting enzyme by the cowpox virus serpin CrmA: an example of cross-class inhibition. *J Biol Chem* 1994;269:19331–19337.

93. Thome M, Schneider P, Hofmann K, et al. Viral FLICE-inhibitory proteins (FLIPs) prevent apoptosis induced by death receptors. *Nature* 1997;386:517–521.

94. Yang X, Stennicke HR, Wang B, et al. Granule mediated apoptosis: granzyme B functions as an apical caspase. *J Biol Chem* 1998;273:34278–34283.

95. Andrade F, Roy S, Nicholson D, Thornberry N, Rosen A, Casciola-Rosen L. Granzyme B directly and efficiently cleaves several downstream caspase substrates: implications for CTL-induced apoptosis. *Immunity* 1998;8:451–460.

96. Joiner KA. Membrane-protein traffic in pathogen-infected cells. *J Clin Invest* 1997;99:1814–1817.

97. Hommel-Berrey G, Bochan MR, Montel AH, Goebel W, Froelich CJ, Brahmi Z. Granzyme B inhibits replication of vesicular stomatitis virus by inducing apoptosis: a novel host defense paradigm. *Cell Immunol* 1997;180:1–9.

98. Wagner RR, Rose JK. Rhabdoviridae: the viruses and replication, In Fields BN, Knupe DM, Howley PM (eds) *Fundamental Virology*. Philadelphia, Lippincott-Raven, 1996, pp 561–575.

99. Isaaz S, Baetz K, Olsen K, Podack ER, Griffiths GM. Serial killing by cytotoxic T lymphocytes: T cell receptor triggers degranulation, re-filling of the

lytic granules and secretion of lytic proteins via a non-granule pathway. *Eur J Immunol* 1995;25: 1071–1079.

100. Spaeny-Dekking EHA, Hanna WL, Wolbink AM, et al. Extracellular granzymes A and B: detection of native species during CTL responses in vitro and in vivo. *J Immunol* 1998;160:1360–1366.

101. Matsumoto R, Sali A, Ghildyal N, Karplus M, Stevens RL. Packaging of proteases and proteoglycans in the granules of mast cells and other hematopoietic cells. *J Biol Chem* 1995;270:19524–19531.

102. Ghildyal N, Friend DS, Stevens RL, et al. Fate of two mast cell tryptases in V3 mastocytosis and normal BALB/c mice undergoing passive systemic anaphylaxis: prolonged retention of exocytosed mMCP-6 in connective tissues, and rapid accumulation of enzymatically active mMCP-7 in the blood. *J Exp Med* 1996;184:1061–1073.

103. Wagner L, Yang OO, Garcia-Zepeda EA, et al. β-Chemokines are released from HIV-1-specific cytolytic T-cell granules complexed to proteoglycans. *Nature* 1998;391:908–911.

104. Masson D, Peters PJ, Geuze HJ, Borst J, Tschopp J. Interaction of chondroitin sulfate with perforin and granzymes of cytolytic T-cells is dependent on pH. *Biochemistry* 1990;29:11229–11235.

105. Toyama-Sorimachi N, Sorimachi H, Tobita Y, et al. A novel ligand for CD44 is serglycin, a hematopoietic cell-lineage-specific proteoglycan. *J Biol Chem* 1995;270:7437–7444.

106. Hanna WL, Zhang X, Turbov J, Winkler U, Hudig D, Froelich CJ. Rapid purification of cationic granule proteases: application to human granzymes. *Protein Purif Exp* 1993;4:398–402.

107. Galvin J, Wang X, Spaenny-Dekking L, Hack CE, Froelich CJ. Apoptosis induced by granzyme B complexed to glycosaminoglycans: implications for granule mediated apoptosis in vivo. *J Immunol* 1999;162:5345–5350.

108. Lee K-D, Oh Y-K, Portnoy DA, Swanson JA. Delivery of macromolecules into cytosol using liposomes containing hemolysin from Listeria monocytogenes. *J Biol Chem* 1996;271:7429–7452.

Cytotoxic Cells: Basic Mechanisms and Medical Applications, edited by Michail V. Sitkovsky and Pierre A. Henkart. Lippincott Williams & Wilkins, Philadelphia © 2000.

Chapter 13

Granzymes: Mediation of Pro-apoptotic and Nonapoptotic Functions of Cytolytic Lymphocytes and Regulation by Endogenous Intracellular and Circulating Inhibitors

Joseph A. Trapani and *Phillip I. Bird

John Connell Laboratory, The Austin Research Institute, Heidelberg, 3084, Australia and;
°Department of Medicine, Monash University, Box Hill Hospital, Victoria, Australia

The cytolytic granules of cytotoxic T lymphocytes (CTLs) and natural killer (NK) cells are specialized organelles housing the principal defense system of higher organisms against abnormal or infected cells. Following stable contact of these cytolytic lymphocytes (CLs) with the target cell (conjugate formation), the granule contents, which include a pore-forming protein (perforin) and a collection of serine proteinases ("granzymes"), are secreted in an orchestrated process (exocytosis) onto the surface of the target cell. Perforin and granzymes then synergize in a calcium-dependent manner, permitting granzymes to enter and kill the target cell.

Investigators are now unraveling the events following the endocytic uptake of granzymes into the target cell cytoplasm and their almost immediate localization in the nucleus. Granzymes (especially the Aspase granzyme B) activate the ubiquitous caspase proteolytic cascade, and this is often sufficient to induce the classic structural and enzymatic changes of apoptotic death. Just as importantly, granzyme B and other granule mediators are also instrumental in circumventing blocks to the caspase pathways set

up by many viruses to prolong the life-span of cells they infect. To date, these caspase-independent pathways remain largely uncharacterized, but they appear to reside principally in the cytoplasm, not the nucleus.

The purpose of this chapter is first to describe the pro-apoptotic and other nonapoptotic functions of granzymes at the molecular and cellular levels; second, to discuss why granzymes are important in our defense against viruses; and third, to describe how potentially lethal toxins such as granzyme B may be regulated to prevent damage to bystander cells and tissue and to the CL itself. Such regulation must be achieved without compromising the homeostatic pro-apoptotic mechanisms that control CL numbers.

GRANZYMES

The principal constituents of cytolytic granules are the granzymes (granule enzymes), a family of closely related, chymotrypsin-like serine proteinases essentially restricted to CLs (1). Granzymes are structurally, functionally, and genetically related to other hematopoietic serine proteinases, especially those of mast cells and monocytes (2), and are the principal constituents of cytolytic granules, comprising up to 90% of their weight (3). Like all serine proteinases, the catalytic activity of granzymes depends on an active site serine residue that is part of a catalytic relay of three amino acids analogous to His[57], Asp[102], and Ser[195] of chymotrypsin (4). The oxyanion hole of granzymes serves to stabilize transitional states following binding of a substrate within the neighboring substrate-binding cleft. The shape, charge, and depth of the cleft confers substrate specificity, allowing cleavage to occur on the carboxyl side of a specific (P1) residue (5).

Granzyme Expression in Health and Disease

Granzyme expression is restricted to activated T lymphocytes, thymocytes, γ/δ T cells, and NK cells (6–8). NK cells and γ/δ T cells synthesize and store granzymes constitutively, but granzyme synthesis must be induced in T cells by antigen or other types of stimulation. Granzymes are expressed by most CD8[+] and some CD4[+] T cells sensitized by antigen or lectin (9). In one extensive study in the mouse, all of the granzyme mRNAs were expressed in alloantigen stimulated CD8[+] and CD4[+] T cells. CD4[−] C8[−] thymocytes (α/β^+ or γ/δ^+) expressed all granzyme mRNAs upon stimulation *in vitro,* and it was suggested that granzyme A expression might be important in T cell development (10). Nonspecific interleukin-2 (IL-2)-stimulated T cells also express granzymes (11,12). Expression of granzyme M is restricted to NK cells, particularly the large granular lymphocyte NK subpopulation (13).

Specific granzyme expression is associated with a number of pathologic conditions, including autoimmune disease, allograft rejection, and infection. For example, granzyme A has been identified in T cell infiltrates in renal allografts (14) and in islet tissue at the onset of type 1 diabetes (15,16). Granzyme A is also present in the granules of infiltrating T cells during viral infection (17) and in skin lesions due to *Leishmania* (18). In one study in the mouse, the number of granzyme A[+] T cells infiltrating cardiac allografts was a sensitive indicator of rejection, and virtually no granzyme A[+] cells were detectable following induction of graft survival with cyclosporin (19,20). The specific expression of granzyme mRNA or protein also occurs in human skin diseases (21), renal allograft rejection (22), rejecting heart grafts (16,23), human immunodeficiency virus (HIV) infection (24), and rheumatoid arthritis (25,26). In arthritic synovial tissue expression of granzymes and perforin is seen in NK cells (27). Thus the patterns of granzyme expression are consistent with a role in inducing tissue damage in viral and autoimmune pathologies. Our understanding of the physiologic significance of these observations has recently been enhanced by the production of granzyme deficient mice, as described in an accompanying chapter.

Physical and Chemical Characteristics of Granzymes

Granzymes have several features that distinguish them from other hematopoietic serine proteinases (Table 13-1). The activation dipeptide, which is cleaved to activate the zymogen, is usually acidic (Glu-Glu or Gly-Glu). The first four residues of the mature enzymes are highly conserved (almost invariably Ile-Ile-Gly-Gly), as are residues 9 to 16 and residues 96 to 102, which comprise a uniformly basic loop of unknown function that is acidic or neutrally charged in mast cell proteinases.

Most granzymes have three conserved disulfide linkages, although granzymes A, M, and -3 have four, like chymotrypsin. Almost all granzymes exist as monomers with a polypeptide backbone of 26 to 28 kDa supplemented with a variable quantity of N-linked glycosylation that can comprise up to 50% of the total weight (e.g., mouse granzyme

TABLE 13-1. *Physical and chemical properties of human and rodent granzymes*

Protease	Species	Enzyme activity	Predicted cleavage	Mr ($\times 10^3$)	Cellular expression
GrA	MHR	Tryptase	Basic	65[a]	CL, γ/δ,[b] thymus
GrB	MHR	Aspase	Acidic, especially Asp	32	CL, γ/δ, thymus
GrC	MR	Unknown	Asn or Ser	27	CTL
GrD	M	Unknown	Hydrophobic	35–50	CTL
GrE	M	Unknown	Hydrophobic	35–45	CTL
GrF	MR	Unknown	Hydrophobic	35–40	CTL
GrG	M	Unknown	Hydrophobic	30	CTL
GrH	H	Unknown		30	CL
GrJ	R	Unknown		30	Unknown
GrM	MHR	Met-ase	Met, Leu, nor-Leu	30	NK

Modified from ref. 54, with permission.
M, mouse; H, human; R, rat; Mr, relative molecular mass; Gr, granzyme.
[a] Homodimer.
[b] γ/δ T cell receptor-positive cell.

D). Granzyme A is the only granzyme known to exist as a disulfide-bonded homodimer of about 65 kDa (3,28). Several other granzymes (including granzyme B) have one unpaired Cys, but do not appear to form homodimers or heterodimers with other granzymes.

Granzymes have unusual substrate preferences. Unlike many of the degradative serine proteinases, granzymes have a far narrower specificity dictated principally, but not exclusively, by the P1 residue of the substrate. As many as four neighboring residues may influence substrate cleavage, which is consistent with a role for granzymes in *processing* rather than degrading target proteins. Granzyme A is trypsin-like in specificity (a "tryptase"), cleaving at basic residues; most of the other granzymes cleave at hydrophobic residues (chymotrypsin-like, or "chymases"). By contrast, granzyme B is distinguished by its unusual ability to cleave after the acidic residue Asp, although some synthetic compounds with Glu or Met at P1 can also be cleaved to a lesser extent (29). The preference for cleavage at Asp explains one key characteristic of granzyme B: a broad ability to activate both proximal (activator) and distal (effector) caspases, leading to apoptotic changes in targeted cells (discussed below). In addition, several of the molecular targets of caspases can also be cleaved directly by granzyme B (30) and (see below).

Biosynthesis, Activation, and Storage of Granzymes

Granzymes are initially synthesized as pre-pro-granzymes but are rapidly activated and stored in an active form complexed with chondroitin sulfate-like proteoglycans (3,12,28). The initial removal of a classic signal (pre) sequence in the endoplasmic reticulum is followed by the pro-enzyme being targeted to the cytolytic granules, where the first two amino acids (the activation dipeptide or pro-sequence) are clipped from the N-terminus by dipeptidylpeptidase 1 (DPP1) during packaging (31).

The granules (or secretory lysosomes) are structurally unique to hematopoietic cells, combining regulated secretion with lysosomal degradation, so CTL-specific proteins, such as perforin and granzymes are located within the granules with typical lysosomal proteins. The granules contain mannose-6-phosphate receptors, which are essential for granzyme trafficking (32); but the other granule constituents, such as perforin and chondroitin sulfate, reach the granules by a separate unknown mechanism. The granules are acidic (pH ~5.5), which promotes DPP1 activity and perforin activation (33) and favors the binding of basic granzymes and perforin to acidic proteoglycans. Proteoglycan binding is thought to reduce the activity of granzymes and perforin and the risk of self-induced damage to the CL (12).

GRANZYME FUNCTIONS

Nonapoptotic Functions of Granzymes

Although it is indisputable that granzymes, particularly granzyme B, are involved in apoptosis induction *within* target cells, it is also clear that granzymes can be detected in extracellular fluids (34). Consistent with this, extracellular functions have also been postulated for granzymes, especially granzyme A. Like other tryptases, including thrombin, purified granzyme A can induce B cell proliferation in the absence of antigenic stimulation (35). It has also been suggested that granzyme A may be involved in regulating B cell proliferation adjacent to inflammatory sites. By cleaving extracellular matrix proteins including proteoglycans, type IV collagens (36), laminin (37), and fibronectin, granzyme A may assist in T and NK cell migration through the subendothelial space (38,39). Interestingly, secretion of granzyme A follows engagement of integrins on CTLs with extracellular matrix proteins (40). In addition, granzyme A can recruit the extracellular matrix degradative capacity of plasmin by activating the pro-urokinase-like plasminogen activator (38,41). Granzymes can also amplify inflammation by directly processing pro-cytokine molecules and by cleaving the thrombin receptor, thereby inducing cytokine secretion. Thrombin receptor activation can result in the release of IL-6 and IL-8 from monocytes and the retraction of neurites in glial cells, particularly oligodendrocytes (42). In addition, granzyme A has recently been shown to activate pro-IL-1β by cleavage at a tryptase site immediately adjacent to the canonical Asp (43).

A direct role for extracellular granzyme A in controlling viral infection has also been postulated. Granzyme A can cleave proteins such as reverse transcriptase and gp70 envelope protein of Moloney murine leukemia virus (38,44). Thus granzyme A secreted into the extracellular space in the vicinity of infected cells might reduce the infectivity of budding virus particles by cleaving viral surface proteins. In support of this hypothesis,

mice deficient in granzyme A expression are profoundly susceptible to infection with the cytopathic orthopox virus ectromelia (45), despite responding normally to other viruses such as lymphocytic choriomeningitis virus (LCMV) (46). Interestingly, *in vitro* cytolytic activity against ectromelia-infected cells is normal in these mice, as are the kinetics of CTL induction *in vivo* (45).

More recently, Simon and colleagues examined the responses of granzyme A-deficient mice to LCMV, ectromelia, and influenza (47). Consistent with the above findings, granzyme A was not essential for recovery from LCMV but was beneficial in protection against ectromelia. By contrast, granzyme A-deficient mice were paradoxically *protected* from intranasal infection with influenza virus. Six days after infection, the knockout mice had an increased viral load, and fewer circulating influenza-specific CTLs were isolated. Despite these deficiencies, survival was improved as the severe inflammatory response seen in the lungs of wild-type mice was far less pronounced. Granzyme A-mediated release and activation of IL-1 (and possibly IL-6 and IL-8) was postulated to reduce alveolar gas transfer in wild-type mice. Thus granzyme functions not apparently central to apoptosis induction can nevertheless be vital to overall survival.

Granzyme B released extracellularly may also directly affect adhesion of surrounding cells to one another and to extracellular matrix proteins via cleavage at Arg-Gly-Asp (RGD) motifs. Cleavage of this type by granzyme B resulted in the release of some tumor cell lines from surface substrata *in vitro,* resulting in cell death (48). Although this type of cleavage might potentially enable disengagement of the effector cell from the target following delivery of the lethal hit, there is currently no direct evidence that granzyme B has this specific extracellular role.

Functions of Granzymes in Apoptosis Induction: Synergy with Perforin

Granzymes must access intracellular substrates to kill a cell, and it has traditionally been accepted that the essential synergistic role of perforin is to provide a passive membrane channel through which granzyme B can enter the cell. The deficiencies of this view are now clear following studies using several experimental systems: (a) The pro-apoptotic functions of perforin cannot be replaced by other membrane-perforating agents, such as complement, or by detergent treatment (49; J.A.T., manuscript in preparation). (b) Granzyme B can enter cells by receptor-mediated endocytosis almost as efficiently in the absence of perforin as in its presence (49–51). (c) The function of perforin in granzyme B-dependent apoptosis can be successfully mimicked by replication-deficient adenovirus particles that act by disrupting endocytic vesicles containing granzyme B (52,53). Thus the key role of perforin is to promote access of pro-apoptotic mediators such as granzymes from a diffusion-limited intracellular compartment of the target cell (i.e., endolysosome) to the cytosol, where target molecules can be freely accessed ("facilitated access" hypothesis) (54).

Perforin-Dependent Pathways to Cell Death: Triggered by Cytolytic Granules?

We and others have recently uncovered hitherto unsuspected layers of complexity in the mechanisms used by CL granule components to destroy target cells, as manifested by the apparent existence of several pathways to cell death (55) (Table 13-2; Fig. 13-1). Pathway 1 is caspase-dependent and operates in the nucleus and cytoplasm. Pathway 2 is caspase-independent and operates principally in the cytoplasm. Further evidence suggests that a third pathway exists that is distinguished from pathways 1 and 2 by its independence from granzyme B.

In the absence of any block to the caspase cascade, caspase activation by granzyme B is sufficient to kill the target cell with a full manifestation of classic cytoplasmic, nuclear, and membrane apoptotic features (pathway 1). *In vitro,* granzyme B has been shown to cleave caspases 2, 3, 6, 7, 8, 9, and 10 but not caspases 1, 4, or 5, which probably have a weak pro-apoptotic function and are more centrally involved in cytokine processing (56–61). One study has suggested that caspases 7 and 10, which are proximal to caspase-3 activation, are crucial upstream targets for granzyme B, but it is not clear whether this holds for all cells (62). Although granzyme B is certainly the major granule activator of caspases, the markedly slowed but not totally abrogated kinetics of apoptosis seen with the CTLs of granzyme B-deficient mice suggests that other granzymes can also activate caspases, albeit with reduced efficiency (63). It is not yet known how caspase activation occurs under these circumstances, but evidence indicates that the serine protease cathepsin G can activate pro-caspase 7 at a Gln-Ala bond adjacent to the favored Asp residue, raising the possibility that targeting of secondary sites by non-Aspase granzymes might circumvent the requirement for granzyme B (64).

It is also likely that granzymes are capable of accessing and cleaving caspase substrates directly, duplicating and amplifying caspase-mediated cell damage. For example, the nu-

TABLE 13-2. *Characteristics of granule-bound cytotoxic pathways*

Pathway	Dependence on caspases	Dependence on GrB	Dependence on perforin	Site of action	Inhibitors
1	Yes	Yes[a]	Yes	N, C	Cr, B
2	No	Yes	Yes	C > N	B
3	No	No	Yes	N, C	Unknown

Modified from ref. 55, with permission.
N, nuclear; C, cytoplasmic; Cr, crmA-like; B, Bcl-2-like.
[a] Pathway 1 can also be triggered via Fas ligation or through activation of intrinsic "programmed cell death."

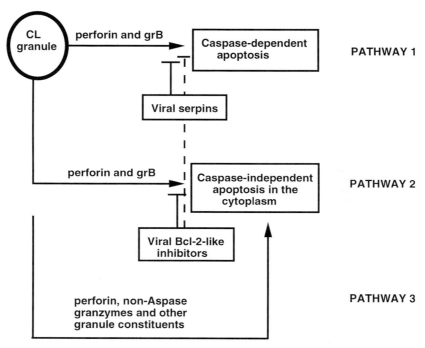

FIG. 13-1. Three putative granule-bound pathways to target cell apoptosis. Pathway 1 involves activation of the caspase-dependent cell suicide pathway by granzyme B (GrB) and perforin, leads to morphologic changes in both the cytoplasm and nucleus, and can be blocked by cytokine response modifier (crmA)-like serine protease inhibitors produced by many viruses, and by Bcl-2-like inhibitors. Pathway 2 is also GrB- and perforin-dependent but involves the caspase-independent triggering of nonnuclear death pathways through cleavage of as yet unrecognized GrB substrates in the cytoplasm. This pathway is not blocked by inhibitors such as crmA or z-VAD-fmk, but is inhibitable by Bcl-2-like molecules. Pathway 3 is also perforin-dependent but is independent of both caspases and grB. As yet uncharacterized granule mediators other than grB are essential for the function of this pathway.

clear caspase substrates poly(ADP-ribose) polymerase (PARP), the catalytic subunit of DNA-dependent protein kinase (DNA-PKcs), and NuMA have all been identified as granzyme B substrates, with cleavage occurring at Asp residues identical to or distinct from those used by caspases (30,65). Additional, noncaspase nuclear ligands for granzyme B have also been identified (66). Based on the fact that granzyme B becomes localized in the target cell nucleus rapidly (50,51), it has been suggested that direct, caspase-independent cleavage of nuclear substrates by granzymes provides the CTL with a mechanism for overcoming viral blocks to caspases (30). However, we view this interpretation with caution, as we have shown that

efficient nuclear targeting of granzyme B is largely *caspase-dependent* (67). Thus granzyme B may not be able to access its nuclear substrates efficiently in the absence of caspase activation. Furthermore, inhibition of caspases with z-VAD-fmk or p35 prevents nuclear damage in response to granzyme B and perforin but does not block apoptotic cell death pathways in the cytoplasm or influence overall cell survival (67,68). These findings indicate that *non* nuclear, caspase-*independent* pathways can be activated by granzyme B and are crucial for CTL-mediated cell death (pathway 2). Supporting this view is the observation that apoptotic death does not rely on the presence of a nucleus, as cytoplasts can be killed in this manner (69).

In other studies we have found that cell death mediated through (purified) granzyme B can be inhibited by Bcl-2 and its analogs (70). As distinct from cells treated with z-VAD-fmk, this inhibition is not limited to nuclear (caspase-dependent) phenomena, and cells expressing Bcl-2 survive indefinitely in culture when exposed to purified perforin and granzyme B (J.A.T., in preparation). However, intact cytolytic granules can overcome this block, indicating that other granule components must be capable of bypassing a Bcl-2-like block of granzyme B (pathway 3). Apart from its dependence on perforin (70), the nature of this third pathway is presently unclear; and although we suspect that non-Aspase granzymes are involved, definitive evidence is lacking.

The characterization of these granzyme-activated, caspase-dependent and caspase-independent cell death pathways remains a key issue in our understanding of granule-dependent cytolysis. To date, little is known of the molecular basis for these pathways or even in which subcellular locations they operate. It is notable that the severity of the immunodeficiency seen in perforin-deficient mice (71,72) is not reflected in any of the granzyme knockouts, implicating perforin as the key to most, if not all, forms of granule-mediated death. With a few exceptions, such as ectromelia infection (45), these studies indicate that given perforin the spectrum of granzyme activities is sufficiently redundant to enable the CTL to achieve target cell destruction, even if absence of the sole Aspase (granzyme B) means that caspase activation is relatively inefficient (63). Some time ago, it was found that inhibitors of caspase-3 and related caspases such as DEVD-CHO had no effect on membrane damage inflicted on target cells by a granule-dependent mechanism but could almost totally block nuclear damage including DNA fragmentation (73). Support for caspase-independent granule-mediated cytolysis has also come from Sarin and her colleagues (68), who showed that cytoplasmic (but not nuclear) damage to cells occurred in response to granule-mediated

cell death despite a blocked caspase cascade. The search for cytosolic and membrane targets of granzyme B is a key area of endeavor and may bring to light hitherto unsuspected pathways to apoptotic death exploited specifically by CL, pathways that may be amenable to manipulation for therapeutic purposes.

REGULATION OF GRANZYMES

Little attention has been paid to the regulation of granzyme-mediated proteolysis despite the long-standing acknowledgment that limiting the activity of serine proteinases is crucial for tissue homeostasis. For example, failure to regulate leukocyte elastase results in the destruction of lung tissue in emphysema, and failure to regulate thrombin results in thrombosis (74). As discussed above, the indications are that granzyme A has many extracellular functions, raising the possibility that it may participate in bystander cell or tissue destruction unless properly controlled. Furthermore, though most attention has focused on the intracellular role of granzyme B, there is evidence that it can hydrolyze extracellular matrix components (75), and it can be detected in plasma by enzyme-linked immunosorbent assay (ELISA)-based techniques (34). Although these observations do not necessarily mean that granzyme B has an additional or specific extracellular role, they do suggest that it may be released as a consequence of target cell or CTL lysis and that rapid inactivation of its proteolytic activity would be required to prevent collateral damage to surrounding tissue.

In addition to control of extracellular granzyme B, studies on the pathways and mechanisms of apoptosis suggest that regulation of granzyme B activity within cells may also occur or be required under certain circumstances. For example, certain viruses have evolved proteins to counter apoptosis induced by infection or CTL attack, and at least one of them is a granzyme B inhibitor. From a physiologic point of view, it may seem desirable that host cells that are targeted by CTLs should not contain endogenous inhibitors of granzyme B that might block cytotoxicity. Yet one exception to this rule may be the CTLs themselves, which may have to control misdirected or inefficiently packaged granzyme B. In this section we describe the known inhibitors of granzymes A and B and discuss how they may function physiologically to contain the activity of these potent serine proteinases.

Granzyme A and B Inhibitors

Like many serine proteinases, granzymes A and B are inactivated by several classes of inhibitor (76,77), includeing small synthetic or microbially derived active site inhibitors such as 3,4-dichloroisocoumarin, phosphoramidon, and chymostatin. A number of other synthetic inhibitors have recently been designed to specifically inhibit these granzymes with a long-term view to therapeutic use, but their description is outside the scope of this review.

Macromolecules that inactive granzymes *in vitro* include the Kunitz-type aprotinin and soybean trypsin inhibitors and the Bowman-Birk-type lima bean trypsin inhibitor. However, there is no evidence to suggest that inhibitors of these latter types control granzyme activity *in vivo*. Potential physiologic inhibitors of the granzymes include the plasma general endoproteinase inhibitor α_2-macroglobulin and several serine proteinase inhibitors (serpins).

α_2-Macroglobulin

α_2-Macroglobulin is a 725-kDa glycoprotein that is present at high concentration ($\sim$2.5 mg/ml) in plasma and is capable of inhibiting a broad range of endoproteinases (78). It consists of four identical subunits linked in pairs by disulfide bonds and acts by forming a 1:1 irreversible complex with the proteinase. Cleavage of α_2-macroglobulin by the proteinase results in a conformational change in the inhibitor that traps and covalently links the

proteinase in a "cage" that is inaccessible to macromolecular substrates but accessible to low-molecular-weight substrates.

Although it appears to be evolutionarily conserved, the physiologic role of α_2-macroglobulin is unclear. Suggested roles range from prevention of tissue injury due to proteases of invading pathogens, parasites, or venoms to the regulation of endogenous plasma proteolytic enzyme pathways. More recent evidence suggests that α_2-macroglobulin–proteinase complexes may modulate the immune response by capturing antigen and binding or degrading cytokines. Finally, it has been demonstrated that α_2-macroglobulin–proteinase complexes are rapidly cleared from the circulation by interaction with a receptor (low density lipoprotein receptor-related protein) present on many cell types; hence it is suggested that the primary role of α_2-macroglobulin is to participate in a protease clearance mechanism.

α_2-Macroglobulin inhibits the proteolytic activity of granzyme A and B *in vitro* (29,76). Although no *in vivo* studies have been done, the efficiency of the *in vitro* interactions suggests that granzymes appearing in the circulation as a result of secretion or CL lysis would eventually be bound and inactivated by α_2-macroglobulin, thereby minimizing proteolytic damage to surrounding tissue. It is also likely that clearance of the granzymes from the circulation is mediated by α_2-macroglobulin.

Serpins

Serpins form a large protein superfamily occurring in higher eukaryotes (79). Most members of the family are inhibitors that inactivate target proteinases by forming tight 1:1 complexes, but their extraordinary molecular flexibility has given rise to several noninhibitory molecules that function as chaperones, hormones, or hormone transporters. Observations that mutations in serpin genes underlie diseases such as thrombosis, liver cirrhosis, emphysema, and hereditary angioedema has led to a concerted effort over many years to establish the structure and mode of action of serpins (74). To date, at least 14 serpin crystal structures have been solved (80), leading to the model for serpin function described below.

As shown in Figure 13-2A, inhibitory serpins have a distinct molecular structure consisting of three β-sheets and nine α-helices that form an essentially globular protein. A distinguishing feature is the presence of an exposed polypeptide loop—the reactive center—which comprises the inhibitory domain of the molecule. The reactive center can be considered a "bait" region for the cognate proteinase and contains a scissile bond between two residues, designated P_1 and P_1'. These residues form part of a sequence resembling a natural cleavage site for the proteinase in which the P_1 residue primarily defines the specificity of the serpin. [The classic example of the importance of the P_1 residue to specificity is the Pittsburgh variant of α_1-proteinase inhibitor, which has a Met to Arg

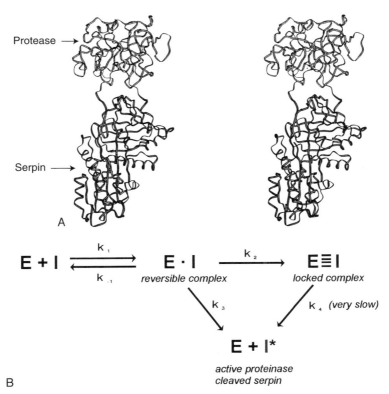

FIG. 13-2. A: Stereo view of a model of a serpin in the initial stages of an interaction with a protease. Human granzyme B (light ribbon structure, modeled on rat mast cell protease) is binding to the intracellular serpin PI-9 (darker ribbon structure, modeled on antithrombin III). Note the exposed, flexible serpin reactive center loop inserted into the active site cleft of the proteinase. Subsequent stages in the interaction require reactive center loop mobility and result in conformational changes to both serpin and proteinase that lock the complex (81,82). **B:** Mechanism of proteinase inhibition by serpins. The generally accepted reaction scheme is shown here. *E*, serine proteinase; *I*, native serpin, *E·I*, reversible Michaelis complex, E $\equiv$ I, locked complex; *I**, cleaved, inactive serpin. Note that some workers propose the existence of a short-lived tetrahedral intermediate between the Michaelis and locked complex (83). The rate of serpin–proteinase complex formation can be estimated by calculating the second constant k_2 according to (84).

mutation at this position, converting it from an inhibitor of neutrophil elastase to a potent inhibitor of thrombin (74).] On binding to cleave the P_1–P_1' bond, the proteinase becomes trapped in an essentially irreversible complex with the serpin. This "locked complex" is formed as a result of a marked conformational change in the serpin triggered by proteinase binding, which probably also causes structural alterations to the proteinase that distort the active site (81,82).

Biochemical evidence (83,84) suggests that the complex formation follows the kinetic pathways outlined in Figure 13-2B, in which serpin—proteinase binding leads to a reversible Michaelis complex that is converted rapidly to the irreversible locked complex (inhibitory pathway). In some cases, a locked complex does not form, leading to breakdown of the Michaelis complex and the release of active proteinase and inactive, cleaved serpin (substrate pathway). The latter pathway usually results from an interaction between a serpin and noncognate proteinase because the exposed nature of the reactive center makes it sensitive to nonspecific proteolysis (cleavage other than between the P_1–P_1' bond). However, some reactions between serpins and cognate proteinases appear to involve competition between the inhibitory and substrate pathways, suggesting that stable complex formation requires rapid isomerization of an intermediate between the initial Michaelis and final locked complexes.

At present there is some debate as to whether the proteinase is covalently attached to the serpin in the locked complex or the interaction results in a tight noncovalent complex consisting of a conformationally altered serpin bound to the proteinase. In the former case it is argued that the complex is trapped in an acyl intermediate analogous to that occurring during substrate hydrolysis; and in the latter, it is argued that proteinase cleavage of the serpin reactive center at the P_1–P_1' bond is required for the conformational changes that lock the complex. Both models are consistent with observations that

the locked complex decays slowly (over days) to release active proteinase and cleaved serpin.

Although a crystal structure of a serpin–proteinase complex is not yet available to distinguish these models, it is clear that the serpin conformational change includes a repositioning of the reactive center strand so that all or part of it is inserted between two strands of one of the β-sheets. The mobility of the reactive center is dependent on other serpin domains, particularly two flanking sequences known as the proximal and distal hinges. In many inhibitory serpins, mutation of a conserved Thr to Arg at P_{14} in the proximal hinge greatly restricts the mobility of the reactive center and results in an inactive inhibitor (74). Mobility of the reactive center and insertion into the β-sheet can also be modulated by binding of cofactors. For example, binding of heparin to antithrombin III increases the association rate constant for the interaction with thrombin by 1,000-fold in a manner that includes a conformational alteration to the reactive center (85).

Serpins and Granzymes

Antithrombin III and Granzyme A

Antithrombin III is a 58-kDa monomeric glycoprotein present in plasma at about 0.15 mg/ml. It is one of the best characterized serpins and is the most important protease inhibitor of the coagulation cascade (86). Mainly because of Arg as the P_1 residue, it is an efficient inhibitor of trypsin-like proteinases such as thrombin, factor Xa, and plasma kallikrein, and the interaction of thrombin and factor Xa with antithrombin III is enhanced 1,000-fold by the cofactor heparin.

Masson and Tschopp (87) have demonstrated that granzyme A is rapidly inactivated in plasma and that antithrombin III is primarily responsible. Granzyme A and antithrombin III form a typical SDS-stable proteinase–serpin complex, and the efficiency of inhibition is accelerated 400-fold by heparin. When antithrombin III is in excess, two molecules of the inhibitor can bind to dimeric granzyme A. Although the exact effects of uncontrolled granzyme A activity on tissue adjacent to degranulating CLs are unknown, it is likely that antithrombin III and heparin represent an efficient mechanism that restricts granzyme A-mediated proteolysis to the target zone.

Protease Nexin-I and Granzyme A

Protease nexin-I is a 43- to 50-kDa glycoprotein that is secreted by many mammalian cells, including platelets, and apparently remains associated with the cell surface (88–90). It is a potent heparin-dependent thrombin and urokinase inhibitor that has a P_1 Arg residue. It promotes neurite outgrowth from a number of neural cell types, and its levels are decreased in a number of neurologic diseases.

Gurwitz et al. (91) have examined the interaction of granzyme A and protease nexin-I and demonstrated a rapid interaction that is accelerated tenfold by heparin. Protease nexin-I is as effective as antithrombin III at inhibiting granzyme A, and it acts by binding to both subunits. At present it is not clear whether protease nexin-I and antithrombin III act in concert to regulate granzyme A, the existence of the two serpins offers a level of redundancy that guards against loss or inactivation of one or the other, or each offers distinct though overlapping tissue-specific protection against granzyme A. (For example, it is conceivable that protease nexin-I offers the primary route of protection in neural tissue.) Answers to these questions require close examination of the effects of granzyme A in mice lacking antithrombin III, protease nexin-I, or both.

α_1-Proteinase Inhibitor and Granzyme B

Formerly known as α_1-antitrypsin, α_1-proteinase inhibitor is a 53-kDa glycoprotein present in plasma at 1.0 to 1.3 mg/ml. It is the major inhibitor of polymorphonuclear leukocyte elastase but has the capacity to inhibit a range of other serine proteinases (86). The P_1 Met of α_1-proteinase inhibitor and the fact that granzyme B can cleave peptide substrates after Met (92) raises the possibility that α_1-proteinase inhibitor inhibits granzyme B.

There is one report in the literature of an interaction between granzyme B and α_1-proteinase inhibitor *in vitro* (29), but the kinetic analysis reported in this study is limited, making it difficult to assess whether the interaction has any physiologic significance. Accordingly, we reexamined the inhibition of human granzyme B by α_1-proteinase inhibitor and estimate that the association rate constant is approximately 10^3 M^{-1} s^{-1} and the inhibitory constant (K_i) is 20 μM (J. Sun and P. Bird, unpublished data). These numbers are well below the figures reported for physiologic serpin–proteinase interactions; for example, the rate constant for leukocyte elastase with α_1-proteinase inhibitor is 10^7 M^{-1} s^{-1} (86), making it unlikely that α_1-proteinase inhibitor regulates granzyme B *in vivo*.

CrmA/SPI-2, a Viral Inhibitor of Granzyme B In Vitro

Poxviruses produce an array of proteins designed to circumvent or suppress host defenses (93). One of them, originally described in cowpox virus, is the cytokine response modifier A (CrmA) protein, also known as serine protease inhibitor 2 (SPI-2) in related poxviruses. Cowpox virus efficiently suppresses the acute inflammatory response in infected chicken embryos, but variants lacking CrmA cannot. CrmA is a 38-kDa intracellular serpin with a conserved proximal hinge domain typical of inhibitory serpins but with an unusual P_1 Asp in the reactive center. In elegant work, Pickup and co-workers showed that the target of CrmA in infected cells is the IL-1β-converting enzyme, a cysteine proteinase that cleaves pro-IL-1β after Asp (94,95). This enzyme is the prototype of the caspase family (it is now known as caspase-1), and many studies have subsequently shown that CrmA is also capable of inhibiting death receptor-mediated apoptosis by inhibiting one or more caspases within cells.

The mechanics of the CrmA–caspase-1 interaction are not yet fully understood, but inhibition apparently requires a mobile reactive center and the P_1 Asp. The fact that CrmA is a functional serpin suggested that it might also inhibit a serine proteinase with a preference for cleaving after Asp. The only known eukaryotic serine proteinase with this specificity is granzyme B, which activates caspases by cleaving after Asp (96). Salvesen's group were subsequently able to demonstrate efficient inhibition of granzyme B activity by CrmA *in vitro* (97).

The ability of CrmA to inhibit caspases and granzyme B *in vitro* suggests that it has multiple biologic roles, including suppression of cytokine processing and inhibition of death receptor- and granzyme B-mediated apoptosis. Although it is clear that CrmA can inhibit death receptor-mediated apoptosis, probably by inactivating the apical caspase-8, it probably does not have the ability to inhibit granzyme B-mediated apoptosis in the context of target cell destruction by CLs. Tewari et al. (98) first examined this issue using cells transfected with CrmA as targets for CTLs. They concluded that CrmA conferred protection against calcium-independent (Fas-mediated) CTL killing but not against calcium-dependent (granzyme B-mediated) killing. These results have recently been repeated using CrmA in transfected cells (99). Although these findings indicate that CrmA is not an effective inhibitor of granzyme B *in vivo*, neither group attempted to isolate and compare transfectants expressing different amounts of CrmA/SPI-2 or to establish whether the levels of CrmA/SPI-2 in the transfectants approach those seen in virally infected cells.

The possibility remains that in these experiments the CrmA level in the transfected cells was not high enough to rapidly counter the incoming granzyme B. A more convincing study has been reported by Macen et al. (100), where cowpox or rabbitpox virus-infected cells were used as targets for cloned CTLs that could kill via the granule-mediated or the Fas-mediated pathway. Cells carrying wild-type virus resisted CTL attack irrespective of the pathway used, whereas those carrying variants lacking the CrmA/SPI-2 gene were killed by Fas-mediated apoptosis but not by granule-mediated apoptosis.

In summary, the results of three studies support the view that although CrmA/SPI-2 may function to control Fas-mediated apoptosis *in vivo*, it is not a physiologic inhibitor of granzyme B.

Proteinase Inhibitor 9: Efficient Inhibitor of Granzyme B In Vivo and In Vitro

Proteinase inbibitor 9 (PI-9) is a 42-kDa human serpin independently discovered by Sprecher et al. (101) and Sun et al. (102). It is also known as cytoplasmic antiproteinase 3 or granzyme B inhibitor. As shown in Figure 13-3, sequence comparisons revealed similarities to CrmA, especially in the reactive center, suggesting that PI-9 may target similar proteinases. Consequently, we demonstrated that PI-9 is a more efficient granzyme B inhibitor than CrmA (association rate constants for complex formation: PI-9 1.7×10^6 M^{-1} s^{-1}; CrmA 2.9×10^5 M^{-1} s^{-1}) and that preincubation with PI-9 inhibits purified granzyme B- and perforin-induced apoptosis of mouse FDC-P1 cells (102). In the same study we showed that PI-9 is intracellular and that it is expressed in immune tissue. In particular, PI-9 expression was noted in cells expressing granzyme B, including lymphokine-activated peripheral blood leukocytes.

In a more recent study we examined the function of PI-9 in greater detail (103). FDC-P1 cells expressing intracellular PI-9 resisted apoptosis induced by purified granzyme B and perforin, and the degree of protection was proportional to the amount of PI-9 expressed. Protection was also observed when

PI-9	..^{320}VEVNEEGTEAAAASSCFVVA**E**=CCMESGPRFCADHPFL..
PI-9 P$_1$ Asp	..^{320}VEVNEEGTEAAAASSCFVVA**D**=CCMESGPRFCADHPFL..
CrmA	..^{284}IDVNEEYTEAAAAT-CALVAD=CASTVTNEFCADHPFI..

FIG. 13-3. Comparison of PI-9, PI-9 P$_1$ Asp mutant, and CrmA reactive centers. The sequences of PI-9 and CrmA were taken from Sun et al. (102) and Ray et al. (94), respectively. Only the portions comprising the hinge and reactive centers of each serpin are shown. A space introduced to optimize sequence alignment is indicated by a *single dash*. Mutated residues are indicated in boldface. The P$_1$-P$_1'$ bond is indicated by a *double dash*.

Fas-negative human MCF-7 cells expressing PI-9 were exposed to CLs, suggesting that PI-9 confers protection even when other cytotoxins are operating and supporting the view that granzyme B is the primary proteinase in granule-mediated apoptosis. Unlike CrmA, PI-9 did not protect cells against Fas-mediated apoptosis.

One key difference between PI-9 and CrmA is the identity of the P$_1$ residue: In PI-9 it is Glu, whereas in CrmA it is Asp. Serpin dogma suggests that the P$_1$ residue should reflect the substrate preference of the target proteinase, and this is certainly true for CrmA, which inhibits Aspases of two distinct classes (caspases and granzyme B). The fact that PI-9 has a P$_1$ Glu and is a better granzyme B inhibitor than CrmA contradicts dogma but is consonant with the fact that granzyme B also cleaves peptide substrates after Glu though less efficiently than after Asp (92).

Given that CrmA is an efficient inhibitor of caspases, the question arises as to whether PI-9 also inhibits caspases. Testing nine of the ten known human caspases, we showed that PI-9 does not interact efficiently with proteinases of this class (103). However, mutation of the P$_1$ Glu to Asp (Fig. 13-3) converted PI-9 from an efficient granzyme B inhibitor but poor caspase inhibitor into a poor granzyme B inhibitor (100-fold less efficient) but effective caspase inhibitor. In addition, the P$_1$ Asp mutant was less protective against granzyme B-mediated apoptosis but protected against Fas-mediated apoptosis. Taken together these results suggest that the P$_1$ Glu makes PI-9 specific for granzyme B and prevents an interaction with caspases.

Based on these studies, our working model for the physiologic role of PI-9 suggests that it is produced by CLs to protect against autolysis produced by ectopic or misdirected granzyme B. Ectopic granzyme B may result from inefficient packaging into granules during biosynthesis or leakage from granules during the professional life of the CL. Misdirection of granzyme B into the CL may occur during killer–target cell conjugation. All of these cases would lead to the appearance of granzyme B in the cytoplasm of the CL and increase the potential for granzyme B-mediated caspase activation and apoptosis. By inactivating any granzyme B appearing in the cytoplasm outside the granules, PI-9 would protect the CL from autolysis. However, the inability of PI-9 to inhibit caspases would allow the CL to be deleted via Fas- or TNF-mediated apoptosis at the conclusion of the immune response. CLs would also be free to respond to stress-mediated apoptotic signals.

This model can be extended to situations where release of granzyme B may threaten other cells of the immune system that attain close proximity to CLs. For example, antigen presenters such as dendritic cells that directly contact CLs during the activation process may be at risk from ectopic granzyme B and may produce PI-9. Further work is required to define the types (leukocyte subsets, dendritic cells) and status (resting or activated) of cells that express PI-9, establish whether the granzyme B–PI-9 interaction is modulated by cofactors, and determine whether extragranular granzyme B or PI-9–granzyme B complexes can be detected within operating CLs.

CONCLUSIONS AND PERSPECTIVES

What is the significance of multiple granule-based cytolytic mechanisms for defense against viruses? Why should a CTL need such a broad array of pro-apoptotic mechanisms comprising granzyme B dependent and independent pathways and caspase dependent and independent pathways—with a wide variety of nuclear or nonnuclear target molecules? The answer to this question is rooted in the co-adaptations of the immune systems of higher organisms and the replicative/invasive mechanisms of countless viruses over eons of evolutionary time. As our knowledge of generic cell death pathways (centered on caspases) has grown, it has become evident that virtually every step of the process can be interfered with by viruses seeking to prolong the life-span of the infected cell. CTL-mediated "altruistic" cell death (also triggered through pathway 1 by CTLs) is a fundamental way of depriving a virus of the metabolic machinery of the infected cell, thereby preventing the spread of the virus. Problems arise if apoptosis of the infected cell is blocked by viral caspase inhibitors such as CrmA or IAPs. In such circumstances the essential role of the immune system is to provide alternative pathways to cell death. In our "three pathway model" [55], pathways 2 and 3 enable the CL to deal with such a viral block by selecting pathways to cytolysis that bypass caspase inhibition and the broader antiapoptotic effects of Bcl-2-like inhibitors, respectively. These contingencies thus provide the CTL with the "final say" over life or death of such an infected cell.

The special ability of CTLs to trigger apoptosis and other effects through the release of these potent proteinases raises the problem of limiting their activity to the target cells without causing damage to the CTL itself or to surrounding tissue. To date, this issue has not been studied extensively, but a number of potential inhibitors of granzymes A and B have been reported. Of these, only α_2-macroglobulin, antithrombin III, protease nexin II, and the intracellular serpin PI-9 are likely to be physiologically relevant, acting to prevent granzyme-mediated collateral damage arising from CL activity. α_2-Macroglobulin has the potential to bind and rapidly remove most granzymes from the circulation. Antithrombin III and protease nexin I are efficient inhibitors of granzyme A. PI-9 is the most efficient and specific granzyme B inhibitor known and may protect the interior of immune cells from extragranular granzyme B, thereby preventing the triggering of unwarranted apoptosis. Because PI-9 does not inhibit caspases, it is restricted to controlling granzyme B and cannot interfere with the Fas-mediated deletion of cells from the immune system.

Acknowledgments

The authors thank the staff of their laboratories, especially Cathy Bird, Jiuru Sun, Mark Smyth, Vivien Sutton, Lisa McDonald, and Kylie Browne, for their support over many years. We also thank our collaborators, particularly Sharad Kumar, David Vaux, Arnold Greenberg, David Jans, Steve Bottomley, and James Whisstock, and their laboratories for sharing their reagents, expertise, and unpublished data. At various times the laboratory of J.A.T. has received generous support from The Wellcome Trust, the National Health and Medical Research Council of Australia, and the Anti-Cancer Council of Victoria. P.I.B. is supported by the National Health and Medical Research Council of Australia.

REFERENCES

1. Tschopp J, Jongeneel CV. Cytotoxic T lymphocyte mediated cytolysis. *Biochemistry* 1988;27:2641–2646.
2. Smyth MJ, Trapani JA. Granzymes: exogenous proteinases that induce target cell apoptosis. *Immunol Today* 1995;16:202–206.
3. Masson D, Tschopp J. A family of serine esterases in lytic granules of cytolytic T lymphocytes. *Cell* 1987;49:679–685.
4. Kraut J. Serine proteases: structure and mechanism of catalysis. *Annu Rev Biochem* 1977;46:331–358.
5. Smyth MJ, O'Connor MD, Trapani JA, Kershaw

MH, Brinkworth RI. A novel substrate-binding pocket interaction restricts the specificity of NK cell-specific proteinase Met-ase-1. *J Immunol* 1996;156:4171–4181.

6. Masson D, Tschopp J. Isolation of a lytic, pore-forming protein (perforin) from cytolytic T-lymphocytes. *J Biol Chem* 1985;260:9069–9072.

7. Garcia-Sanz JA, Plaetinck G, Velotti F, el al. Perforin is present only in normal activated Lyt2[+] T lymphocytes and not in L3T4[+] cells, but the serine protease granzyme A is made by both subsets. *EMBO J* 1987;6:933–938.

8. Ebnet K, Chluba-de Tapia J, Hurtenbach, U, Kramer MD, Simon MM. In vivo primed mouse T cells selectively express T cell-specific serine proteinase-1 and the proteinase-like molecules granzyme B and C. *Int Immunol* 1991;3:9–19.

9. Liu CC, Rafii S, Granelli-Piperno A, Trapani JA, Young JD. Perforin and serine esterase gene expression in stimulated human T cells: kinetics, mitogen requirements, and effects of cyclosporin A. *J Exp Med* 1989;170:2105–2118.

10. Held W, MacDonald HR, Mueller C. Expression of genes encoding cytotoxic cell-associated serine proteases in thymocytes. *Int Immunol* 1990; 2:57–62.

11. Manyak CL, Norton GP, Lobe CG, et al. IL-2 induces expression of serine protease enzymes and genes in natural killer and nonspecific T killer cells. *J Immunol* 1989;142:3707–3713.

12. Trapani JA, Klein JL, White PC, Dupont B. Molecular cloning of an inducible serine esterase gene from human cytotoxic lymphocytes. *Proc Natl Acad Sci USA* 1988;85:6924–6928.

13. Smyth MJ, Wiltrout T, Trapani JA, et al. Purification and cloning of a novel serine protease, RNK-Met-1, from the granules of a rat natural killer cell leukemia. *J Biol Chem* 1992;267:24418–24425.

14. Muller C, Kagi D, Aebischer, T, Odermatt, B, et al. Detection of perforin and granzyme A mRNA in infiltrating cells during infection of mice with lymphocytic choriomeningitis virus. *Eur J Immunol* 1989;19:1253–1259.

15. Held W, MacDonald, HR, Weissman IL, Hess MW, Mueller C. Genes encoding tumor necrosis factor alpha and granzyme A are expressed during development of autoimmune diabetes. *Proc Natl Acad Sci USA* 1990;87:2239–2243.

16. Griffiths GM, Mueller C. Expression of perforin and granzymes in vivo: potential diagnostic markers for activated cytotoxic cells. *Immunol Today* 1991;12:415–419.

17. Kramer MD, Fruth U, Simon HG, Simon MM. Expression of cytoplasmic granules with T cell-associated serine proteinase-1 activity in Ly-2[+] (CD8[+]) T lymphocytes responding to lymphocytic choriomeningitis virus in vivo. *Eur J Immunol* 1989;19:151–156.

18. Moll H, Muller C, Gillitzer R, et al. Expression of T-cell-associated serine proteinase 1 during murine *Leishmania major* infection correlates with susceptibility to disease. *Infect Immun* 1991;59:4701–4705.

19. Mueller C, Shao Y, Altermatt HJ, Hess MW, Shelby J. The effect of cyclosporine treatment on the expression of genes encoding granzyme A and perforin in the infiltrate of mouse heart transplants. *Transplantation* 1993;55:139–145.

20. Chen RH, Ivens KW, Alpert S, et al. The use of granzyme A as a marker of heart transplant rejection in cyclosporine or anti-CD4 monoclonal antibody-treated rats. *Transplantation* 1993;55: 146–153.

21. Wood GS, Mueller C, Warnke RA, Weissman IL. In situ localization of HuHF serine protease mRNA and cytotoxic cell-associated antigens in human dermatoses. a novel method for the detection of cytotoxic cells in human tissues. *Am J Pathol* 1988;133:218–225.

22. Clement MV, Haddad P, Ring GH, Pruna A, Sasportes M. Granzyme B-gene expression: a marker of human lymphocytes "activated" in vitro or in renal allografts. *Hum Immunol* 1990;28: 159–166.

23. Hameed A, Truong LD, Price V, Kruhenbuhl O, Tschopp J. Immunohistochemical localization of granzyme B antigen in cytotoxic cells in human tissues. *Am J Pathol* 1991;138:1069–1075.

24. Devergne O, Peuchmaur M, Crevon MC, et al. Activation of cytotoxic cells in hyperplastic lymph nodes from HIV-infected patients. *AIDS* 1991;5: 1071–1079.

25. Griffiths GM, Alpert S, Lambert E, McGuire J, Weissman IL. Perforin and granzyme A expression identifying cytolytic lymphocytes in rheumatoid arthritis. *Proc Natl Acad Sci USA* 1992;89:549–553.

26. Young LH, Joag SV, Zheng LM, Lee CP, Lee YS, Young JD. Perforin-mediated myocardial damage in acute myocarditis. *Lancet* 1990;336:1019–1021.

27. Tak PP, Kummer JA, Hack CE, et al. Granzyme-positive cytotoxic cells are specifically increased in early rheumatoid synovial tissue. *Arthritis Rheum* 1994;37:1735–1743.

28. Hudig D, Ewoldt GR, Woodard, SL. Proteases and lymphocyte cytotoxic killing mechanisms. *Curr Opin Immunol* 1993;5:90–96.

29. Poe M, Blake JT, Boulton DA, et al. Human cytotoxic lymphocyte granzyme B. its purification from granules and the characterization of substrate and inhibitor specificity. *J Biol Chem* 1991;266:98–103.

30. Andrade F, Roy S, Nicholson D, Thornberry N, Rosen A, Casciola-Rosen, L. Granzyme B directly and efficiently cleaves several downstream caspase substrates: implications for CTL-induced apoptosis. *Immunity* 1998;8:451–460.

31. McGuire MJ, Lipsky PE, Thiele DL. Generation of active myeloid and lymphoid granule serine proteases requires processing by the granule thiol protease dipeptidyl peptidase I. *J Biol Chem* 1993;268:2458–2467.

32. Griffiths GM, Isaaz S. Granzymes A and B are targeted to the lytic granules of lymphocytes by the mannose-6-phosphate receptor. *J Cell Biol* 1993;120:885–896.

33. Uellner R, Zvelebel MJ, Hopkins J, et al. Perforin is activated by proteolytic cleavage during biosynthesis which reveals a phospholipid binding domain. *EMBO J* 1997;16:7287–7296.

34. Spaeny-Dekking EH, Hanna WL, Wolbink AM, et al. Extracellular granzymes A and B in humans:

detection of native species during CTL responses in vitro and in vivo. *J Immunol* 1998;160:3610–3616.

35. Simon MM, Hoschutzky H, Fruth U, Simon HG, Kramer, MD. Purification and characterization of a T cell specific serine proteinase (TSP-1) from cloned cytolytic T lymphocytes. *EMBO J* 1986; 5:3267–3274.

36. Simon MM, Kramer MD, Prester M, Gay S. Mouse T-cell associated serine proteinase 1 degrades collagen type IV: a structural basis for the migration of lymphocytes through vascular basement membranes. *Immunology* 1991;73:117–119.

37. Young JD, Hengartner H, Podack ER, Cohn, ZA. Purification and characterization of a cytolytic pore-forming protein from granules of cloned lymphocytes with natural killer activity. *Cell* 1986; 44:849–859.

38. Simon MM, Kramer MD. Granzyme A. *Methods Enzymol* 1994;244:68–79.

39. Simon MM, Simon HG, Fruth U, Epplen J, Muller-Hermelink HK, Kramer MD. Cloned cytolytic T-effector cells and their malignant variants produce an extracellular matrix degrading trypsin-like serine proteinase. *Immunology* 1987;60:219–230.

40. Takahashi K, Nakamura T, Adachi H, Yagita H, Okumura K. Antigen-independent T cell activation mediated by a very late activation antigen-like extracellular matrix receptor. *Eur J Immunol* 1991;21:1559–1562.

41. Brunner G, Simon MM, Kramer MD. Activation of pro-urokinase by the human T cell-associated serine proteinase HuTSP-1. *FEBS Lett* 1990;260: 141–144.

42. Suidan HS, Bouvier J, Schraer S, Stone SR, Monard D, Tschopp, J. Granzyme A release upon stimulation of cytotoxic T lymphocytes activates the thrombin receptor on neuronal cells and astrocytes. *Proc Natl Acad Sci USA* 1994;91:8112–8116.

43. Irmler M, Hertig S, MacDonald HR, et al. Granzyme A is an interleukin 1 beta-converting enzyme. *J Exp Med* 1995;181:1917–1922.

44. Simon HG, Fruth U, Kramer MD, Simon MM. A secretable serine proteinase with highly restricted specificity from cytolytic T lymphocytes inactivates retrovirus-associated reverse transcriptase. *FEBS Lett* 1987;223:352–360.

45. Mullbacher A, Ebnet K, Blanden RV, et al. Granzyme A is critical for recovery of mice from infection with the natural cytopathic viral pathogen, ectromelia. *Proc Natl Acad Sci USA* 1996;93:5783–5787.

46. Ebnet K, Hausmann M, Lehmann-Grube F, et al. Granzyme A-deficient mice retain potent cell-mediated cytotoxicity. *EMBO J* 1995;14:4230–4239.

47. Simon MM, Hausmann M, Tran T, et al. In vitro- and ex-vivo-derived cytolytic leukocytes from A × B double knockout mice are defective in granule-mediated apoptosis but not lysis of target cells. *J Exp Med* 1998;186:1781–1786.

48. Sayers TJ, Wiltrout TA, Smyth MJ, et al. Purification and cloning of a novel serine protease, RNK-Tryp-2, from the granules of a rat NK cell leukemia. *J Immunol* 1994;152:2289–2297.

49. Shi L, Mai S, Israels S, Browne K, Trapani JA, Greenberg AH. Granzyme B (GraB) autonomously crosses the cell membrane and perforin initiates apoptosis and GraB nuclear localization. *J Exp Med* 1997;185:855–866.

50. Jans DA, Jans P, Briggs LJ, Sutton V, Trapani JA. Nuclear transport of granzyme B (fragmentin-2): dependence of perforin in vivo and cytosolic factors in vitro. *J Biol Chem* 1996;271:30781–30789.

51. Trapani JA, Jans P, Froelich CJ, Smyth MJ, Sutton VR. Jans D. (1998) Perforin-dependent nuclear accumulation of granzyme B precedes apoptosis, and is not a consequence of nuclear membrane dysfunction. *Cell Death Differ* 1998;5:488–496.

52. Froelich CJ, Orth K, Turbov J, et al. New paradigm for lymphocyte granule-mediated cytotoxicity: target cells bind and internalize granzyme B, but an endosomolytic agent is necessary for cytosolic delivery and subsequent apoptosis. *J Biol Chem* 1996;271:29073–29079.

53. Froelich CJ, Dixit VM, Yang X. Lymphocyte granule-mediated apoptosis: matters of viral mimicry and deadly proteases. *Immunol Today* 1998; 19:30–36.

54. Trapani JA, Jans DA, Sutton VR. Lymphocyte granule-mediated cell death. Springer Semin Immunopathol 1998;19:323–343.

55. Trapani JA, Sutton VR, Smyth, MJ. Cytotoxic lymphocyte granules: evolution of vesicles essential for combating virus infections. *Immunol Today* 1999;20:351–356.

56. Darmon AJ, Nicholson DW, Bleackley RC. Activation of the apoptotic protease CPP32 by cytotoxic T-cell-derived granzyme B. *Nature* 1995;377: 446–448.

57. Harvey NL, Trapani JA, Fernandes-Alnemri T, Litwack G, Alnemri ES, Kumar S. Processing of the Nedd2 precursor by ICE-like proteases and granzyme B. *Genes Cells* 1996;1:673–685.

58. Srinivasula SM, Ahmad M, Fernandes-Alnemri T, Litwack G, Alnemri E. Molecular ordering of the Fas-apoptotic pathway: the Fas/APO-1 protease Mch5 is a crmA-inhibitable protease that activates multiple Ced-3/ICE-like cysteine proteases. *Proc Natl Acad Sci USA* 1996;93:14486–14491.

59. Fernandes-Alnemri T, Armstrong RC, Krebs J, et al. In vitro activation of CPP32 and Mch3 by Mch4, a novel human apoptotic cysteine protease containing two FADD-like domains. *Proc Natl Acad Sci USA* 1996;93:7464–7469.

60. Gu Y, Sarnecki C, Fleming MA, Lippke JA, Bleackley RC, Su M. Processing and activation of CMH-1 by granzyme B. *J Biol Chem* 1996;271: 10816–10820.

61. Quan LT, Caputo A, Bleackley RC, Pickup DJ, Salvesen GS. Granzyme B is inhibited by the cowpox virus serpin cytokine response modifier A. *J Biol Chem* 1995;70:10377–10379.

62. Talanian RV, Yang X, Turbov J, et al. Granule-mediated killing: pathways for granzyme B-mediated apoptosis. *J Exp Med* 1997;186:1323–1331.

63. Heusel JW, Wesselschmidt RL, Shresta S, Russell JH, Ley TJ. Cytotoxic lymphocytes require granzyme B for the rapid induction of DNA fragmenta-

tion and apoptosis in allogeneic target cells. *Cell* 1994;76:977–987.

64. Zhou Q, Salvesen G. Activation of pro-caspase-7 by serine proteases includes a non-canonical specificity. *Biochem J* 1997;324:361–364.

65. Froelich CJ, Hanna WL, Poirier GG, et al. Granzyme B/perforin-mediated apoptosis of Jurkat cells results in cleavage of poly(ADP-ribose) polymerase to the 89-kDa apoptotic fragment and less abundant 64-kDa fragment. *Biochem Biophys Res Commun* 1996;227:658–665.

66. Pinkoski MJ, Winkler U, Hudig D, Bleackley RC. Binding of granzyme B in the nucleus of target cells: recognition of an 80-kilodalton protein. *J Biol Chem* 1996;271:10225–10229.

67. Trapani JA, Jans DA, Browne KA, Smyth MJ, Jans PJ, Sutton VR. Efficient nuclear targeting of granzyme B and the nuclear consequences of apoptosis induced by granzyme B and perforin are caspase-dependent, but cell death is caspase-independent. *J Biol Chem* 1998;273:27934–27938.

68. Sarin A, Williams MS, Alexander-Miller MA, Berzofsky JA, Zacharchuk CM, Henkart PA. Target cell lysis by CTL granule exocytosis is independent of ICE/Ced-3 family proteases. *Immunity* 1997;6:209–215.

69. Nakajima H, Golstein P, Henkart PA. The target cell nucleus is not required for cell-mediated granzyme- or Fas-based cytotoxicity. *J Exp Med* 1995;181:1905–1909.

70. Sutton VR, Vaux DL, Trapani JA. Bcl-2 prevents apoptosis induced by perforin and granzyme B, but not that mediated by whole cytotoxic lymphocytes. *J Immunol* 1997;158:5783–5790.

71. Kagi D, Ledermann B, Burki K, et al. Cytotoxicity mediated by T cells and natural killer cells is greatly impaired in perforin-deficient mice. *Nature* 1994;369:31–37.

72. Lowin B, Beermann F, Schmidt A, Tschopp J. A null mutation in the perforin gene impairs cytolytic T lymphocyte- and natural killer cell-mediated cytotoxicity. *Proc Natl Acad Sci USA* 1994;91:11571–11575.

73. Nicholson DW, Ali A, Thornberry NA, et al. Identification and inhibition of the ICE/CED-3 protease necessary for mammalian apoptosis. *Nature* 1995;376:37–43.

74. Stein PE, Carrell RW. What do dysfunctional serpins tell us about molecular mobility and disease? *Struct Biol* 1995;2:96–113.

75. Froelich CJ, Zhang X, Turbov J, Hudig D, Winkler U, Hanna WL. Human granzyme B degrades aggregan proteoglycan in matrix synthesized by chondrocytes. *J Immunol* 1993;151:7161–7171.

76. Simon MM, Kramer MD. Granzyme A. *Methods Enzymol* 1994;244:68–79.

77. Peitsch MC, Tschopp J. Granzyme B. *Methods Enzymol* 1994;244:80–87.

78. Chu CT, Pizzo SV. Alpha2-macroglobulin, complement, and biologic defense: antigens, growth factors, microbial proteases, and receptor ligation. *Lab Invest* 1994;6:792–812.

79. Potempa J, Korzus E, Travis J. The serpin superfamily of proteinase inhibitors: structure, function

and regulation. *J Biol Chem* 1994;269:15957–15960.

80. Whisstock J, Skinner R, Lesk AM. An atlas of serpin conformations. *TIBS* 1998;23:63–67.

81. Wilczynska M, Fa M, Karolin J, Ohlsson P-I, Johansson LB-A, Ny T. Structural insights into serpin–protease complexes reveal the inhibitory mechanism of serpins. *Nat Struct Biol* 1997;4:354–357.

82. Stratikos E, Gettins PW. Major proteinase movement upon stable serpin-proteinase complex formation. *Proc Natl Acad Sci USA* 1997;94:453–458.

83. Patston PA, Gettins PGW, Schapira M. Serpins are suicide substrates: implications for the regulation of proteolytic pathways. *Semin Thromb Hemost* 1994;20:410–416.

84. Beatty K, Beith J, Travis J. Kinetics of association of serine proteinases with native and oxidized alpha-1-proteinase inhibitor and alpha-1-antichymotrypsin. *J Biol Chem* 1980;255:3931–3934.

85. Jin L, Abrahams JP, Skinner R, Petitou M, Pike RN, Carrell RW. The anticoagulant activation of antithrombin by heparin. *Proc Natl Acad Sci USA* 1998;94:14683–14688.

86. Travis J, Salveson GS. Human plasma proteinase inhibitors. *Annu Rev Biochem* 1983;52:655–709.

87. Masson D, Tschopp J. Inhibition of lymphocyte protease granzyme A by antithrombin III. *Mol Immunol* 1988;25:1283–1289.

88. Gronke RS, Bergman BL, Baker JB. Thrombin interaction with platelets: influence of a platelet protease nexin. *J Biol Chem* 1987;262:3030–3036.

89. Gronke RS, Knauer DJ, Veeraraghavan S, Baker JB. A form of protease nexin I is expressed on the platelet surface during platelet activation. *Blood* 1989;73:472–478.

90. Festoff BW, Rao JS, Chen M. Protease nexin I, thrombin- and urokinase-inhibiting serpin, concentrated in normal human cerebrospinal fluid. *Neurology* 1992;42:1361–1366.

91. Gurwitz D, Simon MM, Fruth U, Cunningham DD. Protease nexin-1 complexes and inhibits T cell serine proteinase. *Biochem Biophys Res Commun* 1989;161:300–304.

92. Odake S, Kam CM, Narasimhan L, et al. Human and murine cytotoxic T lymphocyte serine proteases: subsite mapping with peptide thioester substrates and inhibition of enzyme activity and cytolysis by isocoumarins. *Biochemistry* 1991;30:2217–2227.

93. Pickup DJ. Poxviral modifiers of cytokine responses to infection. *Infect Agents Dis* 1994;3:116–127.

94. Ray CA, Black RA, Kronheim SR, et al. Viral inhibition of inflammation: cowpox virus encodes an inhibitor of the interleukin-1-beta converting enzyme. *Cell* 1992;69:597–604.

95. Komiyama T, Ray CA, Pickup DJ, et al. Inhibition of interleukin-1beta converting enzyme by the cowpox virus serpin crmA. *J Biol Chem* 1994;269:19331–19337.

96. Nicholson DW, Thornberry NA. Caspases: killer proteases. *TIBS* 1997;22:299–306.

97. Quan LT, Caputo A, Bleackley RC, Pickup DJ, Salvesen GS. Granzyme B is inhibited by the cow-

pox virus serpin cytokine response modifier A. *J Biol Chem* 1995;270:10377–10379.

98. Tewari M, Dixit VM. Fas- and tumor necrosis factor-induced apoptosis is inhibited by the poxvirus crmA gene product. *J Biol Chem* 1995;270:3255–3260.

99. Atkinson EA, Barry M, Darmon AJ, et al. Cytotoxic T lymphocyte-assisted suicide. caspase 3 activation is primarily the result of the direct action of granzyme B. *J Biol Chem* 1998;273:21261–21266.

100. Macen JL, Garner RL, Musy PY, et al. Differential induction of the Fas- and granule-mediated cytolysis pathways by the orthopoxvirus cytokine response modifier A/SPI-2 and SPI-1 protein. *Proc Natl Acad Sci USA* 1996;93:9108–9113.

101. Sprecher CA, Morgenstern KA, Mathewes S, et al. Molecular cloning, expression, and partial characterization of two novel members of the ovalbumin family of serine proteinase inhibitors. *J Biol Chem* 1995;270:29854–29861.

102. Sun J, Bird CH, Sutton V, et al. A cytosolic granzyme B inhibitor related to the viral apoptotic regulator cytokine response modifier A is present in cytotoxic lymphocytes. *J Biol Chem* 1996;271:27802–27809.

103. Bird CH, Sutton VR, Sun J, et al. Selective regulation of apoptosis: the cytotoxic lymphocyte serpin proteinase inhibitor 9 protects against granzyme B-mediated apoptosis without perturbing the Fas cell death pathway. *Mol Cell Biol* 1998;18:6387–6398.

Cytotoxic Cells: Basic Mechanisms and Medical Applications, edited by Michail V. Sitkovsky and Pierre A. Henkart. Lippincott Williams & Wilkins, Philadelphia © 2000.

Chapter 14

Role of Granzymes in Target Cell Lysis and Viral Infections

Markus M. Simon and °Arno Müllbacher

Max-Planck-Institut für Immunbiologie, Freiburg, Germany; and °Division of Immunology and Cell Biology, John Curtin School of Medical Research, Australian National University, Canberra, Australia

The development of a technique that allows generation of mutant mice with specifically tailored gene deletions (ko mice) promised a clear and definitive means to evaluate the role of the individual products involved in cytolytic effector pathways elicited by cytotoxic T (Tc) cells and natural killer (NK) cells. With the possible exception of the perforin ko mouse (perf$^{-/-}$) (1–3), none of the other relevant mutant mice (i.e., granzyme A or granzyme B ko mice) exhibited the expected clear-cut phenotypes for Tc/NK cell-mediated cytotoxicity (4–8). Even with the perf$^{-/-}$ mouse, its role in the control of certain intracellular pathogens was questioned when antigenic systems of ambiguous biologic relevance were tested (9). One of the main stumbling blocks when testing these granzyme (gzm)-deficient mice was the diverse genetic backgrounds of the animals (129, C57BL/6, or hybrids). It is well established that non-major histocompatibility (MHC) genes play a major role in viral pathogenesis (10,11) including regulation of the Tc cell response (12,13). Evidence for such in gzmA$^{-/-}$ and gzmB$^{-/-}$ mice is presented (see below). Even an analysis of the mechanisms of cytolytic effector function, which at present frequently relies on effector cells generated in *in vitro* allogeneic systems, may ultimately require verification by effector cells induced by biologically relevant pathogens.

ROLE OF GRANZYMES IN Tc/NK CELL-MEDIATED CYTOTOXICITY *IN VITRO*

The discovery of a novel family of serine proteinases in cytoplasmic granules of Tc and NK cells (14–17), synonymously termed T cell specific serine proteinases or granzymes (15,18), came as a surprise to a field that previously considered Tc/NK activity to be mainly executed by perforin and cytokines (19). It is now clear that granzymes play a pivotal role in cytotoxicity and probably other intracellular and extracellular processes *in vivo* after their release from cytotoxic cells.

Expression of Granzymes in Tc and NK Cells

It is known that Tc and NK cells of human, mouse, and rat origin synthesize a number of granzymes, which are stored, together with perforin, within specialized lytic granules (20–23). Upon effector–target cell recognition, granzymes are released into the intercellular space and appear to enter the cytoplasm and nucleus of the target cell and perform their function with the assistance of perforin (24–28). In Tc cells, granzymes are induced only following activation via T cell receptor (TCR) signaling (29–31). To date, eight mouse (A–G, K), six rat, and four human granzymes have been described (20–22). From all the known mouse granzymes, only granzyme A (gzmA) and granzyme B (gzmB), and, if at all, minor amounts of granzyme C (gzmC), have been shown to be expressed in *ex vivo*-derived Tc cells (30,31). However, the tight genetic linkage between gzmA and gzmK on chromosomes 5 and 13 of humans and the mouse, respectively, and between gzmB and gzmsC–G on chromosome 14 in both species (7,32) suggests the possibility that additional granzyme genes are activated owing to putative locus control region elements associated with the two gene clusters; thus they may contribute to the activity(ies) of Tc/NK cells. So far, proteolytic activities have been confirmed only for gzmA and gzmB, using chromogenic compounds and polypeptides as substrates *in vitro* (20,22). Both enzymes exhibit limited proteolysis with distinct requirements for arginine and aspartic acid, respectively, in the substrate P1 position (33–36). This together with the different structures of gzmA and gzmB, the former being a homodimer and the latter a monomer (33,37), suggests that the two granzymes have different substrate specificities and biologic functions. This assumption is supported, at least in part, by recent studies showing that precursor interleukin-1b (IL-1b) is activated by gzmA but not gzmB (38).

Role of Granzymes in the Granule Exocytosis Pathway

Granzymes have been implicated in a variety of T cell-mediated functions, such as detachment of Tc cells from target cells, extravasation, induction of B cell proliferation (20,22), and control of virus replication (39), and also during maturation in the thymus (40). In the past the main emphasis was placed on studies investigating their putative involvement in Tc/NK-mediated cytotoxicity.

It is now clear that Tc cells can kill target cells by at least two independent pathways,

one involving exocytosis of preformed granules and the other requiring ligation of Fas ligand (FasL) on the effector cell with the Fas receptor on target cells (1–3,41–44). Both processes result in target cell apoptosis and lysis by mechanisms that are poorly understood (44). The Fas pathway leads to the assembly of a receptor-associated death-inducing signal complex (45) and subsequent proteolytic activation of members of the caspase family, resulting in apoptosis and necrosis (46,47). Perforin, gzmA, and gzmB have been implicated as main contributors to membrane and nuclear disintegration of target cells by the secretory pathway (44). Using purified proteins, it was found that perforin is critical and sufficient to induce membrane damage of target cells, as measured by chromium 51 (^{51}Cr) release (44,48,49) and that gzmA and gzmB cause DNA fragmentation and apoptotic morphology of target cells, but only in the presence of perforin (23,50,51).

TC/NK Cell-Mediated Cytolysis and Nucleolysis in Granzyme ko Mice

Further information on the involvement of gzmA and gzmB in processes of Tc/NK-mediated cytotoxicity has come from single ko mice with deficiencies for gzmA (gzmA$^{-/-}$) (6,7) and gzmB (gzmB$^{-/-}$) (4,5). Both mutant mice are healthy and show normal hematopoietic and lymphopoietic development. The frequencies of CD4$^+$ and CD8$^+$ T cells from splenocytes responding to mitogens and H-2 alloantigens in primary and secondary mixed lymphocyte cultures with proliferation are comparable to those of normal C57BL/6 (B6) and 129 × B6 mice (4, 6). Most notable, the *in vitro*- and *ex vivo*-derived Tc cells from both ko mice are indistinguishable, in most cases, from those of normal mice in their ability to lyse a variety of target cells as measured by ^{51}Cr release. This indicates that neither gzmA nor gzmB independently is critical for target cell lysis via perforin and contradicts earlier studies indicating that both granzymes are essential for optimal perforin-mediated cytolysis (51,52).

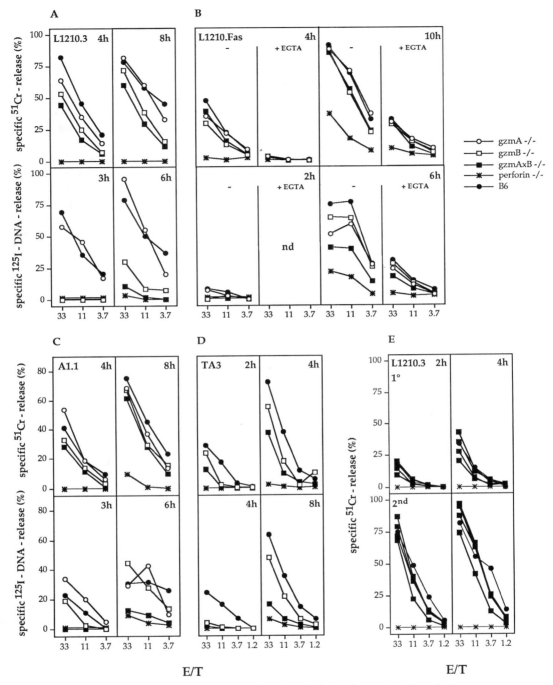

FIG. 14-1. Cytolytic and nucleolytic activities of *in vitro*-derived alloreactive Tc cells from granzymes (*gzmA, gzmB, gzmA × B*) and perforin ko and B6 mice. [51]Cr release (*top panels*) and ^{125}I-DNA release (*lower panels*) of L1210 (**A, E**), L1210.Fas (**B**), A1.1 (**C**), and TA3 (**D**) target cells induced by *in vitro*-derived alloreactive (anti-H-2[d]) Tc cells. Splenocytes from B6 (●), gzmA[−/−] (○), gzmB[−/−] (□), gzmA × B[−/−] (■), and perforin[−/−] (∗) mice (pools of two spleens/mouse strain (**A–D**); spleens of individual mice (**E**) were incubated in primary mixed lymphocyte culture (MLC) (**A–D**) or secondary MLC with irradiated BALB/c stimulator cells (splenocytes) and tested for cytolytic (*top panels*) and nucleolytic (*lower panels*) activities on the allogeneic target cells L1210.3, L1210.Fas, A1.1, and TA3 for the indicated time periods. All values are the mean lysis of triplicate samples at three effector target (E/T) values. SEMs never exceeded 3%.

Studies in which the potential of Tc and NK cells of mice lacking both gzmA and gzmB (gzmA × B$^{-/-}$), were compared with those from single ko mice [i.e., gzmA$^{-/-}$ and gzmB$^{-/-}$ or perforin (perf$^{-/-}$)] to induce lysis of target cells (8) provided a clearer picture. As shown in Figure 14-1 (A–E, top panels), with the exception of perf$^{-/-}$, all alloreactive Tc populations from the granzyme-mutant strains generated against stimulators differing in the whole of the MHC (H-2^d) induced ^{51}Cr release in various target cells, including those that lack or express Fas, at levels and with kinetics similar to those of normal mice. That ^{51}Cr release is a definitive

correlate of cell death with all Tc cell populations tested, including B6, gzmA$^{-/-}$, gzmB$^{-/-}$, gzmA × B$^{-/-}$, perf$^{-/-}$, and perf × A × B$^{-/-}$, is shown by the inverse relation between the amount of ^{51}Cr released from L929 or L929.Fas target cells and the frequency level colony formation by the remaining targets after they were allowed to grow under conditions unsuitable for survival of lymphocytes (Fig. 14-2). Because slight differences in lytic activity of gzmA × B$^{-/-}$ Tc cells occurred between individual sets of experiments, using splenocytes of one or several donors (see also below), *in vitro*-derived primary and secondary H-2^d-reactive

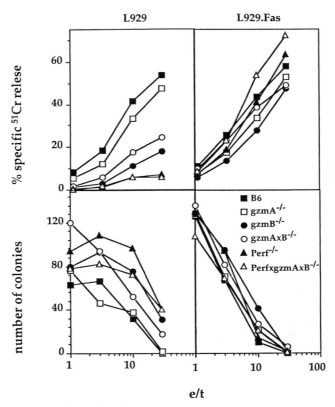

FIG. 14-2. ^{51}Cr release and cell survival (colony forming) assay by alloreactive Tc cells from B6 and ko mice. Splenocytes from B6 (■), gzmA$^{-/-}$ (□), gzmB$^{-/-}$ (●), gzmA × B$^{-/-}$ (○), perf$^{-/-}$ (▲), and perfxgzmA × B$^{-/-}$ (△) mice, were stimulated *in vitro* with B10.A(2R) (K^k) stimulator cells and tested for ^{51}Cr release (*top panels*) on L929 (*left panels*) and L929.Fas (*right panels*) target cells. Cytotoxic assay time was 6 hours. Each point constitutes the mean of percent specific lysis of three separate wells. Spontaneous release was always less than 20%. Cell survival assay (*bottom panels*) of target cells after a 6-hour cytotoxicity assay. Cells from triplicate wells from cytotoxicity assay were pooled and aliquots plated in six well plates and incubated for 8 days. Viable cell colonies were stained with crystal violet and counted.

Tc cell populations from eight (four males, four females) individual gzmA × B$^{-/-}$ mice were tested in addition for their cytolytic activities and compared with those from B6 Tc cells (Fig. 14-1E, shown only for male mice). No differences in lytic activity could be discerned. Similar results were obtained with *ex vivo*-derived H-2^d reactive splenocytes from individual mice of strains B6, gzmA$^{-/-}$, gzmB$^{-/-}$, and gzmA × B$^{-/-}$ (8).

Similar levels of cytolytic activity were also observed with *ex vivo*-derived NK cell populations from gzmA$^{-/-}$, gzmB$^{-/-}$, gzmA × B$^{-/-}$, and B6 mice, when assayed after 2 and 4 hours (Fig. 14-3, top panels). An occasional low level of lytic activity of NK cells from granzyme single or double ko mice (compared to B6 mice) to induce ^{51}Cr release was neither significant nor reproducible (8). On the other hand, no (or only marginal) NK cell-mediated lytic activity can be obtained with splenocytes from perforin$^{-/-}$ mice (1,8).

These findings unequivocally demonstrate that the Tc/NK-mediated exocytosis pathway, leading to ^{51}Cr release, is independent of gzmA and gzmB. However, the participation of other, as yet undefined proteases in perforin-mediated lysis cannot be ruled out. In addition the data do not exclude the possiblity that gzmA and gzmB contribute to cytolysis, as defined by ^{51}Cr release, by inducing apoptotic processes, which finally also lead to disintegration of target cells.

The most important findings with single granzyme ko mice were that gzmB$^{-/-}$, but not gzmA$^{-/-}$, Tc cells are unable to induce rapid DNA fragmentation in target cells, a defect that could be overcome with longer incubation times (4,6). These data were interpreted to mean that gzmB has a nonredundant function in early Tc granule-mediated nucleolysis, but that other mediators, including gzmA or as yet undefined proteases, may be involved in delayed nucleolysis. Independent studies with synthetic inhibitors for gzmA, gzmB, and caspases also implied a role of gzmA in addition to gzmB in target cell nucleolysis but suggested different pathways for the two enzymes (55,56). Definitive evidence for such an interpretation was de-

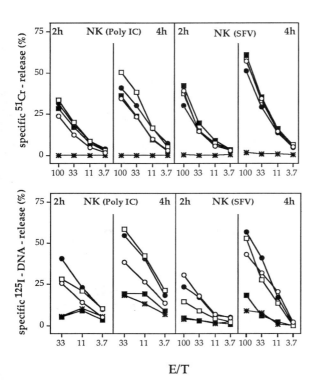

E/T

FIG. 14-3. Cytolytic and nucleolytic activities of *ex vivo*-derived NK cells from B6, gzmA, gzmB, gzmA × B, and perforin ko mice. ^{51}Cr release (*top panels*) and ^{125}I-DNA release (*lower panels*) from YAC-1 target cells by *ex vivo*-derived NK cells from mutant or wt mice. B6 (●), gzmA$^{-/-}$ (○), gzmB$^{-/-}$ (□), gzmA × B$^{-/-}$ (■), and perforin$^{-/-}$ (*) mice were either treated with poly I:C (20 hours) (53) or infected with SFV (2 days) (54) and their splenocytes (*poly I:C,* pool of two spleens; *SFV,* pool of three spleens) were tested for cytolytic (*upper panels*) or nucleolytic (*lower panels*) activities on YAC-1 target cells. Assay times were 2 and 4 hours. All values are the mean lysis of triplicate samples at three or four E/T values. The SEM never exceeded 3%. (From ref. 8, Copyright 1997, The Rockefeller University Press, with permission.)

rived from studies comparing alloreactive Tc cells from gzmA × B$^{-/-}$ with those of gzmA$^{-/-}$ and gzmB$^{-/-}$ mice (Fig. 14-1A–D, bottom panels) (8). Whereas target cell DNA fragmentation was not observed with gzmA × B$^{-/-}$ Tc cells even after extended incubation periods (10 hours), it was normal with gzmA$^{-/-}$ Tc cells and only impaired with gzmB$^{-/-}$ Tc cells in short-term (2–4 hours) but not long-term (4–10 hours) assays. Similarly, *ex vivo*-derived gzmA × B$^{-/-}$ NK cells were defective in nucleolytic activity and caused, if any, only marginal DNA fragmentation when tested on YAC target cells in 2- and 4-hour assays (Fig. 14-3, bottom panels). In contrast, NK cells from gzmA$^{-/-}$ and gzmB$^{-/-}$ mice expressed nucleolytic activities that were already apparent in 2-hour assays and increased in 4-hour assays, reaching lev-

els comparable with those of B6 mice. The combined data lead to the conclusion that gzmA and gzmB are critical for Tc/NK granule-mediated nucleolysis, with gzmB being the main contributor, whereas target cell lysis is due solely to perforin and is independent of both proteases.

The mechanism(s) by which gzmA and gzmB initiate processes leading to nucleolysis of target cells are only beginning to be revealed. Obviously, both granzymes are able to cross the target cell membrane via a still undefined process (24–28) and to exert their proteolytic activities on substrates within the cytoplasm, nucleus, or both (57,58). GzmB was shown to cleave not only most caspase zymogens, though significantly not caspase 1 (i.e., ICE) (47,57–60), but also downstream molecules of the apoptotic path-

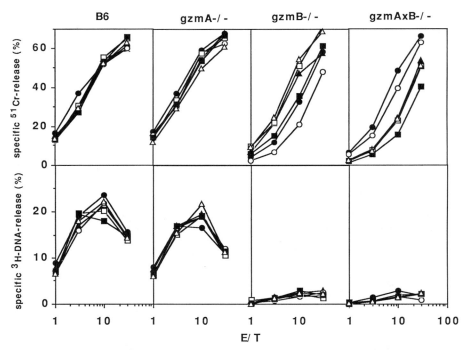

FIG. 14-4. Cytolytic and nucleolytic activities of *in vitro*-derived K^d alloreactive Tc cells from individual B6 and gzmA, gzmB, and gzmA × B ko mice. Splenocytes from six B6 (●), gzmA$^{-/-}$ (○), gzmB$^{-/-}$ (□), and gzmA × B$^{-/-}$ (■) mice were individually incubated with HTG stimulator cells and tested for their ability to induce ^{51}Cr- and [^{3}H]-thymidine release in L1210 target cells. Each point constitutes the mean of the percent specific lysis of three wells. The SEM was always ±3%. Spontaneous release was always less than 20%.

way, such as DNA-dependent protein kinase catalytic subunit (DNA-PK$_{CS}$) and nuclear mitotic apparatus protein (NuMA) (61). The ability of gzmB to cleave death-inducing substrates independent of caspases adds a further dimension to the role of this granzyme in Tc/NK cell-mediated cytolysis and nucleolysis. So far, intracelluar substrates for gzmA are elusive. There is only one report describing the binding of human gzmA to two cytoplasmic and putative HLA-associated proteins and proteolysis of one of them (62). However, their participation in the gzmA pathway of cytotoxicity is unclear.

The conflicting results regarding the cytolytic potential of Tc cells from independently generated gzmA$^{-/-}$ (6,7), gzmB$^{-/-}$ (5,6,8), and gzmA × B$^{-/-}$ (8; and T. Ley, personal communication) need further comment. In fact, in a number of experiments—particularly those in which stimulation was restricted to only part of the MHC locus (i.e., K^d)—we have also observed highly variable cytolytic activities (up to fivefold differences) with alloreactive Tc cells from individual gzmB$^{-/-}$ (129 × B6) (4) and gzmA × B$^{-/-}$ (129 × B6) (8) but not with those of gzmA$^{-/-}$ (B6) (6) and B6 mice (Fig. 14-4: six individual mice/group). As the independent mutations for gzmA [B6 (6); 129 × B6 (7)] and for gzmB [129 × B6 (4)] have been generated in H-2^b haplotype mice, but with different genetic backgrounds (i.e., B6 versus 129 × B6), the latter are of hybrid status; consequently, individual mice are heterogeneous with respect to genes outside the MHC locus. The possibility that exocytosis-mediated induction of ^{51}Cr release by 129 and B6 Tc cells is differentially regulated by granzymes is less likely. This assumption derives from experiments in which the cytolytic potential of allorective 129 and B6 Tc cells was tested in the presence of specific inhibitors for gzmA, gzmB, or caspases (Fig. 14-5). The finding that Tc cells from both mouse strains similarly retained respectable lytic activity upon inactivation of caspases, gzmA, or gzmB and even in the absence of any DNA fragmentation clearly shows that granule exocytosis-mediated lysis can occur in the absence of gzmA, gzmB, and a functinal caspase cascade. Thus it is more likely that the variable cytolytic potential of individual Tc cell populations from such hybrid mice [i.e., gzmA$^{-/-}$ (129 × B6), gzmB$^{-/-}$ (129 × B6), and gzmA × B$^{-/-}$ (129 × B6)] depends on the strength of the antigenic stimulus resulting in differential expression of perforin or other non-MHC genes, such as cytokines or granzymes encoded within the gzmB gene cluster (32). This may falsely implicate the involvement of either of the two granzymes in perforin-mediated ^{51}Cr release. Only a detailed analysis using cloned Tc cell lines, including concomitant quantification of each of the effector molcules known to be involved in the cytolytic machinery of the exocytosis pathway at a given time, can resolve these questions.

ROLE OF GRANULE EXOCYTOSIS PATHWAY IN THE CONTROL OF VIRUS INFECTIONS, WITH SPECIAL EMPHASIS ON POXVIRUSES

The mouse T cell response to the orthopoxvirus ectromelia (Ect), a natural pathogen, has been one of the classic experimental systems for the study of viral pathogenesis (63). It has been especially instrumental in elucidating the role of T cells (64,65), in particular that of CD8$^+$ Tc cells (66,67), in the recovery from primary Ect infections. Only studies on the pathogenesis of lymphocytic choriomeningitis virus (LCMV) have given as much useful insight into the complex interplay between viruses and their natural host, the mouse. This infectious disease model seems to be particularly suitable for dissecting the roles of the individual components of these diverse effector molecules employed by these cytolytic leukocytes. One is mediated by cytokines such as interferon γ (IFN-γ) and interleukins (19) and the other by cytotoxic molecules. In the former instance, data are available from ko mice clearly indicating that lack of IFN-γ results in increased susceptibility to Ect, but that this increased sus-

L1210.3

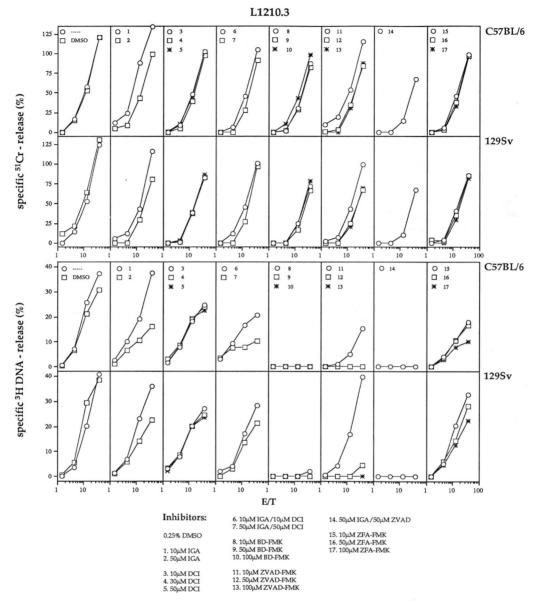

FIG. 14-5. Effect of protease inhibitors on Fas-independent target cell cytolysis and nucleolysis by H-2^d-allorective Tc cells from B6 and 129 mice. Primary *in vitro*-derived K^d,D^d alloreactive Tc cells (anti-BALB/c) from B6 and 129 mice were tested for their cytolytic and nucleolytic activities against L1210 target cells previously incubated with the indicated concentrations of inhibitors for 1 hour. L1210 target cells incubated in medium alone or in the presence of DMSO (0.25%) served as controls. Cytotoxic assay time was 4 hours. Each point constitutes the mean of percent specific lysis of three wells. The SEM was always ±3%. Spontaneous release was always less than 20%.

ceptibility is most likely the effect of regulatory consequences leading to a delay in Tc cell maturation/activation (68,69). With the other type of interplay, the molecules involved in the cytolytic machinery are mediated via the exocytosis pathway. The role of perforin is addressed in another section of this book; data relative to its role in recovery from a primary Ect virus infection have come to light only recently (70; Karupiah, personal communication). From these studies it is evident that perforin is essential in the recovery from Ect virus infection. Virulent Moscow strain Ect at doses as low as 1 to 10 plaque-forming units (PFU) lead to mortality within 8 to 10 days in perf$^{-/-}$ mice when it is given via the footpad. Thus it makes the perf$^{-/-}$ mouse as susceptible as the least resistant mouse strains known (10,11). The wild-type B6 strain, on the other hand, needs more than 10^6 PFU per mouse for mortality to occur (11,70,71). Similar to the nonmouse pathogen vaccinia virus (VV) (9), the absence of perforin does not lead to increased susceptibility to a closely related orthopoxvirus, cowpox (CPV). In the case of CPV a lack of perforin rather than increasing susceptibility has the opposite effect, bestowing some kind of protection (70). The lesson from these experiments is that only natural models molded by evolutionary pressures of survival and dissemination can provide insights into processes of host–parasite relationships and strategies of immune evasion versus immune recovery and elimination.

Role of Granzyme A in Virus Infections

In our initial studies (6) no consistent effect was found in gzmA$^{-/-}$ mice regarding growth of LCMV in liver and spleen, whereas dramatic effects were observed in the perf$^{-/-}$ mouse using the same virus model (1). Similar studies on Ect infections in mice (71) revealed a critical role of gzmA in recovery from this cytopathic viral infection, although no significant differences of cytolytic potential of Tc cells from wild-type B6 or gzmA$^{-/-}$ mice, generated either in *in vitro*

responses to alloantigens (6) or in *in vivo*-activated Tc cells immune to Ect (Fig. 14-6A,B) were observed (71). Similarly, the lytic potential of NK cells, induced *in vivo* by Ect infection, was not affected by a lack of gzmA (Fig. 14-6C) (71). What we did find was an increase in mortality and morbidity, as well as in virus titers and tissue damage in liver and spleen in gzmA$^{-/-}$ mice compared to that in wild-type B6 mice. The role of gzmA in recovery from ectromelia is still elusive, but it probably involves reduction of progeny virus infectivity by its own proteolyic activity or via secondary mediators (71).

An additional role for gzmA in recovery from Ect infection cannot be excluded at this stage and may be masked by the presence of other granzymes, such as gzmB. Such was the case with the observation described above, showing an involvement of gzmA in nucleolytic activity in the absence of gzmB by using double gzmA × B ko mice (8). An additional role for gzmA in recovery from Ect infection cannot be excluded at this stage and may be masked by the presence of other gzms, such as gzmB. Such was the case, with the observation described above, showing an involvement of gzmA in nucleolytic activity in the absence of gzmB by using double gzmA × B ko mice (8). The availability of single and multiple ko mice of granzymes and perforin on the B6 background has clarified some of those important issues. GzmA × perf$^{-/-}$, gzmB × perf$^{-/-}$, and gzmA × B × perf$^{-/-}$ mice did not show an additional effect in the event of Ect infection due to the absolute requirement of perforin in this disease model (see above). However, we found that gzmB$^{-/-}$ mice are more susceptible to Ect than gzmA$^{-/-}$ mice. Most relevant, mice lacking both gzmA and gzmB are as incapable as are perf-deficient mice to control virus infection (Müllbacher et al. submitted). These observations make it clear that gzmB is not inactivated during Ect infection, as proposed previously (72,73; see below) and suggest that perf per se is not the ultimate effector molecule but functions as a means of delivery for other essential effector molecules (i.e., gzms).

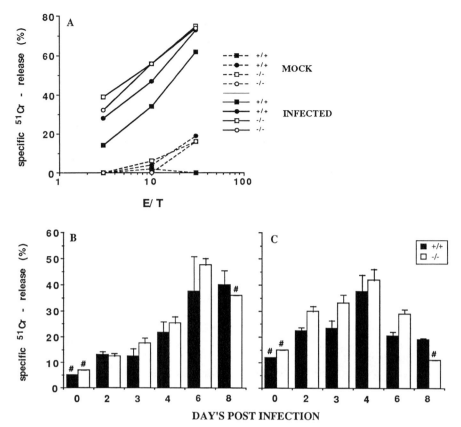

FIG. 14-6. Cytolytic activity of Ect-immune splenocytes and kinetics of induction by gzmA ko mutant mice. **A:** Lytic activity of 6-day immune splenocytes from two individual gzmA$^{-/-}$ (*open symbols*) and two gzmA$^{+/+}$ littermates (*closed symbols*) on H-2-matched, MC57, mock (*broken lines*), or Ect-infected (*solid lines*) target cells. **B:** Mean lytic activity of splenocytes from three individual mice immunized with 10^6 PFU virulent Moscow Ect via the footpad (fp) on Ect-infected MC57 target cells. All values are from a fourfold titration curve and resolved by log regression analysis at an effector/ target ratio of 10:1. *Filled bars,* splenocytes from wild-type mice; *open bars,* −/− animals; #, values from a single animal. The lysis of mock-infected MC57 targets was not significant and is not shown for clarity. **C:** As for **B,** but splenocytes were tested on NK cell-sensitive YAC-1 target cells. (From ref. 71, Copyright 1996, National Academy of Sciences, U.S.A., with permission.)

Role of Poxvirus-Encoded Serpins in Cytolytic Leukocyte-Mediated Nucleolysis and Cytolysis

Serine protease inhibitors or serpins are a large family of proteins involved in the regulation of many normal intra- and extracellular proteolytic enzyme activities (72). Analysis of the genomic sequences of a number of poxviruses revealed that poxviruses encode proteins related to the serpin family of proteinase inhibitors (SPI) (73,74). SPI-2, from

CPV also called cytokine response modifier (crmA), has been shown to inhibit Tc cell-mediated cytotoxic and inflammatory responses by interacting with cellular components involved in the death pathway, such as caspase-3 and caspase-8 (CPP32) (75) and FLICE (76), but also with caspase 1 (IL-I converting enzyme, ICE) (77) and gzmB (78). Serpin-like genes found in VV WR strain (VV-WR), CPV, rabbitpox virus (RPV), variola (73), and Ect (Wallich et al., unpublished observations) exhibit a high homology, which indicates conserved function and evolutionary benefit. The fact that poxviruses encode molecules able to prevent target cell lysis upon delivery of a death signal suggest that serpins evolved to allow infected cells to avoid immune destruction prior to viral replication and virus-induced cytolysis. This is supported by the findings of Tewan et al. (79) and Macen et al. (80), which showed that target cells infected by CPV or RPV were lysed by alloreactive Tc cells to a much lesser extent than mock-infected targets. Infection with virus preparations having mutations within the serpin SPI-1 and SPI-2 genes restored lysis to levels seen with mock-infected targets.

Such inhibition of poxvirus-mediated suppression of alloreactive Tc cell lysis had in fact been reported by Gardner et al. (81) using Ect 20 years earlier. They observed severe inhibition of lysis of Ect-infected target cells by alloreactive Tc cells, whereas the same targets were highly susceptible to lysis by MHC class I (MHC-I)-restricted Ect-immune Tc cells. It was suggested that the inhibition of lysis was due to a decrease in normal MHC-I cell surface expression, a consequence of poxvirus-mediated host protein synthesis inhibition (82). We have recently reinvestigated the role of poxvirus-encoded serpins in light of these findings, taking into account the evidence that functionally active Ect-immune Tc cells are required for recovery from primary Ect infections (83). The main points that emerged from these studies were that (a) poxvirus-immune cytotoxic T cells are cross-reactive at the effector and target cell level between such different viruses as CPV, VV, and the natural mouse pathogen Ect. (b) Despite highly conserved serpins, which are thought to interfere with T cell-mediated cytotoxicity, inhibition of target cell lysis occurred only with Ect and CPV, not with VV. Most importantly, the inhibition is seen predominantly with alloreactive but not MHC-restricted cytotoxic T cells (Fig. 14-7), and inhibition of lysis is target cell type and MHC allotype-dependent. One possible explanation for these findings is that these different Tc cell populations (alloreactive versus MHC-restricted Tc cells) engage target cells with TCRs of differing

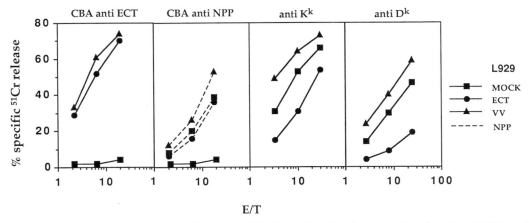

FIG. 14-7. Lysis of poxvirus-infected target by MHC-restricted and alloreactive Tc cells. L929 target cells were mock-infected, infected with ECT or VV for 16 hours and treated with influenza nucleoprotein-derived peptide (NPP) (SDYEGRLI) (*broken lines*) or left untreated (*solid lines*) for 1 hour. They were then tested for lysis by CBA Ect-immune (*first panel*), CBA NPP-immune (*second panel*) MHC-restricted Tc cells, or B6 anti-2R (anti-K^k) and B/c anti-OH (anti-D^k) alloreactive Tc cells (*third and fourth panels*). Cytotoxic assay time was 6 hours. Each point constitutes the mean percent specific lysis of three wells. Spontaneous release was always less than 20%. (From ref. 8, Copyright 1997, The Rockefeller University Press, with permission.)

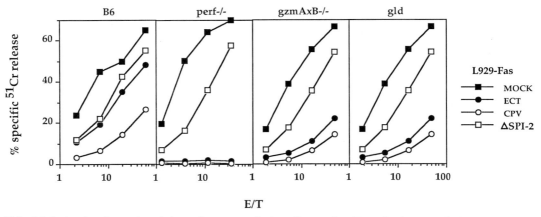

FIG. 14-8. Lysis of poxvirus-infected target cells by alloreactive Tc cells from perforin, granzyme A + B, and fas receptor-deficient mice. L929.Fas target cells were mock-infected (■) or infected with CPV (○) or ECT (●) or with CPV deletion mutant for serpin-2 (crmA) △SPI-2 (□) for 16 hours. They were then tested for lysis by 2R anti-B6 (anti-K^b) alloreactive Tc cells from wild-type B6, perf$^{-/-}$, gzmA × B$^{-/-}$, or gld mice. The cytotoxic assay time was 10 hours. Each point constitutes the mean percent specific lysis of three separate wells. Spontaneous release was always less than 20%.

affinities and thus need different numbers of receptor–ligand interactions to acquire a triggering threshold. Differing TCR affinity interaction may ultimately lead to quantitative differences in granule exocytosis and consequently to varying levels of perforin release. An analysis of the contribution of the two cytolytic mechanisms using mutant mice (gld,Fas-defective; perf$^{-/-}$ and gzmA × B$^{-/-}$ exocytosis-defective) showed that the inhibition of lysis is most pronounced for the fas-mediated pathway (82,83), but it also affects granule exocytosis (Fig. 14-8). The serpin-2 (crmA) gene is responsible for most or all of the inhibition in the absence of either the fas ligand, perforin, or gzmA or gzmB in the effector population. Thus it is unclear to what extent, if at all, poxvirus-encoded serpins are involved in a virus strategy to evade cytolytic effector mechanisms.

Role of gzmA in Other Viral Infection

In addition to Ect and LCMV infections, gzmA$^{-/-}$ mice have been studied in regard to their response to herpes simplex virus (HSV). It has been shown that CD8$^+$ Tc cells are involved in the clearance of HSV from the central nervous system in the absence of overt lysis of neuronal tissue (84). This finding suggested that other effector molecules of CD8$^+$ Tc cells may be involved. Using gzmA$^{-/-}$ ko mice, Pereira and Simmons (personal communications) found that gzmA deficiency was associated with increased clinical disease manifestations and delayed virus clearance. This may yet be an additional example where gzmA reduces virus infectivity possibly by interfering with virus maturation or by inhibiting infection by proteolytic action on the virus particle.

Involvement of gzmA in Other Host–Parasite Interactions

Limited information exists on the role of gzmA in bacterial or parasitic infections, although a role of CD8$^+$ Tc cells has been documented for certain pathogens in both categories. We could not establish a consistent observed defect in gzmA$^{-/-}$ mice to recover from *Listeria monocytogenes* infection (6). However, preliminary evidence in two mouse models of fungal infections— *Candida albicans* (Ashman et al., unpublished data) and *Aspergillus fumigatus*

(Simon and Müllbacher, unpublished observation)—indicates that the absence of gzmA (but not of perforin) enhances the virulence of *C. albicans* and that mice immunocompromised and deficient of gzmA are more apt to succumb to *A. fumigatus* infection than their wild-type equivalent.

Acknowledgments

The authors are grateful to all their colleagues who contributed to the studies on granzymes. We would like to thank in particular Thomas Stehle, Katrin Tertel, Thi-Thanh-Thao Tran, Ron ThaHla, and Melanie Witt for their excellent technical assistance. This work was supported in part by a grant from the Deutsche Forschungsgesellschaft, Si 214/7-1.

REFERENCES

1. Kägi D, Ledermann B, Bürki K, et al. Cytotoxicity mediated by T cells and natural killer cells is greatly impaired in perforin-deficient mice. *Nature* 1994; 369:31–37.
2. Walsh CM, Matloubian M, Liu C-C, et al. Immune function in mice lacking the perforin gene. *Proc Natl Acad Sci USA* 1994;91:10854–10858.
3. Kojima H, Shimohara N, Hanaoka S, et al. Two distinct pathways of specific killing revealed by perforin mutant cytotoxic T lymphocytes. *Immunity* 1994;1:357–364.
4. Heusel JW, Wesselschmidt RL, Shresta S, Russell JH, Ley TJ. Cytotoxic lymphocytes require granzyme B for the rapid induction of DNA fragmentation and apoptosis in allogeneic target cells. *Cell* 1994;76:977–987.
5. Shresta S, MacIvor DM, Heusel JW, Russell JH, Ley TJ. Natural killer and lymphokine-activated killer cells require granzyme B for the rapid induction of apoptosis in susceptible target cells. *Proc Nat Acad Sci USA* 1995;92:5679–5683.
6. Ebnet K, Hausmann M, Lehmann-Grube F, et al. Granzyme A-deficient mice permit cell-mediated cytotoxicity. *EMBO J* 1995;14:4230–4239.
7. Shresta S, Goda P, Wesselschmidt R, Ley TJ. Residual cytotoxicity and granzyme K expression in granzyme A-deficient cytotoxic lymphocytes. *J Biol Chem* 1997;272:20236–20244.
8. Simon MM, Hausmann M, Tran T, et al. In vitro and ex vivo-derived cytolytic leukocytes from granzyme A × B double knockout mice are defective in granule-mediated apoptosis but not lysis of target cells. *J Exp Med* 1997;186:1781–1786.
9. Kägi D, Seiler P, Pavlovic P, et al. The roles of perforin- and fas-dependent cytotoxicity in protection against cytopathic and non cytopathic viruses. *Eur J Immunol* 1995;25:3256–3262.
10. Blanden RV, Deak BD, McDevitt HO. Strategies in virus-host interactions. In: Blanden RV (ed) *Immunology of Virus Diseases,* Canberra, John Curtin School of Medical Research, 1989, pp 125–138.
11. Fenner F, Buller RML. Mousepox. In: Nathanson N (ed) *Viral Pathogenesis.* Philadelphia, Lippincott-Raven, 1997, pp 535–553.
12. Müllbacher A, Brenan M, Bowern N. The influence of non-MHC genes on the cytotoxic T cell response to modified self. *Aust J Exp Biol Med Sci* 1983; 61:57–62.
13. Arora PK, Shearer GM. Non-MHC linked genetic control of murine cytotoxic T lymphocyte response to hapten-modified syngeneic cells. *J Immunol* 1981;127:1822–1827.
14. Pasternack MS, Eisen HN. A novel serine esterase expressed by cytotoxic T lymphocytes. *Nature* 1985; 314:743–745.
15. Kramer MD, Binninger L, Schirrmacher V, et al. Characterization and isolation of a trypsin-like serine protease from a long-term culture cytolytic T cell line and its expression by functional distinct T cells. *J Immunol* 1986;136:4644–4651.
16. Masson D, Zamai M, Tschopp J. Identification of granzyme A isolated from cytotoxic T-lymphocyte-granules as one of the proteases encoded by CTL-specific genes. *FEBS Lett* 1986;208:84–88.
17. Young JD-E, Leong LG, Liu C-C, Damiano A, Wall DA, Cohn ZA. Isolation and characterization of a serine esterase from cytolytic T cell granules. *Cell* 1986;47:183–194.
18. Masson D, Tschopp J. A family of serine esterases in lytic granules of cytolytic T cells. *Cell* 1987;49:679–685.
19. Nabholz M, MacDonald HR, Cytolytic T lymphocytes. *Annu Rev Immunol* 1983;1:273–306.
20. Haddad P, Jenne DE, Kraehenbuehl O, Tschopp J. Structure and possible functions of lymphocyte granzymes. In: Sitkovsky MV, Henkart PA (eds) *Cytotoxic Cells: Effector Function, Generation, Methods.* Boston, Birhaeuser, 1993, pp 251–262.
21. Hudig D, Ewoldt GR, Woodard SL. Proteases and lymphocyte cytotoxic killing mechanisms. *Curr Opin Immunol* 1993;5:90–96.
22. Simon MM, Ebnet K, Kramer MD. Molecular analysis and possible peiotropic function(s) of the T cell-specific serine protease-1 (TSP-1). In: Sitkovsky MV, Henkart PA (eds) *Cytotoxic T cells: Generation, Recognition, Effector Functions, Methods.* Boston, Birkhäuser, 1993, pp 278–294.
23. Shi L, Kam C-M, Powers JC, Aebersold R, Greenberg AH. Purification of three cytotoxic lymphocyte granule serine proteases that induce apoptosis through distinct substrate and target cell interactions. *J Exp Med* 1992;176:1521–1529.
24. Takayama H, Trenn G, Humphrey W Jr, Bluestone JA, Henkart PA, Sitkovsky MV. Antigen receptor-triggered secretion of a trypsin-type esterase from cytotoxic T lymphocytes. *J Immunol* 1987;138: 566–569.
25. Froelich CJ, Orth K, Turbov J, et al. New paradigm for lymphocyte granule-mediated cytotoxicity: target cells bind and internalize granzyme B, but an

endosomolytic agent is necessary for cytosolic delivery and subsequent apoptosis. *J Biol Chem* 1996; 271:29073–29079.

26. Trapani JA, Browne KA, Smyth MJ, Jans DA. Localization of granzyme B in the nucleus: a putative role in the mechanism of cytotoxic lymphocyte-mediated apoptosis. *J Biol Chem* 1996;271:4127–4133.

27. Talanian RV, Yang X, Turbov J, et al. Granule-mediated killing: pathways for granzyme B-initiated apoptosis. *J Exp Med* 1997;186:1323–1331.

28. Shi LF, Mai S, Israels S, Browne K, Trapani JA, Greenberg AH. Granzyme-B (GraB) autonomously crosses the cell-membrane and perforin initiates apoptosis and grab nuclear-localization. *J Exp Med* 1997;185:855–866.

29. Simon H-G, Fruth U, Eckerskorn C, et al. Induction of T cell serine proteinase 1 (TSP-1)-specific mRNA in mouse T lymphocytes. *Eur J Immunol* 1988; 18:855–861.

30. Garcia-Sanz JA, MacDonald HR, Jenne DE, Tschopp J, Nabholz M. Cell specificity of granzyme gene expression. *J Immunol* 1990;145:3111–3118.

31. Ebnet K, Chluba-de Tapia J, Hurtenbach U, Kramer MD, Simon MM. In vivo primed mouse T cells selectively express T cell-specific serine proteinase-1 and the proteinase-like molecules granzyme B and C. *Int Immunol* 1991;3:9–19.

32. Pham CT, Ley TJ. The role of granzyme B cluster proteases in cell-mediated cytotoxicity. *Semin Immunol* 1997;9:127–133.

33. Simon MM, Hoschützky H, Fruth U, Simon H-G, Kramer MD. Purification and characterization of a T cell specific serine proteinase (TSP-1) from cloned cytolytic T lymphocytes. *EMBO J* 1986;5:3267–3274.

34. Odake S, Kam C-M, Narasimhan L, et al. Human and murine cytotoxic T lymphocyte proteases: subsite mapping with thioester substrates and inhibition of enzyme activity and cytolysis by isocoumarins. *Biochemistry* 1991;30:2217–2227.

35. Simon MM, Kramer MD. Granzyme A. *Methods Enzymol* 1994;244:68–79.

36. Tschopp J. Granzyme B. *Methods Enzymol* 1994; 244:80–87.

37. Masson D, Nabholz M, Estrade C, Tschopp J. Granules of cytolytic T-lymphocytes contain two serine esterases. *EMBO J* 1986;5:1595–1600.

38. Irmler M, Hertig S, MacDonald HR, et al. Granzyme A is an interleukin 1b-converting enzyme. *J Exp Med* 1995;181:1917–1922.

39. Simon H-G, Fruth U, Kramer MD, Simon MM. A secretable serine proteinase with highly restricted specificity from cytolytic T lymphocytes inactivates retrovirus associated reverse transcriptase. *FEBS Lett* 1987;223:352–360.

40. Ebnet K, Levelt CN, Tran TT, Eichmann K, Simon MM. Transcription of granzyme A and B genes is differentially regulated during lymphoid ontogeny. *J Exp Med* 1995;181:755–763.

41. Rouvier R, Luciani M-F, Golstein P. Fas involvement in Ca^{2+}-independent T-cell-mediated cytotoxicity. *J Exp Med* 1993;177:195–200.

42. Kägi D, Vignaux F, Ledermann BEA. Fas and perforin pathways as major mechanisms of T cell-mediated cytotoxicity. *Science* 1994;265:528–530.

43. Lowin B, Hahne M, Mattmann C, Tschopp J. Cytolytic T-cell cytotoxicity is mediated through perforin and Fas lytic pathways. *Nature* 1994;370:650–652.

44. Henkart PA. Lymphocyte-mediated cytotoxicity: two pathways and multiple effector molecules. *Immunity* 1994;1:343–346.

45. Nagata S. Apoptosis by death factor. *Cell* 1997;88: 355–365.

46. Boldin MP, Goncharov TM, Goltsev YV, Wallach D. Involvement of Mach, a novel Mort1/Fadd-interacting protease, in Fas/Apo-1- and Tnf receptor-induced cell death. *Cell* 1996;85:803–815.

47. Muzio M, Chinnaiyan AM, Kischkel FC, et al. FLICE, a novel FADD-homologous ICE/CED-3-like protease, is recruited to the CD95 (Fas/APO-1) death-inducing signaling complex. *Cell* 1996;85: 817–827.

48. Henkart PA, Millard PJ, Reynolds CW, Henkart MP. Cytolytic activity of purified cytoplasmic granules from cytotoxic rat large granular lymphocyte tumors. *J Exp Med* 1984;160:75–93.

49. Podack ER, Hengartner H, Lichtenheld MG. A central role of perforin in cytolysis? *Annu Rev Immunol* 1991;9:129–157.

50. Hayes MP, Berrebi GA, Henkart PA. Induction of target cell DNA release by the cytotoxic T lymphocyte granule protease granzyme A. *J Exp Med* 1989;170:933–947.

51. Nakajima H, Park HL, Henkart PA. Synergistic roles of granzymes A and B in mediating target cell death by rat basophilic leukemia mast cell tumors also expressing cytolysin/perforin. *J Exp Med* 1995; 181:1037–1046.

52. Shiver JW, Su L, Henkart PA. Cytotoxicity with target DNA breakdown by rat basophilic leukemia cells expressing both cytolysin and granzyme A. *Cell* 1992;71:315–322.

53. Morelli L, Lusigman Y, Lemieux S. Heterogeneity of natural killer cell subsets in NK-1.1$^+$ and NK-1.1$^-$ inbred mouse strains and their progeny. *Cell Immunol* 1992;141:148–160.

54. Müllbacher A, King NJC. Target cell lysis by natural killer cells is influenced by beta2-microglobulin expression. *Scand J Immunol* 1989;30:21–29.

55. Sarin A, Williams MS, Alexander-Miller MA, Berzofsky JA, Zacharchuk CM, Henkart PA. Target cell lysis by CTL granule exocytosis is independent of ICE/Ced-3 family proteases. *Immunity* 1997;6: 209–215.

56. Anel A, Gamen S, Alava MA, Schmitt-Verhulst AM, Pineiro A, Naval J. Inhibition of CPP32-like proteases prevents granzyme B- and Fas-, but not granzyme A-based cytotoxicity exerted by CTL clones. *J Immunol* 1997;158:1999–2006.

57. Salvesen GS, Dixit VM. Caspases: intracellular signaling by proteolysis. *Cell* 1997;91:443–446.

58. Zhivotovsky B, Burgess DH, Vangs DM, Orrenius S. Involvement of cellular proteolytic machinery in apoptosis. *Biochem Biophys Res Commun* 1997; 230:481–488.

59. Darmon AJ, Ley TJ, Nicholson DW, Bleackley RC. Cleavage of CPP32 by granzyme B represents a critical role for granzyme B in the induction of target cell DNA fragmentation. *J Biol Chem* 1996;271: 21709–21712.

60. Martin SJ, Amarante Mendes GP, Shi L, et al. The cytotoxic cell protease granzyme B initiates apoptosis in a cell-free system by proteolytic processing and activation of the ICE/CED-3 family protease, CPP32, via a novel two-step mechanism. *EMBO J* 1996;15:2407–2416.
61. Andrade F, Roy S, Nicholson D, Thornberry N, Rosen A, Casciola-Rosen L. Granzyme B directly and efficiently cleaves several downstream caspase substrates: implications for CTL-unduced apoptosis. *Immunity* 1998;8:451–460.
62. Beresford PJ, Kam C-MP, Powers JC, Lieberman J. Recombinant human granzyme A binds to two putative HLA-associated proteins and cleaves one of them. *Proc Natl Acad Sci USA* 1997;94:9285–9290.
63. Fenner F, Wittek R, Dumbell KR. *The Orthopoxviruses.* San Diego, Academic Press, 1989.
64. Blanden RV. Mechanisms of recovery from a generalized viral infection: mousepox. I. The effects of anti-thymocyte serum. *J Exp Med* 1970;132:1035–1054.
65. Blanden RV. Mechanisms of recovery from a generalized viral infection: mousepox. II. Passive transfer of recovery mechanisms with immune lymphoid cells. *J Exp Med* 1971;133:1074–1089.
66. Blanden RV. Mechanisms of cell-mediated immunity in viral infection. In: Clinical Aspects. I, vol. 4. Brent L, Holborow J (eds) *Progress in Immunology II.* Amsterdam, North Holland, 1974, pp 117–125.
67. Karupiah GR, Buller ML, van Rooijen N, Duarte CJ, Chen FH. Different roles for CD4+ and CD8+ T lymphocytes and macrophage subsets in the control of a generalized virus infection. *J Virol* 1996;70:8301–8309.
68. Simon MM, Hochgeschwender U, Brugger U, Landolfo S. Monoclonal antibodies to interferon-g inhibit interleukin 2-dependent induction of growth and maturation in lectin/antigen-reactive cytolytic T lymphocyte precursors. *J Immunol* 1986;136:2755–2762.
69. Karupiah G. Type 1 and type 2 cytokines in antiviral defense. *Vet Immunol Immunopathol* 1998;63:105–109.
70. Müllbacher A, Thallea R, Musteanu C, Simon MM. Perforin is essential for the control of ectomelia virus but not related pox viruses in mice. *J Virol* 1999;73:1665–1667.
71. Müllbacher A, Ebnet K, Blanden RV, Stehle T, Museteanu C, Simon MM. Granzyme A is essential for recovery of mice from infection with the natural cytopathic viral pathogen, ectromelia. *Proc Natl Acad Sci USA* 1996;93:5783–5787.
72. Carrel RW, Pemberton PA, Boswell DR. The serpins: evolution and adaptation in a family of protease inhibitors. *Cold Spring Harbor Symp Quant Biol* 1987;52:527–535.
73. Turner PC, Musy PY, Moyer RW. Poxvirus serpins. In: McFadden G (ed) *Viroceptors, Virokines and Related Immune Modulators Encoded by DNA Viruses.* Heidelberg, Springer, 1995, pp 67–88.
74. Buller RML, Palumbo GJ. Poxvirus pathogenesis. *Microbiol Rev* 1991;55:81–122.
75. Tewari M, Quan LT, O'Rourke K, et al. Yama/CPP32 beta, a mammalian homolog of CED-3, is a CrmA-inhibitable protease that cleaves the death substrate poly(ADP-ribose) polymerase. *Cell* 1995;81:801–809.
76. Medema J, Scaffidi C, Kischkel F, et al. FLICE is activated by association with the CD95 death-inducing signaling complex (DISC). *EMBO J* 1997;16:2794–2804.
77. Ray CA, Black RA, Cronheim SR, et al. Viral inhibition of inflammation: cowpox virus encodes an inhibitor of the interleukin-1 beta converting enzyme. *Cell* 1992;69:597–604.
78. Quan LT, Caputo A, Bleackley RC, Pickup DJ, Salvesen GS. Granzyme B is inhibited by the cowpox virus serpin cytokine response modifier A. *J Biol Chem* 1995;270:10377–10379.
79. Tewari M, Telford WG, Miller RA, Dixit VM. CrmA, a poxvirus-encoded serpin, inhibits cytotoxic T-lymphocyte mediated apoptosis. *J Biol Chem* 1995;270:22705–22708.
80. Macen JL, Garner RS, Musy PY, et al. Differential inhibition of Fas- and granule-mediated cytolysis pathways by the orthopoxvirus cytokine response modifier A/SPI-2 and SPI-1 protein. *Proc Natl Acad Sci USA* 1996;93:9108–9113.
81. Gardner I, Bowern NA, Blanden RV. Cell-mediated cytotoxicity against ectromelia virus-infected target cells. III. Role of the H-2 gene complex. *Eur J Immunol* 1975;5:122–127.
82. Moss B. Inhibition of HeLa cell protein synthesis by the vaccinia virion. *J Virol* 1968;2:1028–1037.
83. Müllbacher A, Wallich R, Moyer RW, Simon MM. Poxvirus-encoded serpins do not prevent cytolytic T cell-mediated recovery from primary infections. *J Immunol* 1999;162:7315–7321.
84. Simmons A, Tscharke DC. Anti-CD8 impairs clearance of herpes simplex virus from the nervous system: implication for the fate of virally infected neurons. *J Exp Med* 1992;175:1337–1344.

Cytotoxic Cells: Basic Mechanisms and Medical Applications, edited by Michail V. Sitkovsky and Pierre A. Henkart. Lippincott Williams & Wilkins, Philadelphia © 2000.

Chapter 15

Granulysin and NK-Lysin: Cytotoxic and Antimicrobial Proteins of Cytolytic Lymphocytes

Dennis A. Hanson and Alan M. Krensky

Department of Pediatrics, Division of Immunology and Transplantation Biology,
Stanford University School of Medicine, Stanford, California 94305, USA

Cytotoxic T lymphocytes (CTLs) and natural killer (NK) cells destroy target cells by at least two distinct mechanisms (1–3). Although both mechanisms induce target cell apoptosis specifically and directionally, the initiating molecules involved are completely different. Activation of CTL and NK cells causes release of granules containing effector molecules (perforin, granzymes) that form pores in the target cell membrane and move into the target to activate apoptosis (4,5). In addition, CTL and NK cells express Fas ligand which binds to Fas on the target cell, triggering intracellular signals that result in apoptosis (6,7). Two recently discovered molecules implicated in granule-mediated killing are human granulysin (8) and porcine NK-lysin (9). These molecules are closely related family members or homologs expressed by activated T and NK cells. Granulysin is contained in cytolytic granules and directionally released upon activation of the effector cell receptor (8). Both granulysin and NK-lysin induce target cell lysis and display antimicrobial activity (8–10). This chapter reviews the discovery, structure, and function of these cytolytic molecules.

IDENTIFICATION AND INITIAL CHARACTERIZATION

A cDNA encoded by the human granulysin gene was cloned in 1986 (11) in a search for molecules expressed in T cells 3 to 5 days after activation, a time frame in which T cells attain functional activity. The nucleotide sequence and translated open reading frame (ORF) gave no clues as to what function(s) the molecule might have. Nevertheless, because of an interesting and restricted expression pattern, studies were initiated to characterize the gene product and its regulation.

NK-lysin was isolated in 1994 based on its antibacterial activity as a heat-stable protein from pig intestinal extracts (9). Amino acid sequence analysis followed by cDNA cloning showed that NK-lysin and granulysin share significant sequence homology and belong to the saposin-like protein (SAPLIP) family of distantly related proteins (12) (discussed below).

Identification of the 519 and NKG5 (Granulysin) cDNAs

Jongstra et al. (11) used subtractive hybridization to identify and clone cDNAs expressed by a cultured human T cell line but not by an Epstein-Barr virus (EBV)-transformed B cell line. Seven cross-hybridizing clones from the screen gave an identical DNA sequence. The clone was originally named 519 and encodes the protein later designated granulysin (8) because of its location in granules and its lytic activity.

The 519 cDNA is expressed in both helper and cytotoxic T lymphocytes by Northern blot analysis (11). The message is approximately 900 bp, appearing as a diffuse band owing to the presence of three transcripts of slightly different size (see below). Low levels of the 519 message are present in the T cell tumor HUT78 and an NK tumor line YT (13), but no message is present in EBV-B cell lines or the T cell tumors MOLT-3, MOLT-4, HPB-ALL, or Jurkat (11). Tonsil, placenta, lung, liver, skeletal muscle, smooth muscle, and a primary fibroblast cell line do not express 519 (11). To date, 519 expression appears narrowly restricted to activated T cells and NK cells.

The 519 message is induced more than ten-fold in peripheral blood lymphocytes (PBLs) after mitogenic stimulation with phytohemagglutinin (PHA) or upon allostimulation with an EBV-transformed B cell line (11). Increased expression is first detected 3 days after activation and is maximal by day 5 of culture. These kinetics correspond to the time frame during which T cells attain effector function, such as cytotoxicity. Thus the subtractive hybridization approach yielded a clone with the desired expression pattern.

Sequence analysis of a full-length cDNA clone gives a product of about 850 nucleotides with an ORF of 129 residues (11). The predicted protein does not contain a hydrophobic leader sequence for entry into the secretory pathway nor is the sequence surrounding the presumed start methionine codon a close match to the Kozak consensus for translation initiation. The protein is highly positively charged, is markedly hydrophilic, and does not contain a site for N-linked glycosylation. A database search at the time of these studies did not yield any molecules with significant homology.

Subsequently, Houchins and co-workers used differential hybridization of first strand cDNA probes from NK cells and EBV-B cells on an NK cell cDNA library to isolate NK cell-specific clones (14). They reported a clone, NKG5, with high homology to the previously reported 519 clone. NKG5 contains an ORF of 145 amino acids without N-linked glycosylation sites. The 16 additional amino-terminal residues of the NKG5 predicted protein encode a signal sequence for endoplasmic reticulum insertion and entrance into the secretory pathway (15). The sequence surrounding the predicted start codon closely matches the Kozak consensus sequence.

Southern blot analysis with NKG5 and 519 specific probes suggests that these two messages originate from differential transcription of the same gene (15). Differences in sequence between 519 and NKG5 are attributed to allelic polymorphisms. Northern blots and a library screen with specific probes give a 40:1 estimate for the NKG5/519 relative abundance in NK and T cells (15). The NKG5 message is also restricted to NK and T cells, with no expression in B-LCL, U939, THP-1, K562, HL-60, or Jurkat (15).

A search at the time of publication of these NKG5 data did not reveal any significant homologies to deposited sequences other than 519 (15). Although it did not help in ascertaining a potential function, the higher relative abundance and presence of a consensus Kozak sequence suggest that the major gene product is the larger 145-amino-acid protein. In addition, the presence of a signal sequence in NKG5 places the protein in the secretory pathway.

Purification of NK-Lysin

In a search for antibacterial molecules present in the digestive tract, Andersson et al. isolated a protein with activity against *Escherichia coli* (9). Using a radial diffusion assay to monitor activity during purification, a crude sample of boiled pig intestine was fractionated by ethanol precipitation, ion exchange, and size exclusion chromatography. The sample was further purified by two rounds of reverse-phase chromatography. The insensitivity of the activity to boiling, ethanol precipitation, multiple lyophilizations, extreme changes in pH, and treatment with organic solvents aided in purifying the

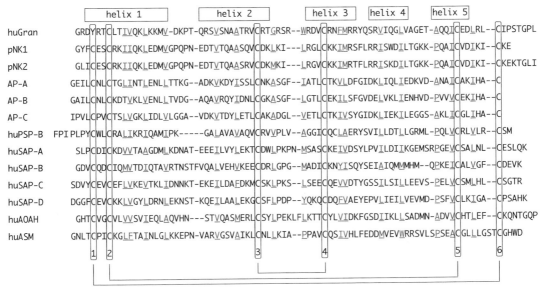

FIG. 15-1. Sequence alignment of SAPLIP family. Conserved cysteine residues, numbered 1–6 at the bottom, are contained within boxes. Lines connecting the numbers demonstrate the disulfide bonding pattern. Conserved hydrophobic residues are underlined and in a lighter typeface. The location of helices 1–5 from the NK-lysin structure (16) are shown at the top. The family members are human granulysin (*huGran*) (11), porcine NK-lysin protein (*pNK1*) and translated cDNA (*pNK2*) (9), amoebapores (*AP*) *A–C* (17), human pulmonary surfactant protein B (*huPSP-B*) (18), human saposins (*huSAP*) *A–D* (19), residues 38–121 of human acyloxyacyl hydrolase (*huAOAH*) (20), and residues 85–169 of human acid sphingomyelinase (*huASM*) (21). (Adapted from ref. 13.)

active protein to apparent homogeneity. The final step resolved the activity into two peaks differing by an amino-terminal glycine residue. Starting from 12 g of material loaded onto the sizing column, the pure peptides yielded 5.1 mg total (0.0425% of the total protein).

Amino-terminal and proteolytic fragment sequences were determined (9). The protein contains 78 residues with a predicted mass (8923.2) similar to that determined by electrospray mass spectrometry (8924.8). The protein contains six cysteines that form three intramolecular disulfide bonds. The pattern of bond formation was elucidated experimentally to be first to sixth, second to fifth, and third to fourth (Fig. 15-1).

A search of the SwissProt database at the time of this work revealed that NK-lysin is homologous to the C-terminal end of the predicted 519 and NKG5 proteins, with

about 33% identity between the pig and human proteins (9). Because of the low identity score it is unclear if granulysin and NK-lysin are strict homologs or represent individual members of a subfamily of lymphocyte-produced, cytotoxic SAPLIPs.

SAPLIP Family

Both NK-lysin and granulysin belong to the SAPLIP family of proteins (12) (Fig. 15-1). The family is named for saposins A to D, four small proteins involved in sphingolipid catabolism (19,22). Other members from mammalian sources include pulmonary surfactant protein-B (SP-B) (23), implicated in lowering surface tension at the liquid–air interface in the lung, and the lipid hydrolases acyloxyacyl hydrolase (20) and acid sphingomyelinase (21). The functions of all these proteins are mediated via interaction with lipids.

More closely related functionally to granulysin and NK-lysin are three lytic SAPLIP members termed amoebapores A, B, and C (17,24). These molecules are present within granules of the protozoan parasite *Entamoeba histolytica*. Many aspects of the killing mechanism used by *E. histolytica* and cytotoxic T and NK cells of mammals are similar. Each kills its target upon contact by the directional release of granules that contain lytic effector molecules, which suggests an ancient yet preserved cytotoxic mechanism related to innate immunity (24,25).

All of the SAPLIP family members identified to date, with the exception of granulysin, share a common spacing of six cysteine residues, with a specific cysteine bonding pattern (12) (Fig. 15-1). Granulysin contains a tyrosine instead of a cysteine at the first position. Also conserved among the family members are hydrophobic residues throughout the sequence. Gaps and insertions within the primary sequence comparison allow the best possible alignment of the cysteines and hydrophobic residues (12) (Fig. 15-1).

The net charges of SAPLIP family members vary: -3 to -6 for saposins, neutral for amoebapore A, $+4$ for PSP-B, $+6$ for NK-lysin protein, $+8$ for the NK-lysin-translated cDNA, and $+11$ for 9-kDa granulysin. Perhaps if all the small SAPLIP members (those whose entire structure consists of the approximately 80-residue SAPLIP domain) have similar folds and bind lipids, their specific functions originate in part from differences in overall charge and the precise placement of these charges (26).

Thus with the discovery of these two molecules and their significant sequence similarities, two research paths have converged. One path used the tools of molecular biology to find a cDNA clone with an interesting expression pattern but no known function for the predicted protein. The other path took a biochemical approach, purifying a protein based on a defined activity but without information as to the cellular source(s) from which the protein originated. Information from both of these approaches provides the basis of our current understanding of these new lytic molecules.

GENES, MESSAGES, AND cDNAs

Granulysin

To understand the difference between the 519 and NKG5 cDNAs and how granulysin gene expression is regulated, a genomic clone for granulysin was isolated (27). The locus spans 3.9 kb, with six exons ranging in size from 95 to 243 bp. Three transcripts termed 519, 520, and 522 were cloned and verified by ribonuclease protection assays (Fig. 15-2). The 520 cDNA and the NKG5 cDNA encode the same predicted protein, differing only in the length of 5′ untranslated sequence. The 519 message contains all of exon II, but because the 5′ end of exon I is truncated it does not encode a start codon until the distal 3′ end of exon II. The 520 message contains all of exon I, with its predicted protein product starting translation within this exon; but it deletes exon II entirely. The 522 message also contains exon I and the start codon, but because of the use of a splice acceptor located internally within exon II it contains a portion of exon II, termed exon IIb. This results in the insertion of 27 amino acids in comparison to the translated product of 520. Only about 4% of granulysin cDNA clones hybridized with an exon II-specific probe, demonstrating that the 520 message is the major transcript of the gene. An identical genomic structure was reported for NKG5 with the exception of the omission of exon II from the 519 study (28). The sequences do, however, contain a small number of single base differences that are attributed to allelic polymorphisms.

The restricted expression of the gene caused both groups that isolated genomic clones to look for and identify potential binding sites for transcription factors (27,28). However, neither TATA or CAAT elements exist in the region located immediately up-

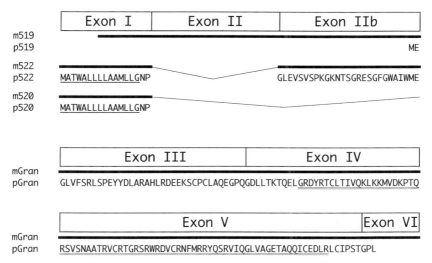

FIG. 15-2. Alternative splicing and predicted proteins of granulysin messages. Messenger RNA (*m*) delineated by *thick lines* and predicted protein (*p*) of 519, 520, and 522 granulysin transcripts are correlated to the six exons of the granulysin gene (27). The length of the boxes depicting exons does not reflect exon size. All transcripts (*mGran/pGran*) are identical in usage for exons III–VI. Excised RNA sequence due to alternative splicing is represented by *thin angled lines*. Signal sequences of p520 and p522 are *single underlined*. The 9-kDa granulysin is *double underlined* and corresponds to the SAPLIP domain of pGran with the exception of the processing of the nine C-terminal residues.

stream from the start site of transcription. Oligonucleotides corresponding to several sites in the putative promoter region bind nuclear factors in electrophoretic mobility shift assays (29). An interesting temporal expression of these activities is present within a time course of PHA activation of PBLs (a known inducer of granulysin expression). Unfortunately, assays using the granulysin "promoter" region to drive transcription/ translation of a heterologous reporter gene give low activity (fivefold or less induction). Therefore putative granulysin transcription factors were not further characterized. This leaves unanswered the question of how granulysin expression is narrowly restricted to T and NK cells.

NK-Lysin

The nucleotide sequence for NK-lysin was obtained using 3'-RACE polymerase chain reaction (PCR) of total RNA from porcine

bone marrow (9). This PCR product was then used to probe a pig bone marrow cDNA library. Two identical clones were isolated that code for NK-lysin but differ at seven residues in comparison to the protein. Six of these differences are compatible with single base changes, and one necessitates a two-base change. The differences in the sequences are ascribed to allelic polymorphisms between the pigs used to isolate the protein and the one of a different breed used to construct the bone marrow cDNA library. Thus it appears that both NK-lysin and granulysin exhibit allelic polymorphism.

The NK-lysin cDNA clone codes for five extra residues at the 3' end of the cDNA that are absent in the isolated protein (9). This implies that the protein is cleaved at the carboxy-terminus and is consistent with data for 9-kDa granulysin (8) (discussed in next section).

The 5' end of the NK-lysin cDNA encodes an additional 46 residues not present in the

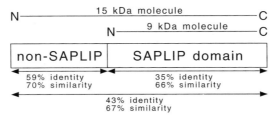

FIG. 15-3. Identity and similarity scores between granulysin and NK-lysin. Scores are reported for the SAPLIP domain, corresponding to the 9-kDa granulysin and the isolated NK-lysin protein; the amino-terminal, non-SAPLIP domain, which is 15-kDa molecule specific; and a combination of the two domains, corresponding to the entire predicted 15-kDa form. (Adapted from ref. 13.)

isolated protein (9). Unlike the SAPLIP domain, which has homology to the other family members, this region has significant homology only to granulysin. Further 5′ in the NK-lysin clone, the ORF does not match granulysin, and an in-frame start codon is not present. Although two out-of-frame ATG codons are postulated to be site(s) of translation initiation (the shift due to a putative error in the cDNA synthesis), these codons do not seem sufficiently far enough 5′ of the granulysin homologous region to allow coding of a signal sequence for entry into the secretory pathway. This suggests that the entire cDNA has not been isolated. There could not be much sequence missing, however, because the size of the clone (approximately 780 bp) is reasonably close to the size of the message on Northern blot (approximately 1,000 nt).

Interestingly, the amino-terminal non-SAPLIP domain in NK-lysin and granulysin has a higher sequence identity (59%) than the SAPLIP domain (35%) (13) (Fig. 15-3). Similarity scores are more closely matched: 70% similarity for the non-SAPLIP domain and 66% for the SAPLIP-homology domain. Studies with PSP-B indicate that the amino-terminal portion of its proprotein is critical for sorting into or retention in a regulated secretory pathway (30). This might explain the higher identity between NK-lysin and granulysin in the amino-terminal domain (i.e., to regulate intracellular trafficking of the protein).

Northern blot analysis of total RNA ex-

tracted from porcine tissues shows expression of NK-lysin in a mixture of T and NK cells (9). NK-lysin expression increases upon culture with interleukin-2 (IL-2), correlating with data for granulysin expression in human T and NK cells. Lower levels of the NK-lysin message are evident in spleen, bone marrow, and colon, with slight expression in blood and small intestine, and none in brain, tongue, liver, thymus, or lymph node. Lack of expression in thymus and lymph node demonstrates that, at least for T cells, differentiation is required for detectable levels of NK-lysin expression.

PROTEIN BIOSYNTHESIS AND LOCALIZATION

Granulysin

Two protein bands of 15 and 9 kDa, equal in intensity, are evident by immunoblot of CTL lysate (8). The amount of these proteins is upregulated 3 to 5 days after activation, in parallel to the message induction. The 15-kDa form of granulysin has not yet been purified to verify the exact amino-terminus, but studies using peptide-specific antisera suggest that it encompasses most of the predicted 520 ORF minus the peptide leader sequence (8,31) (underlined in Fig. 15-2). The experimentally determined termini of 9-kDa granulysin show that granulysin is processed from both ends (8). The residues corresponding to the 9-kDa molecule are double underlined in Figure 15-2.

Pulse chase studies on CTLs were performed to further clarify the relation between the 15- and 9-kDa proteins (8). The 15-kDa protein and two larger proteins of 18 and 22 kDa are immediate products evident after pulse labeling. The amount of these products decreases over 3 hours. The relative amount of 9-kDa protein, present at later time points after pulse labeling, is less than the larger forms over the 3 hours of this experiment. Overnight labeling, however, yields nearly equivalent amounts of steady-state 15- and 9-kDa proteins (31), correlating with immunoblot data. Longer chase times might allow an increase in the 9-kDa label in comparison to that for the 15-kDa protein. These experiments do not demonstrate that the 15-kDa protein is processed to the 9-kDa form. Further complicating this issue is the presence of three transcripts that all could produce granulysin proteins (27). Thus one message might code for one protein and another message for another protein.

To better determine the biosynthetic relation between the forms, transfectants that overexpress granulysin were generated. HUT78, a T cell leukemia line, and YT, an NK cell-like tumor, express endogenous granulysin message (13). Immunoblot analysis shows that the nonlytic, non-granule-containing HUT78 cell line expresses small amounts of 15-kDa granulysin, whereas the lytic YT cell line, which does have granules, makes small amounts of both 15- and 9-kDa proteins (31). Stable transfectants overexpressing the main 520 cDNA were analyzed for the 15- and 9-kDa forms. HUT78.520 transfectants overexpress predominantly 15-kDa granulysin, whereas YT.520 transfectants overexpress equivalent amounts of both 15- and 9-kDa protein (D. A. Hanson and A. M. Krensky, unpublished observation).

Immunoblot analysis of YT.520 cell lysates and supernatants demonstrates that the 9-kDa protein is selectively retained in the cell and not secreted in the culture media, whereas the 15-kDa protein is present in both samples. Preincubation of the cells with 100 nM concanamycin A, an inhibitor of granule acidification, significantly decreases the amount of 9-kDa protein accumulation in the cell with a concomitant increase in intracellular 15-kDa protein. Pulse-chase analysis demonstrates that 15-kDa protein is present in the lysate just after the pulse, but 9-kDa accumulation is detectable only after 2 hours of chase (D. A. Hanson and A. M. Krensky, unpublished observations).

Taken together, these data on YT.520 transfectants indicate that: (a) overexpression of 520 message results in expression of both 15- and 9-kDa proteins; (b) the 15- and 9-kDa molecules are equally abundant at steady state within the cells; (c) the 15-kDa protein can be constitutively secreted, whereas the 9-kDa form is retained within the cell; (d) the 9-kDa form does not appear until 2 hours after biosynthesis; and (e) accumulation of the 9-kDa form is dependent on an acidic cell compartment. Thus the 9-kDa protein is processed from the 15-kDa form in an acidic vesicle, most likely a cytolytic granule compartment.

At present it remains unclear if any proteins are encoded by the relatively minor 519 and 522 transcripts (27). The 519 predicted product does not contain a leader sequence and therefore might not enter the secretory pathway. Furthermore, it does not possess a Kozak sequence for efficient translation initiation and may not contribute significant amounts of protein to the pool of granulysin. The use of the same start codon for the 522 predicted protein as for the 520 predicted protein places the 522 protein in the secretory pathway, but the function or relevance of the extra 27 residues encoded by the 522 message are unknown.

Granulysin is localized to cytolytic vesicles and directionally secreted upon activation of CTLs or NK cells (8). Granulysin-specific antisera stain CTLs in a punctate pattern indicative of vesicle localization. The staining is not present in cells negative for granulysin expression. After conjugation of CTLs with target cells, vesicles containing granulysin reorient to the CTL–target interface.

Following treatment of CTLs with anti-CD3 monoclonal antibody (mAb), there is a marked reduction in staining for granulysin, indicating the regulated secretion of vesicles containing granulysin.

Two color immunofluorescence experiments using CTLs show that granulysin colocalizes with granzyme A (31), perforin (10), and RANTES (31) (separate experiments). The overlap of any two signals is never complete, with some vesicles only singly positive for either molecule. A similar finding was also recently reported for double staining of CD8[+] T cells for RANTES and granzyme A (32).

Granulysin is localized to cytolytic granules by immunogold electron microscopy (Fig. 15-4). The dense cores of the granules contain most of the monoclonal antibody staining. Other cell compartments do not stain positively. There are granule-like vesicles with identical morphology that differ in their granulysin-specific gold labeling. Thus it appears that the granules are heteroge-

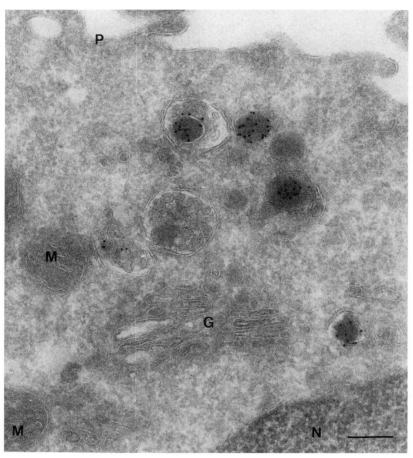

FIG. 15-4. Localization of granulysin to cytolytic granules by immunogold electron microscopy. Ultrathin cryosections of a human T cell cultured with IL-2 and PHA were reacted with a granulysin-specific monoclonal antibody (DH2) followed by protein A–gold conjugate. Nucleus (*N*), mitochondria (*M*), Golgi (*G*) complex, and plasma (*P*) membrane are marked. Bar = 200 nm. (Courtesy of J. Leusen, E. van Donselaar, R. Leckie, and P. J. Peters, University of Utrecht, The Netherlands.)

neous with respect to their contents and that not all granules contain granulysin. This agrees with immunofluorescence data described above.

Subcellular fractionation experiments indicate that granulysin is found in both high- and low-density granules in CTLs (8). The low-density granule fractions contain large amounts of both 15- and 9-kDa granulysin as assayed by immunoblots, whereas the high-density fractions contain only the 9-kDa protein.

NK-Lysin

No studies describing NK-lysin protein biosynthesis have been published. Because of the sequence similarities between the cDNAs of granulysin and NK-lysin, even outside the SAPLIP coding domain, NK-lysin is likely produced as a larger pro-protein and processed to the final product isolated from pig intestine.

CYTOTOXIC ACTIVITIES

NK-Lysin

NK-lysin kills a variety of nucleated mammalian cells including the murine NK target YAC-1 (9), the human NK target K562 (9), EBV-transformed B lymphoblastoid cells (33), and a human histiocytic lymphoma U937 cell line (33). Ninety percent of YAC-1 target cells are lysed by NK-lysin at 50 μg/ml in a 2-hour chromium release assay (9). To date, the only mammalian target cell type resistant to lysis by purified NK-lysin is red blood cells (33).

Flow cytometry using indirect immunofluorescence demonstrates that NK-lysin associates with the target cell surface (9). The staining suggests that NK-lysin physically interacts in a stable manner with the cell membrane.

Purified NK-lysin destabilizes phospholipid vesicles (34). Artificial liposomes prepared from soybean phospholipids were loaded with the fluorescent dye calcein, and

dye release was monitored after the addition of purified NK-lysin 0.1 to 2.0 μg/ml. A dose-dependent release of dye reaches its plateau 10 minutes after NK-lysin addition. NK-lysin at 2.5 μg/ml produces transient electrical conductances across a phospholipid bilayer upon application of 50 mV potential (in either direction). This implies that stable pores are not created in the lipid bilayer by NK-lysin, although macromolecules such as calcein can pass through.

The concentration of NK-lysin used in these noncellular assays is more than one log less than the concentration required for significant chromium 51 (^{51}Cr) release from target cells. Thus the interaction with the phospholipid bilayer and exhibited destabilization effect might be only one activity associated with cytotoxicity. Other activities requiring higher concentrations may be necessary to cause cell death. Alternatively, cell killing may require higher concentrations to overcome cellular repair mechanisms.

Reduction with either dithiothreitol (DTT) or thioredoxin reductase abrogates NK-lysin cytotoxicity (33), implying that intact disulfide bonds are absolutely required for NK-lysin lytic function. It is proposed that thioredoxin reductase physiologically inactivates NK-lysin, thereby controlling unmitigated cytotoxicity.

Granulysin

Purified recombinant 9-kDa granulysin causes dose-dependent lysis of a number of tumor cells in a standard 4-hour chromium release assay (8). Lysis is also observed with purified 9-kDa protein isolated from cells, demonstrating that the lytic activity is not an artifact of recombinant protein (D. A. Hanson and A. M. Krensky, unpublished observations). As for NK-lysin, recombinant 9-kDa granulysin does not lyse human red blood cells (8).

Recombinant 9-kDa granulysin is expressed using the pET28 vector in *E. coli* (8). The 9-kDa, rather than the 15-kDa, form is used because it corresponds to the domain of purified NK-lysin. Induction levels are low in this system, perhaps because granulysin is antibacterial (see below). The amino-terminal His-tag used for purification is removed by thrombin treatment, leaving recombinant 9-kDa granulysin with four extra residues at the N-terminus, GSHM. A quadruple mutant in which all of the cysteines are changed to serines was also created.

Recombinant 9-kDa granulysin exhibits two features suggesting that it is correctly folded in comparison to the cellularly derived 9-kDa form. The first is that a monoclonal antibody (DH2 mAb) recognizes both recombinant and cellular 9-kDa proteins, but boiling the proteins in the presence of DTT destroys this reactivity. Second, both recombinant and cellular 9-kDa granulysin migrate faster on nonreducing sodium dodecyl sulfate-polyacrylamide gel electrophoresis (SDS-PAGE) than do the DTT-reduced samples. Presumably the disruption of intramolecular disulfide bonds unfolds the molecule, destroying the conformational DH2 mAb epitope, making it less compact, and slowing its migration on SDS-PAGE (D. A. Hanson and A. M. Krensky, unpublished observations).

Like NK-lysin, granulysin lytic activity is unaffected by boiling for 10 minutes. However, treatment of granulysin with DTT increases its specific activity, whereas this destroys the lytic activity of NK-lysin (33) and amoebapores (35). Similarly, the quadruple cysteine-to-serine mutant granulysin has a higher specific activity than the wild-type recombinant protein (D. A. Hanson and A. M. Krensky, unpublished observations). These findings indicate that disulfide bonds are not absolutely required for granulysin-mediated cytotoxicity. The mechanism of increased lytic activity associated with reduced or mutant forms of the protein remains unclear.

The type of cell death caused by granulysin was investigated. It induces apoptosis of Jurkat T cells as judged by annexin V staining, nuclear fragmentation, and chromatin condensation (36). Cell death is associated with a significant increase in ceramide and a concomitant decrease in sphingomyelin (SM). A sixfold increase in the ceramide/SM ratio is observed in association with granulysin-mediated cytotoxicity of Jurkat cells. Although exogenous ceramide is known to induce apoptosis (37,38), pretreatment of Jurkat cells with fumonisin-B to deplete cellular ceramide and SM does not affect granulysin-mediated cytotoxicity or nuclear damage (36). Therefore ceramide generation is associated with, but not required for, granulysin-induced lysis and apoptosis.

Caspases have also been implicated in granulysin-mediated cytotoxicity. The granulysin-induced ceramide production pathway uses Z-VAD-fmk-sensitive, Ac-DEVD-CHO-insensitive enzyme(s) (36). Another granulysin-induced cell death pathway does not require ceramide generation or involve either Z-VAD-fmk- or Ac-DEVD-CHO-sensitive enzymes. Both pathways, however, lead to disintegration of the nucleus and death of the cell. The precise enzymes involved in either pathway have not yet been identified.

ANTIMICROBIAL ACTIVITIES

NK-Lysin

NK-lysin kills many, but not all, gram-positive and gram-negative bacteria and yeast (9). The basis for its specificity of lysis remains unknown. NK-lysin protein was isolated based on its ability to inhibit the growth of *E. coli* D21, which it does with a specific activity in the low micromolar range. *Bacillus megaterium* is also highly sensitive, and slightly lower activity is observed against *Candida albicans, Streptococcus pyogenes,* a porcine pathogenic strain of *E. coli,* and *Acinetobacter calcoaceticus.* NK-lysin does not kill *Salmonella typhimurium, Pseudomonas aeruginosa,* or *Staphylococcus aureus.* Reduction by either DTT or mammalian thioredoxin reductase inhibits the anti-*E. coli* activity of NK-lysin (33), again highlighting the importance of disulfide bonds for the active structure.

Granulysin

Granulysin also kills a variety of microbes (10). It exhibits potent antibacterial properties in the range of 1 to 10 μM against *Salmonella typhimurium, Listeria monocytogenes, Escherichia coli,* and *Staphylococcus aureus.* At slightly higher concentration, it kills *Candida albicans, Cryptococcus neoformans,* and the parasite *Leishmania major.*

Mycobacterium tuberculosis (*M. tb.*) is an intracellular pathogen (39). Stenger et al. described two distinct phenotypes of CD1-restricted/*M. tb.*-specific human T cells (40). The CD4$^-$, CD8$^-$ double negative subset kills *M. tb.*-infected macrophages via a Fas–FasL interaction, but the intracellular *M. tb.* remain viable. In contrast, the CD8$^+$ subset kills both the macrophage and the *M. tb.* Although the directed exocytosis of cytolytic granules by CD8$^+$ cells mediates target cell death, lysis of *M. tb.* does not appear to involve either perforin or granzymes. Because of its broad antimicrobial activity, granulysin was evaluated as a potential mediator of granule-dependent *M. tb.* lysis. In support of this hypothesis, CD4$^-$, CD8$^-$ cells, which do not lyse intracellular *M. tb.,* do not express detectable granulysin, whereas CD8$^+$ cells, which kill intracellular *M. tb.,* express high levels of granulysin (10).

Recombinant granulysin kills extracellular *M. tb.* More than 80% of *M. tb.* are killed with 25 μM recombinant granulysin, whereas a control protein has no effect (10). Viability of intracellular *M. tb.,* however, is not affected; and the infected monocytes are only modestly lysed by granulysin at this range. Purified perforin, however, is capable of lysing monocytes. Although neither granulysin nor perforin has any effect on viability of intracellular *M. tb.* alone, the combination eliminates more than 90% of the intracellular *M. tb.* This indicates that granulysin and perforin released from CTLs via granules onto

infected cells may be responsible for the ability of CTLs to kill intracellular *M. tb.*

STRUCTURAL STUDIES

NK-Lysin

The solution phase nuclear magnetic resonance (NMR) structure of NK-lysin is the first solved for a SAPLIP family member (16) (Fig. 15-5). Five amphipathic helices comprise a single globular domain that is held together by the three disulfide bonds. The long helix 1 forms the center of the molecule. Helices 2 and 3 are packed from one side and helices 4 and 5 from the other side. Side chains of residues conserved among family members make up the hydrophobic interior of the NK-lysin structure. Gaps and insertions within the primary sequences of family members, made to allow for best possible alignment of cysteines and conserved

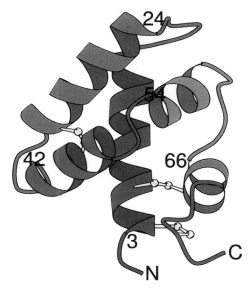

FIG. 15-5. Ribbon diagram of NK-lysin structure. *N,* amino terminus; *C,* carboxy terminus. *Numbers* identify the amino-terminus residues of the five helices. Disulfide bonds are drawn as rods between cysteine residues. (From ref. 16, with permission.)

hydrophobic residues, map to the regions that connect the five amphipathic helices. The bottom of the molecule contains exposed hydrophobic side chains; the middle concentrates many of the positively charged side chains; and the upper half contains more negatively charged residues. A hypothesis on the functional consequences of this observation is outlined in the next section.

The possibility that tertiary but not secondary structure is affected by reduction is raised by circular dichroism (CD) spectra analysis of NK-lysin. Its CD spectra does not change appreciably upon reduction of disulfides (26). Both CD and Fourier transform infrared spectroscopy indicate that NK-lysin structure is also not appreciably different in aqueous solution or when associated with lipid (26,34).

The fluorescence of the single tryptophan in NK-lysin at position 58, located in helix 4 of the NMR structure (Fig. 15-5), shows a shift from a maximum of 350 nm for free NK-lysin to 325 nm for phospholipid vesicle-bound protein (34). This indicates a change to a more hydrophobic environment upon lipid bilayer binding. In addition, fluorescence of this tryptophan is protected from quenching by iodide when bound to lipids but not when free in solution (34), further evidence that the molecule physically inserts into the lipid bilayer upon binding.

Granulysin

A tyrosine residue substitutes for the conserved first cysteine of the SAPLIP domain in the granulysin sequence (Fig. 15-1). Overall structural differences between granulysin and other SAPLIP family members due to this change are unlikely because of the close spacing between the first and second cysteines and the fifth and sixth cysteines of the SAPLIP family. The proteolytic cleavage of the sixth cysteine in purified 9-kDa granulysin (8) also should not affect the structure of granulysin because it lies outside the five

amphipathic helices that shape the molecule (16).

Although no direct biophysical structural studies have been performed on granulysin, a few pieces of data hint at differences between the structures of the 15- and 9-kDa forms. A difference in the amenability of the 9- and 15-kDa protein to reverse-phase chromatography might be due to a difference in solubility at the low pH (D. A. Hanson and A. M. Krensky, unpublished observations). Alternatively, the amino-terminal extension of the 15-kDa form might mask or alter a structure within the 9-kDa SAPLIP domain necessary for retention on the reverse-phase packing. Supporting evidence comes from a deduced differential affinity for the two proteins by the DH2 monoclonal antibody, which has a higher reactivity for the 9-kDa form (D. A. Hanson and A. M. Krensky, unpublished observations). Because the 15-kDa granulysin molecule encompasses the 9-kDa SAPLIP domain, the lower affinity of the DH2 antibody for the 15-kDa protein must be due to the presence of the amino-terminal non-SAPLIP piece. Thus the presence of the non-SAPLIP domain physically alters the 9-kDa structure.

It is attractive to postulate that the altered 15-kDa protein is a nonlytic structure in comparison to the processed 9-kDa molecule. If granulysin were translated directly as the 9-kDa form in the endoplasmic reticulum (ER) of the expressing cell, it could kill the cell by disrupting the ER membrane integrity. If, however, it is made first as a pro-protein in a nonlytic form, then transported to an acidic vesicle for further processing to a lytic form, the cell would be protected from a potentially toxic protein. The cell may be protected from lysis once the protein is contained in cytolytic granules by low pH or association of the positively charged granulysin with sulfated proteoglycans, which would prevent interaction with the lipid bilayer of the granule. This model is analogous to one recently proposed for perforin, which also undergoes processing in cytolytic granules (41).

MODES OF ACTION

The most likely mechanisms by which granulysin and NK-lysin mediate target cell death are membrane disruption (34) and initiation of apoptosis (36). Membrane disruption may involve pore formation as proposed for the amoebapores (42) or electroporation as proposed for NK-lysin (34). In the "barrel stave" pore formation model, amoebapores form a pore through a target cell lipid bilayer, analogous to a barrel, by the self-assembly of bilayer spanning molecules, analogous to the staves of a barrel. Supporting this model are data that chemically crosslinked complexes of amoebapores increase in size upon association with lipids (43). In contrast, NK-lysin appears not to form stable pores.

Ruysschaert et al. proposed a model in which the hydrophobic portion of NK-lysin dips into the lipid portion of the bilayer, allowing the positively charged middle to interact with the negatively charged head groups of the phospholipids, leaving the negatively charged top of the molecule exposed to the outside of the cell (34). By analogy to annexin V, which is also believed to complex superficially with membranes, associated protein(s) can cause an electrostatic field of sufficient potential difference across the bilayer to allow permeabilization via "electroporation" (44). Transient membrane disorder and rearrangement caused by the electric field allow molecules to pass through the membrane. Such a mechanism would account for the variable conductance observed upon NK-lysin addition to a planar phospholipid bilayer. It is of note, however, that these studies were performed at an NK-lysin concentration one log less than that necessary for cell lysis, leaving open the possibility that stable pores may form at higher concentrations.

Additional studies indicate that granulysin induces the target cell to participate in its own death via both activation of the caspase cascade and generation of ceramide from sphingomyelin (36). One unresolved question addresses the mechanism of red blood cell resistance to lysis by either NK-lysin or granulysin. This could be explained by the absence of required apoptotic machinery in red blood cells or attributed to the unique composition of their lipid membrane.

Whatever the precise mechanism of action of the lytic SAPLIP family members, it is clear that they mediate cytolysis via a new pathway shared by CTLs and NK cells with relevance to both innate and adaptive immunity. Although both NK-lysin and granulysin appear relevant to microbial and tumor immunity, future investigations will be required to clarify the physiologic role of these newly recognized granule-associated lytic molecules.

Acknowledgments

This work was supported by NIH grants RO1 DK35008 and AI43348. Dennis A. Hanson was the recipient of a National Science Foundation Graduate Research Fellowship. Alan M. Krensky is a Burroughs Wellcome Scholar in Experimental Therapeutics and the Shelagh Galligan Professor of Pediatrics. The authors thank Carol Clayberger, Allan Kaspar, and Susi Pena for their critical reading of the manuscript.

REFERENCES

1. Henkart PA, Sitkovsky MV. Cytotoxic lymphocytes: two ways to kill target cells. *Curr Biol* 1994; 4:923–925.
2. Podack ER. Execution and suicide: cytotoxic lymphocytes enforce draconian laws through separate molecular pathways. *Curr Opin Immunol* 1995; 7:11–16.
3. Atkinson EA, Bleackley RC. Mechanisms of lysis by cytotoxic T cells. *Crit Rev Immunol* 1995; 15:359–384.
4. Trapani JA, Smyth MJ. Killing by cytotoxic T cells and natural killer cells: multiple granule serine proteases as initiators of DNA fragmentation. *Immunol Cell Biol* 1993;71:201–208.
5. Lowin B, Peitsch MC, Tschopp J. Perforin and granzymes: crucial effector molecules in cytolytic T lymphocyte and natural killer cell-mediated cytotoxicity. *Curr Top Microbiol Immunol* 1995;198:1–24.
6. Berke G. The Fas-based mechanism of lymphocytotoxicity. *Hum Immunol* 1997;54:1–7.

7. Golstein P. Fas-based T cell-mediated cytotoxicity. *Curr Top Microbiol Immunol* 1995;198:25–37.

8. Pena SV, Hanson DA, Carr BA, Goralski TJ, Krensky AM. Processing, subcellular localization, and function of 519 (granulysin), a human late T cell activation molecule with homology to small, lytic, granule proteins. *J Immunol* 1997;158:2680–2688.

9. Andersson M, Gunne H, Agerberth B, et al. NK-lysin, a novel effector peptide of cytotoxic T and NK cells: structure and cDNA cloning of the porcine form, induction by interleukin 2, antibacterial and antitumour activity. *EMBO J* 1995;14:1615–1625.

10. Stenger S, Hanson DA, Teitelbaum R, et al. An antimicrobial activity of cytolytic T cells mediated by granulysin. *Science* 1998;282:121–125.

11. Jongstra J, Schall TJ, Dyer BJ, et al. The isolation and sequence of a novel gene from a human functional T cell line. *J Exp Med* 1987;165:601–614.

12. Munford RS, Sheppard PO, O'Hara PJ. Saposin-like proteins (SAPLIP) carry out diverse functions on a common backbone structure. *J Lipid Res* 1995;36:1653–1663.

13. Pena SV, Krensky AM. Granulysin, a new human cytolytic granule-associated protein with possible involvement in cell-mediated cytotoxicity. *Semin Immunol* 1997;9:117–125.

14. Houchins JP, Yabe T, McSherry C, Miyokawa N, Bach FH. Isolation and characterization of NK cell or NK/T cell-specific cDNA clones. *J Mol Cell Immunol* 1990;4:295–304.

15. Yabe T, McSherry C, Bach FH, Houchins JP. A cDNA clone expressed in natural killer and T cells that likely encodes a secreted protein. *J Exp Med* 1990;172:1159–1163.

16. Liepinsh E, Andersson M, Ruysschaert JM, Otting G. Saposin fold revealed by the NMR structure of NK-lysin [letter]. *Nat Struct Biol* 1997;4:793–795.

17. Leippe M, Andra J, Nickel R, Tannich E, Muller-Eberhard HJ. Amoebapores, a family of membranolytic peptides from cytoplasmic granules of Entamoeba histolytica: isolation, primary structure, and pore formation in bacterial cytoplasmic membranes. *Mol Microbiol* 1994;14:895–904.

18. Jacobs KA, Phelps DS, Steinbrink R, et al. Isolation of a cDNA clone encoding a high molecular weight precursor to a 6-kDa pulmonary surfactant-associated protein. *J Biol Chem* 1987;262:9808–9811.

19. Kishimoto Y, Hiraiwa M, O'Brien JS. Saposins: structure, function, distribution, and molecular genetics. *J Lipid Res* 1992;33:1255–1267.

20. Hagen FS, Grant FJ, Kuijper JL, et al. Expression and characterization of recombinant human acyloxyacyl hydrolase, a leukocyte enzyme that deacylates bacterial lipopolysaccharides. *Biochemistry* 1991;30:8415–8423.

21. Schuchman EH, Suchi M, Takahashi T, Sandhoff K, Desnick RJ. Human acid sphingomyelinase: isolation, nucleotide sequence and expression of the full-length and alternatively spliced cDNAs. *J Biol Chem* 1991;266:8531–8539.

22. O'Brien JS, Kishimoto Y. Saposin proteins: structure, function, and role in human lysosomal storage disorders. *FASEB J* 1991;5:301–308.

23. Whitsett JA, Nogee LM, Weaver TE, Horowitz AD. Human surfactant protein B: structure, function,

24. Leippe M, Muller-Eberhard HJ. The pore-forming peptide of Entamoeba histolytica, the protozoan parasite causing human amoebiasis. *Toxicology* 1994;87:5–18.

25. Leippe M. Ancient weapons: NK-lysin, is a mammalian homolog to pore-forming peptides of a protozoan parasite [letter]. *Cell* 1995;83:17–18.

26. Andersson M, Curstedt T, Jornvall H, Johansson J. An amphipathic helical motif common to tumourolytic polypeptide NK-lysin and pulmonary surfactant polypeptide SP-B. *FEBS Lett* 1995;362:328–332.

27. Manning WC, O'Farrell S, Goralski TJ, Krensky AM. Genomic structure and alternative splicing of 519, a gene expressed late after T cell activation. *J Immunol* 1992;148:4036–4042.

28. Houchins JP, Kricek F, Chujor CS, et al. Genomic structure of NKG5, a human NK and T cell-specific activation gene. *Immunogenetics* 1993;37:102–107.

29. Ortiz BD. Regulation of RANTES and other human late T-cell activation genes: models of temporal regulation and cell-type specific expression [dissertation]. Stanford, Stanford University, 1996.

30. Lin S, Akinbi HT, Breslin JS, Weaver TE. Structural requirements for targeting of surfactant protein B (SP-B) to secretory granules in vitro and in vivo. *J Biol Chem* 1996;271:19689–19695.

31. Pena SV. Characterization of a cytolytic granule-associated lytic protein, granulysin: a human late T cell activation member of the saposin-like protein family [dissertation]. Stanford, Stanford University, 1997.

32. Wagner L, Yang OO, Garcia-Zepeda EA, et al. Beta-chemokines are released from HIV-1-specific cytolytic T-cell granules complexed to proteoglycans. *Nature* 1998;391:908–911.

33. Andersson M, Holmgren A, Spyrou G. NK-lysin, a disulfide-containing effector peptide of T-lymphocytes, is reduced and inactivated by human thioredoxin reductase: implication for a protective mechanism against NK-lysin cytotoxicity. *J Biol Chem* 1996;271:10116–10120.

34. Ruysschaert JM, Goormaghtigh E, Homble F, Andersson M, Liepinsh E, Otting G. Lipid membrane binding of NK-lysin. *FEBS Lett* 1998;425:341–344.

35. Leippe M, Tannich E, Nickel R, et al. Primary and secondary structure of the pore-forming peptide of pathogenic Entamoeba histolytica. *EMBO J* 1992;11:3501–3506.

36. Gamen S, Hanson DA, Kaspar A, Naval J, Krensky AM, Anel A. Granulysin-induced apoptosis. I. Involvement of at least two distinct pathways. *J Immunol* 1998;161:1758–1764.

37. Gamen S, Marzo I, Anel A, Pineiro A, Naval J. CPP32 inhibition prevents Fas-induced ceramide generation and apoptosis in human cells. *FEBS Lett* 1996;390:232–237.

38. Obeid LM, Linardic CM, Karolak LA, Hannun YA. Programmed cell death induced by ceramide. *Science* 1993;259:1769–1771.

39. Schlesinger LS. Entry of Mycobacterium tuberculosis into mononuclear phagocytes. *Curr Top Microbiol Immunol* 1996;215:71–96.

40. Stenger S, Mazzaccaro RJ, Uyemura K, et al. Differential effects of cytolytic T cell subsets on intracellular infection. *Science* 1997;276:1684–1687.

41. Uellner R, Zvelebil MJ, Hopkins J, et al. Perforin is activated by a proteolytic cleavage during biosynthesis which reveals a phospholipid-binding C2 domain. *EMBO J* 1997;16:7287–7296.

42. Keller F, Hanke W, Trissl D, Bakker-Grunwald T. Pore-forming protein from Entamoeba histolytica forms voltage- and pH-controlled multi-state channels with properties similar to those of the barrel-stave aggregates. *Biochim Biophys Acta* 1989; 982:89–93.

43. Leippe M, Ebel S, Schoenberger OL, Horstmann RD, Muller-Eberhard HJ. Pore-forming peptide of pathogenic Entamoeba histolytica. *Proc Natl Acad Sci USA* 1991;88:7659–7663.

44. Huber R, Berendes R, Burger A, et al. Crystal and molecular structure of human annexin V after refinement: implications for structure, membrane binding and ion channel formation of the annexin family of proteins. *J Mol Biol* 1992;223:683–704.

Cytotoxic Cells: Basic Mechanisms and Medical Applications, edited by Michail V. Sitkovsky and Pierre A. Henkart. Lippincott Williams & Wilkins, Philadelphia © 2000.

Chapter 16

TCR-Induced Signaling for Cytotoxicity: Regulation of CD95L (Fas Ligand) Expression in Activated T Lymphocytes

Lyse A. Norian and *Gary A. Koretzky

*Interdisciplinary Graduate Program in Immunology and *Department of Internal Medicine, University of Iowa, Iowa City, Iowa 52242, USA*

T lymphocytes recognize specific peptide–major histocompatibility complex (MHC) complexes and respond by undergoing clonal proliferation and differentiation into effector cells. This expansion of T cell numbers is required for the immune system to combat challenges by viral and intracellular bacterial pathogens. However, once the inciting antigenic stimulus has been cleared, the remaining population of activated T lymphocytes must itself be eliminated to maintain lymphoid tissue homeostasis and decrease chances that circulating cross-reactive T cells could become activated by self antigens. One way in which these cells are eliminated is through a process termed activation-induced cell death (AICD) (1,2). AICD is mediated in part by the interactions of CD95 (Fas) and CD95L (Fas ligand), both of which are upregulated on the surface of activated T cells. These interactions trigger an intracellular cascade involving the caspase family of proteases, which culminates in the apoptotic death of the CD95-bearing cell (3,4). The physiologic activator of CD95, CD95L, is a transmembrane 40-kDa protein belonging to the tumor necrosis factor (TNF) family (5,6). Defects in the expression of either CD95 or CD95L are known to cause lymphoproliferative diseases and autoimmunity in mice and humans, highlighting the important contri-butions of these molecules in the maintenance of immune cell homeostasis (7–9). Therefore the mechanisms controlling CD95L production in activated T cells are critical for understanding the initiation of AICD at the molecular level.

CD95L AS A MEDIATOR OF ACTIVATION-INDUCED CELL DEATH

With appropriate co-stimulation, ligation of the T cell receptor (TCR) leads to cytokine production and proliferation, hallmarks of T lymphocyte activation. However, restimulation of previously activated T cells leads instead to apoptosis (10–13). The function of CD95 as a death-inducer is illustrated by studies demonstrating that engagement of this molecule with antibodies leads to T cell apoptosis (14,15). A direct role for CD95/CD95L regulation of AICD was first implicated in the lpr and gld strains of mice. The lpr strain has defective CD95 expression due to a transposon insertion in the *fas* (CD95) gene (7), and the gld strain has defective CD95L expression due to a point mutation that makes the protein nonfunctional (8). In both murine models, activated T cells are unable to undergo AICD in response to superantigen or anti-CD3 stimulation (16,17).

This inability to maintain homeostasis through AICD likely is responsible for the accumulation of activated T lymphocytes and fatal autoimmunity in both strains of mice. More recently, studies of patients with autoimmune lymphoproliferative syndrome (ALPS), also known as Canale-Smith syndrome, reveal that mutations in CD95 leading to impaired CD95-mediated apoptosis result in autoimmune disease in humans as well (9,18).

The phenomenon of AICD in T cells has been studied extensively. When activated T cells are restimulated via TCR or CD3 ligation, 30% to 70% undergo AICD within 20 hours (10–13,19–22). CD95 and CD95L were shown to be critical mediators of this type of cell death, as blockade of CD95/CD95L interactions markedly decreases apoptosis (19–22). In a comparison between primary and secondary *in vitro* stimulation of murine CD4$^+$ T cells, CD95L-mediated cytotoxicity is augmented in secondary responses (23). This is consistent with the hypothesis that AICD affects restimulated T cells rather than naïve T cells. An interesting observation is that CD95/CD95L interactions can mediate cell suicide and fratricide of neighboring cells (20,22). Initial studies into the regulation of AICD indicated that transcription and de novo protein synthesis were needed for apoptosis to occur (12), and later work demonstrated that both events were needed for CD95L expression and specific cytotoxicity (23). Once on the surface, CD95L is cleaved by a metalloproteinase, but the relative contributions of the soluble versus membrane-bound form of CD95L in AICD remain controversial (24–26).

Early characterization of CD95L expression, as detected by mRNA production, found that it is induced in T cells following a variety of stimuli, including ligation of the TCR, treatment with concanavalin A or high concentrations of interleukin-2 (IL-2), or treatment with pharmacologic agents that activate protein kinase C-dependent and calcium-responsive signaling events [phorbol myristic acetate (PMA) plus ionomycin]

(5,27). Exposure to IL-2 has been shown to enhance AICD of murine T cells by increasing the amount of CD95L mRNA present compared to cells restimulated through the TCRs alone (28). These studies and others have measured CD95L mRNA levels rather than protein. One reason for this is that CD95L protein is present at low levels on the T cell surface, even after upregulated expression, making its detection with antibodies difficult.

The kinetics of CD95L induction following TCR stimulation have also been investigated. CD95L mRNA can be detected within 1 to 6 hours of TCR ligation (20,21). This high level of mRNA is maintained for up to 4 days after stimulation (29). In comparison, CD95L-mediated cytotoxicity is not detectable until 8 to 12 hours after TCR ligation and does not peak until approximately 20 hours after stimulation (20–22).

CD95L is expressed differentially on distinct T cell subsets. Ligation of the TCR on naïve CD4$^+$ cells induces differentiation from T-helper 0 (Th0) cells into Th1 or Th2 populations, an event influenced by the cytokine environment at the time of antigenic exposure. These helper T cells have functions that differ from those of CD8$^+$ cells, which demonstrate most of the T cell cytolytic activity. Activated CD4$^+$ cells express less than 10% of the CD95L mRNA produced by comparably activated CD8$^+$ T cells (27). Initial examination of Th1 and Th2 populations indicated that all Th1 clones but only some Th2 clones express CD95L mRNA (27). However, in other Th2 cell lines, CD95L protein expression is comparable to that observed on Th1 lines (30,31). Although CD4$^+$ cells express less CD95L, they have been utilized in many studies examining the regulation of this molecule. A recent report indicates that CD4 ligation alone is sufficient to upregulate CD95L expression and cell death in primary, unstimulated human peripheral blood T cells (32). It appears that once T cells are activated the reverse effect of CD4 ligation is observed, in that both AICD and CD95L expression are inhibited (33).

From these data it is apparent that expression of CD95L is linked to T cell activation, and that regulation occurs at least partially at the level of transcription. To appreciate the complexity with which CD95L induction is controlled, the intracellular events that couple TCR ligation to transcriptional activation of the CD95L gene must also be examined.

TCR-DEPENDENT SIGNALING EVENTS THAT REGULATE CD95L EXPRESSION

Until recently, little was understood about the intracellular mechanisms that regulate inducible CD95L expression in activated T cells. In contrast, many of the TCR-initiated signal transduction pathways that induce cellular activation are well defined. Phosphorylation and activation of src family protein tyrosine kinases (PTKs) are two of the first intracellular responses to TCR ligation (34,35) and are required for the induction of downstream cellular responses, including the production of IL-2. These kinases are dependent on the phosphatase CD45 for activation. Activated Lck or Fyn, members of the src family PTKs relevant for T cell activation, then leads to the phosphorylation and activation of ZAP-70, a member of the syk family of PTKs. ZAP-70 is recruited to tandem tyrosine-phosphorylated motifs contained within the cytoplasmic tails of the CD3ζ and ε components of the TCR complex. These motifs, known as immunoreceptor-based tyrosine activation motifs (ITAMs), serve as docking sites for activated ZAP-70. Many downstream pathways are dependent on the completion of these TCR-proximal events; activation of the Ras cascade, activation of protein kinase C, and generation of intracellular calcium flux are well characterized examples (34,35). These signal transduction events are commonly used within activated T cells to control the expression of a variety of inducible genes.

Initial studies designed to elucidate which TCR-mediated signal transduction events in-

fluence CD95L expression focused on these pathways. TCR-dependent signaling events known to be required for CD95L expression are shown in Figure 16-1. Studies utilizing the PTK inhibitors genistein and herbimycin A provided the first evidence that PTK activation is required for CD95L induction (36). Administration of either compound inhibits the ability of T cell clones to mediate CD95L-specific lysis of targets (36). Cell lines deficient in either Lck or ZAP-70 provided more direct evidence for the involvement of these specific kinases in the regulation of CD95L expression. The Lck-deficient Jurkat T cell derivative JCaM.1 (37) fails to upregulate CD95L mRNA in response to stimulation through the TCR, but administration of the phorbol ester phorbol myristic acetate (PMA) in conjunction with ionomycin is able to bypass the Lck deficiency and induce CD95L message (38). Similarly, a ZAP-70-deficient Jurkat derivative (39) also fails to induce CD95L mRNA following anti-CD3 stimulation (40). Both cell lines are resistant to AICD, despite the observations that levels of CD95 protein are comparable to the parental Jurkat, and direct ligation of CD95 on either cell line with agonistic antibodies triggers apoptosis (38,40,41). This demonstrates that the defects in AICD are upstream of CD95 signal transduction. Thus, the failure of these mutants to undergo apoptosis following TCR engagement appears to be attributable to the loss of CD95L expression (38,40).

Inducible CD95L expression also requires the association of ZAP-70 with the CD3ζ chain. This was shown in a mutant cell line in which CD3ζ does not associate with the $\alpha\beta$TCR complex (42). This mutation results in an inability of ZAP-70 to associate with the ζ chain, although ZAP-70 is phosphorylated normally in response to TCR ligation. This defect selectively inhibits CD95L mRNA production in activated cells as other functions such as IL-2 production remain unaltered (42,43). These data support a previous model suggesting that the cytoplasmic chain of the CD3ζ chain was responsible for

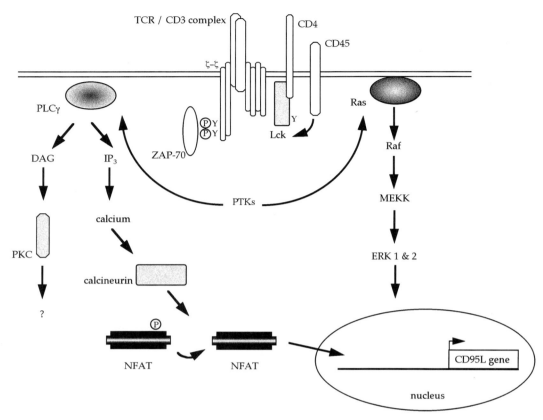

FIG. 16-1. TCR-mediated signaling events known to be required for the transcriptional activation of CD95L. Ligation of the TCR leads to CD45-dependent activation of the src family PTK, Lck. Phosphorylation of CD3ζ chain ITAMs results in the interaction of the syk family PTK, ZAP-70, through its SH2 domains. PTK activity triggers downstream events, such as the Ras cascade, and PLCγ-dependent mobilization of intracellular calcium and PKC activation. The resultant calcium flux in turn activates the serine/threonine phosphatase calcineurin, which dephosphorylates regulatory amino acids on NFAT proteins. Dephosphorylated NFAT is then able to translocate to the nucleus and contribute to CD95L gene transcription. See text for details.

initiating signals that led to an increase in CD95L message (44).

In addition to the involvement of PTKs in regulating activation-induced CD95L expression, calcium mobilization and the serine/threonine phosphatase calcineurin can also influence CD95L expression. Early research indicated that activation of this calcium/calmodulin-dependent phosphatase was needed for optimal induction of CD95L because pretreatment of T cell clones with cyclosporin A, a known inhibitor of calcineurin, decreased CD95L-mediated cyto-

toxicity and CD95L mRNA (36). Further evidence was provided by studies where pretreatment of T cell hybridomas with either cyclosporin A or FK506 blocked CD95L transcription and AICD (45).

Cyclosporin A and FK506 are immunosuppressive drugs that act by inhibiting the activation of calcineurin (46). The most widely recognized substrate for calcineurin is the transcription factor nuclear factor of activated T cells (NFAT). In resting T cells, NFAT proteins are localized to the cytoplasm and are found with key regulatory residues phosphorylated (47). Calcineurin, activated in response to a calcium flux, dephosphorylates these residues. This allows NFAT to translocate into the nucleus where it can bind response elements in the promoters of such genes as IL-2, IL-4, and TNF-α (47). NFAT binding sites are frequently found adjacent to those for the AP-1 family of transcription factors, and association between the two proteins is thought to stabilize NFAT–DNA binding interactions (47). Interestingly, activated T cells from mice made deficient in $NFAT_p$ (one NFAT family member) display greatly reduced levels of CD95L mRNA compared to stimulated cells from wild-type mice (48). Therefore these data implicate NFAT in the control of CD95L expression. Further evidence supporting possible contributions of NFAT in transcriptional regulation of the CD95L gene are discussed later.

TRANSCRIPTIONAL REGULATION OF CD95L

A number of laboratories have made use of reporter constructs to study how transcription of the CD95L gene is regulated. Specific promoter regions, based on the published sequence of the CD95L promoter (49,50), ranging from triplications of 20 basepair (bp) sites to stretches of 2.3 kilobases (kb) of DNA are used to drive expression of heterologous reporter genes (50–55). This model system allows examination of the regions of the CD95L promoter responsible for TCR-mediated induction of transcription and the signaling events that control transcriptional activation through these regions.

We generated a reporter construct in which 486 bp of promoter DNA are used to drive expression of a luciferase reporter gene and used it to study the involvement of several signal transduction mediators in CD95L promoter activation (51). When this construct is transfected transiently into Jurkat cells, reporter activity mimics production of endogenous CD95L mRNA as demonstrated by RNase protection assays. Use of

this construct in a CD45-deficient Jurkat derivative confirmed that CD45 is necessary for TCR-mediated transcriptional activation of the CD95L promoter (51). Reporter activity in these cells is minimal, whereas activation of both the CD45-deficient and parental Jurkat cells with the combination of PMA plus ionomycin produces substantial increases in reporter activity. These results indicate that downstream mediators of CD95L expression are intact in both cell types. This reporter system also illustrates that activation of the Ras pathway is required for optimal CD95L promoter activation, as are the downstream kinases ERK 1 and ERK 2 (51).

Several laboratories have used reporter constructs to investigate the roles of calcineurin and NFAT in the induction of CD95L promoter activation. In agreement with previous observations, pretreatment of transfected T cells with cyclosporin A eliminates inducible reporter construct activity normally detected following T cell stimulation with either TCR ligation or PMA plus ionomycin treatment (50–53). These results again were highly suggestive that NFAT regulated CD95L expression but did not address whether it was due to direct interaction with the promoter or indirect involvement through regulation of other transcription factors. To investigate these possibilities, we demonstrated that overexpression of the $NFAT_c$ protein augmented CD95L promoter activation following TCR ligation (51). Through a combination of techniques, including *in vitro* footprinting and electrophoretic mobility shift assays (EMSAs), we then identified two sites within the first 486 bp of CD95L promoter sequence that are bound by nuclear NFAT proteins in response to T cell activation (51,54). However, only one, located at -277 bases in relation to the translation start site, contributes significantly to inducible promoter activation (54). This finding was corroborated by others who used EMSA super shift analysis to demonstrate that NFAT binding to this site was not accompanied by binding of AP-1, Sp1, or NFκB members to adjacent DNA sequences (50).

Mutation of the sequence at −277 abolishes NFAT binding to this site, and significantly decreases CD95L promoter activity in Jurkat T cells (50,51). Interestingly, crosslinking of CD4 alone leads to NFAT translocation and binding to the −277 response element, accompanied by an increase in luciferase reporter activity (50). Further support for the direct involvement of NFAT proteins in the regulation of CD95L expression was demonstrated recently in human T cell leukemia virus-I (HTLV-I)-infected T cells, which constitutively express CD95L. In this model, the viral Tax protein and $NFAT_p$ are proposed to cooperate in mediating CD95L transcription (55). Taken together, these results indicate that NFAT proteins directly bind to two response elements within the CD95L promoter and contribute to promoter transactivation.

Not all data are consistent with a direct role for NFAT in regulating CD95L expression. One recent finding suggested that the described NFAT binding site at −277 bases within the CD95L promoter is of minimal importance. In this study, deletion of the −277 region had little effect on reporter construct activity in transfected murine T cell hybridomas or human peripheral blood T cell blasts (52). This work identified a single response element bound by the transcription factors Egr-1 and Egr-3, and the authors proposed that Egr-3 is solely responsible for inducible CD95L transcription (52). In contrast to previous data that indicate NFAT directly regulates CD95L expression, this report suggests that the effects of NFAT are indirect, and NFAT functions merely to enhance expression of Egr-3 (52).

The putative Egr response element, located at −214 bases upstream of the translation start site, was also described as contributing to CD95L gene induction by two other laboratories (52,53,56). However, data provided by one of these laboratories indicates that Sp1 binds constitutively to this site and is replaced upon T cell activation by the binding of a protein that is induced following PMA stimulation alone (53). Although NFAT does not bind directly to the −214 site, it is hypothesized that NFAT either interacts with the PMA-sensitive protein that binds to this region, or it mediates its inducible expression (53). At this time, the identity of the PMA-inducible protein is unknown, but it may prove to be an Egr family member.

The Egr family of transcription factors are early response genes that are activated shortly after T cell stimulation. Egr-1 mRNA is transcribed in response to T cell stimulation with PMA alone, but Egr-3 was originally characterized as requiring both PMA and ionomycin-dependent signals for expression (57). Data from our laboratory and others illustrate that the inducible transcription factor that binds to the −214 site can do so in response to PMA-induced signals alone, but that transcriptional activation requires an additional stimulus provided by ionomycin (53,56). Therefore these data do not support a model in which Egr-3 is solely responsible for mediating CD95L promoter activity.

Additional data support the hypothesis that multiple sites contribute to CD95L promoter activity. Mutational analysis of the −214 site alone or in conjunction with the two reported NFAT binding sites (at −277 and −137) suggests that all three reported response elements must be present to achieve maximal CD95L promoter activation in stimulated Jurkat T cells (57). The transcription factor NFκB has been reported to bind two sites within the murine CD95L promoter (58). The more proximal binding site, located at position −132 bases (murine) or −156 bases (human), is fully conserved between the human and murine promoters. Mutation of this conserved NFκB site decreases TCR-inducible murine CD95L promoter activity (58). Therefore it is possible that NFκB also contributes to TCR-mediated induction of CD95L expression in human T cells. The described response elements within the CD95L promoter and the candidate proteins that bind them are summarized in Figure 16-2.

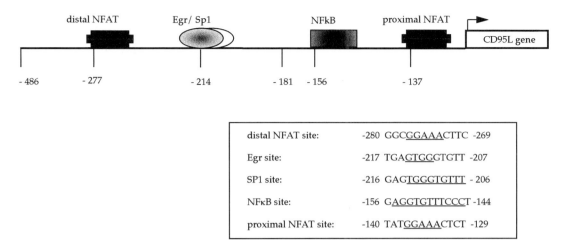

FIG. 16-2. Response elements that regulate TCR-induced CD95L transcription. Two binding sites for NFAT proteins have been identified at −277 and −137 bases 5′ of the translation start site for the CD95L gene. An NFκB site identified in the murine CD95L promoter is fully conserved in the human promoter at −156 bases. Overlapping Sp1 and putative Egr binding sites have been located at −214 bases. The transcription intiation site has been placed at −181 bases. CD95L binding sites for each transcription factor shown are indicated as *underlined sequences* in the box. Other regions of the promoter upstream of the −277 NFAT site have been implicated in stress-induced activation of the CD95L gene.

Another transcription factor has been implicated in the control of CD95L expression, but this protein is proposed to function as a negative regulator. LKLF is a member of the Kruppel family of zinc finger transcription factors, best characterized for their involvement in control of β-globin transcription (59). In mice that contain a homozygous deletion of the gene encoding LKLF, circulating T cells were found to possess an activated phenotype and elevated levels of CD95L surface protein (60). Increased levels of apoptotic lymphocytes were also detected. This led to the conclusion that LKLF functions to maintain T cell quiescence and acts as a negative regulator of CD95L expression, inhibiting CD95L gene transcription in resting cells. LKLF protein is degraded in normal T cells following TCR ligation and would therefore not be present to prohibit CD95L gene transcription by activation-induced transcription factors such as NFAT and Egr. The transcriptional regulation of CD95L

may therefore include positive as well as negative mediators.

NON-TCR-DEPENDENT SIGNALS INDUCING CD95L EXPRESSION

The expression of CD95L can be induced on T cells by a variety of stimuli that do not depend on ligation of the TCR. For example, T cell exposure to agents that cause DNA damage and ultimately result in apoptosis of stressed cells also leads to increased transcription of CD95L (61–63). Such agents include ultraviolet (UV) irradiation and pharmacologic agents such as etoposide and teniposide (61–63). Involvement of the c-Jun N-terminal kinase (JNK) cascade was examined based on prior work illustrating that this pathway was induced in response to cell stress (61). Forced activation of the JNK cascade results in increased transcription and expression of CD95L, as well as increased apoptosis in Jurkat T cells (61). These effects are mediated by a response element located at −338 bases upstream of the translation start site in the human CD95L promoter (62). This response element is bound by two proteins: activating transcription factor-2 (ATF-2) and c-Jun (62).

Two additional stress-sensitive response elements have been identified in the CD95L promoter and were found to be bound by the transcription factors NFκB and AP-1 (63). Both NFκB and AP-1 are activated in Jurkat cells following exposure of the cells to agents that induce DNA damage and apoptosis and bind to more distal regions of the CD95L promoter between −900 and −1,200 bases upstream of the translation start site (63). These results indicate that T cells respond to a variety of stimuli by upregulating the surface expression of CD95L and thus acquire CD95L-mediated cytolytic activity in many circumstances.

CD95L is also expressed constitutively on several tissues including the eye and testis, areas of the body known to have immune privileged status (64). Comparative experiments in our laboratory have suggested differences in the regulation of constitutive versus inducible CD95L expression (51,54,56). In studies using a murine testicular cell line (Sertoli TM4) transfection of our 486-bp reporter construct results in constitutively high levels of promoter activation (51). However, mutation of the −277 NFAT binding site or the −214 Egr/Sp1 site does not diminish reporter activity in the Sertoli TM4 cell line as it does in activated Jurkats (54,57). Thus use of this system can help identify differences and similarities in the ways in which inducible and constitutive expression of CD95L are regulated.

CONCLUSIONS

Activation of T cells results in events that promote cell survival and cell death. The latter occurs through the upregulated surface expression of the AICD-mediator CD95L. The signal transduction pathways that regulate this induced expression of CD95L are incompletely understood at this time. However, recent studies have shown that upon TCR ligation many of the same signal transduction events that mediate cytokine production and cellular activation are also required to induce CD95L expression. Among them are activation of PTKs and the Ras pathway.

The well documented diminution of CD95L expression by treatment with cyclosporin A, a known inhibitor of the calcium-dependent phosphatase calcineurin, is likely due to effects on the transcription factor NFAT. It remains controversial whether NFAT directly or indirectly contributes to CD95L transcription; and there is evidence to suggest that several transcription factors bind to the CD95L promoter and contribute to its transcriptional activation. Although our understanding of the signaling events that control CD95L expression in activated T cells has grown significantly in recent years, there remains much to be learned.

REFERENCES

1. Osborne BA. Apoptosis and the maintenance of homeostasis in the immune system. *Curr Opin Immunol* 1996;8:245–254.
2. Van Parijs L, Abbas AK. Homeostasis and self-tolerance in the immune system: turning lymphocytes off. *Science* 1998;280:243–248.
3. Depraetere V, Golstein P. Fas and other cell death signaling pathways. *Semin Immunol* 1997;9:93–107.
4. Nagata S. Apoptosis by death factor. *Cell* 1997; 88:355–365.
5. Suda T, Takahashi T, Golstein P, Nagata S. Molecular cloning and expression of the Fas ligand, a novel member of the tumor necrosis factor family. *Cell* 1993;75:1169–1178.
6. Suda T, Nagata S. Purification and characterization of the Fas ligand that induces apoptosis. *J Exp Med* 1994;179:873–879.
7. Watanabe-Fukunaga R, Brannan CI, Copeland NG, Jenkins N, Nagata S. Lymphoproliferation disorder in mice explained by defects in Fas antigen that mediates apoptosis. *Nature* 1992;356:314–317.
8. Takahashi T, Tanaka M, Brannan CI, et al. Generalized lymphoproliferative disease in mice, caused by a point mutation in the Fas ligand. *Cell* 1994; 76:969–976.
9. Drappa J, Vaishnaw AK, Sullivan KE, Chu J, Elkon KB. Fas gene mutation in the Canale-Smith syndrome, an inherited lymphoproliferative disorder associated with autoimmunity. *N Engl J Med* 1996; 35:1643–1649.

10. Russell JH, White CL, Loh DY, Meleedy-Rey P. Receptor-stimulated death pathway is opened by antigen in mature T cells. *Proc Natl Acad Sci USA* 1991;88:2151–2155.

11. Wesselborg S, Janssen O, Kabelitz D. Induction of activation-driven death (apoptosis) in activated but not resting peripheral blood T cells. *J Immunol* 1993;150:4338–4345.

12. Rahelu M, Williams GT, Kumararatne DS, Eaton GC, Gaston JSH. Human CD4+ cytolytic T cells kill antigen-pulsed target T cells by induction of apoptosis. *J Immunol* 1993;150:4856–4866.

13. Radvanyi LG, Mills GB, Miller RG. Re-ligation of the T cell receptor after primary activation of mature T cells inhibits proliferation and induces apoptotic cell death. *J Immunol* 1993;150:5704–5715.

14. Yonehara S, Ishii A, Yonehara M. A cell-killing monoclonal antibody (anti-Fas) to a cell surface antigen co-downregulated with the receptor of tumor necrosis factor. *J Exp Med* 1989;169:1747–1756.

15. Itoh N, Yonehara S, Ishii A, et al. The polypeptide encoded by the cDNA for human cell-surface antigen Fas can mediate apoptosis. *Cell* 1991;66: 233–243.

16. Russell JH, Rush B, Weaver C, Wang R. Mature T cells of autoimmune lpr/lpr mice have a defect in antigen-stimulated suicide. *Proc Natl Acad Sci USA* 1993;90:4409–4413.

17. Russell JH, Wang R. Autoimmune gld mutation uncouples suicide and cytokine/proliferation pathways in activated, mature T cells. *Eur J Immunol* 1993;23:2379–2382.

18. Fisher GH, Rosenberg FJ, Straus SE, et al. Dominant interfering Fas gene mutations impair apoptosis in a human autoimmune lymphoproliferative syndrome. *Cell* 1995;81:935–946.

19. Alderson MR, Tough TW, Davis-Smith T, et al. Fas ligand mediates activation-induced cell death in human T lymphocytes. *J Exp Med* 1995;181:71–77.

20. Dhein J, Walczak H, Baumier C, Debatin KM, Krammer PH. Autocrine T cell suicide mediated by APO-1/(Fas/CD95). *Nature* 1995;373:438–441.

21. Brunner T, Mogil RJ, LaFace D, et al. Cell-autonomous Fas (CD95)/Fas-ligand interaction mediates activation-induced apoptosis in T cell hybridomas. *Nature* 1995;373:441–444.

22. Ju ST, Panka DJ, Cul H, et al. Fas (CD95)/FasL interactions required for programmed cell death after T cell activation. *Nature* 1995;373:444–448.

23. Wang JKM, Zhu B, Ju ST, Tschopp J, Marshak-Rothstein A. CD4+ cells reactivated with superantigen are both more sensitive to FasL-mediated killing and express a higher level of FasL. *Cell Immunol* 1997;179:153–164.

24. Martinez-Lorenzo MJ, Alava MA, Anel A, Pineiro A, Naval J. Release of preformed Fas ligand in soluble form is the major factor for activation-induced death of Jurkat T cells. *Immunology* 1996;89:511–517.

25. Oyaizu N, Kayagaki N, Yagita H, Pahwa S, Ikawa Y. Requirement of cell-cell contact in the induction of Jurkat T cell apoptosis: the membrane-anchored but not soluble form of FasL can trigger anti-CD3-induced apoptosis in Jurkat T cells. *Biochem Biophys Res Commun* 1997;238:670–675.

26. Suda T, Hashimoto H, Tanaka M, Ochi T, Nagata S. Membrane Fas ligand kills human peripheral blood T lymphocytes, and soluble Fas ligand blocks the killing. *J Exp Med* 1997;186:2045–2050.

27. Suda T, Okazaki T, Naito Y, et al. Expression of the Fas ligand in cells of T cell lineage. *J Immunol* 1995;154:3806–3813.

28. Refaeli Y, Van Parijs L, London CA, Tschopp J, Abbas AK. Biochemical mechanisms of IL-2-regulated Fas-mediated T cell apoptosis. *Immunity* 1998;8:615–623.

29. Yang Y, Kim D, Fathman CG. Regulation of programmed cell death following T cell activation in vivo. *Int Immunol* 1998;10:175–183.

30. Zhang X, Brunner T, Carter L, et al. Unequal death in T helper (Th) 1 and Th2 effectors: Th1, but not Th2, effectors undergo rapid Fas/FasL-mediated apoptosis. *J Exp Med* 1997;10:1837–1849.

31. Watanabe N, Arase H, Kurasawa K, et al. Th1 and Th2 subsets equally undergo Fas-dependent and -independent activation-induced cell death. *Eur J Immunol* 1997;27:1858–1864.

32. Algeciras A, Dockrell DH, Lynch DH, Paya CV. CD4 regulates susceptibility to Fas ligand- and tumor necrosis factor-mediated apoptosis. *J Exp Med* 1998;187:711–720.

33. Oberg HH, Sanzenbacher R. Langl-Janssen B, et al. Ligation of cell surface CD4 inhibits activation-induced death of human T lymphocytes at the level of Fas ligand expression. *J Immunol* 1997;159:5742–5749.

34. Weiss A, Littman DR. Signal transduction by lymphocyte antigen receptors. *Cell* 1994;75:263–274.

35. Cantrell D. T cell antigen receptor signal transduction pathways. *Annu Rev Immunol* 1996;14: 259–274.

36. Anel A, Buferne M, Boyer C, Schmitt-Verhulst AM, Golstein P. T cell receptor-induced Fas ligand expression in cytotoxic T lymphocyte clones is blocked by protein tyrosine kinase inhibitors and cyclosporin A. *Eur J Immunol* 1994;24:2469–2476.

37. Straus DB, Weiss A. Genetic evidence for the involvement of the lck tyrosine kinase in signal transduction through the T cell antigen receptor. *Cell* 1992;70:585–593.

38. Oyaizu N, Than S, McCLoskey TW, Pahwa S. Requirement of p56lck in T-cell receptor/CD3-mediated apoptosis and Fas-ligand induction in Jurkat T-cells. *Biochem Biophys Res Commun* 1995;213: 994–1001.

39. Williams BL, Schreiber KL, Zhang W, et al. Genetic evidence for differential coupling of Syk family kinases to the T-cell receptor: reconstitution studies in a ZAP-70-deficient Jurkat T-cell line. *Mol Cell Biol* 1998;18:1388–1399.

40. Eischen CM, Williams BL, Zhang W, et al. ZAP-70 tyrosine kinase is required for the up-regulation of Fas ligand in activation-induced T cell apoptosis. *J Immunol* 1997;159:1135–1139.

41. Latinis KM, Koretzky GA. Fas ligation induces apoptosis and Jun kinase activation independently of CD45 and Lck in human T cells. *Blood* 1996; 87:871–875.

42. Sahuquillo AG, Roumier A, Teixeiro E, Bragado R, Alarcon B. T cell receptor engagement in apoptosis-

defective, but interleukin 2 (IL-2)-producing, T cells results in impaired ZAP70/CD3ζ association. *J Exp Med* 1998;187:1179–1192.

43. Rodriguez-Tarduchy G, Sahuquilo AG, Alarcon B, Bragado R. Apoptosis but not other activation events is inhibited by a mutation in the transmembrane domain of T cell receptor β that impairs CD3ζ association. *J Biol Chem* 1996;271:30417–30425.

44. Vignaux F, Vivier E, Malissen B, Depraetere V, Nagata S, Golstein P. TCR/CD3 coupling to Fas-based cytotoxicity. *J Exp Med* 1995;181:781–786.

45. Brunner T, Yoo NJ, LaFace D, Ware CF, Green DR. Activation-induced cell death in murine T cell hybridomas: differential regulation of Fas (CD95) versus Fas ligand expression by cyclosporin A and FK506. *Int Immunol* 1996;8:1017–1026.

46. Clipstone NA, Crabtree GR. Identification of calcineurin as a key signalling enzyme in T-lymphocyte activation. *Nature* 1992;357:695–697.

47. Rao A, Luo C, Hogan P. Transcription factors of the NFAT family: regulation and function. *Annu Rev Immunol* 1997;15:707–747.

48. Hodge MR, Ranger AM, de la Brousse FC, Hoey T, Grusby MJ, Glimcher LH. Hyperproliferation and dysregulation of IL-4 expression in NF-ATp-deficient mice. *Immunity* 1996;4:397–405.

49. Takahashi T, Tanaka M, Inazawa J, Abe T, Suda T, Nagata S. Human Fas ligand: gene structure, chromosomal location and species specificity. *Int Immunol* 1994;6:1567–1574.

50. Holtz-Heppelmann CJ, Algeciras A, Badley AD, Paya CV. Transcriptional regulation of the human FasL promoter-enhancer region. *J Biol Chem* 1998; 273:4416–4423.

51. Latinis KM, Carr LL, Peterson EJ, Norian LA, Eliason SL, Koretzky GA. Regulation of CD95 (Fas) ligand expression by TCR-mediated signaling events. *J Immunol* 1997;158:4602–4611.

52. Mittelstadt PR, Ashwell JD. Cyclosporin A-sensitive transcription factor Egr-3 regulates Fas ligand expression. *Mol Cell Biol* 1998;18:3744–3751.

53. Li-Weber M, Laur O, Hekele A, Coy J, Walczak H, Krammer PH. A regulatory element in the CD95 (APO-1/Fas) ligand promoter is essential for responsiveness to TCR-mediated activation. *Eur J Immunol* 1998;28:2373–2383.

54. Latinis KM, Norian LA, Eliason SL, Koretzky GA.

Two NFAT transcription factor binding sites participate in the regulation of CD95 (Fas) ligand expression in activated human T cells. *J Biol Chem* 1997;272:31427–31434.

55. Rivera I, Harhaj EW, Sun SC. Involvement of NF-AT in type I human T-cell leukemia virus tax-mediated fas ligand promoter transactivation. *J Biol Chem* 1998;273:22382–22388.

56. Norian LA, Latinis KM, Koretzky GA. A newly identified response element in the CD95 ligand promoter contributes to optimal inducibility in activated T lymphocytes. *J Immunol* 1998;161:1078–1082.

57. Mages HW, Stamminger T, Rilke O, Bravo R, Kroczek RA. Expression of PILOT, a putative transcription factor, requires two signals and is cyclosporin A sensitive in T cells. *Int Immunol* 1993;5:63–70.

58. Matsui K, Fine A, Zhu B, Marshak-Rothstein A, Ju ST. Identification of two NFκB sites in mouse CD95 ligand (Fas ligand) promoter: functional analysis in T cell hybridoma. *J Immunol* 1998;161:3469–3473.

59. Anderson KP, Kern CB, Crable SC, Lingrel JB. Isolation of a gene encoding a functional zinc finger protein homologous to erythroid kruppel-like factor: identification of a new multigene family. *Mol Cell Biol* 1995;15:5957–5965.

60. Kuo CT, Veselits ML, Leiden JM. LKLF: a transcriptional regulator of single-positive T cell quiescence and survival. *Science* 1997;277:1986–1990.

61. Faris M, Kokot N, Kasibhatla S, Green DR, Koretzky GA, Nel A. The c-Jun N-terminal kinase cascade plays a role in stress-induced apoptosis in Jurkat cells by up-regulating Fas ligand expression. *J Immunol* 1998;160:134–144.

62. Faris M, Latinis KM, Kempiak SJ, Koretzky GA, Nel A. Stress-induced Fas ligand expression in T cells is mediated through a MEK kinase 1-regulated response element in the Fas ligand promoter. *Mol Cell Biol* 1998;18:5414–5424.

63. Kasibhatla S, Brunner T, Genestier L, Echeverri F, Mahboudi A, Green DR. DNA-damaging agents induce expression of Fas ligand and subsequent apoptosis in T lymphocytes via the activation of NFκB and AP-1. *Mol Cell* 1998;1: 543–551.

64. Griffith TS, Ferguson TA. The role of FasL-induced apoptosis in immune privilege. *Immunol Today* 1997;18:240–244.

Cytotoxic Cells: Basic Mechanisms and Medical Applications, edited by Michail V. Sitkovsky and Pierre A. Henkart. Lippincott Williams & Wilkins, Philadelphia © 2000.

Chapter 17

Transcriptional Regulation of the FasL Gene

Alicia Algeciras-Schimnich and *Carlos V. Paya

*Division of Immunology and *Infectious Diseases, Mayo Clinic, Rochester, Minnesota 55905, USA*

Fas ligand (FasL) is a 40-kDa transmembrane protein member of the tumor necrosis factor (TNF) superfamily whose other members include LTα, LTβ, CD27L, CD30L, CD40L, OX40L, 4-1BBL, and TRAIL (1–4). The active form of FasL, as in TNF, is a membrane-bound trimer that can also be secreted in a soluble molecule (5). Crosslinking of Fas (CD95, Apo-1) by FasL results in the apoptosis of Fas(+) susceptible cells. Cell death by apoptosis mediated by Fas–FasL interactions plays a crucial role in the immune system through its role in the maintenance of T cell homeostasis. Fas–FasL interactions control the induction of peripheral tolerance, lymphocyte cytotoxicity against virus-infected cells and tumors, and the maintenance of "immune privilege" sites (6–10). Dysregulation of Fas–FasL interactions results in disease states characterized by either enhanced lymphocyte apoptosis, as in acquired immunodeficiency syndrome (AIDS) or, by default, in decreased levels of lymphocyte apoptosis, such as in the human autoimmune lymphoproliferative syndrome (ALPS) (11–13). Fas–FasL interactions that lead to cellular apoptosis require two necessary events: (a) a Fas-bearing cell must become susceptible to FasL-mediated apoptosis, and (b) FasL must be expressed in the effector cell. This chapter focuses on the regulation of FasL expression.

The cloning of the murine FasL identified constitutive gene transcription in tissues such as testis and spleen (1). Further investigation identified that FasL gene mRNA can also be induced following lymphoid cell activation and demonstrating that activation-induced cell death (AICD) is dependent on the inducible transcription of FasL (6,14–18). Current knowledge indicates that FasL expression is highly regulated in a cell- and environment-specific manner. Its expression is absent in certain lymphoid and non-lymphoid cells but can be rapidly induced following the immune response (6,14). Alternatively, in other cell types and tissues FasL expression is constitutively present but can also be further upregulated by certain stimuli such as human immunodeficiency virus (HIV) infection of human macrophages (19–26).

Despite the relevance of FasL expression in the immune system, little is known as to what controls the inducible and basal levels of expression in a cell-specific manner. At least two mechanisms have been identified to regulate FasL expression: transcriptional and posttranslational. The latter involves cleavage of the membrane-bound FasL by matrix metalloproteases (14–18,27). Their function and activation by extracellular stimuli are poorly understood, and to date there is no link between FasL expression and metalloprotease regulation, especially as it pertains to the immune system. On the contrary, there is a more direct *in vivo* correlation between FasL expression and levels of FasL mRNA, suggesting that the transcriptional control of FasL gene may be the major form of FasL regulation.

The initial studies addressing the transcriptional regulation of FasL are based on mRNA analysis in a variety of primary and transformed lymphocytes (1,7,8,14,15). Altogether, such studies demonstrate absent FasL mRNA levels in cells under resting conditions but its rapid and transient induction by a variety of extracellular stimuli. Combination of pharmacologic agents such as phorbol myristica acetate (PMA) and ionomycin or crosslinking of CD3, CD4, FcγRI, or lectins have all been shown to transiently increase FasL mRNA levels (17,18–30). In addition, a number of tissues and cell types (both transformed and primary) have been shown to constitutively express detectable FasL mRNA. Due to the relevance of FasL, the apparent differences in its transcriptional regulation has made the need to identify and functionally characterize the enhancer promoter region of this gene an important priority.

The initial cloning of the murine and human FasL genes included a 400-basepair (bp) sequence upstream from the translation codon in which putative *cis*-acting factors were noted (31). However, a functional characterization of the transcription factors that control FasL expression was lacking until recently. Several groups have cloned and initially characterized the human FasL enhancer promoter region (32,33). In this chapter we discuss recent findings by several groups including ours on the studies addressing transcriptional regulation of FasL in both an inducible and a constitutive fashion.

ROLE OF NFAT IN THE INDUCIBLE FASL TRANSCRIPTION IN T CELLS

Using commercially available techniques for cDNA amplification our group isolated a 2.3-kb genomic region located 5' upstream of the FasL translation initiation site (32). This region extended the previously identified 486 bp upstream the FasL translational start site (31). Several transcription *cis*-acting motifs such as Sp1/Ets, NFAT, NFκB-like, and MEKK-1 RE were identified in the proximal −486 bp to the transcription initiation site (Fig. 17-1). In addition, experiments using different truncations of the 2.3-kb promoter region demonstrated the presence of negative regulatory elements (NRE) located within −2365 and −454 and within −373 and −318, as deletions of these regions significantly increase the basal activity of the FasL promoter (see below). The inducible responsive element was located between −260 and −300; and using a variety of cell types of the many stimuli tested, only ionomycin and anti-CD3 crosslinking of T cells were shown

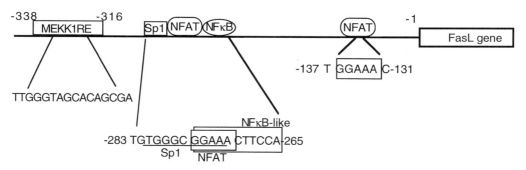

FIG. 17-1. Fas ligand (FasL) promoter region. Transcription factors DNA binding site within the FasL promoter region. The DNA nucleotide sequence and their position in respect to the transcription initiation site are illustrated.

to upregulate the FasL promoter enhancer region. This observation led to a search for the *cis*-acting motifs and transcription factors that would respond to T cell activation-dependent upregulation of FasL (32).

A common feature of ionomycin- and anti-CD3-initiated signal transduction is the increase in intracellular Ca^{2+}, which leads to activation of the serine phosphatase calcineurin, a main effector of the activation of NFAT (34–36). Two NFAT binding sites are present within the FasL promoter, and previous studies demonstrated that the CD3-dependent induction of FasL mRNA in T cells is inhibited by cyclosporin A and FK506, immunosuppressive drugs that inhibit calcineurin and hence NFAT activity (14,17,37). Transient overexpression of NFATc1 and NFATc2 in conjunction with luciferase reporter construct containing full length or truncations of the FasL promoter or a triplicate version of the FasL NFAT was sufficient to induce transcription of the FasL promoter (32,33). NFAT transcriptional activity was observed only in the truncations containing nucleotides -318 to -237. Likewise, overexpression of a constitutive active form of calcineurin induced the transcriptional activity of the FasL promoter constructs containing nucleotides -318 to -237 (32). As expected, the transcriptional activity mediated by both NFAT overexpression and constitutive active calcineurin were blocked by treatment with cyclosporin A or FK506.

Further studies demonstrated [by mutational analysis of the two NFAT sites designated NFAT distal (nt. -272 to -276) and NFAT proximal (nt. -134 to -138) relative to the TATA box] that only the distal NFAT site plays a major role in FasL promoter activity (38). Latinis et al. demonstrated that a triplicate version of the distal and proximal NFAT sites can function independently to drive transcription in activated T cells. However mutations of each site in the -486-bp FasL promoter showed that mutations of the distal NFAT site completely abolish the induction of promoter activity following TCR stimulation of Jurkat T cells. In contrast, mu-

tations of the proximal NFAT sites have a minimum effect on the transcriptional activity of the FasL promoter (38). These results are in agreement with our observations where truncations of the region that contained the distal NFAT site decrease the transcriptional activity of a luciferase reporter construct to background levels.

Interestingly, NFAT is also involved in virus-induced FasL expression. Expression of human T cell leukemia virus-I (HTLV-I) Tax transactivator induces FasL expression in Jurkat T cells (39). Co-transfection experiments demonstrated that Tax upregulates the FasL promoter activity, and mutations of the NFAT binding site abolish Tax-induced activation of the FasL promoter (40). Mice deficient in NFATp (NFATc2, NFAT1) and NFAT4 (NFATc3, NFATx) support our observation of a major role of NFAT in the regulation of the FasL promoter. These mice display defects in the expression of FasL and of cytokines known to be regulated by NFAT, such as interleukin-4 (IL-4), IL-13, granulocyte/macrophage colony-stimulating factor (GM-CSF), and tumor necrosis factor-α (TNF-α), but these mice also lack FasL expression and exhibit lymphocyte hyperproliferation (41,42).

NFAT has been generally described as a transcription factor that interacts with related (NF-κB) or unrelated (AP-1) transcription factors to drive the transcription of a variety of cytokine genes (43). The putative sequence in the FasL promoter containing the NFAT site is flanked and overlapped with Sp1 and NF-κB sites. Overexpression of these other transcription factors does not enhance the transcriptional activity mediated by NFAT. Moreover, antibodies against various NF-κB subunits, c-Fos, c-Jun, or Sp-1 do not modify the DNA binding characteristic of the NFAT complex. Therefore the NFAT binding site in the FasL promoter does not require the interaction of NFAT within other transcription factors to drive FasL gene transcription and, similarly, TNF-α promoter and in the enhancer region of the IL-3 gene (44,45).

NEGATIVE REGULATORY ELEMENTS

Our group (32) and Li-Weber et al. (46) reported that deletions of the region containing nt. -2365 to -454 increases the basal and inducible activity of the promoter. These observations suggested the presence of possible silencer or repressor binding sites in this region. Two potential transcription factors have been identified as possible negative regulators of the FasL promoter. First, the lung Kruppel-like factor (LKLF) is a gene related to the erythroid-specific zinc finger transcription factor that binds to a CACCC sequence in the promoter of the β-globin genes and regulates erythroid development (47–50). LKLF mRNA is present in resting single positive thymocytes and splenocytes. Following T cell receptor (TCR)-mediated activation of splenic T cells, LKLF protein and mRNA levels are significantly decreased (51). T cells from LKLF knockout mice contain a spontaneously activated T cell phenotype. FasL expression on LKLF T cells is equal or higher than that observed after TCR-mediated activation of T cells of WT animals (51). These findings suggest that LKLF negatively regulate the FasL promoter.

Another potential negative regulator of the FasL promoter is the transcription factor glucocorticoid-induced leucine zipper (GILZ). The GILZ gene is induced in T cells after dexamethasone treatment (52). GILZ expression protects T cells from anti-CD3-induced apoptosis but not from apoptosis induced by other apoptotic stimuli such as serum starvation, anti-Fas treatment, and ultraviolet (UV) irradiation. The ability of GILZ to inhibit cell death correlates with the inhibition of anti-CD3-induced upregulation of FasL mRNA expression as determined by RNase protection assays (52). More detailed studies of the function of LKLF and GILZ in the regulation of the FasL promoter are necessary to confirm whether any of these proteins are involved in FasL gene repression. In addition it will be interesting to see whether these transcription factors are absent in those cell types that constitutively express FasL.

AP1, NF-κB, AND CHEMOTHERAPEUTIC AGENTS

One of the mechanisms by which cells respond to cytotoxic stress and DNA damage is by undergoing apoptosis. Studies have provided evidence that anticancer chemotherapeutic agents that lead to cell stress and DNA damage mediate apoptosis by the induction of FasL expression (53). In contrast to TCR-induced FasL expression, FasL expression by chemotherapeutic agents is NFAT-independent. Stimulation of T cell lines with DNA damaging agents such as teniposide, etoposide, and ultraviolet B (UVB) irradiation induce apoptosis and increase FasL mRNA levels. DNA damage induced FasL promoter activity requires activation of the SAPK/JNK signaling pathway. T cell lines transfected with a dominant active MEKK1 undergo apoptosis that is dependent on constitutive JNK pathway activation and FasL expression (54). Transfection of a dominant active MEKK-1 (DA-MEKK1) under the control of a tetracycline-regulated system results in a tenfold increase in the FasL promoter basal activity. In contrast, overexpression of a dominant negative MEKK1 (DN-MEKK1) completely blocks the increase in FasL promoter activity following UV irradiation, gamma irradiation, or anisomycin treatment. The effect of the JNK pathway in FasL upregulation following DNA damage is dependent on an MEKK-1-regulated response element located on position -338 to -316 of the FasL promoter (55). Mutation of this response element abrogates DA-MEKK1-mediated FasL promoter activation and interferes with stress-induced activation of the promoter. EMSA analysis demonstrated that the AP-1 binding proteins ATF-2 and c-jun bind to the MEKK-1 response element. Mutants of these two proteins, which lack the consensus JNK phosphorylation sites, abrogate the transcriptional activation of the FasL promoter (55). In addition, an AP-1 binding site present between nt. −1043 to −1050 on the FasL promoter has been implicated in FasL expression following DNA damage (56). In fact, mutations of the AP-1 binding site in the FasL promoter abrogate teniposide-induced FasL promoter activity; and overexpression of the AP-1 components, cFos and cJun, is sufficient to induce FasL promoter activity (56). Altogether these results suggest that activation of the JNK pathway results in activation of AP-1 transcription factors followed by FasL upregulation and apoptosis.

Evidence suggests that the role of NF-κB in FasL expression is based mainly on inhibition of NF-κB by its natural inhibitor IκB. Overexpression of a wt or mutant IκB inhibits activation of the FasL promoter induced by DNA, damaging inducing agents, and it inhibits basal promoter activity (56). Consistent with these observations, overexpression of the NF-κB subunit p65 upregulates FasL promoter activity. In addition, a single nucleotide substitution of the NFκB DNA binding site in the FasL promoter is no longer activated by etoposide or teniposide treatment. In addition, oxidative stress induced by hydrogen peroxide upregulates FasL mRNA levels (57). This is associated with activation of NF-κB, and its inhibition by a transdominant IκB mutant attenuated FasL gene transcription (57).

Sp1 AND CONSTITUTIVE FasL EXPRESSION IN IMMUNE PRIVILEGED SITES

The Fas ligand is constitutively expressed in cells of immune privileged sites such as testicles, placenta, eye, and brain (9,19,22, 50,58,59). Moreover, several malignant cell lines and cell types express FasL, and its expression has been attributed as a mechanism to escape immune destruction and to contribute to invasive growth of the tumor (60–67). How the constitutive expression of FasL is regulated in such immune privileged sites and in malignancies is currently unknown.

Our group has studied transcriptional regulation of the FasL in Sertoli cells, known to have constitutive FasL expression (19). Using various truncations of the FasL promoter constructs fused to a luciferase reported gene, a region between nt. −318 and −237 relative to the transcription initiation site was found to be responsible for promoting transcription in Sertoli cells (68). This region contains DNA binding sites for NF-κB, NFAT, and Sp1. Point mutation analysis of these DNA binding sites indicates that the Sp1 DNA binding site is important for the FasL promoter activity observed in Sertoli cells. In contrast, mutations within the NF-κB-like and NFAT binding sites do not have a major effect in the constitutive FasL promoter activity. Sp1 and Sp3 are transcription factors mainly involved in the regulation of housekeeping genes (69). Sp1 is an activator of transcription (69,70), whereas Sp3 has been reported to function as an activator or an inhibitor of transcription (70–73). EMSA analysis demonstrated that the transcription factors Sp1 and Sp3 bind to the Sp1 binding site in the promoter. More important, overexpression of Sp1 further enhances transcriptional activity of a wt type but not of an Sp1 mutated FasL promoter construct in Sertoli cells. However, overexpression of Sp3 does not increase the basal FasL promoter activity in Sertoli cells, nor does it inhibit the transcriptional activity triggered by the overexpression of Sp1.

Our group further investigated the role of Sp1 in the basal FasL promoter activity using T cell lines. Transient transfection into Jurkat T cells of different FasL promoter constructs demonstrated that mutations of the Sp1 DNA binding site diminished the basal promoter activity. Similarly, overexpression of Sp1 increases the promoter basal transcriptional levels, whereas it has no effect on the inducible TCR-mediated upregulation of FasL. Based on these results, it can be hypothesized that constitutive expression of

TABLE 17-1. *Regulation of FasL expression*

Expression	Stimuli	Transcription factor (s)	Cell type	Role	References
Inducible	TCR activation PMA/Ionomycin	NFAT	Jurkat T cells	AICD	32, 33, 38
Inducible	HTLV-1 tax	NFAT	Jurkat T cells	Immune evasion?	40
Inducible	H_2O_2 Etoposide Teniposide γ-Irradiation UVB	NF-κB, cJUN, ATF-2, cFOS	Microgial cells Jurkat T cells	Apoptosis	51, 54
Constitutive		Sp-1	Sertoli cells	Immune privileged sites	68

FasL is at least regulated by the levels of Sp1 present in cells. Whether Sp1 is involved in the constitutive expression of FasL in other cells from immune privilege sites or malignancies warrants further study.

AREAS OF FUTURE STUDY

In view of the relevance of FasL to the immune system, other areas that require further study include understanding the transcriptional regulation of FasL in antigen-presenting cells, such as dendritic cells and differentiated macrophages. Previous data from our group indicating constitutive FasL mRNA in human macrophages and its further upregulation by HIV infection (*in vitro* and *in vivo*) suggest that both constitutive and inducible FasL transcription can be observed within the same cell (23,25,26). Whether different mechanisms or the degree of activity of the same mechanism regulate FasL expression in HIV-infected macrophages needs further study. A second area that can benefit from a detailed analysis of the transcriptional regulation of FasL is in intestinal epithelial cells (IECs). The recent observation that nonlymphoid cells such as IECs can de novo express FasL through transcriptional mechanisms following an immune response is relevant to T cell homeostasis (74).

CONCLUSIONS

Expression of death-inducing molecules, such as FasL, must be tightly regulated to maintain cellular homeostasis. FasL can be constitutively or inducibly expressed depending on the cell type (Table 17-1). The constitutive expression of FasL may be controlled at least by Sp1-type transcription factors. On the other hand, inducible FasL expression is regulated depending on the stimulus and in a cell-specific manner. TCR induced FasL expression in T cells is mainly controlled by NFAT, whereas DNA damage induced FasL expression is regulated by the JNK pathway through the activation of AP1 and NF-κB transcription factors. These initial observations highlight the plasticity of the transcriptional regulation of this gene. Moreover, they argue for a more detailed analysis of the role of the various transcription factors that regulate FasL in a cell- and environment-specific manner and their impact on disease states characterized by FasL dysregulation.

REFERENCES

1. Suda T, Takahashi T, Goldstein P, Nagata S. Molecular cloning and expression of the Fas ligand, a novel member of the tumor necrosis factor family. *Cell* 1993;75:1169–1178.
2. Suda, T, Nagata S. Purification and characterization of the Fas-ligand that induces apoptosis. *J Exp Med* 1994;179:873–879.
3. Gruss HJ, Dower SK. Tumor necrosis factor ligand superfamily: involvement in the pathology of malignant lymphomas. *Blood* 1995;85:3378–3404.
4. Wiley SR, Schooley K, Smolak PJ, et al. The novel receptor TRAIL-R4 induces NF-kappaB and protects against TRAIL-mediated apoptosis yet retains an incomplete death domain. *Immunity* 1995;3:673–682.
5. Tanaka M, Suda T, Takahashi T, Nagata S. Expres-

sion of the functional soluble form of human Fas ligand in activated lymphocytes. *EMBO J* 1995; 14:1129–1135.

6. Singer GG, Abbas AK. The Fas antigen is involved in peripheral but not thymic deletion of T lymphocytes in T cell receptor transgenic mice. *Immunity* 1994;1:365–371.

7. Hanabuchi S, Koyanagi M, Kawasaki A, et al. Fas and its ligand in a general mechanism of T-cell-mediated cytotoxicity. *Proc Natl Acad Sci USA* 1994;91:4930–4934.

8. Arase H, Arase N, Saito T. Fas-mediated cytotoxicity by freshly isolated natural killer cells. *J Exp Med* 1995;181:1235–1238.

9. Griffith TS, Brunner T, Fletcher SM, Green DR, Ferguson TA. Fas ligand-induced apoptosis as a mechanism of immune privilege. *Science* 1995;270: 1189–1193.

10. Griffith TS, Ferguson, TA. The role of FasL onduced apoptosis if immune privilege. *Immunol Today* 1997;18:240–244.

11. Fisher GH, Rosenberg FJ, Straus SE, et al. Dominant interfering Fas gene mutations impair apoptosis in a human autoimmune lymphoproliferative syndrome. *Cell* 1995;81:935–946.

12. Rieux-Laucat F, Le Deist F, Hivroz, C, et al. Mutations in Fas associated with human lymphoproliferative syndrome and autoimmunity. *Science* 1995; 268:1347–1349.

13. Oyaizu N, Pahwa S. Role of apoptosis in HIV disease pathogenesis. *J Clin Immunol* 1995;15:217–231.

14. Dhein J, Walczak H, Baümler, C, Detatin K-M. Autocrine T-cell suicide mediated by APO-1/(Fas/ CD95). *Nature* 1995;373:438–441.

15. Brunner T, Mogil RJ, LaFace D, et al. Cell-autonomous Fas (CD95)/Fas-ligand interaction mediates activation-induced apoptosis in T-cell hybridomas. *Nature* 1995;373:441–444.

16. Ju S-T, Panka DJ, Cui H, et al. Fas(CD95)/FasL interactions required for programmed cell death after T-cell activation. *Nature* 1995;373:444–448.

17. Alderson MR, Tough TW, Davis-Smith T, et al. Fas ligand mediates activation-induced cell death in human T lymphocytes. *J Exp Med* 1995;181:71–77.

18. Yang Y, Mercep M, Ware CF, Ashwell JD. Fas and activation-induced Fas ligand mediate apoptosis of T cell hybridomas: inhibition of Fas ligand expression by retinoic acid and glucocorticoids. *J Exp Med* 1995;181:1673–1682.

19. Bellgrau D, Gold D, Selawry H, Moore J, Franzusoff A, Duke RC. A role for CD95 ligand in preventing graft rejection. *Nature* 1995;377:630–632.

20. Twigg HD III, Iwamoto GK, Soliman DM. Role of cytokines in alveolar macrophage accessory cell function in HIV-infected individuals. *J Immunol* 1992;149:1462–1469.

21. Liles WC, Kiener PA, Ledbetter JA, Aruffo A, Klebanoff SJ. Differential expression of Fas (CD95) and Fas ligand on normal human phagocytes: implications for the regulation of apoptosis in neutrophils. *J Exp Med* 1996;184:429–440.

22. Hunt JS, Vassmer D, Ferguson TA, Miller L. Fas ligand is positioned in mouse uterus and placenta to prevent trafficking if activated leukocytes between the mother and the conceptus. *J Immunol* 1997;58:4122–4128.

23. Badley AD, McElhinny JA, Leibson PJ, Lynch DH, Alderson MR, Paya CV. Upregulation of FasL expression by human immunodeficiency virus in human macrophages mediates apoptosis of uninfected T lymphocytes. *J Virol* 1996;70:199–206.

24. Badley AD, Dockrell D, Simpson M, et al. Macrophage-dependent apoptosis of CD4$^+$ T lymphocytes from HIV-infected individuals is mediated by FasL and tumor necrosis factor. *J Exp Med* 1997; 185:55–64.

25. Mitra, D, Steiner, M, Lynch, DH, Staiano-Coico L, Laurence J. HIV-1 upregulates Fas ligand expression in CD4$^+$ T cells in vitro and in vivo: association with Fas-mediated apoptosis and modulation by aurintricarboxylic acid. *Immunology* 1996;87: 581–585.

26. Dockrell DH, Badley AD, Villacian JS, et al. The expression of FasL by macrophages and its upregulation by human immunodeficiency virus infection. *J Clin Invest* 1998;101:2394–2405.

27. Kayagaki N, Kawasaki, A, Ebata T, et al. Metalloproteinase-mediated release of human Fas ligand. *J Exp Med* 1995;182:1777–1783.

28. Eischen CM, Schilling JD, Lynch DH, Krammer PH, Leibson PJ. Fc receptor-induced expression of Fas ligand on activated NK cell facilitates cell-mediated cytotoxicity and subsequent autocrine NK cell apoptosis. *J Immunol* 1996;156:2693–2699.

29. Oyaizu N, Adachi Y, Hashimoto F, et al. Monocytes express Fas ligand upon CD4 cross-linking and induced CD4$^+$ T cell apoptosis. *J Immunol* 1997;158: 2456–2463.

30. Westendorp MO, Frank R, Ochsenbauer C, et al. Sensitization of T cells to CD95-mediated apoptosis by HIV-1 Tat and gp120. *Nature* 1995;375:497–500.

31. Takahashi T, Tanaka M, Inazawa, J, Abe T, Suda, T, Nagata S. Human Fas ligand: gene structure, chromosomal location and species specificity. Int Immunol 1994;6:1567–1574.

32. Holtz-Heppelmann CJ, Algeciras A, Badley AD, Paya CV. Transcriptional regulation of the human FasL promoter-enhancer region. *J Biol Chem* 1998;273:4416–4423.

33. Latinis KM, Carr LL, Peterson EJ, Norian LA, Eliason SL, Koretzky GA. Regulation of CD95 (Fas) ligand expression by TCR-mediated signaling events. *J Immunol* 1997;158:46093–4611.

34. Clipstone NA, Crabtree GR. Identification of calcineurin as a key signalling enzyme in T-lymphocyte activation. *Nature* 1992;357:695–697.

35. Liu J, Farmer JD, Lane WS, Friedman J, Wiessman I, Schreiber SL. Calcineurin is a common target of cyclophilin-cyclosporin A and FKBP-FK506 complexes. *Cell* 1991;49:806–815.

36. O'Keefe SJ, Tamura J, Kincaid RL, Tocci MJ, O'Neill EA. FK-506- and CsA-sensitive activation of the interleukin-2 promoter by calcineurin. *Nature* 1992;357:692–694.

37. Brunner T, Yoo NJ, LaFace, D, Mare CF, Green DR. Activation-induced cell death in murine T cell hybridomas: differential regulation of Fas (CD95) versus Fas ligand expression by cyclosporin A and FK506. *Int Immunol* 1996;8:1017–1026.

38. Latinis KM, Norian LA, Eliason SL, Koretzky GA. Two NFAT transcription factor binding sites participate in the regulation of CD95 (Fas) ligand expression in activated human T cells. *J Biol Chem* 1997;272:31427–31334.

39. Chen X, Zachar V, Zdravkovic M, Guo M, Ebbesen P, Liu X, Role of Fas/FasL pathway in apoptotic cell death induced by human T cell lymphotropic virus type I Tax transactivator. *J Gen Virol* 1997; 78:3277–3285.

40. Rivera I, Harhaj EW, Sun S-C. Involvement of NFAT in type I human T cell leukemia virus Tax-mediated Fas ligand promoter transactivation. *J Biol Chem* 1998;273:22382–22388.

41. Hodge MR, Ranger AM, Charles de la Brousse F, Hoey T, Grusby MJ, Glimcher LH. Hyperproliferation and dysregulation of IL-4 expression in NF-ATp-deficient mice. *Immunity* 1995;4:397–405.

42. Ranger AM, Oukka M, Rengarajan J, Glimcher LH. Inhibitory function of two NFAT family members in lymphoid homeostasis and Th2 development. *Immunity* 1998; 9:627–635.

43. Rao A. NF-ATp: a transcription factor required for the co-ordinate induction several cytokine genes. *Immunol Today* 1994;15:274–281.

44. Tsai EY, Yie J, Thanos D, Goldfeld AE. Cell-type-specific regulation of the human tumor necrosis factor alpha gene in B cells and T cells by NFATp and ATF-2/JUN. *Mol Cell Biol* 1996;16:5232–5244.

45. Duncliffe KN, Bert AG, Vadas MA, Cockerill PN. A T cell-specific enhancer in the interleukin-3 locus is activated cooperatively by Oct and NFAT elements within a DNase I-hypersensitive site. *Immunity* 1997;6:175–185.

46. Li-Weber M, Laur O, Hekele A, Coy J, Walczak H, Krammer PH. A regulatory element in the CD95 (Apo-1/Fas) ligand promoter is essential for responsiveness to TCR-mediated activation. *Eur J Immunol* 1998;28:2373–2383.

47. Shields JM, Yang VW. Identification of the DNA sequence that interacts with the gut-enriched Kruppel like factor. *Nucleic Acids Res* 1998;26:796–802.

48. Shields JM, Yang VW. Two potent nuclear translocation signals in the gut-enriched Kruppell-like factor define a subfamily of closely related Kruppel proteins. *J Biol Chem* 1997;272:18504–18507.

49. Anderson KP, Kern CB, Crable SC, Lingrel JB. Isolation of a gene encoding a functional zinc finger protein homologous to erythroid Kruppel like factor: identification to a new multigene family. *Mol Cell Biol* 1995;15:5957–5967.

50. Miller IJ, Bieker JJ. A novel, erythroid cell-specific murine transcription factor that binds to the CACCC element and its related to the Kruppel family of nuclear proteins. *Mol Cell Biol* 1993; 13:2776–2786.

51. Kuo CT, Veselits ML, Leiden JM. LKLF: a transcriptional regulator of single-positive T cell quiscence and survival. *Science* 1997;277:1986–1990.

52. D'Adamio F, Zollo O, Moraca R, et al. A new dexamethasone-induced gene if the leucine zipper family protects T lymphocytes from TCR/CD3-activated cell death. *Immunity* 1997;7:803–812.

53. Friesen C, Herr I, Krammer PH, Debatin K-M. Involvement of the CD95 (Apo-1/Fas) receptor/ligand system in drug induced apoptosis in leukemia cells. *Nat Med* 1996;2:574–577.

54. Faris M, Kokot N, Latinis K, et al. The c-Jun N-terminal kinase cascade plays a role in stress-induced apoptosis on Jurkats cells by up-regulating Fas ligand expression. *J Immunol* 1998;160:134–144.

55. Faris M, Latinis KM, Kempiak SJ, Koretzky GA, Nel A. Stress-induced Fas ligand expression in T cells is mediated through a MEK kinase 1- regulated response element in the Fas ligand promoter. *Mol Cell Biol* 1998;18:5414–5424.

56. Kasibhatla S, Brunner T, Genestier L, Echeverri F, Mahboubi A, Green DR. DNA damaging agents induce expression of Fas ligand and subsequent apoptosis in T lymphocytes via the activation of NF-κB and AP-1. *Mol Cell* 1998;1:543–551.

57. Vogt M, Bauer MK, Ferrari D, Schulze-Osthoff K. Oxidative stress and hypoxia/reoxigenation trigger CD95 (APO-1/Fas) ligand expression in microgial cells. *FEBS lett* 1998;429:67–72.

58. Xerri L, Devilard E, Hassoun J, Mawas C, Birg F. Fas ligand is not only expressed in immune privileged human organs but is also coexpressed with Fas in various epithelial tissues. *Mol Pathol* 1997; 50:87–91.

59. Saas P, Walker P, Hahne M, et al. Fas ligand expression by astrocytoma in vivo: maintaining immune privilege in the brain? *J Clin Invest* 1997;99:1173–1178.

60. Yano H, Fukuda K, Haramaki M, et al. Expression of Fas and anti-Fas-mediated apoptosis in human hepatocellular carcinoma cell lines. *J Hepatol* 1996;25:454–464.

61. Tanaka M, Suda T, Haze K, et al. Fas ligand in human serum. *Nat Med* 1996;2:317–322.

62. Sugihara A, Saiki S, Tsuji M, et al. Expression of Fas and Fas ligand in the testes and testicular germ cell tumors: an immunohistochemical study. *Anticancer Res* 1997;17:3861–3865.

63. Strand S, Hofmann WJ, Hug H, et al. Lymphocyte apoptosis induced by CD95 (APO-1/Fas) ligand-expressing tumor cells—a mechanism of immune evasion? *Nat Med* 1996;2:1361–1366.

64. Xerri L, Devilard E, Hassoun J, Haddad P, Birg F. Malignant and reactive cells from human lymphomas frequently express Fas ligand but display a different sensitivity to Fas-mediated apoptosis. *Leukemia* 1997;11:1868–1877.

65. Perzova R, Loughran TP. Constitutive expression of Fas ligand in large granular lymphocyte leukemia. *Br J Haematol* 1997;97:123–126.

66. O'Connell J, O'Sullivan GC, Collins JK, Shanahan F. The Fas counterattack: Fas-mediated T cell killing by colon cancer cells expressing Fas ligand. *J Exp Med* 1996;184:1075–1082.

67. Hahne M, Rimoldi D, Schroter M, et al. Melanoma cell expression of Fas(Apo-1/CD95) ligand: implications for tumor immune escape. *Science* 1996; 274:1363–1366.

68. McClure RF, Heppelmann CJ, Paya CV. Constitutive Fas ligand gene transcription in Sertoli cells is regulated by Sp1. *J Biol Chem* 1999;274:7756–7762.

69. Saffer JD, Jackson SP, Annarella MB. Developmental expression of Sp1 in the mouse. *Mol Cell Biol* 1991;11:2189–219.

70. Look DC, Pelletier MR, Tidwell RM, Roswit WT, Holtzman MJ. Stat1 depends on transcriptional synergy with Sp1. *J Biol Chem* 1995;270:30264–30267.

71. Hagen G, Muller S, Beato M, Susuke G. Sp1-mediated transcriptional activation is repressed by Sp3. *EMBO J* 1994;13:3843–3851.

72. Conn KJ, Rich CB, Jensen DE, et al. Insulin-like growth factor-I regulates transcription of the elastin gene through a putative retinoblastoma control ele-ment: a role for Sp3 acting as a repressor of elastin gene transcription. *J Biol Chem* 1996;271:28853–28860.

73. Ihn H, Trojanowska M. Sp3 is a transcriptional acti-vator of the human alpha 2(I) collagen gene. *Nucleic Acids Res* 1997;15:3712–3717.

74. Bonfoco E, Stuart PM, Brunnr T, et al. Inducible nonlymphoid expression of Fas ligand is responsible for superantigen-induced peripheral deletion of T cells. *Immunity* 1998;9:711–720.

Cytotoxic Cells: Basic Mechanisms and Medical Applications, edited by Michail V. Sitkovsky and Pierre A. Henkart. Lippincott Williams & Wilkins, Philadelphia © 2000.

V / CYTOTOXIC LYMPHOCYTES *IN VIVO*

Chapter 18

Perforin-Dependent Cytotoxicity in Autoimmunity and Antiviral Resistance

David Kägi

Ontario Cancer Institute, Amgen Institute, Toronto, Ontario M5G 2M9, Canada

Infection with a number of viruses leads to potent major histocompatibility complex class I (MCH-I)-restricted cytotoxic T cell responses (1,2). The finding that CD8$^+$ T cells not only mediate this cytotoxic activity *in vitro* but also protect animals from virus infection *in vivo* suggested that lysis of infected cells by cytotoxic T lymphocytes (CTLs) is an important effector mechanism of viral clearance. In autoimmune diseases, on the other hand, specific destruction of certain cell types in the target organs of the disease and the presence of CD8$^+$ T cells in the inflammatory infiltrates in these organs also led to the conclusion that the cytotoxic activity of T cells may account for the pathogenic tissue damage. In both cases, however, the evidence for a crucial role of cytotoxicity versus cytokines secreted by T cells was often circumstantial, resulting in controversial discussions of this issue (3–5). Because it is now generally accepted that T cells mediate their cytotoxic activity via a perforin and a Fas-dependent mechanism (6–10) it is possible to address the role of T cell-mediated cytotoxicity *in vivo* more directly than before. In this chapter the recent progress in understanding the role of the cytotoxic activity of T cells in controlling viral replication and causing tissue damage in autoimmune disease is summarized.

AUTOIMMUNE DISEASES

The pathology of many autoimmune diseases is characterized by mononuclear infiltrates with activated T cells and destruction of target tissue. To classify the various autoimmune diseases and in the hope of interfering with disease progression it was always of high interest to define the molecular mechanisms that cause the depletion of target cells. Many autoimmune diseases are thought to be caused by lytic autoantibodies or CD4$^+$ T cell-mediated delayed type hypersensitivity (DTH)-like inflammatory responses. The involvement of autoreactive CTLs in causing tissue damage is discussed in only a few instances. In Hashimoto's thyroiditis, perforin-expressing CD8$^+$ T cells are found in higher proportions in thyroid infiltrates than in peripheral blood (11), and infiltrating CD8$^+$ T cells were found to express perforin (12). The infiltration of CD8$^+$ T cells was also observed in a mouse model of Hashimoto's disease (13). In multiple sclerosis in humans the cytotoxicity of human myelin basic protein-specific CD4$^+$ T cells via the perforin- and the Fas-dependent pathway, expression of Fas on MHC-II-negative oligodendrocytes, and Fas ligand (FasL) expression on infiltrating lymphocytes has suggested that CD4$^+$ T cells may damage oligodendrocytes by noncognate bystander cytotoxicity (14–16). Findings in experimental encephalitis, a model system for multiple sclerosis in humans, however, failed to confirm such a mechanism (17). Coxsackie virus-induced myocarditis has certain aspects of an autoimmune disease; after infection with the virus, CD8[+] T cells develop that lyse infected and uninfected myocardial cells (18). It is thought that the virus-specific CTLs initiate the lesions in the heart and that the consequential release of myocardial antigens leads to the propagation of heart disease by autoreactive T cells. Perforin expression has been found in heart-infiltrating cells from coxsackie virus-infected mice (19), and circular lesions formed by perforin were described in the membranes of cardiac myocytes (20).

The autoimmune disease for which most evidence of an involvement of T cell-mediated cytotoxicity in pathogenesis exists is insulin-dependent autoimmune diabetes mellitus (IDDM) type I. This disease is characterized by the loss of insulin-producing pancreatic β cells. During its early and clinically silent phase, T cells and other inflammatory cells infiltrate the islets causing a progressive loss of β cells. When most of the β cells have disappeared, the lack of insulin secretion leads to a failure of blood glucose homeostasis and diabetes. Although there is a consensus that IDDM is caused by autoreactive T cells, many other aspects of the disease are still poorly understood, including the breakdown of tolerance against islet cell antigens, the failure of mechanisms controlling self-reactive T cells, genetic and environmental susceptibility factors, and the molecular effector mechanisms that are responsible for the elimination of β cells.

In the past this last point has been addressed by defining the role of the CD4[+] (helper) T cells versus the CD8[+] (cytotoxic) T cell subset. In these studies, the NOD mouse strain has proved useful because it models quite well the spontaneous initiation and chronic progressive course of the disease and the polygenic inheritance of susceptibility genes (21). A number of studies

have shown that adoptive transfer with primary cells taken directly *ex vivo* requires CD4[+] and CD8[+] T cells (22,23). Cloned islet cell-reactive NOD CD4[+] T cells, however, were able to induce diabetes in NOD-scid mice in the absence of CD8[+] T cells (24,25), arguing for a contact-independent mechanism of beta cell destruction because β cells appear not to express MHC-II. At the time, these findings were taken as evidence that both T cell subsets are required for the transfer of diabetes with polyclonal primary T cells but that cloned CD4[+] T cells are able to induce diabetes in the absence of CD8[+] T cells, given high numbers and specificity.

On the other hand, a study using flow cytofluorometry of islet-infiltrating leukocytes has shown that CD8[+] T cells infiltrated the pancreas of young, prediabetic NOD mice earlier than CD4[+] T cells and B cells (26). Similarly, in a pancreas from a patient who had died only a month after diagnosis of diabetes, the islet-infiltrating T cells consisted mainly of the CD8[+] subset (27). Several studies have further supported the crucial role of CD8[+] T cells in diabetes of NOD mice: β_2-Microglobulin-negative and hence CD8[+] T cell-deficient NOD mice developed neither insulitis nor diabetes (28–31). Also, depletion of CD8[+] T cells by antibody treatment 2 to 5 weeks after birth prevented the development of insulitis and also abrogated the ability of CD4[+] T cells to induce insulitis (32). Finally, CD8[+] T cell clones from NOD mice that were generated by restimulation with transgenic islet cells expressing the costimulatory molecule B7.1 were able to transfer diabetes to irradiated NOD and NOD-scid mice (33). These findings clearly demonstrated that CD8[+] T cells are not only responsible for the lysis of β cells in the late effector phase, but that they also may have a role in the early induction phase by affecting the properties of autoreactive CD4[+] T cells.

Perforin-deficient mice lack a major pathway of T cell-mediated cytotoxicity and natural killer (NK) cell-mediated cytotoxicity

(6–10). Because perforin-deficient mice have no defect in activation or proliferation of T cells and generate normal B cell responses (6), they are well suited to directly address the role of cytotoxicity *in vivo*. We first studied diabetes in a mouse model system using transgenic mice expressing glycoprotein of lymphocytic choriomeningitis virus (LCMV-GP) in the pancreas. Expression of the LCMV-GP transgene does not induce T cell tolerance; instead, LCMV-GP-specific T cells are present in a state of "ignorance" in these mice (34). Infection with LCMV triggers an acute virus-specific immune response that induces insulitis and diabetes in perforin-expressing transgenic mice by day 10 after infection. LCMV-GP transgenic perforin-deficient mice, in contrast, did not develop diabetes, although they developed marked insulitis (35). Because perforin-deficient mice are unable to clear an LCMV infection (6), which is eliminated in wild-type C57BL/6 mice by day 8 after infection, diversion of LCMV-GP-specific T cells by abundant virus-infected cells in perforin-deficient mice could have accounted for the failure of perforin-deficient LCMV-GP transgenic mice to develop diabetes. To exclude this possibility we avoided LCMV infection by using an experimental approach in which LCMV-GP-specific T cells are activated by infection with an LCMV-GP-recombinant vaccinia virus strain (vacc-LCMV-GP). The main advantage of this experiment was that the virus load in normal control and perforin-deficient mice did not vary significantly because perforin-deficient mice have an intact ability to control a number of cytopathic viruses, including vaccinia virus (36). The adoptive transfer of LCMV-GP-specific T cell receptor (TCR) transgenic, perforin-deficient T cells activated by LCMV-GP-recombinant vaccinia virus led to marked insulitis with infiltration of CD4[+] and CD8[+] T cells without the development of diabetes. These findings indicate that perforin-dependent cytotoxicity is not required for the initiation of insulitis but is crucial for the destruction of β cells in the later effector phase.

There was a possibility that these findings were specific to this model system, as LCMV induces a strong cytotoxic immune response, and the diabetes develops, unlike human diabetes, acutely without chronic long-term insulitis. It was therefore of interest to test the role of perforin-dependent cytotoxicity in the NOD mouse model, where the spontaneous onset and the chronic inflammation of the pancreatic islets are more similar to the human disease. In addition, we surmised that the slower course of diabetes in the NOD mouse may reveal additional perforin-independent effector mechanisms, which may have been masked during the acute progression of diabetes in the LCMV-GP transgenic model.

In perforin-deficient NOD mice, diabetes developed only with greatly reduced incidence and delayed onset, despite the development of insulitis with infiltration of CD4[+] and CD8[+] T cells that was comparable to normal control NOD mice (37). This shows that perforin-dependent cytotoxicity is a crucial effector mechanism for β cell elimination by CTLs in autoimmune diabetes. The observation that perforin-deficient mice developed diabetes at low frequency pointed also to the existence of one or several additional diabetogenic effector mechanisms that can cause diabetes during the chronic inflammation of the islets in the absence of perforin. Combinations of tumor necrosis factor (TNF) and lymphotoxin-α (LT-α) with interleukin-1 (IL-1) and interferon-γ (IFN-γ) (38–40) have been shown previously to have potent toxic effects on β cells. We recently have obtained evidence that diabetes induction by perforin-deficient T cells *in vivo* is dependent on TNF receptor 1 (p55) expression on β cells (66). This finding suggests that the diabetes induced by the transfer of cloned CD4[+] T cells and the delayed diabetes developing in perforin-deficient NOD mice is induced by the local secretion of synergistic cytokines including TNF and LT-α, which are selectively toxic to β cells and probably function without direct cell-to-cell contact.

Immunohistologic analysis of islets from diabetic NOD mice have shown that 60% to 70% of the infiltrating T cells were CD4$^+$ and only 30% to 40% CD8$^+$. In human diabetes, in contrast, two independent reports have shown that the infiltrate is dominated by CD8$^+$ T cells with only a few CD4$^+$ T cells present. These analyses were performed with the pancreas of a 12-year-old girl who died from ketoacidotic coma after having symptoms of diabetes for only a month (27) and by a second group investigating disease recurrence in three diabetic patients who had received pancreas grafts from their corresponding identical twins and one patient whose graft was from an HLA identical sibling (41). In all of these cases, the islet infiltrating CD8$^+$ T cells outnumbered the CD4$^+$ T cells by far. These findings raise the question of whether in human diabetes, CD8$^+$ T cell-mediated β cell lysis via perforin-dependent cytotoxicity may play an even more important role than in NOD mice.

ANTIVIRAL RESISTANCE

Protection against infectious diseases is the most important task that drove the development of the immune system during evolution. The ability to recognize peptides derived from intracellular antigens in association with MHC-I molecules on virtually any cell of the same individuum underscores the central role that CD8$^+$ T cells have in the immune response against intracellular pathogens, especially against viruses. Although these notions are widely accepted, we are still just beginning to understand how CD8$^+$ T cells are able to control infections with viruses that differ greatly in their strategy of replication, susceptibility to effector mechanisms, and interaction with the host organism. Indirect evidence that CD8$^+$ T cells exert their antiviral effect by contact-dependent lysis of infected cells was provided by studying the adoptive transfer of a CTL clone specific for one influenza A virus subtype in mice that were simultaneously infected with two subtypes (42). The finding

that only replication of that particular subtype and not of the second subtype was reduced indicated that CTLs control virus replication by a strictly contact-dependent mechanism, but it could not rule out completely noncytotoxic secreted cytokines such as IFN-γ and TNF with an effect over a very short range. The difficulty of detecting morphologic evidence for CTL-induced necrosis during antiviral immune responses *in vivo* and other arguments added to the controversy about the role of contact-dependent cytotoxicity in the control of virus infection (3,4,43,44).

The availability of mice deficient for the effector molecules involved in T cell-mediated cytotoxicity has helped to overcome the difficulty of distinguishing between contact-dependent cytotoxicity and short-range cytokines *in vivo*. The perforin-deficient mouse is especially suitable because its defect in the main mechanism of CTL-mediated cytotoxicity does not affect the proliferation and activation of CD8$^+$ T cells, its ability to secrete cytokines, and the induction of B cell responses (6–10). The observation that perforin-deficient mice failed to clear infection with lymphocytic choriomeningitis virus (LCMV) (6) established the concept that cytotoxic activity is a crucial factor in the control of primary viral infection. Surprisingly, perforin-deficient mice were resistant against vesicular stomatitis (VSV), Semliki Forest (SFV), and vaccinia viruses despite of the vigorous primary CTL response that the latter virus induces in normal mice (36). The most striking difference between these two groups was that LCMV is a noncytopathic virus that can chronically infect immune-suppressed animals without causing disease, whereas vesicular stomatitis, Semliki Forest, and vaccinia virus are cytopathic; that is, they kill the host cell during infection. These findings led us to postulate that the nature of the interaction of a virus with the infected host cell is a crucial factor in determining the effectivity of cytotoxic activity in curtailing viral replication. Our somewhat reductionistic hypothesis was that T cell-mediated cytotoxicity is more effective in controlling infections with viruses that are noncytopathic (i.e., that do not kill the host cell during infection) than against cytopathic viruses (for a more detailed description see ref. 45). This is consistent with the idea that after infection with a noncytopathic virus, infected cells could persist and continue to produce infectious virus unless they are eliminated by a cytolytic immune response, given that antiviral cytokines may be able to reduce, but not completely abrogate, intracellular viral replication.

In the case of cytopathic viruses, on the other hand, elimination of infected cell is not absolutely required because they will die due to the cytotoxicity of the virus. Lysis by CTLs could nevertheless reduce viral proliferation by killing infected cells in midcycle before assembly of a full yield of infectious virions is completed. This requires the expression and presentation of viral antigens at this point of the viral life cycle. *In vitro* experiments with vaccinia virus have indeed shown that vaccinia-specific CTLs were able to reduce viral replication only when added to infected cells 1 hour, but not 4 hours, after infection (46). The time window during which lysis can reduce viral proliferation is much shorter for cytopathic than for noncytopathic viruses, where lysis at any point after infection is protective. If recognition and lysis of an infected cell are relatively slow in respect to the viral infectious cycle, T cell-mediated cytolysis is primarily effective in controlling infections with noncytopathic viruses. Limited accessibility of infected cells *in vivo* (47) and the delay of 3 to 4 hours between CTL–target cell conjugation and membrane disruption during *in vitro* cytotoxicity assays indicates that kinetic restraints of the $CD8^+$ T cell response may prevent the timely killing of cells infected with cytopathic viruses in midcycle. Certain viruses may be cytopathic to certain cells and noncytopathic to others infected *in vivo*. Because nonlytically infected cells are potentially able to form a persisting virus reservoir it is expected that their elimination by CTL-mediated lysis would be essential for clearance of a virus that is noncytopathic only in a subset of infected cells.

It is important to recognize that T cell-mediated cytotoxicity may be necessary but not sufficient for clearance of noncytopathic virus infections. Lysis of infected cells inevitably leads to release of infectious virus. Activated phagocytic cells and the prevention of virus spreading to uninfected cells and tissues by interferons, TNF, or neutralizing antibodies play an important role not only in the control of cytopathic viruses such as vaccinia virus (44), VSV (48), and SFV (49) but also against noncytopathic viruses. This point is supported by the increased titers of LCMV that develop after administration of IFN-γ-specific antibodies (50) and in IFN-γ receptor- or IFN-α/β receptor-deficient mice (48).

Meanwhile, perforin-deficient mice have been infected with a number of additional viruses. Two recent reports confirmed the importance of perforin-dependent cytotoxicity in controlling noncytopathic virus infections. Perforin-deficient mice failed to eliminate a recombinant E1-deleted adenovirus from the liver (51). The persistent infection with almost no signs of liver pathology that develops in rag2-deficient mice shows the low cytopathogenicity of this virus (52). Infection of perforin-deficient mice with Theiler's virus also resulted in unrestricted replication death from viral encephalomyelitis (53).

Rotavirus infection, on the other hand, is cytopathic in enterocytes, and the time course of shedded viral antigen in the feces was similar in normal control and perforin-deficient mice (54). JHMV, a neurotropic member of the mouse hepatitis group of coronaviruses, cannot readily be classified as either cytopathic or noncytopathic. As with many viruses, it lyses cell lines *in vitro*; but whether it is cytopathic to the various cell types it infects *in vivo* is not clear. When injected into perforin-deficient mice, JHMV was cleared, but with delayed kinetics (55).

Perforin-deficient mice were highly susceptible to ectromelia, which is generally regarded as a cytopathic virus (56). Liver damage is thought to be the main cause of death in ectromelia infection; and replication in macrophages, especially in Kupffer cells, is a crucial step in the subsequent infection of hepatocytes (57). One report indicated that infectious ectromelia virus can persist for at least 60 days in splenic dendritic cells and macrophages from acutely infected mice (57). This raises the question whether ectromelia virus may be less cytopathic to macrophages and dendritic cells *in vivo* than to hepatocytes and other infected host cell types. If this is the case, cytotoxic activity may be the crucial effector mechanism that eliminates persisting ectromelia infection in antigen-presenting cells and prevents fatal spreading of the virus to the liver. Perforin-deficient mice, even when depleted of CD4$^+$ T cells, resolved influenza A virus infection similarly to that in normal control mice (58), in line with the lytic infection this virus causes in epithelial cells of the respiratory tract and the prominent role that antibodies play in the clearance of influenza virus infection.

Although interpretation of these findings is limited by our incomplete understanding of the interaction of many viruses with the host organism, it can be concluded that perforin-dependent cytotoxicity is essential for the control of all tested noncytopathic viruses. The results obtained with the viruses that are generally regarded as cytopathic are more difficult to interpret because it is often not known whether these viruses indeed are cytopathic to all cell types they infect *in vivo*. Nevertheless, the experimental evidence clearly indicates that cytotoxic T cell responses play a much more prominent role in controlling infections with cytopathic than noncytopathic viruses. It is conceivable that a cytopathic virus that is lytic only in a delayed fashion is susceptible to control by T cell-mediated cytotoxicity, and it remains to be seen whether an example for such a virus can be identified.

In vitro chromium 51(^{51}Cr)-release assays have shown that in addition to the perforin-mediated pathway, CTLs lyse target cells by a second pathway that is mediated by the interaction of FasL on the CTLs and Fas on the target cell (7,59,60). The contribution of this pathway to overall lysis is dependent on the level of Fas expression on the surface of the target cell (61). For typical Fas-expressing target cells it is estimated that the pathway contributes about 30% to overall cytotoxic activity. It was therefore expected that this pathway would also contribute to clearance of LCMV, which has been shown to depend on perforin-dependent cytotoxicity. Surprisingly, no protective effect of Fas-dependent cytotoxicity was measured in an adoptive transfer system in which perforin-dependent cytotoxicity reduced LCMV titers more than 1,000-fold (36). This may be explained by the expression of factors that inhibit Fas-mediated apoptosis in infected cells. Such mechanisms have been demonstrated for other viruses. The product of the *crmA* gene from cowpox virus has been shown to inhibit Fas-mediated apoptosis (62–64). Also, adenovirus is able to induce internalization and subsequent lysosomal degradation of Fas in infected cells by the viral RID–protein complex (65).

CONCLUSIONS

The current data indicate that T cell-mediated cytotoxic activity is involved in clearance of primary infections with only some and not all viruses that generate measurable cytotoxic responses. There is a clear correlation between the cytopathogenicity of a virus and the involvement of perforin-dependent cytotoxicity in clearance. One of the main questions that remains to be answered is whether the strong cytotoxic immune responses that develop after infection with some noncytopathic viruses, such as vaccinia virus, are merely by-products of CD8$^+$ T cell activation or if this activity serves a purpose that has yet to be defined.

REFERENCES

1. Marker O, Volkert M. Studies on cell-mediated immunity to lymphocytic choriomeningitis virus in mice. *J Exp Med* 1973;137:1511–1525.

2. Zinkernagel RM, Doherty PC. Restriction of in vitro T cell mediated cytotoxicity in lymphocytic choriomeningitis within a syngeneic or semiallogeneic system. *Nature* 1974;248:701–702.

3. Lehmann-Grube F, Moskophidis D, Löhler J. Recovery from acute virus infection: role of cytotoxic T lymphocytes in the elimination of lymphocytic choriomeningitis virus from spleens of mice. *Ann NY Acad Sci* 1988;532:238–256.

4. Martz E, Howell DM. CTL: virus control cells first and cytolytic cells second? DNA fragmentation, apoptosis and the prelytic halt hypothesis. *Immunol Today* 1989;10:79–86.

5. Benoist C, Mathis D. Cell death mediators in autoimmune diabetes: no shortage of suspects. *Cell* 1997;89:1–3.

6. Kägi D, Ledermann B, Bürki K, et al. Cytotoxicity mediated by T cells and natural killer cells is greatly impaired in perforin-deficient mice. *Nature* 1994; 369:31–37.

7. Kägi D, Vignaux F, Ledermann B, et al. Fas and perforin pathways as major mechanisms of T cell-mediated cytotoxicity. *Science* 1994;265:528–530.

8. Kojima H, Shinohara N, Hanaoka S, et al. Two distinct pathways of specific killing revealed by perforin mutant cytotoxic T lymphocytes. *Immunity* 1994;1:357–364.

9. Lowin B, Beermann F, Schmidt A, Tschopp J. A null mutation in the perforin gene impairs cytolytic T lymphocyte- and natural killer cell-mediated cytotoxicity. *Proc Natl Acad Sci USA* 1994;91:11571–11575.

10. Walsh CM, Matloubian M, Liu C-C, et al. Immune function in mice lacking the perforin gene. *Proc Natl Acad Sci USA* 1994;91:10854–10858.

11. Iwatami Y, Hidaka Y, Matsuzuka F, Kuma K, Amino N. Intrathyroidal lymphocyte subsets, including unusual CD4+CD8+ cells and CD3lo TCR alpha betalo/CD4− CD8− cells in autoimmune thyroid disease. *Clin Exp Immunol* 1993;93:430–436.

12. Wu Z, Podack ER, McKenzie JM, Olsen KJ, Zakarija M. Perforin-expression by thyroid-infiltrating T cells in autoimmune thyroid disease. *Clin Exp Immunol* 1994;98:470–477.

13. Many MC, Maniratunga S, Varis I, Dardenne M, Drexhage HA, Denef JF. Two-step development of Hashimoto-like thyroiditis in genetically autoimmune prone non-obese diabetic mice: effects on iodine induced cell necrosis. *J Endocrinol* 1995; 147:311–320.

14. Vergelli M, Hemmer B, Muraro PA, et al. Human autoreactive CD4+ T cell clones use perforin- or Fas/Fas ligand-mediated pathways for target cell lysis. *J Immunol* 1997;158:2756–2761.

15. D'Souza SD, Bonetti B, Balasingam V, et al. Multiple sclerosis: Fas signalling in oligodendrocyte cell death. *J Exp Med* 1996;184:2361–2370.

16. Dowling P, Shang G, Raval S, Menonna J, Cook S, Husar W. Involvement of the CD95 (Apo-1/Fas) receptor/ligand system in multiple sclerosis brain. *J Exp Med* 1996;184:1513–1518.

17. Malipiero U, Frei K, Spanaus KS, et al. Myelin oligodendrocyte glycoprotein-induced autoimmune encephalomyelitis is chronic/relapsing in perforin knockout mice, but monophasic in Fas- and Fas

18. ligand-deficient lpr and gld mice. *Eur J Immunol* 1997;27:3151–3160.

18. Schwimmbeck PL, Badorff C, Rohn G, Schulze K, Schultheiss HP. The role of sensitized T cells in myocarditis and dilated cardiomyopathy. *Int J Cardiol* 1996;54:117–125.

19. Seko Y, Shinkai Y, Kawasaki A, et al. Expression of perforin in infiltrating cells in murine hearts with acute myocarditis caused by coxsackievirus B3. *Circulation* 1991;84:788–795.

20. Seko Y, Shinkai Y, Kawasaki A, Yagita H, Okumura K, Yazaki Y. Evidence of perforin-mediated cardiac myocyte injury in acute murine myocarditis caused by coxsackie virus B3. *J Pathol* 1993; 170:53–58.

21. Makino S, Kunimoto K, Muraoka Y, Mizushima Y, Katagiri K, Tochino Y. Breeding of a non-obese diabetic strain of mice. *Exp Anim* 1980;29:1–13.

22. Bendelac A, Carnaud C, Boitard C, Bach JF. Syngeneic transfer of autoimmune diabetes from diabetic NOD mice to healthy neonates: requirement for both L3T4+ and Lyt-2+ T cells. *J Exp Med* 1987; 166:823–832.

23. Miller BJ, Appel MC, O'Neil JJ, Wicker LS. Both the Lyt-2+ and L3T4+ T cell subsets are required for the transfer of diabetes in nonobese diabetic mice. *J Immunol* 1988;140:52–58.

24. Bradley BJ, Haskins K, La Rosa FG, Lafferty KJ. CD8 T cells are not required for islet destruction induced by a CD4-positive islet-specific T cell clone. *Diabetes* 1992;41:1603–1608.

25. Katz JD, Benoist C. T helper cell subsets in insulin-dependent diabetes. *Science* 1995;268:1185–1188.

26. Jarpe AJ, Hickman MR, Anderson JT, Winter WE, Peck AB. Flow cytometric enumeration of mononuclear cell populations infiltrating the islets of Langerhans in prediabetic NOD mice: development of a model of autoimmune insulitis for type I diabetes. *Reg Immunol* 1991;3:305–317.

27. Bottazzo GF, Dean BM, McNally JM, MacKay EH, Swift PGF, Gamble DR. In situ characterization of autoimmune phenomena and expression of HLA molecules in the pancreas in diabetic insulitis. *N Engl J Med* 1985;313:353–360.

28. Katz J, Benoist C, Mathis D. Major histocompatibility complex class I molecules are required for the development of insulitis in non-obese diabetic mice. *Eur J Immunol* 1993;23:3358–3360.

29. Wicker LS, Leiter EH, Todd JA, et al. Beta2-microglobulin-deficient mice do not develop insulitis or diabetes. *Diabetes* 1994;43:500–504.

30. Sumida T, Furukawa M, Sakamoto A, et al. Prevention of insulitis and diabetes in beta 2-microglobulin-deficient non-obese diabetic mice. *Int Immunol* 1994;6:1445–1449.

31. Serreze DV, Leiter E, Christianson J, Greiner D, Roopenian DC. Major Histocompatibility complex class I-deficient NOD-*B2m*null mice are diabetes and insulitis resistant. *Diabetes* 1994;43:505–509.

32. Wang B, Gonzalez A, Benoist C, Mathis D. The role of CD8+ T cells in the initiation of insulin-dependent diabetes mellitus. *Eur J Immunol* 1996; 26:1762–1769.

33. Wong FS, Visintin I, Wen L, Flavell RA, Janeway CA. CD8 T cell clones from young nonobese dia-

betic (NOD) islets can transfer rapid onset of diabetes in NOD mice in the absence of CD4 cells. *J Exp Med* 1996;183:67–76.

34. Ohashi PS, Oehen S, Bürki K, et al. Ablation of "tolerance" and induction of diabetes by virus infection in viral antigen transgenic mice. *Cell* 1991; 65:305–317.

35. Kägi D, Odermatt B, Ohashi PS, Zinkernagel RM, Hengartner H. Development of insulitis without diabetes in transgenic mice lacking perforin-dependent cytotoxicity. *J Exp Med* 1996;183:2143–2152.

36. Kägi D, Seiler P, Pavlovic J, et al. The roles of perforin- and Fas-dependent cytotoxicity in protection against cytopathic and noncytopathic viruses. *Eur J Immunol* 1995;25:3256–3262.

37. Kägi D, Odermatt B, Seiler P, Zinkernagel RM, Mak TW, Hengartner H. Reduced incidence and delayed onset of diabetes in perforin-deficient NOD mice. *J Exp Med* 1997;186:989–997.

38. Mandrup-Poulsen T, Bendtzen K, Dinarello CA, Nerup J. Human necrosis factor potentiates human interleukin-1 mediated rat pancratic beta-cell cytotoxicity. *J Immunol* 1987;139:4077–4082.

39. Campbell IL, Iscaro A, Harrison LC. IFN-gamma and tumor necrosis factor-alpha cytotoxicity to murine islets of Langerhans. *J Immunol* 1988;141:2325–2329.

40. Pukel H, Baquerizo H, Rabinovitch A. Destruction of rat islet cell monolayers by cytokines: synergistic interactions of interferon-gamma, tumour necrosis factor, lymphotoxin and interleukin 1. *Diabetes* 1988;37:133–136.

41. Sibley RK. Recurrent diabetes mellitus in the pancreas iso- and allograft: a light and electron microscopic analysis of four cases. *Lab Invest* 1985; 53:132–144.

42. Lukacher AE, Braciale VL, Braciale TJ. In vivo effector function of influenza virus-specific cytotoxic T lymphocyte clones is highly specific. *J Exp Med* 1984;160:814–825.

43. Oldstone MBA, Blount P, Southern PJ, Lampert PW. Cytoimmunotherapy for persistent virus infection reveals a unique clearance pattern from the central nervous system. *Nature* 1986;321:239–243.

44. Ramsay AJ, Ruby J, Ramshaw IA. The case for cytokines as effector molecules in the resolution of virus infection. *Immunol Today* 1993;14:155–157.

45. Kägi D, Hengartner H. Different roles for cytotoxic T cells in the control of infections with cytopathic versus noncytopathic viruses. *Curr Opin Immunol* 1996;8:472–477.

46. Zinkernagel RM, Althage A. Antiviral protection by virus-immune cytotoxic T cells: infected target cells are lysed before infectious virus progeny is assembled. *J Exp Med* 1977;145:644–651.

47. Ando K, Guidott LG, Cerny A, Ishikawa T, Chisari FV. CTL access to tissue antigen is restricted in vivo. *J Immunol* 1994;153:482–488.

48. Müller U, Steinhoff U, Reis LFL, et al. Functional role of type I and type II interferons in antiviral defense. *Science* 1994;264:1918–1921.

49. Hwang SY, Hertzog PJ, Holland KA, et al. A null mutation in the gene encoding a type I interferon receptor component eliminates anti-proliferative responses to interferon alpha and beta and alters

macrophage responses. *Proc Natl Acad Sci USA* 1995;92:11284–11288.

50. Wille A, Gessner A, Lother H, Lehmann-Grube F. Mechanism of recovery from acute virus infection. VIII. Treatment of lymphocytic choriomeningitis virus-infected mice with interferon-gamma monoclonal antibody blocks generation of virus-specific cytotoxic T lymphocytes and virus elimination. *Eur J Immunol* 1989;19:1283–1288.

51. Yang Y, Xiang Z, Ertl H, Wilson JM. Upregulation of class I major histocompatibility complex antigens by interferon gamma is necessary for T cell-mediated elimination of recombinant adenovirus-infected hepatocytes in vivo. *Proc Natl Acad Sci USA* 1995;92:7257–7261.

52. Yang Y, Ertl HCJ, Wilson JM. MHC class I-restricted cytotoxic T lymphocytes to viral antigens destroy hepatocytes in mice infected with E1-deleted recombinant adenoviruses. *Immunity* 1994; 1:433–442.

53. Pena Rossi C, McAllister A, Tanguy M, Kägi D, Brahic M. Theiler's virus infection of perforin-deficient mice. *J Virol* 1998;72:4515–4519.

54. Franco MA, Tin C, Rott LS, VanCott JL, McGhee JR, Greenberg HB. Evidence for CD8+ T cell immunity to murine rotavirus in the absence of perforin, Fas and gamma interferon. *J Virol* 1997;71:479–486.

55. Lin MT, Stohlman SA, Hinton DR. Mouse hepatitis virus is cleared from the central nervous systems of mice lacking perforin-mediated cytolysis. *J Virol* 1997;71:383–391.

56. Ramshaw IA, Ramsay AJ, Karupiah G, Rolph MS, Mahalingam S, Ruby JC. Cytokines and immunity to viral infections. *Immunol Rev* 1997;159:119–135.

57. Mims CA. Aspects of the pathogenesis of virus diseases. *Bacteriol Rev* 1964;28:30–71.

58. Topham DJ, Tripp RA, Doherty PC. CD8+ T cells clear influenza virus by perforin or Fas-dependent processes. *J Immunol* 1997;159:5197–5200.

59. Rouvier E, Luciani MF, Golstein P. Fas involvement in Ca2+-independent T cell mediated cytotoxicity. *J Exp Med* 1993;177:195–200.

60. Lowin B, Hahne M, Mattmann C, Tschopp J. Cytolytic T-cell cytotoxicity is mediated through perforin and Fas lytic pathways. *Nature* 1994;370:650–652.

61. Kägi D, Ledermann B, Bürki K, Zinkernagel RM, Hengartner H. Lymphocyte-mediated cytotoxicity in vitro and in vivo: mechanisms and significance. *Immunol Rev* 1995;146:95–115.

62. Ray CA, Black RA, Kronheim SR, et al. Viral inhibition of inflammation: cowpox virus encodes an inhibitor of the interleukin-1 beta converting enzyme. *Cell* 1992;69:597–604.

63. Enari M, Hug H, Nagata S. Involvement of an ICE-like protease in Fas-mediated apoptosis. *Nature* 1995;375:78–80.

64. Los M, van de Craen M, Penning LC, et al. Requirement of an ICE/CED-3 protease for Fas/Apo-1-mediated apoptosis. *Nature* 1995;375:81–83.

65. Tollefsen AE, Hermiston TW, Lichtenstein DL, et al. Forced degradation of Fas inhibits apoptosis in adenovirus-infected cells. *Nature* 1998;392:726–730.

66. Kägi D, Ho A, Odermatt B, et al. TNF receptor 1-dependent beta cell toxicity as an effector pathway in autoimmune diabetes. *J Immunol* 1999;162:4598–4605.

Cytotoxic Cells: Basic Mechanisms and Medical Applications, edited by Michail V. Sitkovsky and Pierre A. Henkart. Lippincott Williams & Wilkins, Philadelphia © 2000.

Chapter 19

Cytotoxic Lymphocytes in Hepatitis B

Barbara Rehermann

Liver Diseases Section, NIDDK, National Institutes of Health, Bethesda, Maryland 20892-1800, USA

The hepatitis B virus (HBV) is a parenterally transmitted, hepatotropic virus that causes inflammatory liver disease. Hepatitis can present as acute disease with a self-limited course or as chronic infection with continuing intrahepatic inflammation that may eventually cause liver cirrhosis and hepatocellular carcinoma. The outcome of infection depends on the kinetics of the virus–host interaction and in particular on the strength of the immune response. If infection occurs in immunocompetent adults, HBV can be cleared in most cases, while infection early or late in life results in a high incidence of viral persistence (1). Similarly, the response rate to hepatitis B surface antigen (HBsAg) vaccination decreases with age. This is presumably due to a decreased immune response state.

In addition to antibody and T helper (Th) cell responses, cytotoxic T cells (CTLs) play a particularly important role in the immune response to HBV because these are the main effector cells that recognize and eliminate HBV from infected hepatocytes. The CTL response to HBV is multispecifically targeted against epitopes in all viral proteins and can exert varying, even opposing effects: On one hand, it can mediate viral clearance and long-lasting immune memory that contributes to protection against reinfection; on the other hand, it can mediate chronic, intrahepatic inflammation, the precondition for the development of hepatocellular carcinoma (HCC).

Various CTL functions have also been demonstrated at the molecular level: CTLs can cure HBV-infected cells by secretion of cytokines that inhibit viral gene expression and replication, but they can also kill infected cells via fas- and granzyme-mediated pathways. These different aspects of the CTL response to HBV are presented in this chapter. Knowledge of CTLs and their role in viral clearance and immunopathogenesis may contribute to the development of rationally designed immunotherapies for chronically infected patients.

ACTIVATION AND FUNCTION OF CYTOTOXIC T CELLS

$CD8^+$ T cells represent the main effector limb during many viral infections. They recognize endogenously synthesized viral peptides in the antigen-binding groove of HLA class I molecules on the surface of virus-infected cells. These peptides, which are generated from endogenously synthesized viral antigens within the cell, are typically 8 to 11 amino acids long and contain an HLA-specific binding motif. Recognition of the peptide–major histocompatibility complex (MHC) by the T cell receptor–CD8 complex results in activation of CTLs to either kill or cure virus-infected cells: "Death" of infected cells can be induced as apoptosis via the Fas or tumor necrosis factor receptor (TNF-R) pathway or via granzyme-mediated lysis.

"Cure" of infected cells is induced via secreted cytokines such as TNF-α, interferon-γ (IFN-γ) and interleukin-2 (IL-2), which suppress viral gene expression and replication (2–4). In addition, cytotoxic T cells may also exert immune regulatory functions (5–7); for example, it is known that hepatitis B envelope (HBeAg)-specific CD8$^+$ T cells suppress the proliferative response of intrahepatic CD4$^+$ cells in patients with chronic hepatitis (8).

ANALYSIS OF THE CTL RESPONSE IN HBV-INFECTED PATIENTS

Acute Self-Limited Hepatitis B

Most patients with acute hepatitis B who are able to clear the infection mount a vigorous HLA class I restricted CTL response that is detectable in the peripheral blood early after infection, simultaneously with or even prior to the humoral immune response (9). It correlates with the rise in serum alanine aminotransferase (ALT) levels and persists for decades after recovery (10). In contrast, the same response is not readily detectable in the blood of chronically infected patients.

The CTL response is targeted against multiple epitopes that are located in all viral proteins and restricted by many different HLA alleles. Interestingly, even patients who share a given HLA allele may mount CTL responses against different HBV epitopes within the panel of peptides that exhibit a high binding affinity to this allele, indicating that many variables within the complexity of virus–host interactions can influence the immune response.

The kinetics of the CTL response during the acute phase of infection is not well characterized. For example, chronically infected patients, even those who acquire HBV infection during adulthood, display only infrequent and weak CTL responses in the blood. At this time, it is not known whether these patients never mounted a strong response during the acute phase of infection, whether their initial CTL response was restricted to a small panel of epitopes or whether to subdominant instead of dominant epitopes, or whether the CTL response underwent early downregulation. More sensitive methods that allow quantitative detection of peptide-specific CTLs with labeled peptide–MHC tetrameric complexes via FACS analysis (11) have proven that HBV-specific CTLs are not completely absent, but are present at low numbers in the blood of chronically infected patients (12). This new technique should help to elucidate the kinetics of the virus–host interaction and its association with the outcome of infection when used in prospective analyses of the HBV-specific immune response from the acute stage of infection to recovery or persistent infection with chronic liver disease.

Indirect conclusions on the kinetics of the CD8$^+$ CTL response may also be drawn from the analysis of the CD4$^+$ T cell response. Prospective analyses of patients who were able to clear the infection revealed that the HBcore-specific T cell response decreases in the peripheral blood 4 to 8 weeks after acute hepatitis B (13). Hepatitis B core antigen (HBcAg)-specific T cell clones that were predominantly of the Th0 (30%) or Th1 phenotype (70%) could be isolated at these time points but did not produce IL-2 upon antigen-specific stimulation and inhibited antigen-specific proliferation of the identical responsive clones isolated from earlier time points. Anergy induction may therefore be involved in the downregulation of the virus-specific immune response after viral clearance (13). Despite this downregulation of antigen-specific T cells early after clearance of the HBV, strong memory responses of predominantly Th0-like cells are detectable in the peripheral blood several years after virus elimination (14).

Similar kinetics have been reported for CD8$^+$ T cells in a different viral infection. In acute LCMV infection, up to 40% of CD8$^+$ T cells can be stained with a GP33 tetramer. These antigen-specific CD8$^+$ T cells then undergo an anergic state with absent cytotoxicity and reduced interferon production before most of these cells are finally deleted (15). Whether the same kinetics of the CD8$^+$ CTL response is also present in acute, self-limited HBV infection still needs to be evaluated.

Recovery from Hepatitis B

Recovery from hepatitis B is characterized by a balance between the persistence of CTLs and low levels of replicating virus. CTL and Th lymphocyte responses are readily detectable in the peripheral blood of most patients even decades after complete clinical and serologic recovery from acute hepatitis B. Whether the persistence of these HBV-specific CTLs requires the presence of antigen or replicating virus is still a controversial point. Whereas specific CD4$^+$ Th cells can be stimulated by antigen trapped on and presented by follicular dendritic cells in the regional lymph nodes, this is generally not possible for CTLs, as most soluble antigens can only enter the class II, not the class I processing pathway. Interestingly, the hydrophobic HBsAg is a notable exception because it has been demonstrated to be processed via the endosomal pathway (16,17). Accordingly, processing can be inhibited by reagents that prevent acidification of endosomes or interfere with acid proteases (16,17).

Vaccination with HBsAg does induce HBs-specific CTLs in mice (16,17) and in humans (Rehermann et al., unpublished observation); it may therefore represent an example that CTLs can be induced by soluble protein in the absence of replicating virus. However, there are also differences between the HBV-specific CTL response of HBsAg vaccinees and patients who recovered from natural HBV infection, indicating that remaining HBV proteins are not sufficient to maintain the HBV-specific CTL response after clinical recovery. In vaccinees, the HBsAg-induced peripheral blood CTL response declines below the threshold of detectability in the peripheral blood a few weeks after vaccination, whereas it persists at high levels in the blood of patients who recovered from hepatitis B. Moreover, the CTL response of recovered patients is not only targeted against epitopes within HBsAg but also against epitopes within HBV polymerase, a protein that is not secreted and present only in minute amounts during HBV replication in infected cells. In addition, cytotoxic T cells detected in the blood of recovered patients do not display the phenotype of resting memory cells but that of recently activated cells; that is, they express the activation markers DR and CD69 on their surface, indicating stimulation within the 24 to 48 hours prior to analysis. Moreover, patients who maintain a CTL response up to 30 years after recovery from acute hepatitis B and antigen clearance are characterized by the persistence of low levels of HBV-DNA in serum or lymphocytes (10). Therefore, transcriptionally active HBV seems to maintain the HBV-specific immune response via de novo induction of HBV-specific CTLs, whereas the latter control the viral load. Similar observations of persisting CTLs and low levels of replicating virus have also been made in patients with a sustained response to IFN therapy, indicating that similar mechanisms of viral clearance and immunosurveillance contribute to the recovery from both acute and chronic HBV infection (19).

Specifically, these CTLs appear to control and limit viral load and, together with the HBV-specific antibody and T helper responses, seem to protect from viral reinfection and from reactivation of hepatitis. Accordingly, it has also been reported that organs from HBsAg-negative, anti-HBs-positive donors can transmit HBV infection when the recipient is immunosuppressed (20,21).

In which organs and tissues HBV persists after recovery from hepatitis B is not known. In chronic hepatitis B, replicative forms of the virus have been detected in bile duct epithelium and smooth muscle cells (22), in pancreas, kidney, and skin (23), in brain, endocrine tissues, and lymph nodes (24,25), and nonreplicative forms in cells of the immune system. Experiments in transgenic mice have shown that some of these sites (e.g., the renal tubular epithelium and the choroid plexus) are not readily accessible to the CTLs (26) because of a closed basal membrane and could therefore represent immunoprivileged sites.

Chronic Hepatitis B

It is generally assumed that in chronic HBV infection the CTL response is too weak to clear the infection but strong enough to mediate liver injury. As described above, HBV-specific CTLs are detected only rarely in the blood of chronically infected patients but can be readily isolated from liver biopsy samples.

At the site of inflammation (i.e., within the liver) HBV-specific CD8$^+$ and CD4$^+$ T cells contribute to the intrahepatic inflammatory infiltrate (27). In addition, B cells form lymphoid follicles in the portal tracts and sinusoids that function as peripheral lymphoid organs (28,29). These HBV-specific cells initiate immune-mediated liver disease that can be profoundly amplified by antigen-nonspecific cells recruited to the site of infection. In chronic active hepatitis, for example, the intrahepatitic infiltrate reaches from the portal fields through the liver parenchyma toward the central veins, a feature characterized as piecemeal necrosis.

Analysis of transgenic mice that express HBsAg intrahepatically has shown that injected HBsAg-specific, CD8$^+$ T cell clones attach to HBsAg-positive hepatocytes in the space of Disse and trigger them to undergo apoptosis (30). In addition, analysis of liver infiltrating lymphocytes in hepatitis C has demonstrated that these highly activated, intrahepatic lymphocytes then undergo programmed cell death themselves (31). Hence in hepatitis C and presumably also hepatitis B, the liver-infiltrating lymphocytes do not expand but undergo apoptosis in the liver and are replaced by a continuous stream of new lymphocytes that infiltrate the liver from the blood.

Potential Mechanism of HBV Persistence and Escape from Immunosurveillance

Various mechanisms of HBV persistence may apply according to the age and immune response state of the individual at the time of HBV infection. Most chronically infected patients acquire HBV infection through vertical transmission from mother to child. This is particularly true for countries in Central Africa and Southeast Asia, where the prevalence of chronic hepatitis B is 8% to 15% (32,33). This high incidence of chronic HBV infection associated with vertical transmission of the HBV may be due to the tolerance of the neonatal immune system at the time of infection.

In fact, most neonates who develop persistent infection are born to HBsAg- and HBeAg-positive mothers; and the small, secreted HBeAg is thought to act as a tolerogen. Because of its small size it is able to cross the placental membrane (34,35) and reach the thymus of the unborn child, where it is recognized as self-antigen, and causes HBeAg-specific tolerance. Interestingly, T cell tolerance is more complete in Th1 cells than in Th2 cells; and T cell tolerance induced in utero therefore affects the Th1/Th2 balance toward a predominance of Th2 cells. Th2 cells support the development of HBV antibodies rather than CTLs, and therefore there is generally no evidence of immune-mediated liver injury during the first 1.5 decades of life. When the thymus involutes, however, tolerance can no longer be maintained, resulting in immune-mediated liver injury initiated by antigen-specific CTLs. Obviously, the age of the child at the time of infection is crucial for the development of an HBV carrier state and correlates inversely with the rate of chronic infections (36).

This hypothesis has been supported by reports that nontransgenic progeny of HBeAg transgenic mice display weak cellular responses to both HBeAg and HBcAg (37). This effect is due to tolerance rather than deletion or anergy of antigen-specific T cells, as immunization with an HBeAg-derived peptide (aa 129-140) induces Th cells that then stimulate autoantibody production by HBeAg-specific B cells.

Hypothetically, the weak or missing HBV-specific Th cell response can affect and diminish the induction of HBV-specific cytotoxic T cells in at least two ways: First, it has been shown that Th cells are necessary to activate professional antigen-presenting cells, such as dendritic cells (38). Only activated dendritic cells express the cytokines and co-stimulatory molecules that are required for efficient induction of CTLs. Second, early exposure to the tolerogenic HBeAg may skew the balance between HBcAg- and HBeAg-specific Th1 and Th2 cells toward a Th2 profile as described above. This, however, favors the induction of humoral rather than cellular immune responses, as generation of CTLs is supported by Th1 cytokines.

Different mechanisms, however, may contribute to the development of chronic hepatitis B in immunocompetent adults. It is possible that consistently high serum levels of HBsAg anergize or exhaust envelope-specific CD4 cells early in the infection because there have been coincidental reports that an antienvelope T cell response may occur during the preclinical incubation period of disease (39). CTLs could contribute to this downregulation of the HBV-specific Th cell response, as CD4$^+$ and CD8$^+$ T cells have been shown to recognize a sequence between amino acids 133 and 145 of the envelope antigen (40). Because CD4$^+$ T cells can internalize and process hepatitis B envelope antigen via the transferrin receptor and also express MHC-II molecules they could become targets for HBV-specific class II-restricted cytotoxic T cells. The lysis of antigen-presenting CD4$^+$ cells could then downregulate the class II-restricted CD4$^+$ T cell response, decrease the activation of dendritic cells (38), and consequently prevent an efficient induction of CTLs.

Finally, it is also possible that CTLs present in the intrahepatic infiltrate and, at low precursor frequency, in the peripheral blood of patients with chronic hepatitis B are not sufficiently activated to induce viral clearance. For example, it has been noted that CTLs specific for nondominant epitopes are predominant in chronic viral infections (41), whereas CTLs specific for dominant epitopes are found in acute, self-limited viral infections. CTLs specific for nondominant epitopes frequently display a high affinity for their target antigens and limited T cell receptor (TCR) usage (41), indicating that they may not be able to adjust to viral variants that emerge in chronic infection (see below).

In addition, there is emerging evidence that the effects of cytokines such as IFN-γ and TNF-α rather than the cytotoxic function of CTLs are required to mediate viral clearance (12). Importantly, elicitation of T cell effector functions follows a certain hierarchy: Low peptide concentrations can induce cytotoxic effector functions of CTLs, whereas higher peptide concentrations are required to induce IFN-γ production and responsiveness to IL-2, and the highest stimulation is required to amplify virus-specific T cells (43). It is therefore possible that insufficiently activated CTLs may not be able to clear the infection via cytokine-mediated mechanisms but may still be able to induce immunologically mediated liver injury via cytotoxic effects.

Another candidate mechanism proposed to contribute to viral persistence is viral escape from immune recognition by mutations in CTL epitopes. Although it has not been shown that CTL escape variants develop during acute hepatitis B and contribute to a chronic outcome of infection, viral variations within CTL epitopes have been demonstrated in chronic HBV infection (44,45) and in HLTV, HIV, and HCV infections (46–51). In several cases mutations resulted in the generation of antagonist epitopes that inhibited the immune response against the original epitope either completely (52,53) or partially by affecting certain T cell functions such as proliferation or cytokine secretion (54).

To assess the pathogenic potential of these variants and their influence on the outcome of infection, it must be considered that the cellular immune response in acute HBV infection is not focused on single epitopes but is rather multispecifically targeted against many epitopes within highly conserved DNA sequences (9,55–58). HBV would therefore have to mutate in many epitope regions to establish immune escape variants. Because several epitopes are conserved even in the evolutionarily related retroviruses (59), mutations in at least some epitopes do not seem to be compatible with the viral life cycle (44,45). Instead, viral mutations may also emerge because of molecular rather than immunologic advantages for the virus. For example, mutations in the precore protein of HBV occur in well defined sites (i.e., in matching pairs on each site of the stem-loop structure of the pregenomic viral RNA) (60,61) to improve the basepairing, thereby stabilizing the stem loop structure. These mutations might confer a replication advantage for HBV, as this region contains the origin of replication and the packaging signal. In summary, HBV variants that escape from immunosurveillance and even antagonize the CTL response against wild-type sequences have been demonstrated in chronic HBV infection; but it is still not known whether viral escape plays a role during acute infection or is the consequence rather than the cause of persistent infection (62).

ANALYSIS OF THE HBV-SPECIFIC CTL RESPONSE IN TRANSGENIC MOUSE MODELS

Models for Acute Hepatitis

Studies on the role of the MHC-restricted immune response to HBV have long been hampered by the fact that the necessary reagents and experimental systems were not available. Apart from humans, chimpanzees are the only natural hosts for HBV; and the limited availability and outbred nature of these animals and the missing immunologic reagents render immune response and vaccination studies difficult. The generation of mice transgenic for individual or all HBV proteins and even replicate HBV and produce infectious virus has therefore contributed much to the current knowledge on HBV immunopathogenesis. The following paragraphs describe studies and observations that are relevant for our understanding of the antiviral and pathogenic effects of cytotoxic T cells.

Adoptive transfer of HBV-specific CTLs into transgenic mice that express HBsAg in hepatocytes revealed that the initiation of liver disease in acute hepatitis is based on antigen-specific recognition by $CD8^+$ lymphocytes, which attach to HBsAg-positive hepatocytes and trigger them to undergo apoptosis (30). Microscopically, apoptotic hepatocytes appear as acidophilic Councilman bodies. During the first few hours after onset of acute hepatitis CTLs recruit antigen-nonspecific inflammatory host cells into the liver, and they finally outnumber the HBV-specific CTLs by at least a factor of 100. This efficient, antigen-independent amplification cascade mediated by antigen-nonspecific T cells and inflammatory cytokines causes most of the histopathologic manifestations of liver disease and can be prevented by neutralizing antibodies to IFN-γ or by inactivation of macrophages.

In addition, recent experiments with transgenic mice that replicate the HBV genome (63) have demonstrated that cytokines produced by cytotoxic T cells can also "cure" hepatocytes from the HBV without killing the cells. These effects are mediated by cytokines such as IFN-γ and TNF-α and cause posttranscriptional downregulation of all viral gene products including the intrahepatic nucleocapsid and the viral replicative intermediates. It is not yet known which of the described mechanisms (i.e., destruction of HBV-infected cells or suppression of viral gene expression and replication) dominates in certain forms of liver disease.

Models for Chronic Hepatitis and Hepatocellular Carcinoma

The risk of developing hepatocellular carcinoma (HCC) is at least 200-fold greater for persons with chronic hepatitis B than for uninfected persons. The lifetime risk of death from HCC or cirrhosis is 40% to 50% for men and 15% for women.

Molecular and immunologic factors have been discussed in regard to their contribution to carcinogenesis. Integrated, transcriptionally active HBV DNA sequences are present in hepatoma cells, even in patients without serologic markers for HBV infection (64). It has therefore often been suggested that integration of HBV DNA, deletions in the flanking sequences of the host genomic DNA, or effects of individual HBV gene products may play a role in the development of HCC. In particular, the HBx protein, a nuclear and cytoplasmic protein with trans-activating abilities, has been linked with hepatocarcinogenesis, as it activates transcription factors such as NF-kB, AP-1, and c/EBV, as well as cytoplasmic signal transduction cascades, such as the Ras-Raf-MAPK cascade. It has also been shown to inhibit *p53* gene function *in vitro* (65–68).

Chronic inflammatory liver injury has long been discussed as a procarcinogenic process, and accumulation of large amounts of HBV large envelope proteins in the endoplasmic reticulum (ER) of ground-glass hepatocytes has been shown to trigger severe chronic inflammatory processes, resulting in hepatocellular injury, regenerative hyperplasia, DNA damage, and aneuploidy (69–72). Nevertheless, the effects of CTLs as initiators of inflammatory liver disease have been difficult to analyze. The main reason is that hepatitis induced by adoptive transfer of CTLs into HBsAg transgenic mice is transient and nonfatal, precluding analysis of the effects of chronic inflammatory liver disease. Presumably, adoptively transferred CTLs have a limited life-span and cannot be regenerated in this model.

A recently reported mouse model for chronic hepatitis has permitted analysis of long-term effects of chronic inflammatory liver injury (73). Specifically, transgenic mice that were tolerant for the intrahepatically expressed HB envelope proteins were thymectomized, lethally irradiated, and reconstituted with T cell-depleted bone marrow from nontransgenic mice. The adoptive transfer of splenocytes from nontransgenic mice immunized with HBsAg resulted in acute hepatitis due to HBsAg-specific CTLs and the disappearance of HBsAg from the serum due to the transferred HBsAg-specific B cells (73). Importantly, however, HBsAg-specific CTLs were not able to downregulate HBV gene expression completely, and the mice developed chronic hepatitis. HBsAg-specific CTL responses were still present in the spleens 17 months after adoptive transfer, and all animals developed multiple, large hepatocellular carcinomas at this time. In contrast, mice substituted with bone marrow and splenocytes from transgenic (i.e., tolerant) mice displayed a lower degree of serologic and histologic evidence of chronic hepatitis throughout the observation period and only one mouse developed HCC or benign adenoma, respectively, at the time of autopsy (73). The results of this study demonstrate clearly that chronic inflammatory liver injury and continuing liver regeneration constitutes a main factor in the process of hepatocarcinogenesis.

THERAPEUTIC APPROACHES TO ENHANCE THE HBV-SPECIFIC CTL RESPONSE

Though vaccines to prevent HBV infection have been available for about 20 years and the recent vaccination of all infants will ultimately decrease the incidence of de novo infection, there is still no causal and successful therapy for the treatment of most chronically infected persons. The ability of the vaccine to induce HBV-specific CTLs that kill or cure

HBV-infected host cells is particularly important if it should be considered for the treatment of these chronically infected patients.

Specifically, the selective stimulation and expansion of HBV-specific CTLs in the blood of patients with chronic HBV or the de novo induction of CTLs against multiple immunodominant epitopes might facilitate viral clearance. Importantly, the concept of degenerate peptide-binding motifs has been extended from class II to class I binding (74), indicating that a peptide-based vaccine may be feasible despite the wide variety of MHC haplotypes. Along this line, a lipopeptide-based vaccine has been developed that consists of an HLA-A2-restricted HBV CTL epitope linked to a Th epitope derived from tetanus toxoid and two molecules of palmitic acid (75). Although a phase I clinical trial has shown that this vaccine can induce a dose-dependent HBV-specific CTL response (a) that is comparable in strength to memory responses against influenza virus, (b) that recognize endogenously processed antigen *in vitro,* and (c) that persists for more than 9 months in the peripheral blood (76), the response was obviously not strong enough to mediate viral clearance. It may therefore be more feasible to design vaccines that present multiple epitopes (77,78) to induce long-lasting and effective antibody and CTL responses (79). This would also decrease the risk of emerging CTL escape mutants that may result in a more rapid course of disease as reported for a human immunodeficiency virus (HIV)-infected person (80).

Rapid induction of CTL and high-avidity antibody responses can be achieved efficiently with DNA immunization (81). Intramuscular or intradermal administration of DNA expression vectors encoding sequences of the desired immunogenic protein under the control of an appropriate promoter has been shown to induce a strong immune response at the T and B cell level in mice (82). Especially intradermal injection can induce stronger and earlier CTL responses due to direct transfection of professional antigen-presenting cells (e.g., Langerhans cells) (81).

Vaccination with DNA has the advantage that DNA vectors are less expensive and easier to produce than antigenic proteins used in the current vaccines. Moreover, DNA immunization induces a strong CTL response and a Th cell and antibody response to the expressed protein (82); and finally, the antigenic proteins are expressed *in vivo* in transfected cells and yield naturally (i.e., endogenously) processed epitopes. It therefore carries the efficacy of live attenuated vaccines without the risk of an infection of the vaccinee. Moreover, it has been shown in the murine model that DNA vaccination can enlarge the number of responding haplotypes for CTL induction (83).

Indeed, in animals, DNA-mediated immunization has been shown to induce a CTL and antibody response against a broad variety of pathogens, such as influenza (84), HIV-1 (85,86), and rabies virus (87). Immunization of mice with a DNA vaccine encoding the three envelope proteins induced immunoglobulins M and G (IgM, IgG) HBs-specific antibodies; and the humoral immune response that was first present 1 to 2 weeks after infection was maintained for at least 6 months (88). Transgenic mice that express the whole HBV genome except for the core gene and secret HBsAg in the serum, have also been immunized with a plasmid expressing the small and middle forms of the HBenv proteins. After a single DNA immunization, HBsAg was cleared from the serum, and HBVmRNA was downregulated in the liver for 5 months of follow-up (89,90), an effect that can be attributed to the function of the CTLs. These mice are a model for chronic hepatitis B, so DNA immunization might also represent a valuable approach to treat chronically infected patients. Immunization of two chimpanzees with a plasmid encoding the major and middle HBV envelope proteins also induced anti-HBs antibodies; and the observed IgM to IgG (mainly IgG1) class switch indicates the induction of a Th2-type cellular immune response.

The type of immune response induced by DNA vaccination can also be modulated by the addition of cytokines such as IL-12, which mediates Th1 and CTL induction and stimulates the production of IFN-γ and TNF from natural killer (NK) and T cells. Certain CpG motifs in bacterial DNA can even function as adjuvants and bias the immune response toward a Th1 profile by induction of endogenous production of IL-12 (91).

DNA sequences that code for the desired antigens can also be delivered orally by live, attenuated *Salmonella* or *Shigella* vaccine strains. These bacteria invade the gastrointestinal mucosa, which represents a much greater surface area than the quadriceps muscle used for DNA injection; they persist in M cells in the Peyer plaques of the intestinal mucosa and are eventually phagocytosed by macrophages and dendritic cells, which then become activated and migrate into lymph nodes and the spleen (92). In addition to the ease of vaccine delivery, antigen presentation for induction of CTLs may be more efficient than by intramuscularly delivered DNA vaccines (93). Ultimately, a strong humoral and cellular, mucosal, and systemic immune response is induced (94).

CONCLUSIONS

The strategy of boosting the HBV-specific CTL immune response in patients with chronic hepatitis by synthetic peptide, DNA-based, or other vaccine strategies might strengthen the cellular immune response and tip the balance between virus and host. Hopefully, a new treatment that combines immunotherapeutic and antiviral approaches and aims at the induction or enhancement of a cellular Th1 and cytotoxic T cell response may become available for chronically infected patients. It would ultimately decrease morbidity and mortality due to HCC and other risks of chronic hepatitis B.

REFERENCES

1. Chiaramonte M, Floreani A, Naccarato R. Hepatitis B virus in the elderly: an underestimated problem. *Biomed Pharmacother* 1987;41:121–123.

2. Guidotti LG, Ando K, Hobbs MV, et al. Cytotoxic T lymphocytes inhibit hepatitis B virus gene expression by a noncytolytic mechanism in transgenic mice. *Proc Natl Acad Sci USA* 1994;91:2764–3768.

3. Gilles PN, Fey G, Chisari FV. Tumor necrosis factor-alpha negatively regulates hepatitis B virus gene expression in transgenic mice. *J Virol* 1992;66:3955–3960.

4. Guidotti LG, Guilhot S, Chisari FV. Interleukin 2 and interferon alpha/beta downregulate hepatitis B virus gene expression in vivo by tumor necrosis factor dependent and independent pathways. *J Virol* 1994;68:1265–1270.

5. Bloom BR, Salgame P, Diamond B. Revisiting and revising suppressor T cells. *Immunol Today* 1992;13:131–136.

6. Seder RA, Boulay J-L, Finkelman F, et al. CD8+ T cells can be primed in vitro to produce IL-4. *J Immunology* 1992;148:1652–1656.

7. Salgame P, Abrams JS, Clayberger C, et al. Differing lymphokine profiles of functional subsets of human CD4 and CD8 T cell clones. *Science* 1991;254:279–282.

8. Ferrari C, Penna A, Giuberti T, et al. Intrahepatic, nucleocapsid antigen-specific T cells in chronic active hepatitis B. *J Immunol* 1987;139:2050–2058.

9. Rehermann B, Fowler P, Sidney J, et al. The cytotoxic T lymphocyte response to multiple hepatitis B virus polymerase epitopes during and after acute viral hepatitis. *J Exp Med* 1995;181:1047–1058.

10. Rehermann B, Ferrari C, Pasquinelli C, Chisari FV. The hepatitis B virus persists for decades after patients' recovery from acute viral hepatitis despite active maintenance of a cytotoxic T-lymphocyte response. *Nat Med* 1996;2:1104–1108.

11. Altman J, Moss PAH, Goulder PJR, et al. Phenotypic analysis of antigen specific T lymphocytes. *Science* 1996;274:94–96.

12. Maini MK, Ogg S, Boni C, et al. Direct visualisation of hepatitis B virus (HBV)-specific cytotoxic T cells with an human leucocyte antigen (HLA) class I-peptide tetrameric complex allows a new insight into their actual frequency [abstract]. *Hepatology* 1998;28:485A.

13. Diepolder HM, Jung MC, Wierenga E, et al. Anergic TH1 clones specific for hepatitis B virus (HBV) core peptides are inhibitory to other HBV core-specific CD4+ T cells in vitro. *J Virol* 1996;70:7540–7548.

14. Penna A, Artini M, Cavalli A, et al. Long lasting memory T cell responses following self-limited acute hepatitis B. *J Clin Invest* 1996;11566:30575–22828.

15. Gallimore A, Glithero A, Godkin A, et al. Induction and exhaustion of lymphocytic choriomeningitis virus-specific cytotoxic T lymphocytes visualized using soluble tetrameric major histocompatibility complex class I-peptide complexes. *J Exp Med* 1998;187:1383–1393.

16. Schirmbeck R, Melber K, Kuhröber A, Janowicz ZA, Reimann J. Immunization with soluble hepatitis B virus surface protein elicits murine H-2 class I-restricted CD8+ cytotoxic T lymphocyte responses in vivo. *J Immunol* 1994;152:1110–1119.

17. Schirmbeck R, Melber K, Mertens T, Reimann J. Antibody and cytotoxic T-cell responses to soluble hepatitis B virus (HBV) S antigen in mice: implication for the pathogenesis of HBV-induced hepatitis. *J Virol* 1994;68:1418–1425.

18. Safrit JT, Andrews CA, Zhu T, Ho DD, Koup RA. Characterization of human immunodeficiency virus type I-specific ctotoxic T lymphocyte clones isolated during acute seroconversion: recognition of autologous virus sequences within a conserved imunodominant epitope. *J Exp Med* 1994;179:463–472.

19. Rehermann B, Lau D, Hoofnagle J, Chisari FV. Cytotoxic T lymphocyte responsiveness after resolution of chronic hepatitis B virus infection. *J Clin Invest* 1996;97:1655–1665.

20. Thiers V, Nakajima E, Kremsdorf D, et al. Transmission of hepatitis B from hepatitis B-seronegative subjects. *Lancet* 1988;2:1273–1276.

21. Wachs ME, Amend WJ, Ascher NL, et al. The risk of transmission of hepatitis B from HBsAg(−), HBcAb(+), HBIgM(−) organ donors. *Transplantation* 1995;59:230–234.

22. Blum HE, Stowring L, Figus A, Montgomery CK, Haase AT, Vyas GN. Detection of hepatitis B virus DNA in hepatocytes, bile duct epithelium and vascular elements by in situ hybridization. *Proc Natl Acad Sci USA* 1983;80:6682–6685.

23. Dejean A, Lugassy C, Zafrani S, Tiollais P, Brechot C. Detection of hepatitis B virus DNA in pancreas, kidney and skin of two human carriers of the virus. *J Gen Virol* 1984;65:651–655.

24. Yoffe B, Burns DK, Bhatt HS, Combes B. Extrahepatic hepatitis B virus DNA sequences in patients with acute hepatitis B infection. *Hepatology* 1990; 12:187–192.

25. Beasley RP, Hwang LY, Stevens CE, et al. Efficacy of hepatitis B immune globulin for prevention of perinatal transmission of the hepatitis B virus carrier state: final report of a randomized double-blind, placebo-controlled trial. *Hepatology* 1993;3:135–141.

26. Ando K, Guidotti LG, Cerny A, Ishikawa T, Chisari FV. Access to antigen restricts cytotoxic T lymphocyte function in vivo. *J Immunol* 1994;153:482–489.

27. Barnaba V, Franco A, Alberti A, Balsano C, Benvenuto R, Balsano F. Recognition of hepatitis B envelope proteins by liver-infiltrating T lymphocytes in chronic HBV infection. *J Immunol* 1989; 143:2650–2655.

28. Badardin KA, Desmet VJ. Interdigitating and dendritic reticulum cells in chronic active hepatitis. *Histopathology* 1984;8:657–667.

29. Dienes HP, Hütteroth T, Hess G, Meuer SC. Immunoelectron microscopic observations on the inflammatory infiltrates and HLA antigens in hepatitis B and non-A, non-B. *Hepatology* 1987;7:1317–1325.

30. Ando K, Guidotti LG, Wirth S, et al. Class I restricted cytotoxic T lymphocytes are directly cytopathic for their target cells in vivo. *J Immunol* 1994;152:3245–3253.

31. Nuti S, Rosa D, Valiante NM, et al. Dynamics of intra-hepatic lymphocytes in chronic hepatitis C: enrichment for Valpha24+ T cells and rapid elimination of effector cells by apoptosis. *Eur J Immunol* 1998;28:3448–3455.

32. Margolis HS, Alte MJ, Hadler SC. Hapatitis B: evolving epidemiology and implications for control. *Semin Liver Dis* 1991;11:84–92.

33. Maynard JE. Hepatitis B: global importance and need for control. *Vaccine* 1990;8(Suppl):185–200.

34. ArakawaK, Tsuda F, Takahashi K, et al. Materno-fetal transmission of IgG-bound hepatitis B e antigen. *Pediatr Res* 1982;16:247–250.

35. Lee JKSD, Lo KJ, Wu JC, et al. Prevention of maternal-infant hepatitis B virus transmission by immunization: the role of serum hepatitis B virus DNA. *Hepatology* 1986;6:369–373.

36. Beasley RP, Hwang L. Postnatal infectivity of hepatitis B surface antigen-carrier mothers. *J Infect Dis* 1983;147:185–190.

37. Milich DR, Jones JE, Hughes JL, Price J, Raney AK, McLachlan A. Is it a function of the secreted hepatitis B e antigen to induce immunologic tolerance in utero? *Proc Natl Acad Sci USA* 1990; 87:6599–6603.

38. Ridge JP, Di Rosa F, Matzinger P. A conditioned dendritic cell can be a temporal bridge between a cD4+ T-helper and a T-killer cell. *Nature* 1998; 393:474–478.

39. Vento S, Rondanelli EG, Ranieri S, O'Brien CJ, Williams R, Eddleston ALWF. Prospective study of cellular immunity to hepatitis B virus antigens from the early incubation phase of acute hepatitis B. *Lancet* 1987;2:119–122.

40. Franco A, Paroli M, Testa U, et al. Transferrin receptor mediates uptake and presentation of hepatitis B envelope antigen by T lymphocytes. *J Exp Med* 1992;175:1195–1205.

41. Van der Most RG, Sette A, Oseroff C, et al. Analysis of cytotoxic T cell responses to dominant and subdominant epitopes during acute and chronic lymphocytic choriomeningitis virus infection. *J Immunol* 1996;157:5543–5554.

42. Demkowicz WE Jr, Littaua RA, Wang J, Ennis FA. Human cytotoxic T-cell memory: long-lived responses to vaccinia virus. *J Virol* 1996;70:2627–2631.

43. Valitutti S, Müller S, Dessing M, Lanzavecchia A. Different responses are elicited in cytotoxic T lymphoytes by different levels of T cell receptor occupancy. *J Exp Med* 1996;183:1917–1921.

44. Bertoletti A, Sette A, Chisari FV, et al. Natural variants of cytotoxic epitopes are T-cell receptor antagonists for antiviral cytotoxic T cells. *Nature* 1994;369:407–410.

45. Bertoletti A, Constanzo A, Chisari FV, et al. Cytotoxic T lymphocyte response to a wild-type hepatitis B virus epitope in patients chronically infected by variant viruses carrying substitutions within the epitope. *J Exp Med* 1994;180:933–943.

46. Klenerman P, Rowland-Jones S, McAdams S, et al. Cytotoxic T-cell activity antagonized by naturally occurring HIV-1 Gag variants. *Nature* 1994;369: 403–407.

47. Borrow P, Wei X, Horwitz MS, et al. Antiviral pressure exerted by HIV-1-specific cytotoxic T lymphocytes (CTLs) during primary infection demonstrated by rapid selection of CTL escape virus. *Nat Med* 1997;3:212–217.

48. Chang KM, Rehermann B, McHutchison JG, et al. Immunological significance of cytotoxic T lympho-

cyte epitope variants in patients chronically infected by the hepatitis C virus. *J Clin Invest* 1997;100:2376–2385.

49. Kaneko T, Moriyama T, Udaka K, et al. Impaired induction of cytotoxic T lymphocytes by antagonism of a weak agonist borne by a variant hepatitis C virus epitope. *Eur J Immunol* 1997;27:1782–1787.

50. Goulder PJ, Phillips RE, Colbert RA, et al. Late escape from an immunodominant cytotoxic T-lymphocyte response associated with progression to AIDS. *Nat Med* 1997;3:212–217.

51. Niewiesk S, Daenke S, Parker CE, et al. Naturally occurring variants of human T-cell leukemia virus type I Tax protein impair its recognition by cytotoxic T lymphocytes and the transactivation function of Tax. *J Virol* 1995;69:2649–2653.

52. Lanzavecchia A. Understanding the mechanisms of sustained signaling and T cell activation. *J Exp Med* 1997;185:1717–1719.

53. Evavold BD, Allen PM. Separation of IL-4 production from Th cell proliferation by an altered T cell receptor ligand. *Science* 1991;252:1308–1310.

54. Sloan-Lancaster J, Evavold B, Allen P. Induction of T-cell anergy by altered T-cell-receptor ligand. *Nature* 1993;363:156–159.

55. Eckhardt SG, Milich DR, McLachlan A. Hepatitis B virus core antigen has two nuclear localization sequences in the arginine-rich carboxyl terminus. *J Virol* 1991;65:575–582.

56. Nassal M. The arginine-rich domain of the hepatitis B virus core protein is required for pregenome encapsidation and productive viral positive-strand DNA synthesis but not for virus assembly. *J Virol* 1995;66:4107–4116.

57. Nayersina R, Fowler P, Guilhot S, et al. HLA A2 restricted cytotoxic T lymphocyte responses to multiple hepatitis B surface antigen epitopes during hepatitis B virus infection. *J Immunol* 1993;150: 4659–4671.

58. Eble BE, MacRae DR, Lingappa VR, Ganem D. Multiple topogenic sequences determine the transmembrane orientation of hepatitis B surface antigen. *Mol Cell Biol* 1987;7:3591–3601.

59. Miller RH, Robinson WS. Common evolutionary origin of hepatitis B virus and retroviruses. *Proc Natl Acad Sci USA* 1986;83:2531–2535.

60. Lok ASF, Akarca U, Greene S. Mutations in the precore region of hepatitis B virus serve to enhance the stability of the secondary structure of the pregenome encapsidation signal. *Proc Natl Acad Sci USA* 1994;91:4077–4081.

61. Borysiewicz LK, Morris S, Page J, Sissons JGP. Human cytomegalovirus-specific cytotoxic T lymphocytes: requirements for in vitro generation and specificity. *Eur J Immunol* 1983;13:804–809.

62. Chisari FV, Ferrari C. Hepatitis B virus immunopathogenesis. *Annu Rev Immunol* 1995;13:29–60.

63. Guidotti LG, Matzke B, Schaller H, Chisari FV. High-level Hepatitis B virus replication in transgenic mice. *J Virol* 1995;69:6158–6169.

64. Paterlini P, Gerken G, Nakajima E, et al. Polymerase chain reaction to detect hepatitis B virus DNA and RNA sequences in primary liver cancers from patients negative for hepatitis B surface antigen. *N Engl J Med* 1990;323:80–85.

65. Beg AA, Ruben SM, Scheinman RI, Haskill S, Rosen CA, Baldwin AS Jr. I kappa B interacts with the nuclear localization sequences of the subunits of NF-kappa B: a mechanism for cytoplasmic retention. *Genes Dev* 1992;6:1899–1913. Erratum: *Genes Dev* 1992;6:2664–2665.

66. Ganchi PA, Sun SC, Greene WC, Ballard DW. I kappa B/MAD-3 masks the nuclear localization signal of NF-kappa B p65 and requires the transactivation domain to inhibit NF-kappa B p65 DNA binding. *Mol Biol Cell* 1992;3:1339–1352.

67. Grilli M, Chiu JJ, and Lenardo MJ. NF-kappa B and Rel: participants in a multiform transcriptional regulatory system. *Int Rev Cytol* 1993;143:1–62.

68. Su F, Schneider RJ. Hepatitis B virus HBx protein activates transcription factor NF-kappaB by acting on multiple cytoplasmic inhibitors of rel-related proteins. *J Virol* 1996;70:4558–4566.

69. Huang SN, Chisari FV. Strong, sustained hepatocellular proliferation precedes hepatocarcinogenesis in hepatitis B surface antigen transgenic mice. *Hepatology* 1995;21:620–626.

70. Chisari FV, Filippi P, Buras J, et al. Structural and pathological effects of synthesis of hepatitis B virus large envelope polypeptide in transgenic mice. *Proc Natl Acad Sci USA* 1987;84:6909–6913.

71. Chisari FV, Klopchin K, Moriyama T, et al. Molecular pathogenesis of hepatocellular carcinoma in hepatitis B virus transgenic mice. *Cell* 1989;59:1145–1156.

72. Dunsford HA, Sell S, Chisari FV. Hepatocarcinogenesis due to chronic liver cell injury in hepatitis B virus transgenic mice. *Cancer Res* 1990;50:3400–3407.

73. Nakamoto Y, Guidotti LG, Kuhlen CV, Fowler P, Chisari FV. Immune pathogenesis of hepatocellular carcinoma. *J Exp Med* 1998;188:341–350.

74. Doolan DL, Hoffman SL, Southwood S, et al. Degenerate cytotoxic T cell epitopes from P. falciparum restricted by multiple HLA-A and HLA-B supertype alleles. *Immunity* 1997;7:97–112.

75. Vitiello A, Ishioka G, Grey HM, et al. Development of a lipopeptide-based therapeutic vaccine to treat chronic HBV infection. 1. Induction of a primary cytotoxic T lymphocyte response in humans. *J Clin Invest* 1995;95:341–349.

76. Livingston BD, Crimi C, Grey H, et al. The hepatitis B virus-specific CTL responses induced in humans by lipopeptide vaccination are comparable to those elicited by acute viral infection. *J Immunol* 1997; 159:1383–1392.

77. Tam JP, Lu YA. Vaccine engineering: enhancement of immunogenicity of synthetic peptide vaccines related to hepatitis in chemically defined models consisting of T- and B-cell epitopes. *Proc Natl Acad Sci USA* 1989;86:9084–9088.

78. Tam JP. Synthetic peptide vaccine design: synthesis and properties of a high-density multiple antigenic peptide system. *Proc Natl Acad Sci USA* 1988; 85:5409–5413.

79. Nardelli B, Defoort JP, Huang W, Tam JP. Design of a complete synthetic peptide-based AIDS vaccine with a built-in adjuvant. *AIDS Res Hum Retroviruses* 1992;8:1405–1407.

80. Koenig S, Conley AJ, Bewah YA, et al. Transfer of

HIV-1-specific cytotoxic T lymphocytes to an AIDS patient leads to selection for mutant HIV variants and subsequent disease progression. *Nat Med* 1995; 1:330–336.

81. Boyle JS, Silva A, Brady JL, Lew AM. DNA immunization: induction of higher avidity antibody and effect of route on T cell cytotoxicity. *Proc Natl Acad Sci USA* 1997;94:14626–14631.

82. Davis HL, Michel M-L, Whalen RG. DNA-based immunization induces continuous secretion of hepatitis surface antigen and high levels of circulating antibody. *Hum Mol Genet* 1993;2:1847–1851.

83. Schirmbeck R, Bohm W, Ando K, Chisari FV, Reimann J. Nucleic acid vaccination primes hepatitis B virus surface antigen-specific cytotoxic T lymphocytes in nonresponder mice. *J Virol* 1995;69:5929–5934.

84. Ulmer JB, Donnelly JJ, Parker SE, et al. Heterologous protection against influenza by injection of DNA encoding a viral protein. *Science* 1993; 259:1745–1749.

85. Wang B, Boyer J, Srikantan V, et al. DNA inoculation induces neutralizing immune responses against human immunodeficiency virus type 1 in mice and nonhuman primates. *DNA Cell Biol* 1993; 12:799–805.

86. Wang B, Ugen KE, Srikantan V, et al. Gene inoculation generates immune responses against human immunodeficiency virus type 1. *Proc Natl Acad Sci USA* 1993;980:4156–4160.

87. Xiang ZQ, Spitalnick S, Tran M, Wunner WH, Cheng J, Ertl HCJ. Vaccination with a plasmid vector carrying the rabies virus glycoprotein gene induces protective immunity against rabies virus. *Virology* 1994;199:132–140.

88. Michel ML, Davis HL, Schleef M, Mancini M, Tiollais P, Whalen RG. DNA-mediated immunization to the hepatitis B surface antigen in mice: aspects of the humoral response mimic hepatitis B viral infection in humans. *Proc Natl Acad Sci USA* 1995;92:5307–5311.

89. Mancini M, Hadchouel M, Davis HL, Whalen RG, Tiollais P, Michel ML. DNA-mediated immunization in a transgenic mouse model of the hepatitis B surface antigen chronic carrier state. *Proc Natl Acad Sci USA* 1996;93:12496–12501.

90. Mancini M, Hadchsuel M, Tiollais P, Pourcel C, Michel ML. Induction of anti-hepatitis B surface antigen (HBsAg) antibodies in HBsAg producing transgenic mice: a possible way of circumventing "nonresponse" to HBsAg. *J Med Virol* 1993; 39:67–74.

91. Pan ZK, Ikonomidis G, Lazenby A, Pardoll D, Paterson Y. A recombinant Listeria monocytogenes vaccine expressing a model tumour antigen protects mice against lethal tumour cell challenge and causes regression of established tumours. *Nat Med* 1995; 1:471–477.

92. Darji A, Guzman CA, Gerstel B, et al. Oral somatic transgene vaccination using attenuated S. typhimurium. *Cell* 1997;91:765–775.

93. Rescigno M, Citterio S, Thery C, et al. Bacteria-induced neo-biosynthesis, stabilization, and surface expression of functional class I molecules in mouse dendritic cells. *Proc Natl Acad Sci USA* 1998; 95:5229–5234.

94. Schodel F, Kelly SM, Peterson DL, Milich DR, Curtiss R. Hybrid hepatitis B virus core-pre-S proteins synthesized in avirulent Salmonella typhimurium and Salmonella typhi for oral vaccination. *Infect Immun* 1994;62:1669–1676.

*Cytotoxic Cells: Basic Mechanisms and
Medical Applications,* edited by Michail V.
Sitkovsky and Pierre A. Henkart. Lippincott
Williams & Wilkins, Philadelphia © 2000.

Chapter 20

Cytotoxic T-Cell Responses to Intracellular Pathogens

Steffen Stenger and *Robert L. Modlin

*Institut fuer Klinische Mikrobiologie, Immunologie, und Hygiene, Universitaet Erlangen,
D-91054 Erlangen, Germany; and *Division of Dermatology, Department of Microbiology and
Immunology, and the Molecular Biology Institute, University of California,
Los Angeles, California 90095, USA*

Host defense against intracellular pathogens is traditionally believed to be dominated by CD4$^+$ T cells. Recently it has become clear that CD8$^+$ T cells are another crucial component of protective immunity against infection with intracellular organisms. Protection mediated by CD8$^+$ T cells is due not only to their ability to secrete T helper-1 (Th1) cytokines (e.g., interferon-γ) but also to their ability to lyse host cells infected with the pathogen. Lysis of infected host cells releases intracellular bacteria, thereby reducing the reservoir of infected cells. The bacteria are dispersed and taken up at low multiplicities of infection by activated infiltrating macrophages, which can kill them. In addition, the process of lysing the infected target cell may directly or indirectly result in the death of the bacteria. The identification of two mechanisms of lysis induced by cytotoxic T lymphocytes (CTLs)—the granule exocytosis pathway and the Fas–Fas ligand (FasL) interaction—have provided new insights into the role of CTLs in immunity to infection.

INTRODUCTION

Cytotoxic T cell activity has been detected in multiple T cell subsets: principally CD8$^+$

T cells which recognize 9- and 10-amino-acid peptide antigens presented by major histocompatibility complex class I (MHC-I) molecules, but also CD4$^+$ T cells that recognize 15-amino-acid peptides presented by MHC-II molecules. Another CTL population whose recognition mechanism is less well understood is represented by T cell receptor (TCR)$\gamma\delta^+$ T cells (1). Recently a novel subset of human CTLs has been characterized that recognizes mycobacterial lipid and lipoglycan antigens presented by the nonpolymorphic molecule CD1 (2–4). The murine homolog to CD1, termed CD1d, has also been implicated in presenting synthetic (5) and naturally occurring peptides (6) and glycolipids (7) to CTLs.

The CTL has long been recognized as a central effector cell in the immune response to viruses. Work over the past decade has expanded our knowledge about the spectrum of pathogens that can induce a CTL response such that it includes intracellular bacteria and parasites.

To outline the principles of CTL responses in intracellular infection we focus on five prototypic intracellular pathogens. Because of the availability of appropriate mouse models, much of our understanding about the mechanisms of CTL responses has been

made in infections with *Leishmania major,*
Toxoplasma gondii, Listeria monocytogenes,
Trypanosoma cruzi, and *Mycobacterium tu-*
berculosis. L. major and *M. tuberculosis* are
obligate intracellular pathogens residing primarily within the phagolysosomes of host
macrophages. Whereas *L. major* has adapted
to survive in the acidic environment of the
phagolysosome (8), *M. tuberculosis* avoids
destruction by inhibiting acidification (9) and
arresting the appropriate development of
phagolysosomes (10). *L. monocytogenes, T.*
gondii, and *T. cruzi* have a broader host cell
spectrum and escape the hostile environment
of the phagolysosome into the cytoplasm to
ensure their survival.

The investigation of human T cell responses to intracellular pathogens is complex
and relies mainly on the *in vitro* analysis of
samples derived from patients. Given the
high morbidity and mortality of tuberculosis,
this disease has drawn most attention for
studying the role of human CTLs.

CONTRIBUTION OF CD8+ T CELLS TO IMMUNITY IN MURINE MODELS OF INTRACELLULAR INFECTION

Evidence implicating CD8+ T cells in immunity against intracellular pathogens has
been derived from various experimental approaches. Initial studies investigating the
contribution of CD8+ T cells to immunity
against intracellular pathogens depleted
CD8 cells by the injection of antibodies prior
to infection. Elimination of CD8 cells by this
method aggravated the course of a cutaneous
infection with *L. major* in a resistant mouse
strain, even though the final outcome of the
infection was not altered (11,12). Resistance
to reinfection and an efficient maintenance
of immunity against infection with *L. major,*
however, required the presence of CD8+ T
cells (12–14). Experiments, in which CD8+
cells were shown to be responsible for the
conversion of susceptible BALB/c mice into
a resistant phenotype after depletion of CD4+

cells confirmed the contribution of CD8+ T
cells to immunity against *L. major* (15). In tuberculosis deletion of CD8+ CTLs by antibody treatment resulted in marked aggrava-
tion of the disease (16,17). A substantial role
for CTLs in host defense against intracellular
pathogens has been derived from studies of
listeriosis, toxoplasmosis, and trypanosomia-
sis in mouse models. Depletion of CD8+ T
cells exacerbated disease, indicating an essential contribution of this subtype to the resistance to infection with *L. monocytogenes*
(18), *T. gondii* (19), and *T. cruzi* (20).

An alternative approach to investigate the
differential contribution of T cell subsets to
immunity in intracellular infection is the
transfer of immunity by injecting antigen-
specific T cells into irradiated recipient animals prior to infection. In listeriosis, transfer
of long-lasting immunity requires exclusively
MHC-I-compatible CD8+ T cells (21). Similarly, CD8+ cytotoxic T cell lines specific for
trypanosomal *trans*-sialidase are sufficient to
transfer a high degree of protection against
a subsequent challenge with *T. cruzi* (22). In
toxoplasmosis the combined action of CD8+
T cells and CD4+ T cells is required for the
transfer of protective immunity. In these experiments CD8+ T cells contribute to immunity by the production of interferon-γ (IFN-
γ) but not by cytolysis of infected cells
(23,24). In animal models of tuberculosis,
CD8+ T cells have been shown to be weakly
protective in transfer assays. The local immune response in the lung was particularly
dependent on the presence of CD8+ T
cells (25).

More recently, gene-targeted mice with
disrupted expression of key immunologic
targets have provided new insight into the
role of T cell subsets known to contain CTLs
in host defense against intracellular pathogens. For example, β_2-microglobulin knockout ($\beta_2 m^{-/-}$) mice are unable to express
MHC-I or MHC-I-like molecules and therefore cannot generate CD8+ CTLs, NK1.1 T
cells, or CD1-restricted T cells. Infection of
$\beta_2 m^{-/-}$ mice with *T. cruzi* demonstrated dis-

tinct effects on the immunologic response. Even though production of the immuno-protective Th1-type cytokines interleukin-2 (IL-2) and IFN-γ was increased, mice suffered from severe parasitemia and died earlier than the control animals. These data indicate that CD8$^+$ T cells, NK1.1 T cells, or CD1-restricted T cells exert their protective activity by a distinct pathway than by the secretion of Th1-type cytokines, possibly by lysis of parasite-infected target cells (26–28). More specifically, mice with a defined mutation in the CD8 gene displayed striking increases in mortality to infection with *T. cruzi*. In β_2m$^{-/-}$ mice, infection with *L. monocyto-genes* was contained but not resolved, whereas in littermate controls infection was progressively cleared (30). These findings were extended by a study demonstrating that β_2m$^{-/-}$ mice not only developed exacerbated disease and delayed clearance of *Listeria* in the primary immune response but also upon secondary challenge (31). These data provided proof for an important contribution of CD8$^+$ T cells in primary and secondary infection with *L. monocytogenes*. Similarly, β_2m$^{-/-}$ mice succumb to *M. tuberculosis* infection (32). Although IFN-γ production in tissues and granuloma formation were evident, tenfold higher numbers of bacilli were found in infected tissues. Reminiscent of the data obtained from the adoptive transfer experiments, the predominant site of disease exacerbation was the lung.

Together these studies indicate a substantial role for CD8$^+$ T cells and, by inference, CTLs in host defense against intracellular pathogens. CD8$^+$ T cells likely complement other components of the immune system to mount an efficient and long-lasting immune response to these intracellular bacteria.

On the other hand, a critical role for CD8$^+$ T cells is not universal for all intracellular pathogens. β_2m$^{-/-}$ mice were found to be as resistant as their littermate controls to a cutaneous *L. major* infection (33). These results were confirmed by infection of mice with disruption in the CD8α-gene, which in con-

trast to β_2m$^{-/-}$ mice lack only CD8$^+$ cells, not NK1.1 or CD1-restricted T cells (34). Despite the absence of MHC-I molecules and peripheral CD8$^+$ T lymphocytes, β_2m$^{-/-}$ mice survived a lethal challenge with tachyzoites of *T. gondii* following vaccination with an attenuated parasite mutant. Protection was dependent on the emergence of a population of NK1.1$^+$ cells, which lack cytolytic activity but produce IFN-γ (35). These data do not exclude that other T cell subsets with cytolytic capacity play a critical role in these infections.

CD8$^+$ CTLs IN HUMAN TUBERCULOSIS

In tuberculosis, the absence of CD8$^+$ T cells leads to a complete switch from a resistant to a susceptible phenotype. Accordingly, strong efforts have been undertaken to generate and characterize cytolytic T cell lines specific for *M. tuberculosis*. Although it remains difficult to generate CTLs from mice infected with virulent strains of *M. tuberculosis*, progress has been made in characterizing CTLs from humans with tuberculosis.

Clinical evidence for a role of CD8$^+$ cells in the protective immune response against *M. tuberculosis* came from a patient who was human immunodeficiency virus (HIV)-negative with relapsing episodes of pulmonary tuberculosis (36). A strikingly reduced number of CD8$^+$ T cells was the only abnormal immunologic parameter and was thus suggestive of being causative for the persistence of tubercle bacilli. A more direct approach demonstrated *M. tuberculosis*-reactive CTLs in the lungs of patients with tuberculosis (37). Furthermore, CD8$^+$ CTLs that produce high levels of IFN-γ can be derived from tuberculosis patients in high frequency (38). These MHC-I-restricted T cells recognized a well defined early secreted antigen of *M. tuberculosis* (ESAT6). Clones isolated from these cells exert strong cytolytic activity against ESAT6 pulsed targets, supporting the hypothesis that CD8$^+$ CTLs are involved in host defense against *M. tuberculosis.*

Cytotoxic T lymphocytes that recognize nonpeptide antigens of *M. tuberculosis* in the context of human CD1 molecules have been derived from normal individuals (39), patients with tuberculosis (4), and patients co-infected with *M. tuberculosis* and HIV (40). Not only can these CTLs recognize antigen-pulsed targets, they also recognize and lyse *M. tuberculosis*-infected macrophages (4,41). Finally, human CD8$^+$ CTLs that are *M. tuberculosis*-specific, but not restricted by MHC-I or CD1, were detected at high frequency in tuberculosis-infected individuals, suggesting a novel nonpolymorphic MHC-Ib antigen-presenting pathway involved in immunity to tuberculosis (42).

EFFECTOR FUNCTIONS OF CD8$^+$ T CELLS

The effector function by which CD8$^+$ T cells contribute to protective immunity against intracellular pathogens can be threefold: (a) The first is secretion of IFN-γ, which is known to be a major activator of the defense mechanisms of the host cells in mice. (b) CTL-mediated lysis of the target cells results in release of the pathogen into the extracellular environment. The bacteria could then be taken up by freshly recruited macrophages, which can kill them (43). Alternatively, CD8$^+$ T cells might directly recognize and kill the microrganisms present in the extracellular environment. Microbial pathogens that can be killed directly by T cells include fungi such as *Candida albicans* (44) and *Cryptococcus neoformans* (45) and parasites such as *Schistosoma mansoni* (46), *Entamoeba histolytica* (47), and *T. gondii* (48). Moreover, antigen-specific CD8$^+$ T cells secrete a bactericidal factor with the capacity to inhibit the growth of *Pseudomonas aeruginosa*, *Escherichia coli,* and *Staphylococcus aureus* (49,50). (c) CTL-mediated lysis and simultaneous killing of the intracellular pathogen as detailed in the following section.

IMPACT OF CTLs ON VIABILITY OF THE PATHOGEN

Learning about the fate of the intracellular pathogen after CTL-mediated host cell lysis requires us to study the interaction of the effector cell with the infected target cell. CD8$^+$ T cell lines that can detect antigen on the surface of cells infected with *Leishmania, Toxoplasma, Listeria, Trypanosoma,* and *Mycobacterium* in the context of MHC-I have been derived. In the case of mycobacteria a unique subset of T cells, recognizing nonprotein antigens in the context of CD1, has been introduced. Most studies that have analyzed antigen-specific CD8$^+$ T cells found that the lines are potent producers of IFN-γ and are highly cytolytic against infected host cells (4,51–56). When determining the functional impact of the interaction between CTLs and the target cell, several studies demonstrated reduced viability of the pathogen. Whether the death of the microorganisms is a result of the action of IFN-γ, as demonstrated for leishmania (52), or an immediate event associated with cell-to-cell contact, as indicated in studies with mycobacteria (4,57,58) and listeria (55), varies with the experimental set up and the pathogen under investigation. These studies have provided evidence that CTLs play a prominent role, particularly in the protective immune response to intracellular pathogens, by their ability to kill the intracellular invader directly.

TWO CYTOTOXICITY PATHWAYS

The increasing amount of evidence showing that CTLs are important effector cells in host defense against intracellular pathogens has initiated an exciting field of investigation that focuses on elucidating the mechanisms of cytotoxicity. Mechanistic studies were pioneered by investigators who defined two virtually independent pathways involved in T cell-mediated cytotoxicity.

The granule exocytosis pathway is characterized by secretion of the lytic protein perforin, which may polymerize to form a pore in the host cell, allowing entry of the co-secreted granule contents (e.g., granzymes), leading to apoptosis of the target cell. The second mechanism is nonsecretory and involves crosslinking of a surface membrane ligand present on some antigen-activated CTLs (FasL) and a death receptor on the target cell (Fas), which initiates a cascade of proteolytic enzymes ultimately resulting in target cell lysis and apoptosis.

The generation of perforin-deficient mice yielded the first definitive evidence for the relevance of perforin in the clearance of viral infections *in vivo* and *in vitro* (59,60). Nevertheless, carefully conducted *in vitro* analyses detected remaining lytic activity against some lymphohematopoietic targets (59), natural killer (NK) cell targets, and fibroblasts (60) despite the absence of perforin. Shortly after this observation two simultaneously published studies identified the Fas cytolytic pathway as the second mechanism of cytotoxicity in perforin-deficient CTLs (61,62). These studies indicated that CTLs from perforin-deficient mice lysed Fas-expressing target cells but could not lyse Fas-deficient targets or targets expressing mutant Fas molecules. Taken together these data not only confirmed the primary role of perforin but simultaneously revealed a major contribution of the perforin-independent Fas-mediated pathway in antigen-specific cytolysis. Based on the lysis of the limited selection of target cells, it was estimated that the perforin mechanism is responsible for approximately two-thirds of the killing activity, one-third being contributed by Fas (62). Thus, two complementary, specific cytotoxic mechanisms are functional in CTLs, one based on the secretion of lytic proteins and one that depends on cell surface ligand–receptor interaction.

The two pathways of cytotoxicity can be distinguished not only by the interaction of molecules at the contact zone between CTLs and the target but also by the initiation of distinct downstream events that are initiated in the target cell. Previous studies had impli-cated caspases in rapid target cell death induced by the granule exocytosis and Fas–FasL pathways. Sarin et al. (63) confirmed this notion by showing that apoptotic nuclear damage induced by both pathways is blocked by caspase inhibitors. However, the two pathways differ in their requirement for caspases for target cell lysis. Only Fas-mediated cytolysis is dependent on the proteolytic action of caspases, whereas lysis via the granule exocytosis does not require caspases. The finding that the two CTL pathways initiate distinct molecular events in target cells is likely relevant for some of the differential effects of Fas/FasL- and perforin-mediated cytolysis in host responses to microbial pathogens described below.

ROLE OF PERFORIN-MEDIATED CYTOTOXICITY IN INTRACELLULAR INFECTION

The granule exocytosis pathway does not seem to be involved in immunity to *L. major*. Gene-targeted knockout mice that do not express perforin, a major effector molecule of the granule-exocytosis pathway, did not have an altered course of infection after a cutaneous infection with *L. major* (64). An earlier finding had already indicated that granzyme A, a molecule co-injected with perforin into the target cell and believed to contribute to cytotoxicity mediated by the granule exocytosis pathway (65), was expressed more prominently in a susceptible mouse strain than in a resistant strain (66). These data imply that the granule exocytosis pathway facilitates tissue destruction rather than contributing to protective immunity.

Analyzing the contribution of the mechanisms of cytotoxicity, two laboratories infected perforin-deficient mice with *L. monocytogenes*. The first study showed delayed clearance of the pathogen from the spleen, but the overall susceptibility induced by a primary challenge was not decreased (67). In contrast, protection against a secondary infection was drastically impaired. The capability of transferring protective immunity by perforin-deficient CD8⁺ T cells was reduced 10-fold (liver) to 100-fold (spleen), underlining the relevance of perforin-mediated cytotoxicity in secondary infection with *L. monocytogenes*.

A second laboratory investigated whether specific antilisterial immunity can be provided by transfer of listeriolysin-specific CD8⁺ T cell lines derived from perforin-deficient mice (68). In contrast to the initial study, immunity to a subsequent challenge with *L. monocytogenes* could be transferred to normal mice by CD8⁺ T cells from perforin- or FasL-deficient mice and IFN-γ-depleted hosts. Only mice depleted of tumor necrosis factor-α (TNF-α) failed to convert to an immune phenotype. These data suggest that CD8⁺ T cell-mediated immunity to an intracellular bacterial pathogen can function independently of perforin and FasL, which define the two major pathways of cell-mediated cytolysis. A possible explanation for these discordant results could be that one group (67) transferred polyclonal antigen-specific CD8⁺ T cells, whereas the other group (68) had immunized the donor mice with listeriolysin, a single well defined immunodominant antigen.

Upon challenge with *T. cruzi,* mice with disruption in the genes controlling either perforin or granzyme B, both critical components of the granule exocytosis pathway of cytotoxicity, had mortality rates similar to those of wild-type mice. However, peak parasitemia was elevated during the acute stage of infection, suggesting a complementary but not crucial contribution of perforin to protective immunity. In addition, protection from secondary infection by prior exposure to an avirulent strain of trypanosomes was maintained in the absence of perforin (69).

The role of the granule exocytosis pathway in immunity to toxoplasmosis was addressed *in vivo* by immunizing perforin-deficient mice and subsequently infecting with a virulent strain of *T. gondii*. Even though *in vitro* cytotoxicity against tachyzoite-infected targets was severely reduced, the mice were completely resistant to the infection *in vivo*. In contrast, a strain with low virulence that progresses to a chronic cyst-forming stage induced accelerated mortality after 75 days in the absence of perforin despite normal IFN-γ production. These data show that perforin-dependent cytolytic function is not required for host resistance to lethal acute infection in preimmunized animals but contributes to the control of infection during the chronic stage (70).

The course of infection with virulent *M. tuberculosis* in perforin-deficient mice was independently investigated by two laboratories. Perforin deficiency did not influence the bacterial burden or the histologic appearance of organs during the early course of disease induced by intravenous infection (71) or aerosol challenge (72). Similarly, lack of an additional granule-component, granzyme B, which is a nonredundant component in the rapid induction of target cell DNA fragmentation (73), also did not have an impact on disease throughout the observation period (72). However, at late stages of infection the number of bacteria in liver, lung, and spleen of perforin-deficient mice is significantly higher than in control animals (A. O. Sousa and B. R. Bloom, personal communication). Therefore, CTLs may be important in the control of persisting bacteria during the chronic stage of infection.

The granule exocytosis pathway of cytotoxicity does not seem to contribute to immunity against intracellular pathogens during the acute stage of infection. However, in toxoplasmosis and tuberculosis (both prototypic diseases in which acute infection is followed by an asymptomatic, chronic stage with perhaps lifelong persistence of the pathogen), the presence of perforin-containing cytotoxic granules may be necessary for containment of the disease. The susceptibility of perforin-deficient mice against a secondary, but not a primary, challenge with *L. monocytogenes* is also compatible with a role of cytotoxic granules in the long-term maintenance of a protective immune response against intracellular pathogens.

ROLE OF FAS–FASL-MEDIATED CYTOTOXICITY IN INTRACELLULAR INFECTION

The Fas–FasL pathway of cytotoxicity, however, seems to be required for the resolution of lesions induced by *L. major* but not other intracellular pathogens. Fas- or FasL-deficient mice develop progressive lesions, which in the case of FasL deficiency can be cured if exogenous recombinant FasL is administered (64). Susceptibility in Fas- deficient mice is surprisingly accompanied by elevated levels of IL-12, strong Th1 responses, and enhanced nitric oxide production, all parameters usually associated with clearance of the parasite (74). It remains to be resolved by which mechanism Fas–FasL-mediated cytotoxicity contributes to the resolution of cutaneous leishmaniasis. The apoptotic death of parasite-harboring macrophages could limit the number of host cells for the parasite at the site of disease and increase the ratio between IFN-γ producing Th1 cells and infected cells. Also the apoptotic death of infected macrophages reduces the extent of tissue injury at the site of lesions, as cells undergoing apoptosis are rapidly ingested and removed by phagocytosis while still intact before their toxic content is released (75). In addition, the uptake of apoptotic cells containing parasites by dendritic cells could facilitate generation of additional CTLs to combat the infection (76). Studies of patients with American cutaneous leishmaniasis indicate that CTLs could contribute to tissue injury; only CTLs derived from patients with the tissue-destructive mucocutaneous form, but not the localized form, showed significant cytotoxicity against autologous infected macrophages (77).

The Fas/FasL pathway is not critical to host defense against *L. monocytogenes*. After intraperitoneal infection of Fas-deficient mice, there was no decrease in resistance to listerial infection as assessed by bacterial growth (78). Similarly, these mice do not show increased susceptibility to an aerosol or intravenous infection with *M. tubercu-*

losis (71,72). It is somewhat paradoxical that only with leishmania infections, where depletion of perforin had no effect, is the outcome impaired in Fas/FasL-deficient mice. Additional studies would be needed to clarify whether the Fas–FasL pathway perhaps supplements the perforin pathway of cytotoxicity during the late stages of toxoplasmosis and tuberculosis. However, Fas- and FasL-deficient mice do not provide an appropriate model to investigate the chronic stages of disease, as they spontaneously develop a lymphoproliferative disorder, which excludes long-term studies.

MECHANISM AND FUNCTIONAL RELEVANCE OF CTLs IN HUMANS

Two approaches have been undertaken to analyze the functional relevance of lysis of human macrophages infected with mycobacteria.

First, lysis of infected cells was induced by exogenously adding stimuli that mimic effector mechanisms of CTL-mediated lysis. Apoptosis of *M. tuberculosis*-infected human macrophages induced by extracellular adenosine triphosphate, a component of the cytolytic granules of CTLs, killed the host cell as well as the bacteria (79,80). On the other hand, purified perforin, a major effector molecule of CTL-induced lysis, or granulysin, a recently identified granule component that has bactericidal activity, did not reduce the viability of intracellular *M. tuberculosis* (81). In contrast, a combination of perforin and granulysin, which co-localize in T cell cytotoxic granules, resulted in macrophage lysis and decreased viability of intracellular mycobacteria. These data indicate that granulysin is a mycobactericidal agent but may not effectively be delivered to the phagolysosomal compartment. In contrast, perforin is an ineffective antimicrobial agent, although it has the capacity to lyse infected target cells. Thus granulysin could kill intracellular *M. tuberculosis* if perforin, or possibly other pore-forming molecules of T cell granules, provided access to the intracellular compartment. The studies on the effect of FasL-induced apoptosis are conflicting. Although FasL ligation by anti-CD95 treatment has no effect on the viability of intracellular *M. bovis* BCG (80), apoptosis induced by soluble recombinant FasL was associated with a substantial reduction in mycobacterial viability (82).

Second, the effects of CTL-mediated lysis on bacterial viability were examined more directly by co-incubation of infected cells with antigen-specific CTLs. *In vivo* cytolysis of infected target cells is the result of an intimate interaction of the macrophage with the CTL. It was recently demonstrated that, in CD1-restricted CTLs reactive to *M. tuberculosis,* the mechanism of target cell lysis could be correlated with the cell surface phenotype (4). Two subsets were identified: CD4$^-$CD8$^-$ (double negative) T cells and CD8$^+$ T cells efficiently lysed macrophages infected with *M. tuberculosis*. The cytotoxicity of CD4$^-$CD8$^-$ T cells was mediated by Fas/FasL interaction and had no effect on the viability of the mycobacteria. The CD8$^+$ T cells lysed infected macrophages by a Fas-independent, granule-dependent mechanism that simultaneously resulted in killing the intracellular bacteria. In addition, the presence of granulysin and perforin was demonstrated in cytotoxic granules of CD8$^+$, but not DN CTLs (81). The role of CD8$^+$ CTLs in protection against intracellular pathogens might therefore not merely be to lyse target cells and disperse the intracellular pathogens but in addition to deliver granulysin, a lethal weapon by which CTLs can directly reduce the viability of a variety of intracellular pathogens attempting to evade host defense. These data indicate that two phenotypically distinct subsets of human CTLs use different mechanisms to kill infected cells and contribute in different ways to host defense against intracellular infection. CTLs that lyse targets by the Fas/FasL pathway might contribute to immunity by preventing tissue injury by depleting antigen-expressing and antigen-processing cells, thereby effectively down-regulating the immune response.

CONCLUSIONS

The identification of CTLs as a component of immunologic defense against intracellular pathogens has spurred efforts to develop vaccines that stimulate this T cell subset. For the most part, it involves identification of the microbial antigens and peptides that stimulate CD8$^+$ MHC-I-restricted T cell responses. An example is the successful vaccination of mice with listeriolysin, which was delivered into the cytoplasm by a bacterial vector (83). Protection against a lethal challenge with *L. monocytogenes* was mediated by CD8$^+$ CTLs, which were specific for an immunodominant peptide from listeriolysin.

A new generation of efforts involves the development of DNA-based vaccines. Vaccination of mice by injection of tumor cells expressing the *M. leprae* gene for heat shock protein 65 are protected against a subsequent challenge with virulent *M. tuberculosis* (84). This efficient treatment elicits CD8$^+$ T cells, which are cytolytic and more importantly reduce the viability of intracellular *M. tuberculosis* (85). Vaccination with plasmid DNA encoding for a 38-kDa glycolipoprotein (86) or antigen 85 (87,88) of *M. tuberculosis* also induces CD8$^+$ CTLs, which are likely to be involved in the induction of protective immunity by this regimen.

The identification of antigens that stimulate CTLs and the mechanism of delivery in vaccines, together with further insight into the mechanism by which CTLs lead to immunity against microbial pathogens, should lead to new immunoprophylactic and immunotherapeutic options in the fight against infectious disease.

REFERENCES

1. Kaufmann SH. Role of T-cell subsets in bacterial infections. *Curr Opin Immunol* 1991;3:465–470.
2. Porcelli S, Brenner MB, Greenstein JL, Balk SP, Terhorst C, Bleicher PA. Recognition of cluster of differentiation 1 antigens by human CD4-CD8-cytolytic T lymphocytes. *Nature* 1989;341:447–450.
3. Sieling PA, Chatterjee D, Porcelli SA, et al. CD1-restricted T cell recognition of microbial lipoglycans. *Science* 1995;269:227–230.

4. Stenger S, Mazzaccaro RJ, Uyemura K, et al. Differential effects of cytolytic T cell subsets on intracellular infection. *Science* 1997;276:1684–1687.
5. Castano AR, Tangri S, Miller JEW, et al. Peptide binding and presentation by mouse CD1. *Science* 1995;269:223–226.
6. Lee DJ, Abeyratne A, Carson DA, Corr M. Induction of an antigen-specific, CD1-restricted cytotoxic T lymphocyte response In vivo. *J Exp Med* 1998; 187:433–438.
7. Joyce S, Woods AS, Yewdell JW, et al. Natural ligand of mouse CD1d1: cellular glycosylphosphatidylinositol. *Science* 1998;279:1541–1544.
8. Bogdan C, Rollinghoff M. The immune response to Leishmania: mechanisms of parasite control and evasion. *Int J Parasitol* 1998;28:121–134.
9. Sturgill-Koszycki S, Schlesinger PH, Chakraborty P, et al. Lack of acidification in Mycobacterium phagosomes produced by exclusion of the vesicular proton-ATPase. *Science* 1994;263:678–681.
10. Clemens DL, Horwitz MA. Characterization of the Mycobacterium tuberculosis phagosome and evidence that phagosomal maturation is inhibited. *J Exp Med* 1995;181:257–270.
11. Farrell JP, Muller I, Louis JA. A role for Lyt-2+ T cells in resistance to cutaneous leishmaniasis in immunized mice. *J Immunol* 1989;142:2052–2056.
12. Muller I, Pedrazzini T, Kropf P, Louis J, Milon G. Establishment of resistance to Leishmania major infection in susceptible BALB/c mice requires parasite-specific CD8+ T cells. *Int Immunol* 1991; 3:587–597.
13. Muller I. Role of T cell subsets during the recall of immunologic memory to Leishmania major. *Eur J Immunol* 1992;22:3063–3069.
14. Muller I, Kropf P, Etges RJ, Louis JA. Gamma interferon response in secondary Leishmania major infection: role of CD8+ T cells. *Infect Immun* 1993; 61:3730–3738.
15. Hill JO, Awwad M, North RJ. Elimination of CD4+ suppressor T cells from susceptible BALB/c mice releases CD8+ T lymphocytes to mediate protective immunity against Leishmania. *J Exp Med* 1989; 169:1819–1827.
16. Muller I, Cobbold SP, Waldmann H, Kaufmann SHE. Impaired resistance to Mycobacterium tuberculosis infection after selective in vivo depletion of L3T4+ and Lyt-2+ T cells *Infect Immun* 1987;55: 2037–2041.
17. Leveton C, Barnass S, Champion B, et al. T-cell-mediated protection of mice against virulent Mycobacterium tuberculosis. *Infect Immun* 1989; 57:390–395.
18. Czuprynski CJ, Brown JF. Effects of purified anti-Lyt-2 mAb treatment on murine listeriosis: comparative roles of Lyt-2+ and L3T4+ cells in resistance to primary and secondary infection, delayed-type hypersensitivity and adoptive transfer of resistance. *Immunology* 1990;71:107–112.
19. Suzuki Y, Remington JS. Dual regulation of resistance against Toxoplasma gondii infection by Lyt-2+ and Lyt-1+, L3T4+ T cells in mice. *J Immunol* 1988;140:3943–3946.
20. Tarleton RL. Depletion of CD8+ T cells increases susceptibility and reverses vaccine-induced immunity in mice infected with Trypanosoma cruzi. *J Immunol* 1990;144:717–724.
21. Bishop DK, Hinrichs DJ. Adoptive transfer of immunity to Listeria monocytogenes: the influence. *J Immunol* 1987;139:2005–2009.
22. Wizel B, Nunes M, Tarleton RL. Identification of Trypanosoma cruzi trans-sialidase family members as targets of protective CD8+ TC1 responses. *J Immunol* 1997;159:6120–6130.
23. Gazzinelli RT, Hakim FT, Hieny S, Shearer GM, Sher A. Synergistic role of CD4+ and CD8+ T lymphocytes in IFN-gamma production and protective immunity induced by an attenuated Toxoplasma gondii vaccine. *J Immunol* 1991;146:286–292.
24. Khan IA, Ely KH, Kasper LH. Antigen-specific CD8+ T cell clone protects against acute Toxoplasma gondii infection in mice. *J Immunol* 1994;152:1856–1860.
25. Orme IM. The kinetics of emergence and loss of mediator T lymphocytes acquired in response to infection with Mycobacterium tuberculosis. *J Immunol* 1987;138:293–298.
26. Tarleton RL, Koller BH, Latour A, Postan M. Susceptibility of beta 2- microglobulin-deficient mice to Trypanosoma cruzi infection "see comments". *Nature* 1992;356:338–340.
27. Nickell SP, Stryker GA, Arevalo C. Isolation from Trypanosoma cruzi-infected mice of CD8+, MHC-restricted cytotoxic T cells that lyse parasite-infected target cells. *J Immunol* 1993;150:1446–1457.
28. Low HP, Santos MA, Wizel B, Tarleton RL. Amastigote surface proteins of Trypanosoma cruzi are targets for CD8+ CTL. *J Immunol* 1998;160:1817–1823.
29. Rottenberg ME, Bakhiet M, Olsson T, et al. Differential susceptibilities of mice genomically deleted of CD4 and CD8 to infections with Trypanosoma cruzi or Trypanosoma brucei. *Infect Immun* 1993; 61:5129–5133.
30. Roberts AD, Ordway DJ, Orme IM. Listeria monocytogenes infection in beta 2 microglobulin-deficient mice. *Infect Immun* 1993;61:1113–1116.
31. Ladel CH, Flesch IE, Arnoldi J, Kaufmann SH. Studies with MHC-deficient knock-out mice reveal impact of both MHC I- and MHC II-dependent T cell responses on Listeria monocytogenes infection. *J Immunol* 1994;153:3116–3122. Erratum: *J. Immunol* 1995;154:4223.
32. Flynn JL, Goldstein MM, Triebold KJ, Koller B, Bloom BR. Major histocompatibility complex class I-restricted T cells are required for resistance to Mycobacterium tuberculosis infection. *Proc Natl Acad Sci USA* 1992;89:12013–12017.
33. Wang Z-E, Reiner SL, Hatam F, et al. Targeted activation of CD8+ cells and infection of β_2-microglobulin deficient mice fail to confirm a primary protective role for CD8+ cells in experimental leishmaniasis. *J Immunol* 1993;151:2077–2086.
34. Huber M, Timms E, Mak TW, Rollinghoff M, Lohoff M. Effective and long-lasting immunity against the parasite Leishmania major in CD8-deficient mice. *Infect Immun* 1998;66:3968–3970.
35. Denkers EY, Gazzinelli RT, Martin D, Sher A. Emergence of NK1.1+ cells as effectors of IFN-gamma dependent immunity to Toxoplasma gondii

in MHC class I-deficient mice. *J Exp Med* 1993; 178:1465–1472.

36. Bothamley GH, Festenstein F, Newland A. Protective role for CD8 cells in tuberculosis "letter". *Lancet* 1992;339:315–316.

37. Tan JS, Canaday DH, Boom WH, Balaji KN, Schwander SK, Rich EA. Human alveolar T lymphocyte responses to Mycobacterium tuberculosis antigens: role for CD4⁺ and CD8⁺ cytotoxic T cells and relative resistance of alveolar macrophages to lysis. *J Immunol* 1997;159:290–297.

38. Lalvani A, Brookes R, Wilkinson RJ, et al. Human cytolytic and interferon gamma-secreting CD8⁺ T lymphocytes specific for Mycobacterium tuberculosis. *Proc Natl Acad Sci USA* 1998;95:270–275.

39. Porcelli S, Morita CT, Brenner MB. CD1b restricts the response of human CD4-8⁻ T lymphocytes to a microbial antigen. *Nature* 1992;360:593–597.

40. Gong J, Stenger S, Zack JA, et al. Isolation of Mycobacterium-reactive CD1-restricted T cells from patients with human immunodeficiency virus infection. *J Clin Invest* 1998;101:383–389.

41. Jackman RM, Stenger S, Lee A, et al. The tyrosine-containing cytoplasmic tail of CD1b is essential for its efficient presentation of bacterial lipid antigens. *Immunity* 1998;8:341–351.

42. Lewinsohn DM, Alderson MR, Briden AL, Riddell SR, Reed SG, Grabstein KH. Characterization of human CD8⁺ T cells reactive with Mycobacterium tuberculosis-infected antigen-presenting cells. *J Exp Med* 1998;187:1633–1640.

43. Kaufmann SHE. CD8⁺ T lymphocytes in intracellular microbial infections. *Immunol Today* 1988; 9:168–174.

44. Beno DW, Stover AG, Mathews HL. Growth inhibition of Candida albicans hyphae by CD8⁺ lymphocytes. *J Immunol* 1995;154:5273–5281.

45. Levitz SM, Dupont MP. Phenotypic and functional characterization of human lymphocytes activated by interleukin-2 to directly inhibit growth of Cryptococcus neoformans in vitro. *J Clin Invest* 1993; 91:1490–1498.

46. Ellner JJ, Olds GR, Lee CW, Kleinhenz ME, Edmonds KL. Destruction of the multicellular parasite Schistosoma mansoni by T lymphocytes. *J Clin Invest* 1982;70:369–378.

47. Salata RA, Cox JG, Ravdin JI. The interaction of human T-lymphocytes and Entamoeba histolytica. *Parasite Immunol* 1987;9:249–261.

48. Khan IA, Smith KA, Kasper LH. Induction of antigen-specific parasiticidal cytotoxic T cell splenocytes by a major membrane protein (P30) of Toxoplasma gondii. *J Immunol* 1988;141:3600–3605.

49. Markham RB, Goellner J, Pier GB. In vitro T cell-mediated killing of Pseudomonas aeruginosa. I. Evidence that a lymphokine mediates killing. *J Immunol* 1984;133:962–968.

50. Markham RB, Pier GB, Goellner JJ, Mizel SB. In vitro T cell-mediated killing of Pseudomonas aeruginosa. II. The role of macrophages and T cell subsets in T cell killing. *J Immunol* 1985;134:4112–4117.

51. Kaufmann SH, Rodewald HR, Hug E, de Libero G. Cloned Listeria monocytogenes specific non-MHC-restricted Lyt-2⁺ T cells with cytolytic and protective activity. *J Immunol* 1988;140:3173–3179.

52. Smith LE, Rodrigues M, Russell DG. The interaction between CD8⁺ cytotoxic T cells and Leishmania-infected macrophages. *J Exp Med* 1991; 174:499–505.

53. Subauste CS, Koniaris AH, Remington JS. Murine CD8⁺ cytotoxic T lymphocytes lyse Toxoplasma gondii-infected cells. *J Immunol* 1991;147:3955–3959.

54. Curiel TJ, Krug EC, Purner MB, Poignard P, Berens RL. Cloned human CD4⁺ cytotoxic T lymphocytes specific for Toxoplasma gondii lyse tachyzoite-infected target cells. *J Immunol* 1993;151:2024–2031.

55. Jiang X, Gregory SH, Wing EJ. Immune CD8⁺ T lymphocytes lyse Listeria monocytogenes-infected hepatocytes by a classical MHC class I-restricted mechanism. *J Immunol* 1997;158:287–293.

56. Kima PE, Ruddle NH, McMahon-Pratt D. Presentation via the class I pathway by Leishmania amazonensis-infected macrophages of an endogenous leishmanial antigen to CD8⁺ T cells. *J Immunol* 1997;159:1828–1834.

57. DeLibero G, Flesch I, Kaufmann SHE. Mycobacteria-reactive Lyt-2⁺ T cell lines. *Eur J Immunol* 1988;18:59–66.

58. Silver RF, Li Q, Boom WH, Ellner JJ. Lymphocyte-dependent inhibition of growth of virulent Mycobacterium tuberculosis H37Rv within human monocytes: requirement for CD4⁺ T cells in purified protein derivative-positive, but not in purified protein derivative-negative subjects. *J Immunol* 1998; 160:2408–2417.

59. Kagi D, Ledermann B, Burki K, et al. Cytotoxicity mediated by T cells and natural killer cells is greatly impaired in perforin-deficient mice [see comments]. *Nature* 1994;369:31–37.

60. Lowin B, Beermann F, Schmidt A, Tschopp J. A null mutation in the perforin gene impairs cytolytic T lymphocyte- and natural killer cell-mediated cytotoxicity. *Proc Natl Acad Sci USA* 1994;91:11571–11575.

61. Kojima H, Shinohara N, Hanaoka S, et al. Two distinct pathways of specific killing revealed by perforin mutant cytotoxic T lymphocytes. *Immunity* 1994;1:357–364.

62. Lowin B, Hahne M, Mattmann C, Tschopp J. Cytolytic T-cell cytotoxicity is mediated through perforin and Fas. *Nature* 1994;370:650–652.

63. Sarin A, Williams MS, Alexander-Miller MA, Berzofsky JA, Zacharchuk CM, Henkart PA. Target cell lysis by CTL granule exocytosis is independent of ICE/Ced-3 family proteases. *Immunity* 1997; 6:209–215.

64. Conceicao-Silva F, Hahne M, Schroter M, Louis J, Tschopp J. The resolution of lesions induced by Leishmania major in mice requires a functional Fas (APO-1, CD95) pathway of cytotoxicity. *Eur J Immunol* 1998;28:237–245.

65. Shresta S, Goda P, Wesselschmidt R, Ley TJ. Residual cytotoxicity and granzyme K expression in granzyme A-deficient cytotoxic lymphocytes. *J Biol Chem* 1997;272:20236–20244.

66. Frischholz S, Rollinghoff M, Moll H. Cutaneous leishmaniasis: co-ordinate expression of granzyme A and lymphokines by CD4⁺ T cells from susceptible mice. *Immunology* 1994;82:255–260.

67. Kagi D, Ledermann B, Burki K, Hengartner H, Zinkernagel RM. CD8$^+$ T cell-mediated protection against an intracellular bacterium by perforin-dependent cytotoxicity. *Eur J Immunol* 1994;24:3068–3072.

68. White DW, Harty JT. Perforin-deficient CD8$^+$ T cells provide immunity to Listeria monocytogenes by a mechanism that is independent of CD95 and IFN-gamma but requires TNF-alpha. *J Immunol* 1998;160:905.

69. Kumar S, Tarleton RL. The relative contribution of antibody production and CD8$^+$ T cell function to immune control of Trypanosoma cruzi. *Parasite Immunol* 1998;20:207–216.

70. Denkers EY, Yap G, Scharton-Kersten T, et al. Perforin-mediated cytolysis plays a limited role in host resistance to Toxoplasma gondii. *J Immunol* 1997;159:1903–1908.

71. Laochumroonvorapong P, Wang J, Liu CC, et al. Perforin, a cytotoxic molecule which mediates cell necrosis, is not required for the early control of mycobacterial infection in mice. *Infect Immun* 1997;65:127–132.

72. Cooper AM, D'Souza C, Frank AA, Orme IM. The course of Mycobacterium tuberculosis infection in the lungs of mice lacking expression of either perforin- or granzyme-mediated cytolytic mechanisms. *Infect Immun* 1997;65:1317–1320.

73. Heusel JW, Wesselschmidt RL, Shresta S, Russell JH, Ley TJ. Cytotoxic lymphocytes require granzyme B for the rapid induction of DNA fragmentation and apoptosis in allogeneic target cells. *Cell* 1994;76:977–987.

74. Huang FP, Xu D, Esfandiari EO, Sands W, Wie XQ, Liew FY. Mice defective in Fas are highly susceptible to Leishmania major infection despite elevated IL-12 synthesis, strong Th1 responses, and enhanced nitric oxide production. *J Immunol* 1998;160:4143–4147.

75. Savill J, Fadok V, Henson P, Haslett C. Phagocyte recognition of cells undergoing apoptosis. *Immunol Today* 1993;14:131–136.

76. Albert ML, Sauter B, Bhardwaj N. Dendritic cells acquire antigen from apoptotic cells and induce class I-restricted CTLs. *Nature* 1998;392:86–89.

77. Brodskyn CI, Barral A, Boaventura V, Carvalho E, Barral-Netto M. Parasite- driven in vitro human lymphocyte cytotoxicity against autologous infected macrophages from mucosal leishmaniasis. *J Immunol* 1997;159:4467–4473.

78. Fuse Y, Nishimura H, Maeda K, Yoshikai Y. CD95 (Fas) may control the expansion of activated T cells after elimination of bacteria in murine listeriosis. *Infect Immun* 1997;65:1883–1891.

79. Burk MR, Mori L, de Libero G. Human V gamma 9-V delta 2 cells are stimulated in a cross- reactive fashion by a variety of phosphorylated metabolites. *Eur J Immunol* 1995;25:2052–2058.

80. Altare F, Durandy A, Lammas D, et al. Impairment of mycobacterial immunity in human interleukin-12 receptor deficiency. *Science* 1998;280:1432–1435.

81. Stenger S, Hanson DA, Teitelbaum R, et al. An antimicrobial activity of cytolytic T-cells mediated by granulysin. *Science* 1998;282:121–125.

82. Oddo M, Renno T, Attinger A, Bakker T, MacDonald HR, Meylan PR. Fas ligand-induced apoptosis of infected human macrophages reduces the viability of intracellular Mycobacterium tuberculosis. *J Immunol* 1998;160:5448–5454.

83. Sirard JC, Fayolle C, de Chastellier C, Mock M, Leclerc C, Berche P. Intracytoplasmic delivery of listeriolysin O by a vaccinal strain of Bacillus anthracis induces CD8-mediated protection against Listeria monocytogenes. *J Immunol* 1997;159:4435–4443.

84. Tascon RE, Colston MJ, Ragno S, Stavropoulos E, Gregory D, Lowrie DB. Vaccination against tuberculosis by DNA injection. *Nat Med* 1996;2:888–892.

85. Silva CL, Silva MF, Pietro RC, Lowrie DB. Characterization of T cells that confer a high degree of protective immunity against tuberculosis in mice after vaccination with tumor. *Infect Immun* 1996;64:2400–2407.

86. Zhu X, Venkataprasad N, Thangaraj HS, et al. Functions and specificity of T cells following nucleic acid vaccination of mice against Mycobacterium tuberculosis infection. *J Immunol* 1997;158:5921–5926.

87. Huygen K, Content J, Denis O, et al. Immunogenicity and protective efficacy of a tuberculosis DNA vaccine. *Nat Med* 1996;2:893–898.

88. Denis O, Tanghe A, Palfiet K, et al. Vaccination with plasmid DNA encoding mycobacterial antigen 85A stimulates a CD4$^+$ and CD8$^+$ T-cell epitopic repertoire broader than that stimulated by H37Rv infection. *Infect Immun* 1998;66:1527–1533.

Cytotoxic Cells: Basic Mechanisms and Medical Applications, edited by Michail V. Sitkovsky and Pierre A. Henkart. Lippincott Williams & Wilkins, Philadelphia © 2000.

Chapter 21

Tumor Surveillance *In Vivo* Depends on Perforin-Mediated Cytolysis

Maries F. van den Broek, David Kägi, and Hans Hengartner

Institute of Experimental Immunology, University Hospital, Zürich, CH8091 Zürich, Switzerland

Natural killer (NK) cells contribute to the host defense mechanism by lysing virus-infected cells or tumor cells in an antigen-nonspecific way. In contrast to cytotoxic lymphocytes (CTLs), which need several days to be activated, NK cells can be activated within hours by interferon (IFN) α/β or by interleukin-12 (IL-12). The lytic activity of NK cells is regulated both by activating and inhibitory molecules (1–3). Self-major histocompatibility complex class I (MHC-I) molecules on target cells have been shown to bind to NK inhibitory receptors (KIRs), thereby preventing the lytic activity of NK cells (4–6). Recently, these inhibitory receptors of mice and humans have been cloned and identified as members of the Ly-49 family (7) and the killer cell inhibitory gene family (8,9), respectively. NK-specific triggering molecules are less well defined.

Because viral infection of cells often inhibits protein synthesis in general or interferes with the export of MHC-I molecules (10,11), virus-infected cells may become resistant to CTL-dependent lysis and become susceptible to NK-dependent lysis instead. Also tumors are known to downregulate the expression of MHC-I molecules to escape immune surveillance, thereby making themselves a target for NK cells (12–14).

As has been described for CTLs (15–20), NK cells also may theoretically use perforin and Fas/Fas ligand (FasL) interactions to lyse target cells *in vivo* and *in vitro.* Using perforin-deficient (PKO), Fas-deficient (*lpr/lpr*) and FasL-deficient (*gld/gld*) mice, we and others could demonstrate that, similar to CTLs, NK cells use predominantly perforin for their effector function *in vivo* and *in vitro* (17,21–23). We activated NK cells in C57BL/6 mice, PKO mice, and *gld* mice by injection of 200 μg poly-IC or of 10^6 pfu lymphocytic choriomeningitis virus (LCMV), both of which are known to induce IFN-α. Subsequent analysis of lytic activity in the spleen toward MHC-I$^+$/Fas^{low} (RMA), MHC-I$^-$/Fas^{low} (RMA-S), and MHC-I$^-$/Fas^{high} (YAC-1) targets showed that absence of FasL (*gld* mice) did not influence the level of killing of MHC-I$^-$ targets, whereas the absence of perforin (PKO) abolished all lytic activity toward MHC-I$^-$ targets, even if the latter expressed high levels of Fas and were shown to be susceptible to FasL-mediated lysis (22,24) (Fig. 21-1). Thus NK cells use perforin as the main mechanism and do not use Fas/FasL as an alternative lytic pathway, even if perforin is lacking. Over the past years, some papers have been published that suggest a significant role for FasL in NK-mediated target cell lysis (27–30), which seems to be in conflict with our findings. The differences may be explained by the use of different effector populations used in differ-

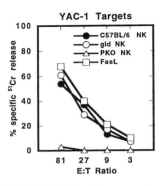 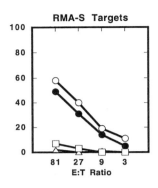 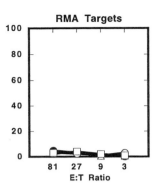

FIG. 21-1. NK cells use perforin and not FasL to lyse MHC-I⁻ target cells. NK cells were generated *in vivo* by intravenous injection of 10^6 pfu lymphocytic choriomeningitis virus (LCMV), strain WE, into C57BL/6, C57BL/6-*gld/gld* (FasL-deficient), or C57BL/6-PKO (perforin-deficient), mice 48 hours before isolation of splenocytes. Lytic activity was determined in a 5-hour ^{51}Cr-release assay. Spontaneous release of target cells was less than 18%. The percentage of FasL-mediated lysis (□) was determined in a 5-hour ^{51}Cr-release assay using vaccinia virus–FasL-infected (3 hours, MOI 3) MC57G (H-2^b) fibroblasts as effectors (25,26). The expression of MHC-I and of Fas of the target cells was measured by FACS analysis and was (in arbitrary units) as follows: *RMA* MHC-I, 1,300; Fas, 30; *RMA*-S MHC-I, 20; Fas, 30; *YAC-1* MHC-I, 20; Fas, 150; *MBL-2*. Fas MHC-I, 1,200; Fas, 350. RMA and RMA-S (TAP-deficient subclone of RMA) are Rauscher leukemia virus-induced B cell lymphoma cells of C57BL/6 origin; YAC-1 is a Moloney leukemia virus-induced B cell lymphoma of A/Sn origin; and MBL-2.Fas is a Fas-transfected, Moloney leukemia virus-induced B cell lymphoma of C57BL/6 origin.

ent studies: Arase et al. (27) showed that freshly isolated murine NK1.1⁺CD3⁻ cells were able to lyse MRL$^{+/+}$, but not MRL$^{lpr/lpr}$ thymocytes in a 12-hour assay, suggesting a major role for FasL. They could not explain, however, why perforin, which was presumably present in the NK effectors, was not able to lyse MRL$^{lpr/lpr}$ targets. In addition, it has been shown that NK1.1⁺CD3⁻ effectors from FasL-deficient *gld* mice are equally effective in lysing Fas⁺ targets as NK1.1⁺CD3⁻ effectors from normal mice. Eischen et al. (28) described that human CD3⁻CD16⁺ clones transcribe FasL mRNA after CD16 crosslinking and that they were able to lyse Fas⁺ target cells (Fas-transfected P815 cells). The use of clones cultured *in vitro* for a long time as a representation of an *in vivo* situation is doubtful, however. Liu et al. (29) used lymphokine-activated killer (LAK) cells from perforin-deficient mice that expressed FasL mRNA to lyse Fas⁺ target cells *in vitro*. The LAK cells were probably derived from a mixture of CTLs and NK cells, which

makes it difficult to determine the exact effector population. Moreover, the Fas⁺ targets were Fas-transfected P815 cells, which are known to express considerable levels of MHC-I molecules, probably making them unsuitable targets for classic NK cells (6). Finally, Oshimi et al. (30) showed that freshly isolated human CD3⁻CD16⁺ cells use FasL to lyse a variety of target cells after CD16 crosslinking. This type of cytotoxicity, however, is not the classic NK-mediated cytolysis but, rather, antibody-dependent cell-mediated cytotoxicity (ADCC). Obviously, the effector pathways used by NK cells may vary depending on the method of activation.

In vivo, NK cells are thought to form the first line of defense against MHC-I$^{low/-}$ aberrant cells, such as some tumor cells or virus-infected cells. Functional *in vivo* data on effector mechanisms of NK cells are still rather scarce, but the present data support a role for perforin and not for additional or alternative lytic mechanisms. To analyze the mechanism of cytolytic activity of NK cells *in vivo*, we

TABLE 21-1. *Control of a syngeneic, MHC-class I⁻ lymphoma: dependence on perforin*

Inoculated tumor	Time until weight increase >15% (days)	
	C57BL/6	C57BL/6-PKO
10^2 RMA-S	>80	20 ± 4
10^4 RMA-S	41 ± 4	17 ± 2
10^6 RMA-S	19 ± 3	16 ± 3

Male C57BL/6 or C57BL/6-PKO mice were injected intraperitoneally with different numbers of live RMA-S cells in 0.25 ml PBS. Mice were observed daily for tumor growth by monitoring the weight of the mice. They were killed when the weight had increased >15% compared to a control group consisting of age- and sex-matched, noninjected animals, which is obligatory according to Swiss federal and cantonal laws on animal protection. C57BL/6 mice injected with 10^2 RMA-S cells did not show any signs of tumor growth by the time the experiment was stopped (day 80). Three mice were injected per group.

injected various amounts of the syngeneic, MHC-I⁻ lymphoma RMA-S into C57BL/6 or PKO mice that had been or not injected with 200 μg poly-IC 48 hours previously; we found that C57BL/6 mice controlled the tumor at least 100 times better than the PKO mice (23) (Table 21-1). Because RMA-S cells do not express sufficiently high levels of Fas, this experiment does not allow any conclusions on the role of Fas/FasL interactions. In addition, we injected C57BL/6, C57BL/6-PKO, and C57BL/6-CD8-deficient (31) mice subcutaneously with various doses (25–400 μg) of the chemical carcinogen methylcholanthrene (MCA) in corn oil and followed the kinetics and incidence of fibrosarcoma development in the individual mice (25) (Table 21-2). The absence of perforin increased

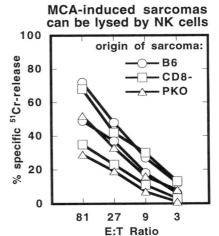

MCA-induced sarcomas can be lysed by NK cells

FIG. 21-2. MCA-induced fibrosarcomas are susceptible to NK-mediated cytolysis. Mice [C57BL/6 (B6), CD8⁻/⁻, PKO] were injected subcutaneously with 100 μg MCA, and the resulting fibrosarcomas ($n = 6$) were isolated and cultured. These cultured fibrosarcoma cell lines were used as targets for poly-IC-induced (200 μg i.v. at −48 hours) splenic NK cells of C57BL/6 mice in a 5-hour ^{51}Cr-release assay. Spontaneous release of target cells was (depending on the target) 12% to 17%.

both the incidence and the kinetics of sarcoma development, whereas the absence of CD8⁺ cells had no effect. Thus MCA-induced sarcomas are controlled by NK cells in a perforin-dependent fashion. We isolated six different MCA-induced tumors (two different tumors from each strain), put them into culture, and used them as targets for NK cells in a ^{51}Cr-release assay. All six tumor

TABLE 21-2. *Methylcholanthrene-induced sarcomas: control by NK cells in a perforin-dependent fashion*

MCA dose (μg)	No. of mice with sarcoma/total		
	C57BL/6	CD8⁻/⁻	PKO
25	1/6 (day 200)	1/6 (day 200)	6/6 (day 75)
100	8/10 (day 200)	7/10 (day 200)	10/10 (day 60)
400	5/5 (day 120)	Not done	5/5 (day 48)

Mice were injected subcutaneously with MCA in corn oil and were observed daily for sarcoma development by palpation. If tumors were >15 mm in diameter, the mice were killed. The experiment was ended at day 200.

Differences between PKO and C57BL/6 or PKO and CD8⁻/⁻ were statistically significant ($p < 0.01$, unpaired Mann-Whitney U-test), whereas differences between C57BL/6 and CD8⁻/⁻ were not.

lines were susceptible to lysis by C57BL/6 NK cells (Fig. 21-2) but not by PKO NK cells (data not shown). In addition, all cell lines were resistant to CTL-mediated lysis (data not shown). All six cell lines expressed low levels of MHC-I (arbitrary units in FACS: 10–50) and of Fas (arbitrary units in FACS: 12–30). As a comparison, NK-sensitive RMA-S cells and YAC-1 cells expressed 420 arbitrary units and 160 arbitrary units of MHC-I, respectively. Also other studies, using syngeneic (17) or allogeneic (32,33) tumors showed a major role for perforin, although in allogeneic systems an additional role for FasL and tumor necrosis factor-α (TNF-α) could be demonstrated (32,33): these studies did not, however, dissect the effector population further into CTLs and NK cells.

TUMOR SURVEILLANCE BY CYTOTOXIC T LYMPHOCYTES

Tumor cells can develop in all individuals as a result of exposure to irradiation, oncogenic viruses, or mutagenic reagents; or they may be due to spontaneous mutations. The balance between the growth kinetics and metastatic capacity of the tumor and the ability of the host to control the tumor determines finally whether the host survives. Control of tumor growth is mediated by two arms of the immune response: the innate (e.g., NK cells) and the acquired [e.g., CTLs, T-helper (Th) cells, and antibodies] immunity. To prime acquired immunity, the tumor must present tumor-specific antigens in the context of MHC-I or MCH-II antigens to the host's CD8+ and CD4+ cells, respectively (34–36). Under pressure of the immune response, tumor escape variants may arise that lack MHC molecules, co-stimulatory molecules, or tumor-specific antigens (12–14,37,38). It has been shown that MHC-I− tumor variants can be controlled *in vivo* by NK cells (23,25,38; see above).

To investigate the role of perforin in the control of syngeneic tumors *in vivo*, we performed three sets of experiments: We in-

jected perforin-deficient (PKO) and immunocompetent (C57BL/6 = B6) mice with (a) titrated amounts of syngeneic tumor cell lines with or without previous priming, (b) mutagenic chemicals, or (c) oncogenic viruses. We then compared tumor incidence, kinetics, and the ability to eliminate the tumor between PKO and B6 mice (25).

Injection of B6 and PKO mice with syngeneic tumor cell lines revealed that, depending on the tumor cell line used, B6 mice were able to control 10 to 100 times more cells than PKO mice in an unprimed situation, and up to 10,000 times more cells in a primed situation (25) (Table 21-3). Therefore, even without previous priming, perforin-mediated cytotoxicity seems to be a crucial effector mechanism in the control of tumor cells of both lymphoid [MBL-2 (B cell lymphoma), EL-4 (thymoma)] and non-lymphoid [MC57G (fibrosarcoma)] origin. After priming, the difference between PKO and B6 mice was even more pronounced, suggesting that priming of CD8+ rather than of CD4+ cells is responsible for resistance against high tumor loads. RMA (B cell lymphoma) and SR23B (adenovirus + *ras*-transformed embryonic fibroblasts) (39) were controlled to a similar extent in both mouse strains. Because MBL-2 and RMA are related lymphomas and express comparable levels of MHC molecules, this finding was unexpected but may be explained by different growth kinetics or by different efficiencies of CD4+ priming (not studied here) of the two cell lines. SR23B cells could be controlled to a similar extent in both strains as far as the size of "inoculum" is considered. The sarcomas in PKO mice, however, were significantly smaller than those in B6 mice, which may be due to increased basal levels of macrophage activation, serum TNF-α, and serum IFN-γ (40). B16 melanomas could not be controlled by either strain, even at low numbers, probably because the extremely low levels of MHC-I and MHC-II molecules on the surface. Comparison of the control of Fas-transfected and mock-transfected MBL-2 cells in B6 and PKO mice revealed

TABLE 21-3. *Control[a] of syngeneic tumor cell lines by primed and unprimed PKO and B6 mice* in vivo

Tumor	MHC		Susc. to FasL-mediated lysis[c]	Unprimed		Primed[d]	
	CI.I[b]	CL.II[b]		B6	PKO	B6	PKO
MC57G	330	3	0	10^6	10^5	ND	ND
MBL-2	1100	3	0	10^4	$<10^2$	$>10^6$	10^5
MBL-2Fas	1200	3	54	10^5	10^3	$<10^6$	$10^{6\,e}$
RMA	1300	3	6	10^4	10^4	$<10^6$	$<10^6$
EL-4	1500	3	4	10^4	$<10^2$	$>10^6$	$<10^2$
B16	40	3	0	10^2	10^2	ND	ND
SR23B	75	3	0	10^6	10^6	ND	ND

[a] The cell numbers represent the lowest number of tumor cells that could *not* be controlled *in vivo*. The number of tumor cells injected ranged from 10^2 to 10^6 in tenfold steps. Data result from two independent experiments using groups of two or three mice each (total number of mice per group was four to six). Unless otherwise stated, groups were homogeneous; that is, none of the mice within a group could control the amount of cells listed in the table.

[b] As determined by FACS analysis. All cell lines were measured in one and the same experiment, and the values represent arbitrary units of fluorescence.

[c] Percentage specific killing by vaccinia virus–FasL-infected MC57G effector cells at an E/T ratio of 10:1 in a 5-hour ^{51}Cr release assay (33).

[d] Mice were primed by intraperitoneal injection of 5×10^6 irradiated tumor cells on days -14 and -7 followed by a challenge with live tumor cells on day 0 (MBL-2, MBL-2Fas, RMA). Alternatively, mice were infected with 10^6 pfu recombinant vaccinia virus expressing the vesicular stomatitis virus nucleoprotein (VSV-NP) on day -14 followed by challenge with VSV-NP transfected or of mock transfected EL-4 cells (EL-4).

[e] Only two of four mice controlled this amount of MBL-2Fas cells.

that Fas$^+$ MBL-2 cells were controlled ten times better in both strains than the Fas$^-$ cells, although the amount of controllable cells was 100-fold lower in PKO mice. After priming PKO mice, the resistance against MBL-2Fas and MBL-2 was increased 100-fold to 10^5 and 10^4 cells, respectively, suggesting the priming of perforin-independent effector pathways. Priming of B6 mice, however, resulted in resistance to more than 10^6 cells independent of the presence of Fas, stressing the need for perforin-dependent and perforin-independent effector mechanisms. Taken together, we could not demonstrate a major role for Fas in the eradication of a tumor cell line, but neither could we exclude a minor role.

A more physiologic method for studying tumor surveillance *in vivo* is the induction of primary tumors *in vivo* by viruses or carcinogens instead of injection of rather large amounts of *in vitro* cultured tumor cell lines. We used subcutaneous injection of 25 to 400 μg MCA to induce sarcomas, chronic skin application of 10 nmol 12-*O*-tetradecanoyl-phorbol-13-acetate (TPA) + 3 nmol 7,12-

dimethylbenzanthracen (DMBA) to induce papillomas (41), or subcutaneous injection of 10^3 focus forming units of Moloney murine sarcoma and leukemia virus (MoMSV) complex to induce sarcomas (42). PKO mice appeared to be more susceptible to the development of MCA-induced sarcomas at all doses of MCA tested (25) (Table 21-2) compared to B6 and CD8-deficient mice, pointing toward crucial, perforin-dependent involvement of NK cells in sarcoma control (see above). In contrast, TPA + DMBA induced papillomas with similar kinetics, size, and incidence in B6 and PKO mice, demonstrating no role for perforin in this tumor model.

MoMSV-induced sarcomas usually are rejected by immunocompetent mice within 3 weeks in a H-2D^b-restricted CTL-dependent way (42), whereas lethal tumors develop in *nu/nu* or CD4$^+$-depleted mice. PKO and B6 mice developed sarcomas with similar incidence (100%) and kinetics (maximal tumor size between days 9 and 14). On the other hand, although 100% of the PKO and B6 mice rejected the tumor, they did it with slightly different kinetics: B6 mice were tumor-free by day 30, whereas PKO mice needed 55 days. In addition, the maximal size of the sarcomas in B6 mice was somewhat smaller (150 ± 50 mm^3) compared to that in PKO mice (280 ± 65 mm^3). CD8-depleted mice were comparable to PKO mice in all aspects of the MoMSV tumor model, showing involvement of CTLs and not of NK cells in the control of MoMSV-induced sarcomas. Long-term follow-up (more than 7 months) of B6 and PKO mice after rejection of the primary local sarcoma allowed us to make the interesting observation that all B6 mice remained healthy and tumor-free as checked by autopsy, whereas all PKO mice developed lymphomas in several lymphoid organs, resulting in death 9 to 12 months after MoMSV inoculation (F. Ossendorp, M. van den Broek, unpublished observations). These data clearly show that perforin-dependent CTLs seem to be of minor importance for acute control of the primary sarcoma, but they are crucial for control of secondary, lethal lymphomas. At this time, we do not know whether the secondary lymphomas resulted from metastases of the primary sarcoma or they were newly induced by persisting MoMVS in PKO mice.

Finally, we have never observed spontaneous malignancies of any kind in PKO mice that were kept over 1 year in our facilities (about 100 mice over a period of 5 years). This, however, does not bagatellize the physiologic role of perforin in tumor control because mouse facilities are a relatively protected environment devoid of irradiation, toxins, mutagens, and exogenous oncogenic viruses; and the spontaneous development of perforin-only controllable tumors may have an incidence of less than 1% and therefore are too rare to be observed in 100 mice.

Taken together, we could show that both CTLs (for MHC-I$^+$ tumors) and NK cells (for MHC-I$^-$ tumors) use a perforin-mediated cellular effector mechanism as the major cytotoxic mechanism to control the growth of syngeneic tumors *in vivo*. A significant contribution of FasL-Fas interactions or of TNF-α to the control of syngeneic tumors *in vivo* could not be demonstrated until now.

REFERENCES

1. Gumperz JE, Parham P. The enigma of natural killer cells. *Nature* 1995;378:245–248.
2. Raulet DH. Recognition events that inhibit and activate natural killer cells. *Curr Opin Immunol* 1996;8:372–377.
3. Moretta A, Bottino C, Vitale M, et al. Receptors for HLA class I molecules on human NK cells. *Annu Rev Immunol* 1996;14:619–648.
4. Ljunggren HC, Kärre K. Host resistance directed selectively against H-2 deficient lymphoma variants: analysis of the mechanisms. *J Exp Med* 1985;162:1745–1759.
5. Yokoyama WM, Seaman WE. The Ly-49 and NKR-PI gene family encoding lectin-like receptors on natural killer cells. *Annu Rev Immunol* 1993;11:613–635.
6. Kärre K. Express ourself or die: peptides, MHC molecules and NK cells. *Science* 1995;276:978–979.
7. Colonna M, Samaridis J. Cloning of immunoglobulin superfamily members associated with HLA-C and HLA-B recognition by human NK cells. *Science* 1996;268:405–408.
8. Wagtman N, Biassoni R, Cantoni C, et al. Molecular clones of the p58 NK cell receptor reveal immunoglobulin-related molecules with diversity in both intracellular and extracellular domains. *Immunity* 1995;2:439–449.
9. Lanier LL, Philips JH. Inhibitory MHC class I receptors on NK cells and T cells. *Immunol Today* 1996;17:86–91.
10. Hill A, Barnett BC, McMichael AJ, McGeoch DJ. HLA class I molecules are not transported to the cell surface in cells infected with herpes simplex virus type 1 and type 2. *J Immunol* 1994;152:22736–22741.
11. DelVal M, Hengel H, Hacker H, et al. Cytomegalovirus prevents antigen presentation by blocking the transport of peptide-loaded MHC class I molecules to the medial Golgi compartment. *J Exp Med* 1992;176:729–737.
12. Schrier PJ, Bernards R, Vaessen TMJ, Houweling A, van der Eb A. Expression of class I MHC antigens switched off by highly oncogenic adenovirus 12 in transformed cells. *Nature* 1983;305:776–779.
13. Uyttenhove C, Maryanski J, Boon T. Escape of mouse mastocytoma P815 after nearly complete rejection is due to antigen-loss variants rather than to immunosuppression. *J Exp Med* 1983;157:1040–1052.
14. Smith MEF, Marsh SCE, Bodmer JG, Gelsthorpe K, Bodmer WF. Loss of HLA-A, -B, -C allele products and LFA-3 in colorectal neoplasia. *Proc Natl Acad Sci USA* 1989;86:5557–5561.
15. Henkart P. Mechanisms of lymphocyte-mediated cytotoxicity. *Annu Rev Immunol* 1985;3:31–58.

16. Podack ER, Hengartner H, Lichtenheld MG. A central role of perforin in cytolysis? *Annu Rev Immunol* 1991;9:129–151.

17. Kägi D, Ledermann B, Bürki K, et al. Cytotoxicity mediated by cytotoxic T cells and natural killer cells is greatly impaired in perforin-deficient mice. *Nature* 1994;369:31–37.

18. Kägi D, Vignaux F, Leerman B, et al. Fas and perforin pathways as major mechanisms of T cell mediated cytotoxicity. *Science* 1994;265:528–230.

19. Lowin B, Hahne M, Matzmann C, Tschopp J. Cytolytic T cell cytotoxicity is mediated through the perforin and Fas lytic pathways. *Nature* 1994;370:650–652.

20. Kojima H, Shinohara N, Hanaoka S, et al. Two pathways of specific killing revealed by perforin mutant cytotoxic T lymphocytes. *Immunity* 1994;1:357–364.

21. Walsh CM, Matloubian M, Lui CC, et al. Immune function in mice lacking the perforin gene. *Proc Natl Acad Sci USA* 1994;91:10854–10858.

22. Kägi D, Ledermann B, Bürki K, Zinkernagel R, Hengartner H. Lymphocyte-mediated cytotoxicity in vitro and in vivo: mechanisms and significance. *Immunol Rev* 1995;146:95–116.

23. Van den Broek MF, Kägi D, Zinkernagel R, Hengartner H. Perforin dependence of natural killer cell-mediated tumor control in vivo. *Eur J Immunol* 1995;25:3514–3516.

24. Van den Broek MF, Kägi D, Hengartner H. Effector pathways of natural killer cells. *Curr Top Microbiol Immunol* 1998;230:123–131.

25. Van den Broek MF, Kägi D, Ossendorp F, et al. Decreased tumor surveillance in perforin-deficient mice. *J Exp Med* 1996;184:1781–1790.

26. Ehl S, Hoffmann-Rohrer U, Nagata S, Hengartner H, Zinkernagel R. Different susceptibility of cytotoxic T cells to CD95 (Fas/Apo-1)-ligand mediated cell death after activation in vivo versus in vitro. *J Immunol* 1996;156:2357–2360.

27. Arase H, Arase N, Saito T. Fas-mediated cytotoxicity by freshly isolated NK cells. *J Exp Med* 1995;181:1235–1238.

28. Eischen C, Schiling J, Lynch D, Krammer P, Leibson P. Fc receptor induced expression on activated NK cells facilitates cell-mediated cytotoxicity and subsequent autocrine NK cell apoptosis. *J Immunol* 1996;156:2693–2699.

29. Liu CC, Walsh C, Eto N, Clarke W, Young D. Morphologica and functional characterization of perforin-deficient lymphokine-activated killer cells. *J Immunol* 1995;155:602–608.

30. Oshimi Y, Oda S, Honda Y, Nagata S, Miyazaki S. Involvement of Fas ligand and Fas-mediated pathway in the cytotoxicity of human natural killer cells. *J Immunol* 1996;157:2909–2915.

31. Fung-Leung W, Schilham M, Rahemtulla A, et al. CD8 is needed for development of cytotoxic but not for helper cells. *Cell* 1992;65:443–451.

32. Walsh C, Hayashi F, Saffran D, Ju S, Berke G, Clark W. Cell-mediated cytotoxicity results from, but may not be critical for, primary allograft rejection. *J Immunol* 1996;156:1436–1441.

33. Braun M, Lowin B, French L, Acha-Orbea H, Tschopp J. Cytotoxic T cells deficient in both functional Fas ligand and perforin show residual cytolytic activity yet lose their capacity to induce lethal graft-versus-host disease. *J Exp Med* 1996;183:657–661.

34. Greenberg P. Adoptive T cell therapy of tumors: mechanisms operative in the recognition and elimination of tumor cells. *Adv Immunol* 1991;49:281–355.

35. Melief C. Tumor eradication by adoptive transfer of cytotoxic T lymphocytes. *Adv Cancer Res* 1992;58:281–355.

36. Van Pel A, van der Bruggen P, Coulie P, et al. Genes coding for tumor antigens recognized by cytotoxic T lymphocytes. *Immunol Rev* 1995;145:229–250.

37. Zijlstra M, Melief C. Tumourigenicity of cells transformed by adenovirus type 12 by evasion of T cell immunity. *Nature* 1983;305:776–779.

38. Kärre K, Ljunggren H, Piontek G, Kiessling R. Selective rejection of H-2-deficient lymphoma variants suggests alternative immune strategy. *Nature* 1986;319:675–678.

39. Toes R, Offringa R, et al. An Adenovirus type 5 early region 1B CTL epitope mediating tumor eradication by CTL clones is downmodulated by an activated *ras* oncogene. *J Immunol* 1995;154:3396–3405.

40. Kägi D, Ledermann B, Bürki K, Hengartner H, Zinkernagel R. CD8+ T cell mediated protection against an intracellular bacterium by perforin-dependent cytotoxicity. *Eur J Immunol* 1994;24:3068–3072.

41. Fischer W, Beland P, Lutz W. DNA adducts, cell proliferation and papilloma latency time in mouse skin after repeated application of DMBA and TPA. *Carcinogenesis* 1993;14:1285–1288.

42. Stukart M, Vos A, Melief C. Cytotoxic T cell response against lymphoblasts infected with Moloney (Abelson) murine leukemia virus: methodological aspects and H-2 requirements. *Eur J Immunol* 1981;11:251–257.

Cytotoxic Cells: Basic Mechanisms and Medical Applications, edited by Michail V. Sitkovsky and Pierre A. Henkart. Lippincott Williams & Wilkins, Philadelphia © 2000.

Chapter 22

Role of Fas-Dependent Lytic Function in *In Vivo* Immune Regulation and Pathogenesis

Kimberly A. Sabelko-Downes, Anja R. B. Thilenius, Kathleen A. Kelly, and John H. Russell

Department of Molecular Biology and Pharmacology, Washington University School of Medicine, St. Louis, Missouri 63110, USA

Fas (CD95/APO-1) is a death receptor, and lytic interactions between Fas and its ligand (FasL/CD95L) have been associated with several immune-related processes. Included among them are immune privilege (1,2), in which FasL would provide a barrier to prevent autoreactive Fas$^+$ lymphocytes from entering privileged sites, and peripheral T cell tolerance (3). Fas and FasL, which are type I and type II transmembrane proteins and members of the tumor necrosis factor (TNF)/ nerve growth factor (NGF)-receptor and TNF families of proteins, respectively (4), can also serve as a cytotoxic mechanism between FasL-bearing T cells and Fas-expressing targets (5). This Fas-dependent lytic mechanism, which culminates in the apoptotic destruction of the Fas-expressing targets, is especially important with CD4$^+$ effectors that are principally of the T-helper-1 (Th1) subset (6,7). Such a lytic interaction between antigen-specific T cells and anergic B cells has been proposed as one mechanism for the elimination of anergic B cells *in vivo* (8,9).

In contrast to CD4$^+$ effector T cells, CD8$^+$ cytotoxic lymphocytes (CTLs) primarily use a granule exocytosis pathway to lyse antigen-bearing target cells (10). This mechanism requires direct contact between effector and target and involves polarization of pre-formed cytotoxic granules toward the site of interaction and release of the granule components into the small gap between the two cells. Furthermore, the extracellular Ca^{+2} instantaneously inactivates any perforin that might escape the zone of contact between the CTL and the target. Consequently, although the lethal hit results from a secretory process, there is little damage to bystander targets. However, when a T cell (either CD4$^+$ or CD8$^+$) uses a Fas-dependent lytic mechanism, both direct and bystander targets may be killed (11). During direct lysis, the antigen-presenting cell (APC) is also the Fas$^+$ target. It presents antigen to and thereby activates the T cell, which induces expression of FasL and enables the T cell to lyse the APC. For bystander lysis, the APC again activates the T cell, inducing expression of FasL, but the target is a third, Fas$^+$ cell that may lack the appropriate major histocompatibility complex (MHC)-restricting element to activate the T cell.

The role of Fas and its ligand in the regulation of autoimmune disease has been extensively studied in *lpr* and *gld* mice, which carry autosomal recessive mutations and consequently lack functional expression of Fas or FasL, respectively (12–14). Defective expression of these molecules in *lpr* and *gld* mice is associated with a lymphoproliferative disease that is largely of T cell origin and a spontaneous autoimmune disease with similarities to the nephritis associated with the human disease systemic lupus erythematosus (12–14). The severity of both syndromes varies depending on the genetic background (12), suggesting that endogenous antigens are important in the maintenance or initiation (or both) of disease. The lymphoproliferative phenotype coupled with the observation that T cells from these mice are defective in antigen-driven cell death of mature, peripheral T cells is in accord with the hypothesis that Fas and FasL are important for regulating the expansion of lymphocyte populations.

This chapter summarizes results from a series of experiments designed to better define the role of Fas and FasL in immune responses *in vivo* and determine the effect of deficient Fas and FasL expression on the severity and regulation of two autoimmune diseases, collagen-induced arthritis and experimental allergic encephalomyelitis. These studies have revealed a role for Fas-dependent lytic interactions in regulating the expansion of lymphocytes during chronic inflammation, with minimal involvement of Fas-mediated lysis in the regulation of acute immune responses involving either Th1 effectors or T-dependent B cell responses. We also describe a potential physiologic role for Fas-mediated bystander lysis as a novel mechanism of destruction of MHC class II⁻ (MHC-II⁻) cells in CD4⁺ T cell-mediated diseases.

FAS-DEPENDENT LYSIS IN *IN VIVO* IMMUNE RESPONSES

The magnitude of an immune response is generally thought to be regulated, at least in part, by the degree of effector cell clonal expansion in response to antigen. Our working hypothesis for the experiments described here was that if Fas- and FasL-dependent control of population expansion is an important, primary mechanism limiting the response to various challenges, the magnitude

and duration of the responses should be increased in Fas- or FasL-deficient mice. The effect of the *lpr* and *gld* mutations were initially examined on the C57BL/6 or B10.PL backgrounds, as the slow progression of the lymphoproliferative disease with few autoimmune sequelae allowed us to examine more prolonged immune challenges with animals having a less compromised lymphoid compartment (12).

Delayed-Type Hypersensitivity Response

The first test of this hypothesis was to determine the effects of the *lpr* and *gld* mutations on a Th1 cytokine-driven delayed-type hypersensitivity (DTH) response. Mice were immunized with guinea pig myelin basic protein (gpMBP) in complete Freund's adjuvant and subsequently challenged with either purified protein derivative (PPD, a component of the adjuvant) or gpMBP. Figure 22-1 illustrates the responses measured by comparing the thickness of the experimental footpad with the contralateral footpad challenged with vehicle alone. The result demonstrates essentially concordant responses to either antigen in both magnitude and duration between wild-type B10.PL mice and either congenic mutant strain. These data indicate that Fas and its ligand are not necessary for the development or resolution of this Th1-dependent inflammatory response.

T-Dependent B Cell Response

The lupus-like autoimmune syndrome most closely associated with the *lpr* mutation is caused by immune complex deposition in the glomerulus. Although the effector antibody is a B cell product, the disease requires that both T and B cells contain the *lpr* mutation (15,16). We have tested the effects of the *lpr* and *gld* mutations in a well characterized T-dependent B cell response to determine if Fas-dependent function altered not only the quantitative aspects but also the qualitative aspects of the reaction. We chose the response to the nitrophenyl (NP) hapten,

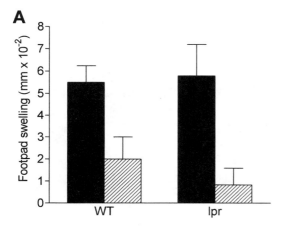

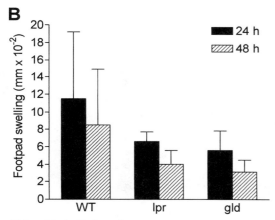

FIG. 22-1. Delayed-type hypersensitivity responses are similar in magnitude and kinetics in wild-type and congenic *lpr* and *gld* animals. **A:** B10.PL (*n* = 4) and B10.PL.*Fas*[lpr] (*n* = 7) mice were primed subcutaneously with guinea pig myelin basic protein (gpMBP) in complete Freund's adjuvant (CFA). Three weeks later the mice were injected in the hind footpad with 12.5 μg purified protein derivative (PPD) or vehicle. Footpad thickness was measured at 24 hours (*solid bars*) and 48 hours (*hatched bars*). The difference between control and experimental measurements is reported as the mean ± SD. **B:** EAE was induced in B10.PL (*n* = 7), B10.PL.*Fas*[lpr] (*n* = 5), and B10.PL.*Fasl*[gld] (*n* = 8) mice as described in Table 22-2. Control mice were injected with CFA rather than gpMBP emulsified in CFA. Thirty days later the mice were challenged with 50 μg gpMBP or vehicle. Footpad thickness was measured at 24 and 48 hours. The difference between control and experimental measurements is reported as the mean ± SD.

which in C57BL/6 mice is characterized by somatic mutation, affecting antibody affinity.

Mice were primed, boosted (NP-OVA), and bled at the indicated times; and high- and low-affinity antibodies were measured by enzyme-linked immunosorbent assay (ELISA) on plates coated with bovine serum albumin (BSA) conjugated at low and high ratios of NP to measure high- and low-affinity antibodies, respectively (Fig. 22-2). The kinetics and magnitude of the development of high-affinity antibodies was essentially concordant in wild-type and mutant mice. We and others (17) have also compared qualitative histologic characteristics (number, location, and size) of germinal center (GC) formation and cellular composition during GC development in response to NP-OVA and found no notable differences between C57BL/6 and B6.*lpr* mice in any of these parameters. This similarity in the formation of GCs and overall development of antibody titer and affinity indicates that Fas and FasL are not important primary regulators that limit this T-dependent B cell response.

Murine Acquired Immunodeficiency Syndrome

The development of murine acquired immunodeficiency syndrome (MAIDS), a disease characterized by massive lymphocyte proliferation, hypergammaglobulinemia, and immunodeficiency in both T and B cell functions, requires the presence of mature CD4+ T cells and B lymphocytes (18–20). MAIDS is initiated by a defective leukemia retrovirus, with the characteristic hyperaccumulation of CD4+ T cells likely resulting from an interaction of a large number of T cells with a MAIDS-associated superantigen (21,22). These reactive T cell populations eventually become anergic and die by apoptosis.

We and our colleagues used this model to examine the role of Fas-dependent lysis during a more chronic antigenic stimulation *in vivo* (23). When disease was induced in congenic *lpr* or *gld* mice, there was a greatly

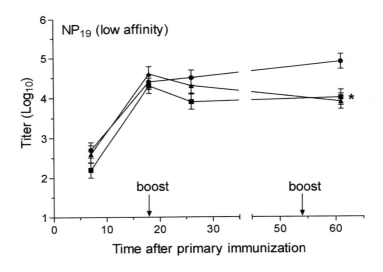

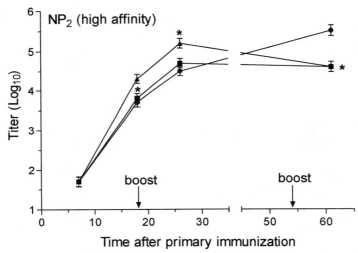

FIG. 22-2. Antinitrophenyl (NP) hapten responses are similar in wild-type and congenic *lpr* and *gld* animals. Wild-type (B6, *circles*), B6.*lpr* (*squares*), and B6.*gld* (*triangles*) mice were injected with NP-OVA in alum and bled at the indicated times. Anti-NP antibodies were measured by ELISA on plates coated with NP_{19}-BSA (*top panel*) or NP_2-BSA (*bottom panel*) to estimate the titers of low- and high-affinity antibodies, respectively. Statistically significant differences are indicated (*).

accelerated accumulation of $CD4^+$ cells, but not of the $CD4^-CD8^-$ cells that characterize the lymphoproliferative disease associated with these two mutations, compared to that seen in susceptible C57BL/6 animals. This exacerbation of the course of disease was apparently due to a greatly reduced rate of $CD4^+$ cell death in the absence of Fas or FasL. Interestingly, the $CD4^+$ cells did become anergic at a similar time, suggesting that Fas is not involved in the induction of anergy. The absence of a role for Fas in anergy induction was also observed by van Parijs et al. (24).

Fas-DEPENDENT LYSIS IN AUTOIMMUNE DISEASE

Lytic interactions between Fas and FasL could influence the regulation or pathology (or both) of autoimmune disease through several mechanisms. Fas and its ligand could play a role in regulating the immune response by interacting on or between T cell elements, limiting autoreactive clonal expansion or selection of pathogenic CD4$^+$ phenotypes. FasL expressed on cells in the target organ may contribute to the immune privileged status of the organ, providing a barrier to prevent autoreactive, Fas$^+$ lymphocytes from entering or surviving within this site. Disruption of immune privilege may result in an influx of autoreactive lymphocytes into privileged organs, whereas defects in peripheral tolerance may promote the expansion of autoreactive T cells, either of which would exacerbate autoimmune disease. Alternatively, expression of Fas in the target organ could render cells within this site as targets for a lytic interaction with FasL that has been transiently induced on T cells by contact with self-peptides on cellular elements expressing major histocompatibility proteins. If this were the case, defective expression of either Fas or its ligand should suppress the development or severity of disease.

We have tested this hypothesis by comparing the immune responses to the autoimmune-inducing antigens chick type II collagen and gpMBP in congenic mice carrying the *lpr* or *gld* mutation with those observed in wild-type animals. These induced responses culminate in collagen-induced arthritis or experimental allergic encephalomyelitis, respectively.

Collagen-Induced Arthritis

Collagen-induced arthritis (CIA) can be actively induced in susceptible mice by injection of the T-dependent antigen type II collagen (25). Weak or transient disease (or both) can be transferred with either serum or immunized T cells; but progressive, persistent disease requires that both T cells and serum be transferred (26). Recently, a role for CD8$^+$ T cells in the initiation and regulation of recovery from CIA has been described (27). As with human rheumatoid arthritis, susceptibility to murine collagen-induced arthritis is linked with specific MHC-II haplotypes (28). Several MHC haplotypes produce responses to heterologous type II collagen, but the H-2^q haplotype produces the highest titers of specific or cross-reactive antibodies to the autologous protein, and this haplotype is most associated with CIA (29,30). The H-2^b haplotype is relatively resistant to CIA and produces a modest antibody titer.

It was of interest to determine if a deficiency in Fas would alter this MHC-associated regulation and produce a more robust antibody response or convert a disease-resistant haplotype to disease-sensitive. We compared both antibody responses and disease in wild-type and *lpr* mice (H-2^b) to that observed in animals with a sensitive haplotype (H-2^q) and found that the *lpr* mutation does not overcome the MHC-defined limits of a response in either antibody titer or disease susceptibility (Table 22-1, experiment 1). Therefore to examine the effect of the *lpr* mutation on the severity of CIA, we introduced the mutation onto the B10.Q background. Again we found that the *lpr* mutation did not enhance the incidence or severity of CIA, a disease dependent on B cell and CD8$^+$ T cell effectors, on the susceptible MHC haplotype (Table 22-1, experiment 2).

Experimental Allergic Encephalomyelitis

Experimental allergic encephalomyelitis (EAE), an animal model of the autoimmune demyelinating disease multiple sclerosis (MS), is characterized by central nervous system (CNS) inflammation and demyelination that manifests clinically as a predictable course of ascending paralysis and subsequent remission. EAE can be induced in several rodent species by active immunization with

TABLE 22-1. *Comparison of responses to chick type II collagen in H-2^b and H-2^q mice*

Mouse strain[a]	MHC haplotype	Disease incidence[b]	Mean clinical score	Antibody titer[c]
Experiment 1				
B10.Q	H-2^q	4/7	ND	23.0 ± 7.9 (n = 3)
B6	H-2^b	0/9	—	2.80 ± 0.84 (n = 8)
B6.*lpr*	H-2^b	0/6	—	2.00 ± 0.94 (n = 4)
Control B6.*lpr*[d]	H-2^b	0/5	—	0.30 ± 0.11 (n = 5)
Experiment 2				
B10.Q	H-2^q	2/5 (2,2)	2.0 ± 0	ND
+/+	H-2^q	3/4 (1,2,2)	1.33 ± 0.58	ND
+/*lpr*	H-2^q	8/10 (1,2,2,2,2,2,3,3)	2.13 ± 0.64	ND
lpr/lpr	H-2^q	2/5 (2,2)	2.0 ± 0	ND

MHC, major histocompatibility complex; ND, not determined.

[a] The indicated 8-week-old male mice were injected at the base of the tail (100 μl) with 50 μg of chick type II collagen in complete Freund's adjuvant (CFA) on day 0 and boosted by a similar injection with an additional 50 μg of collagen in incomplete Freund's adjuvant (IFA) on day 21. Animals were monitored up to 3 months for clinical signs of arthritis and graded as follows: 0 = normal; 1 = swollen toe or knuckle; 2 = swollen paw or deformity; 3 = ankylosis. Scoring was done with coded mice so the genotype was not known until the experiments were concluded. Some of the animals were bled on day 29 for determination of antibody titer to type II collagen.

[b] Incidence of animals with swelling and loss of movement in hind feet 21 to 72 days after primary injection. Maximum clinical score for individual mice are shown in parentheses.

[c] Antibody titer to type II collagen determined by ELISA expressed as arbitrary units.

[d] Age- and sex-matched controls that were not injected.

myelin components such as gpMBP or passive transfer of activated, MBP-specific, CD4$^+$ T cells (31,32) of the Th1 but not Th2 subset (33,34) into naive mice. CD8$^+$ T cells are not primary effectors in the initiation or recovery from acute EAE, although they have been implicated as major participants in the resistance to spontaneous relapses (35,36). As with MS, susceptibility to EAE is genetically linked to the MHC locus, rendering some murine strains including B10.PL (H-2^u) susceptible and others such as C57BL/6 (H-2^b) relatively resistant to the induction of EAE (37,38).

To determine the effect of a deficiency in Fas or FasL on the Th1-dependent response to MBP, we initially examined the active induction of EAE in mice carrying the *lpr* or *gld* mutation on the relatively resistant B6 (H-2^b) background and found that the *lpr* and *gld* mutations again could not overcome the MHC-defined limits of

disease in that they did not exacerbate the incidence or severity of EAE in H-2^b mice (39). We then introduced both mutations onto the susceptible B10.PL (H-2^u) background and were surprised to find that defective expression of Fas or FasL dramatically ameliorated clinical signs of actively induced EAE in otherwise susceptible mice (Table 22-2) without affecting the production of MBP-specific Th1 T cells, the development of a Th1-mediated immune response *in vivo* (Fig. 22-1), or the infiltration of inflammatory cells into the CNS (39). Considerably fewer Tunel-positive, apoptotic cells were detected in inflammatory lesions of *lpr* mice when compared to wild-type lesions of similar severity in both the upper and lower spinal cord (data not shown) (39). These data are consistent with the hypothesis that a Fas-mediated lytic interaction necessary for the progression of EAE is reduced in the *lpr* animals and thus

TABLE 22-2. *Effect of the* lpr *and* gld *mutations on experimental allergic encephalomyelitis in H-2ᵘ mice*

Mouse genotype[a]	Mean day of onset of clinical signs of EAE	Mean duration of clinical signs (days)	Incidence of clinical signs[b]	Mean peak clinical score[c,d]	Mean peak disease severity[d,e]
B10.PL	12.2 ± 2.8	9.7 ± 5.1	30/40 (75%)	2.3 ± 1.7	3.0 ± 1.2
+/+	11.5 ± 2.4	10.6 ± 3.6	20/26 (77%)	2.8 ± 1.8	3.6 ± 1.0
+/lpr	11.9 ± 2.6	9.1 ± 4.3	19/29 (66%)	2.1 ± 1.8	3.2 ± 1.2
lpr/lpr	10.7 ± 2.6	3.8 ± 3.1	13/35 (37%)	0.63 ± 0.86	1.50 ± 0.78
gld/gld	12.6 ± 0.9	7.8 ± 2.4	5/24 (21%)	0.33 ± 0.70	1.60 ± 0.55

EAE, experimental allergic encephalomyelitis.

[a] EAE was actively induced in 6- to 8-week old mice backcrossed one, three, or six generations by immunization with 200 μg guinea pig myelin basic protein (gpMBP) in incomplete Freund's adjuvant (IFA) supplemented with 4 mg/ml *M. tuberculosis* (H37RA) via hind footpad or subcutaneous injections on day 0. Control mice were injected with IFA supplemented with *M. tuberculosis*. Pertussis toxin 100 to 200 ng was administered intravenously 24 and 72 hours later. Clinical signs of disease were monitored daily beginning on day 7 and were graded as follows: 0 = normal, 0.5 = partial loss of tail tonicity, 1 = complete loss of tail tonicity, 2 = ataxia, 3 = partial hindlimb paralysis, 4 = full hindlimb paralysis, 5 = moribund. Moribund animals were sacrificed. Scoring was done with coded mice so the genotype was not known until the experiments were concluded. Data were pooled from seven experiments.

[b] Incidence was defined as a clinical score of $\geq$ grade 1. Control mice did not develop disease.

[c] Mean peak clinical score was determined using the maximal clinical score for each mouse of a given genotype. Scores were compared between genotypes by analysis of variance (ANOVA). *Lpr* versus +/+, $p = 6.6 \times 10^{-8}$; versus B10.PL, $p = 1.5 \times 10^{-6}$. *Gld* versus B10.PL, $p = 1.2 \times 10^{-6}$.

[d] Mean peak clinical scores and mean peak disease severity for males versus females were not statistically different.

[e] Mean peak disease severity was calculated using only those mice with clinical signs $\geq$ grade 1. *Lpr* versus +/+, $p = 9.6 \times 10^{-7}$; versus B10.PL, $p = 3.9 \times 10^{-4}$. *Gld* versus B10.PL, $p = 0.02$.

implicated a role for Fas in the pathogenesis of this Th1 cell-mediated disease.

Fas-DEPENDENT BYSTANDER LYSIS

Although it is generally agreed that EAE is autoimmune in nature, the precise mechanism(s) of myelin disruption remain unknown. The MHC-II⁻ oligodendrocyte and its associated myelin have been identified as principal targets of destruction in EAE and MS (40–43); and herein lies the conundrum as to how the CD4⁺ T cells that mediate EAE can induce damage in a disease where the major targets of destruction lack the appropriate MHC-restricting elements. Fas-dependent bystander lysis would provide a mechanism of CD4⁺ T cell mediated killing that is completely independent of the MHC haplotype and, instead, relies on expression of Fas by potential target cells such as oligodendrocytes.

With both Fas-dependent direct and by-stander lysis, an antigen-presenting cell (APC) activates the T cell, inducing expression of FasL, which enables the T cell to lyse its target(s). However, whereas the APC is the Fas⁺ target during direct lysis, during bystander killing a third, Fas⁺ cell is lysed. Figure 22-3 demonstrates some of the salient features of both Fas-dependent direct and bystander lysis using I-Aᵇ-restricted, pigeon cytochrome *c* (PCC)-specific Th1 T cell effectors and H-2ᵇ-expressing macrophages as APCs. We found that macrophage APCs can stimulate wild-type T cells to lyse direct or bystander targets and do so in an effector/target (E/T) and antigen dose-dependent manner. The *gld* T cells lacking functional FasL were unable to lyse any targets, although they did produce cytokines at levels comparable to those seen with wild-type cells (11). Likewise, although Fas-deficient *lpr* macrophages could stimulate T cells for bystander lysis, neither they nor Fas⁻ bystander targets were killed (Fig. 22-3A and data not

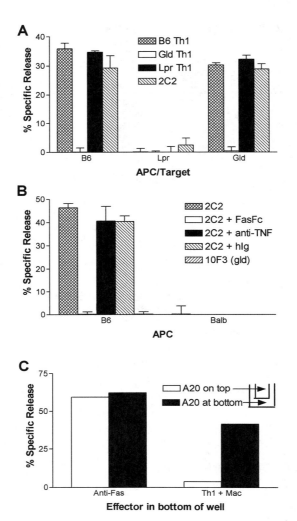

FIG. 22-3. Fas-dependent direct and bystander lysis by antigen-stimulated Th1 cells. **A:** Direct lysis: I-A^b-restricted wild-type (B6) (*cross-hatched bars*), *gld* (*open bars*), and *lpr* (*solid bars*) Th1 cell lines or clones (2C2, *hatched*) were added to wells containing ^{51}Cr-labeled, H-2^b-expressing wild-type (B6) *lpr* or *gld* macrophages and pigeon cytochrome *c* (PCC) 20 μg/ml. After 18 hours supernatants were harvested to determine ^{51}Cr release. Spontaneous release was 18% for B6, *lpr,* and *gld* targets. **B:** Bystander lysis: The I-A^b-restricted Th1 clones 2C2 (wild-type) (*cross-hatched bar*) or 10F3 (*gld*) (*hatched left bar*) were added to wells containing unlabeled B6 (H-2^b) or Balb (H-2^d) macrophages, ^{51}Cr-labeled A20 cells (H-2^d lymphoma), and PCC 20 μg/ml. Cultures were incubated for 18 hours alone or in the presence of Fas-Fc 20 μg/ml (*open bar*), human IgG 20 μg/ml (*hatched right bar*), or anti-TNF 50 μg/ml (*solid bar*). Spontaneous release from the A20 target cells was 31%. **C:** Anti-Fas (Jo2, 1 μg/ml) or I-A^b-restricted Th1 cells plus H-2^b macrophages and PCC 10 μg/ml were added to the lower chamber of Transwells. ^{51}Cr-labeled A20 cells were added to the same chamber (*solid bars*) or the upper chamber (*open bars*) separated 1 mm from the lower chamber by a semipermeable membrane (0.4-μm pores). After 16 hours the membrane was ruptured, and the total contents (1.1 ml) of both chambers were harvested and quantitatively transferred to a test tube. The tube was centrifuged to pellet the cells, and the fraction of ^{51}Cr remaining in the supernatant was determined. Spontaneous release was 30%.

shown). As we have previously shown, by-stander activity is TNF-independent (Fig. 22-3B) and requires close proximity between the T cell, the APC, and the bystander target, as bystander targets were not lysed during co-culture in Transwells (Fig. 22-3C) (11). Furthermore, bystander killing is not MHC-restricted, as MHC-mismatched bystander targets were lysed (Fig. 22-3B,C).

Professional versus Nonprofessional APCs

All the professional APCs we have tested [macrophages, B cell lymphomas, fresh lipo-polysaccharide (LPS)-activated B cells] were extremely efficient at stimulating both Fas-dependent bystander and direct killing. This is in contrast to some "nonprofessional" epi-thelial line APCs, which were unable to stim-ulate bystander lysis, even though they them-selves were killed in a Fas-dependent process while serving as APCs (Fig. 22-4) (11). In an effort to better understand the role of accessory proteins in both direct and by-stander lysis, we have genetically modified the previously described bladder cell line (257CL3) that expresses Fas and MHC-II but lacks most co-stimulatory molecules by transfecting the bladder cells with either ICAM-1 (CD54) or B7-1 (CD80).

In Figure 22-5, these bladder cells were used as APCs to activate I-A^b-restricted, PCC-specific Th1 cell effectors. In a direct killing assay where the bladder cells were also the Fas$^+$, ^{51}Cr-labeled targets, we found that both the intercellular adhesion mole-cule-1 (ICAM-1) and B7-1 transfectants were more efficient than the parental 257CL3 cells at stimulating their own lysis. However, only the B7 transfected cells were able to stimulate the T cells to lyse a third, Fas$^+$ target (EL4-Fas). We believe that ICAM-1 affects direct lysis by augmenting adhesion between the CD4$^+$ T cell and the APC, whereas an increase in FasL expres-sion on T cells following a B7–CD28 interac-tion is likely to be one of the important mech-anisms that APCs transfected with B7-1 use to stimulate bystander lysis (44).

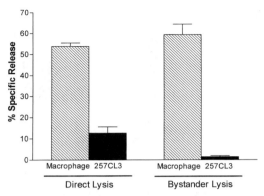

FIG. 22-4. Stimulation of direct and bystander lysis by professional and nonprofessional anti-gen-presenting cells (APCs). Direct lysis: An I-A^b-restricted Th1 cell line was added to wells containing ^{51}Cr-labeled, H-2^b-expressing profes-sional (macrophages) (*hatched bars*) or nonpro-fessional (IFN-γ-pretreated 257CL3) (*solid bars*) APCs/targets and 10 μM pigeon cytochrome *c* (PCC). After 18 hours supernatants were har-vested to determine ^{51}Cr release. Spontaneous release results were 30% (macrophages) and 49% (257CL3). Bystander lysis: The same Th1 cell line was added to wells containing H-2^b-ex-pressing APCs (IFN-γ-pretreated 257CL3 or macrophages), 10 μM PCC, and ^{51}Cr-labeled by-stander targets (EL4 or EL4-Fas, H-2^b) for 18 hours. Spontaneous release was 27% (EL4-Fas) and 39% (EL4).

These experiments suggest that the inter-actions between the T cell and the APC, not the T cell and the target, are critical for stim-ulating any kind of killing in that the target in CD4$^+$ T cell-mediated, Fas-dependent by-stander lysis plays little role in determining specificity beyond expressing Fas on its sur-face. Instead, the APC seems to regulate the ability of CD4$^+$ T cells to mediate bystander killing through its expression of accessory molecules. In contrast, we have found that Fas-dependent bystander lysis mediated by CD8$^+$ T cells is enhanced when the target cell (in contrast to the APC) expresses an adhesion molecule such as ICAM-1 (45). Thus, whereas CD4$^+$ T cells may regularly use the Fas-dependent pathway to kill direct or bystander targets when they are stimu-lated by the proper APCs, CD8$^+$ T cells may

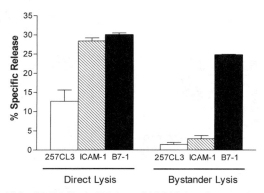

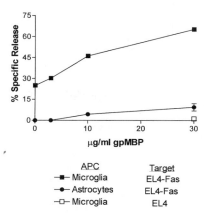

FIG. 22-5. Both B7-1 and ICAM-1 enhance the capacity of 257CL3 cells to stimulate direct lysis, whereas only B7-1 can stimulate Fas-dependent bystander killing. Direct lysis: An I-A^b-restricted Th1 cell line was added to wells containing ^{51}Cr-labeled, H-2^b-expressing 257CL3 (*open bars*), 257CL3-B7 (*solid bars*), or 257CL3-ICAM (*hatched bars*) APCs/targets pretreated with IFN-γ for 48 hours and 10 μM pigeon cytochrome *c* (PCC). After 18 hours supernatants were harvested to determine ^{51}Cr release. Spontaneous release results were 49% (257CL3), 46% (B7-1), and 28% (ICAM-1). Bystander lysis: The same Th1 T cell line was added to wells containing H-2^b-expressing, IFN-γ pretreated APCs (257CL3, 257CL3-B7, or 257CL3-ICAM), 10 μM PCC, and ^{51}Cr-labeled bystander targets (EL4 or EL4-Fas, H-2^b) for 18 hours. Spontaneous release results were 26% (EL4-Fas) and 30% (EL4). Percent specific release of EL4 cells with all APCs was zero.

FIG. 22-6. Microglia, but not astrocytes, can stimulate T cells to lyse Fas$^+$ bystander targets. An I-A^u-restricted T cell line was added to wells containing H-2^u-expressing microglia (*squares*) or astrocyte (*circles*) APCs pretreated with IFN-γ for 5 days, guinea pig myelin basic protein (gpMBP), and ^{51}Cr-labeled, H-2^b-expressing EL4 (*open symbols*) or EL4-Fas (*solid symbols*) bystander targets for 18 hours. Spontaneous release results were 33% (EL4) and 29% (EL4-Fas).

use only a Fas-mediated lytic mechanism under limited conditions in which they receive a signal from both the APC and the target.

Role of Fas-Dependent Bystander Lysis in EAE

The fact that CD4$^+$ T cells determine which targets to kill through interactions with the APC raises the question as to which cells in the CNS would be capable of stimulating CNS-reactive T cells to lyse Fas$^+$ bystander targets. Because both microglia and astrocytes are potential APCs in the CNS (46–49), we have examined the ability of these two cell types to stimulate Fas-dependent bystander lysis *in vitro*. Microglia and astrocytes pretreated with 100 U/ml IFN-γ

expressed MHC-II and ICAM-1, but only microglia expressed B7-1 and rather low levels of Fas (44). When we tested the ability of these IFN-γ pretreated microglia and astrocytes to serve as APCs to activate I-A^u-restricted, MBP-specific T cell effectors to lyse ^{51}Cr-labeled, MHC-mismatched, Fas$^+$ bystander targets, we found that microglia, but not astrocytes, were able to stimulate the T cells to kill the bystander targets (Fig. 22-6).

DISCUSSION

Fas-Dependent Lysis in *In Vivo* Immune Responses

The severe, spontaneous autoimmune syndromes associated with the *lpr* and *gld* mutations clearly demonstrate the importance of Fas and FasL in regulating lymphocyte homeostasis (12). However, the results discussed here demonstrate that these mutations in Fas and FasL neither qualitatively nor quantitatively affect a variety of nominal immune responses involving either Th1 effectors or T-dependent B cell responses. The normal development and affinity maturation of the T-dependent B cell response to the NP hapten (Fig. 22-2) extends earlier work demonstrating a normal idiotypic response to the arsenate hapten (50) and normal germinal center development in response to the NP hapten (17) in *lpr* mice. The lack of a modulation of a CD4$^+$ effector function (i.e., DTH response) extends the observation that the *lpr* allele does not modulate the acute response to lymphocytic choriomeningitis virus, largely a function of CD8$^+$ cells (51). Thus it appears that Fas-dependent lysis does not play a prominent role in regulating acute responses to nominal antigens. The elimination of the antigen, production of negative regulatory cytokines such as IL-10 and transforming growth factor-β (TGF-β), and growth factor withdrawal are probably more important mechanisms for the termination of most normal immune responses. During a more chronic exposure to antigen, such as that encountered in the CD4$^+$ lymphoproliferative disease associated with MAIDS virus infection, Fas becomes an important regulatory molecule limiting the immune response.

These studies have also examined the role of Fas and FasL in immune responses to the autoimmune inducing antigens chick type II collagen and gpMBP. We have demonstrated that the *lpr* mutation does not override the limits placed on effector cell responses by MHC or affect disease on a sensitive haplotype in the CIA model. These mutations do not overcome MHC-defined limits of effector cell function in EAE either, although both mutations dramatically ameliorate clinical signs of EAE on a sensitive haplotype. Nevertheless, it is clear that mutations affecting either protein do accelerate at least some forms of spontaneous autoimmune disease (12), and we have found that the two mutations dramatically exacerbate the course of the chronic CD4$^+$ lymphoproliferative disease associated with MAIDS virus infection (23).

It appears that the effect of the *lpr* and *gld*

mutations on a given autoimmune disease depends on the effector mechanism(s) involved in the pathogenesis of the disease. Thus, Fas does not seem to play a primary role in regulating CIA, a disease in which B cells and CD8$^+$ T cells are the likely effectors. This is consistent with our data indicating a nominal role for Fas in T-dependent B cell responses and the fact that Fas-mediated death is not the only, or primary, lytic mechanism in the arsenal of a CD8$^+$ cytolytic cell. In contrast, CD4$^+$ T cells of the Th1 subset are the primary effector cells in EAE; and in this system we have found that Fas and FasL enhance progression of the acute phase of disease. This is in accord with studies demonstrating that a Fas-dependent lytic mechanism is especially important in CD4$^+$ Th1 cells (6,7). A similar pathogenic role for Fas-dependent lysis has been described during the initiation of diabetes, a T cell-mediated disease, in nonobese diabetic (NOD) mice (52,53). Thus the role of Fas may be a function of both the duration of exposure to the eliciting antigen(s) and the type of effector cells elicited. This model has important therapeutic implications, as it may be possible to manipulate chronic regulatory pathways without creating a situation of general immunocompromise.

FasL and Immune Privilege in the CNS

There has been interest in the potential role of FasL as a mechanism of enforcing immune privilege, as suggested by the experiments in testes and corneal epithelium (1,2). Here we have determined that defective expression of FasL or its receptor does not affect the ability of potentially autoreactive cells to infiltrate the CNS, nor does it exacerbate the incidence or severity of the Th1 response to the autoimmune inducing antigen gpMBP. Therefore it appears that FasL is not an instrumental component of immune privilege, in the most strict definition of the term, in the CNS. However, using the adoptive transfer model of EAE we found that FasL induced on CNS cells by inflammation may play a role in recovery from the primary insult by limiting the expansion of activated T cell populations in the CNS (54).

Fas-Dependent Bystander Lysis in EAE

We (39) and others (55,56) have demonstrated that the *lpr* and *gld* mutations ameliorate the clinical symptoms of myelin basic protein or myelin oligodendrocyte glycoprotein (MOG)-induced EAE in B10.PL or C57BL/6 mice, respectively. We have found that both the *lpr* and *gld* mutations dramatically ameliorate clinical signs of EAE without affecting the development of a Th1 response or the level of inflammatory cell infiltration into the CNS. The inflammatory cell types entering the CNS were not altered in *lpr* mice either (unpublished observation). However, the extent of apoptotic cell death was diminished in lesions from *lpr* animals. These data suggest that whereas the induction of disease-producing elements is normal, severe damage in the CNS is limited in the absence of Fas or FasL, which implicates a role for an interaction between Fas expressed on CNS cells with FasL in the pathogenesis of EAE.

If the death of Fas[+] targets in the CNS contributes to the pathogenesis of EAE; and if the effectors of EAE are indeed CD4[+] T cells, lytic function may rely on Fas-dependent bystander lysis, a process we previously demonstrated can occur (11). Through bystander lysis, any Fas[+] cells including oligodendrocytes could serve as targets for FasL[+] effector T lymphocytes activated by nearby MHC-II-expressing APCs. We found that microglia, but not astrocytes, were able to stimulate MBP-specific T cells to kill Fas[+] bystander targets. Presumably, *lpr* mice are lacking these Fas[+] bystander targets and therefore are protected from developing severe clinical signs of EAE.

Although Fas mRNA is not expressed in normal CNS tissue, its expression may be induced during inflammation by TNF-α or interferon-γ (IFN-γ), cytokines found in EAE (57) and MS (58) lesions and known to upregulate Fas expression (59) and sensi-

tivity to Fas agonists (60). Indeed, recent studies indicate that Fas expression is induced on oligodendrocytes in MS lesions, whereas microglial cells in these lesions express substantial amounts of FasL (61). Taken together with the results we have reported here, it appears that Fas and its ligand are effector molecules that dramatically enhance the progression of EAE. Fas-mediated bystander lysis would be a novel mechanism of destruction of MHC-II[−] oligodendrocytes in a CD4[+] T cell-mediated disease and could provide important clues to understanding the mechanism of autoimmune demyelination.

Acknowledgments

The authors are grateful to Julie Ritchey for technical assistance with the delayed-type hypersensitivity experiments and Ruduan Wang for her contributions in the bystander lysis experiments. This work was supported in part by grants from the NCI (CA28533) and the MS Society (RG2835).

REFERENCES

1. Bellgrau D, Gold D, Selawry H, Moore J, Franzusoff A, Duke RC. A role for CD95 ligand in preventing graft rejection [see comments]. *Nature* 1995;377: 630–632.
2. Griffith TS, Brunner T, Fletcher SM, Green DR, Ferguson TA. Fas ligand-induced apoptosis as a mechanism of immune privilege [see comments]. *Science* 1995;270:1189–1192.
3. Russell JH. Activation-induced death of mature T cells in the regulation of immune responses. *Curr Opin Immunol* 1995;7:382–388.
4. Nagata S, Golstein P. The Fas death factor. *Science* 1995;267:1449–1456.
5. Rouvier E, Luciani MF, Golstein P. Fas involvement in Ca^{2+}-independent T cell-mediated cytotoxicity. *J Exp Med* 1993;177:195–200.
6. Stalder T, Hahn S, Erb P. Fas antigen is the major target molecule for CD4[+] T cell-mediated cytotoxicity. *J Immunol* 1994;152:1127–1133.
7. Ju ST, Cui H, Panka DJ, Ettinger R, Marshak-Rothstein A. Participation of target Fas protein in apoptosis pathway induced by CD4[+] Th1 and CD8[+] cytotoxic T cells. *Proc Natl Acad Sci USA* 1994;91:4185–4189.
8. Rathmell JC, Cooke MP, Ho WY, et al. CD95 (Fas)-dependent elimination of self-reactive B cells upon

interaction with CD4$^+$ T cells. *Nature* 1995;376: 181–184.

9. Rathmell JC, Townsend SE, Xu JC, Flavell RA, Goodnow CC. Expansion or elimination of B cells in vivo: dual roles for CD40$^-$ and Fas (CD95)-ligands modulated by the B cell antigen receptor. *Cell* 1996;87:319–329.

10. Henkart MP, Henkart PA. Lymphocyte mediated cytolysis as a secretory phenomenon. *Adv Exp Med Biol* 1982;146:227–247.

11. Wang R, Rogers AM, Ratliff TL, Russell JH. CD95-dependent bystander lysis caused by CD4$^+$ T helper 1 effectors. *J Immunol* 1996;157:2961–2968.

12. Cohen PL, Eisenberg RA. *Lpr and gld:* single gene models of systemic autoimmunity and lymphoproliferative disease. *Annu Rev Immunol* 1991;9: 243–269.

13. Watanabe-Fukunaga R, Brannan CI, Copeland NG, Jenkins NA, Nagata S. Lymphoproliferation disorder in mice explained by defects in Fas antigen that mediates apoptosis. *Nature* 1992;356:314–317.

14. Takahashi T, Tanaka M, Brannan CI, et al. Generalized lymphoproliferative disease in mice, caused by a point mutation in the Fas ligand. *Cell* 1994;76: 969–976.

15. Sobel ES, Katagiri T, Katagiri K, Morris SC, Cohen PL, Eisenberg RA. An intrinsic B cell defect is required for the production of autoantibodies in the *lpr* model of murine systemic autoimmunity. *J Exp Med* 1991;173:1441–1449.

16. Sobel ES, Cohen PL, Eisenberg RA. *lpr* T cells are necessary for autoantibody production in lpr mice. *J Immunol* 1993;150:4160–4167.

17. Smith KG, Nossal GJ, Tarlinton DM. FAS is highly expressed in the germinal center but is not required for regulation of the B-cell response to antigen. *Proc Natl Acad Sci USA* 1995;92:11628–11632.

18. Yetter RA, Buller RM, Lee JS, et al. CD4$^+$ T cells are required for development of a murine retrovirus-induced immunodeficiency syndrome (MAIDS). *J Exp Med* 1988;168:623–635.

19. Mosier DE, Yetter RA, Morse HCd. Functional T lymphocytes are required for a murine retrovirus-induced immunodeficiency disease (MAIDS). *J Exp Med* 1987;165:1737–1742.

20. Cerny A, Hugin AW, Hardy RR, et al. B cells are required for induction of T cell abnormalities in a murine retrovirus-induced immunodeficiency syndrome. *J Exp Med* 1990;171:315–320.

21. Selvey LA, Morse HC, Granger LG, Hodes RJ. Preferential expansion and activation of V beta 5$^+$ CD4$^+$ T cells in murine acquired immunodeficiency syndrome. *J Immunol* 1993;151:1712–1722.

22. Hugin AW, Vacchio MS, Morse HC. A virus-encoded "superantigen" in a retrovirus-induced immunodeficiency syndrome of mice. *Science* 1991; 252:424–427.

23. Kanagawa O, Vaupel BA, Korsmeyer SJ, Russell JH. Apoptotic death of lymphocytes in murine acquired immunodeficiency syndrome: involvement of Fas-Fas ligand interaction. *Eur J Immunol* 1995;25:2421–2427.

24. van Parijs L, Ibraghimov A, Abbas AK. The roles of costimulation and Fas in T cell apoptosis and peripheral tolerance. *Immunity* 1996;4:321–328.

25. Holmdahl R, Jansson L, Gullberg D, Rubin K, Forsberg PO, Klareskog L. Incidence of arthritis and autoreactivity of anti-collagen antibodies after immunization of DBA/1 mice with heterologous and autologous collagen II. *Clin Exp Immunol* 1985; 62:639–646.

26. Seki N, Sudo Y, Mizuhara H, et al. Type II collagen-induced murine arthritis: induction of arthritis depends on antigen-presenting cell function as well as susceptibility of host to an anticollagen immune response. *J Immunol* 1992;148:3093–3099.

27. Tada Y, Ho A, Koh DR, Mak TW. Collagen-induced arthritis in CD4$^-$ or CD8-deficient mice: CD8$^+$ T cells play a role in initiation and regulate recovery phase of collagen-induced arthritis. *J Immunol* 1996;156:4520–4526.

28. Wooley PH, Luthra HS, Stuart JM, David CS. Type II collagen-induced arthritis in mice. I. Major histocompatibility complex (I region) linkage and antibody correlates. *J Exp Med* 1981;154:688–700.

29. Holmdahl R, Klareskog L, Andersson M, Hansen C. High antibody response to autologous type II collagen is restricted to H-2q. *Immunogenetics* 1986;24:84–89.

30. Holmdahl R, Jansson L, Andersson M, Larsson E. Immunogenetics of type II collagen autoimmunity and susceptibility to collagen arthritis. *Immunology* 1988;65:305–310.

31. Panitch HS, McFarlin DE. Experimental allergic encephalomyelitis: enhancement of cell-mediated transfer by concanavalin A. *J Immunol* 1977;119: 1134–1137.

32. Mokhtarian F, McFarlin DE, Raine CS. Adoptive transfer of myelin basic protein-sensitized T cells produces chronic relapsing demyelinating disease in mice. *Nature* 1984;309:356–358.

33. Ando DG, Clayton J, Kono D, Urban JL, Sercarz EE. Encephalitogenic T cells in the B10.PL model of experimental allergic encephalomyelitis (EAE) are of the Th-1 lymphokine subtype. *Cell Immunol* 1989;124:132–143.

34. Baron JL, Madri JA, Ruddle NH, Hashim G, Janeway CA Jr. Surface expression of alpha 4 integrin by CD4 T cells is required for their entry into brain parenchyma. *J Exp Med* 1993;177:57–68.

35. Jiang H, Zhang SI, Pernis B. Role of CD8$^+$ T cells in murine experimental allergic encephalomyelitis. *Science* 1992;256:1213–1215.

36. Koh DR, Fung-Leung WP, Ho A, Gray D, Acha-Orbea H, Mak TW. Less mortality but more relapses in experimental allergic encephalomyelitis in CD8$^{-/-}$ mice. *Science* 1992;256:1210–1213.

37. Zamvil SS, Steinman L. The T lymphocyte in experimental allergic encephalomyelitis. *Annu Rev Immunol* 1990;8:579–621.

38. Fritz RB, Skeen MJ, Chou CH, Garcia M, Egorov IK. Major histocompatibility complex-linked control of the murine immune response to myelin basic protein. *J Immunol* 1985;134:2328–2332.

39. Sabelko KA, Kelly KA, Nahm MH, Cross AH, Russell JH. Fas and Fas ligand enhance the pathogenesis of experimental allergic encephalomyelitis, but are not essential for immune privilege in the central nervous system. *J Immunol* 1997;159:3096–3099.

40. Prineas JW. The *Neuropathology of Multiple Sclerosis*. Amsterdam, Elsevier Science, 1985.
41. Raine CS. *Experimental Allergic Encephalomyelitis and Experimental Allergic Neuritis*. Amsterdam, Elsevier Science, 1985.
42. Raine CS. The Norton lecture: a review of the oligodendrocyte in the multiple sclerosis lesion. *J Neuroimmunol* 1997;77:135–152.
43. Raine CS. Biology of disease: analysis of autoimmune demyelination: its impact upon multiple sclerosis. *Lab Invest* 1984;50:608–635.
44. Thilenius ARB, Sabelko-Downes KA, Russell JH. The role of the antigen presenting cell in Fas-mediated direct and bystander killing: potential *in vivo* function of Fas in experimental allergic encephalomyelitis. *J Immunol* 1998;162:643–650.
45. Rogers AM, Thilenius AR, Russell JH. Cyclosporine-insensitive partial signaling and multiple roles of Ca^{2+} in Fas ligand-induced lysis. *J Immunol* 1997;159:3140–3147.
46. Williams K Jr, Ulvestad E, Cragg L, Blain M, Antel JP. Induction of primary T cell responses by human glial cells. *J Neurosci Res* 1993;36:382–390.
47. Rott O, Tontsch U, Fleischer B. Dissociation of antigen-presenting capacity of astrocytes for peptide-antigens versus superantigens. *J Immunol* 1993;150:87–95.
48. Nikcevich KM, Gordon KB, Tan L, et al. IFN-gamma-activated primary murine astrocytes express B7 costimulatory molecules and prime naive antigen-specific T cells. *J Immunol* 1997;158:614–621.
49. Dhib-Jalbut S, Gogate N, Jiang H, Eisenberg H, Bergey G. Human microglia activate lymphoproliferative responses to recall viral antigens. *J Neuroimmunol* 1996;65:67–73.
50. Very DL Jr, Panka DJ, Weissman D, Wysocki L, Manser T, Marshak-Rothstein A. Lack of connectivity between the induced and autoimmune repertoires of *lpr/lpr* mice. *Immunology* 1993;80:518–526.
51. Razvi ES, Jiang Z, Woda BA, Welsh RM. Lymphocyte apoptosis during the silencing of the immune response to acute viral infections in normal, *lpr*, and Bcl-2-transgenic mice. *Am J Pathol* 1995;147:79–91.
52. Itoh N, Imagawa A, Hanafusa T, et al. Requirement of Fas for the development of autoimmune diabetes in nonobese diabetic mice. *J Exp Med* 1997;186:613–618.
53. Chervonsky AV, Wang Y, Wong FS, et al. The role of Fas in autoimmune diabetes. *Cell* 1997;89:17–24.
54. Sabelko-Downes KA, Cross AH, Russell JH. Dual role for Fas ligand in the initiation of and recovery from experimental allergic encephalomyelitis. *J Exp Med* 1999;189:1195–1205.
55. Waldner H, Sobel RA, Howard E, Kuchroo VK. Fas- and FasL-deficient mice are resistant to induction of autoimmune encephalomyelitis. *J Immunol* 1997;159:3100–3103.
56. Malipiero U, Frei K, Spanaus KS, et al. Myelin oligodendrocyte glycoprotein-induced autoimmune encephalomyelitis is chronic/relapsing in perforin knockout mice, but monophasic in Fas- and Fas ligand-deficient *lpr* and *gld* mice. *Eur J Immunol* 1997;27:3151–3160.
57. Olsson T. Critical influences of the cytokine orchestration on the outcome of myelin antigen-specific T-cell autoimmunity in experimental autoimmune encephalomyelitis and multiple sclerosis. *Immunol Rev* 1995;144:245–268.
58. Cannella B, Raine CS. The adhesion molecule and cytokine profile of multiple sclerosis lesions [see comments]. *Ann Neurol* 1995;37:424–435.
59. Moller P, Koretz K, Leithauser F, et al. Expression of APO-1 (CD95), a member of the NGF/TNF receptor superfamily, in normal and neoplastic colon epithelium. *Int J Cancer* 1994;57:371–377.
60. Yonehara S, Ishii A, Yonehara M. A cell-killing monoclonal antibody (anti-Fas) to a cell surface antigen co-downregulated with the receptor of tumor necrosis factor. *J Exp Med* 1989;169:1747–1756.
61. Dsouza SD, Bonetti B, Balasingam V, et al. Multiple sclerosis-Fas signaling in oligodendrocyte cell death. *J Exp Med* 1996;184:2361–2370.

Cytotoxic Cells: Basic Mechanisms and Medical Applications, edited by Michail V. Sitkovsky and Pierre A. Henkart. Lippincott Williams & Wilkins, Philadelphia © 2000.

Chapter 23
Helping Killers

John Paul Ridge, Francesca Di Rosa, and Polly Matzinger

Ghost Lab, Laboratory of Cellular and Molecular Immunology, National Institute of Allergy and Infectious Diseases, National Institutes of Health, Bethesda, Maryland 20892, USA

Faced with the near impossibility of bringing together two rare migratory cells that cannot detect each other's presence (the T-helper and the T-killer) the immune system builds a link using a dendritic cell. Dendritic cells are thought to exist in two states: resting (or immature) and activated (mature). We have found a third state (superactivated). In the activated state a dendritic cell can present antigen and activate T-helper cells but not T killers. However, a T helper can induce the dendritic cell to become superactivated and gain the ability to stimulate a killer.

HISTORY

The mature, circulating, antigen-specific cells of the immune system face a challenge that does not trouble most other cells of the body. They must find each other, and they must do it often and quickly each time there is need of an immune response. The problem is compounded by the rarity of the communicating partners, as only about 1 in 10^5 or 10^6 circulating lymphocytes can react to any particular antigen. Thus a rare T helper cell specific for a particular pathogen needs to find an equally rare B cell specific for the same antigen. That these encounters occur at all is due to the circulation patterns of these cells in lymph nodes and other specialized organs, as well as to the B cell's ability to act as an antigen-presenting cell (APC) and attract the appropriate helper by creating a surface display of major histocompatibility complex class II (MHC-II) molecules loaded with peptides from the antigen the B cell has captured (1,2). Once a B cell has attracted the right T-helper cell, it uses a family of receptor–ligand pairs, such as B7, CD40, and various cytokine receptors, to stimulate the T cell and receive stimuli in turn (3).

The T killer cells cannot do this; and if the two-cell exchange between rare T and B cells seems challenging enough, the problem is far worse for communication between T-helpers and T-killer cells, where the interaction requires a third cell, the APC, which brings the two together by displaying antigens to both (4,5). The problem is twofold. First there is the challenge of bringing together three rare, circulating cells. Second, because T-killers do not express the sorts of co-stimulatory molecules expressed by B cells and APCs (and, in mice, do not express MHC-II molecules with which to present antigen to helper T cells) there is the question of how help is stimulated and delivered.

Keene and Forman (4) suggested that the presenting cell has a rather passive relationship with the killer, and that, like a B cell, it functions mainly to stimulate the helper cell, which then secretes cytokines necessary for the growth of the neighboring killer. For several reasons we do not find this picture completely satisfying. First, there is no guarantee that a rare T-helper and an equally rare T-killer should find the same APC at the same time. Because killers recognizing antigen become tolerant if there is no help available (4,6–9), many potentially useful killers would be rendered useless by the lack of immediate help. Second, the T-helper must wastefully secrete its cytokines into an environment that may contain no killers to receive them. Third, killer responses to certain viruses are unimpaired by the absence of helper cells (10–14), suggesting that the immune system has found a way to circumvent the need for help in some situations. The three-cell interaction above offers no explanation for the existence of these helper-independent killer responses.

A decade ago,[1] Lafferty and his colleagues suggested the alternative view that help for cytotoxic lymphocytes (CTLs) may be routed through the APC rather than supplied directly (15). They suggested that the antigen-specific T-helper stimulates the APC, rather than the killer, and that the APC now becomes able to activate the CD8 killer cell directly. In this way, rare antigen-specific T-helpers would be able to make up for their scarcity by inducing the differentiation of several APCs and thus assist many CTL precursors without needing to see the antigen at precisely the same time. In addition, helper-independent killer responses to certain viruses might be explained if an infected APC responds to intracellular viral signals by undergoing superactivation.

In the study reported here, we set out to determine if help for killers is delivered directly or through the APC and found that CD4$^+$ T-helpers can indeed route their activity through dendritic cells, the best professional (16,17) APCs. We found that enriched and activated dendritic cells cannot activate killers, though they can present antigen and activate CD4$^+$ T-helpers to proliferate and produce cytokines. After an interaction with

a helper T cell, antibodies to the surface molecule CD40, or a virus infection, they can differentiate into a second, superactivated state in which they are able to stimulate killers in the absence of any further need for T help.

EXPERIMENTAL SYSTEM

Helper Dependence of Killer CD8 Cells

We chose to study the response to the male antigen H-Y for several reasons. First, unlike killers to many viruses (10–14), killers of H-Y have long been known to be dependent on T help (7,18,19). Second, there are few, if any, environmental antigens that cross react with H-Y (20); and third, T cells from normal virgin female mice do not respond to H-Y *in vitro* unless they have first been primed *in vivo* (21), allowing us to differentiate easily between primary and secondary responses.

Figure 23-1 illustrates the helper dependence of the memory CD8 T killer response and shows that T help can be delivered by soluble factors. Normal female C57BL/6 (B6) mice, primed *in vivo* with an injection of male spleen cells, were able to generate good killer responses against male spleen stimulators *in vitro* (Fig. 23-1a). The response disappeared if we depleted CD4 helpers from the responding populations just before the *in vitro* culture (Fig. 23-1b) and reappeared with the addition of interleukin-2 (IL-2)-containing supernatant (Fig. 23-1c). These data document the helper dependence of the memory anti-H-Y response and lend some support to Keene and Forman's view that help can be delivered by soluble factors (4).

Stimulatory Capacity of Activated Dendritic Cells

Under normal *in vivo* conditions, dendritic cells residing in tissues are in a resting state (sometimes called "immature") wherein they express very low surface MHC-II, CD40, and the B7 co-stimulatory molecules.

---

[1]In 1992 we also suggested this (7). Having not seen Lafferty's work we did not refer to it in earlier papers. With apologies we now remedy this oversight.

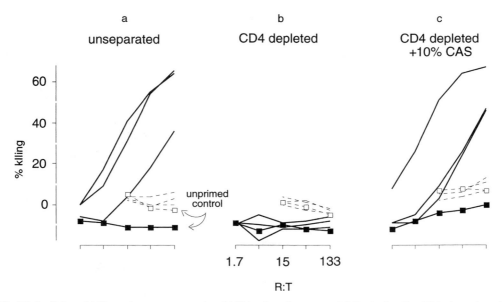

FIG. 23-1. Primed killers do not respond to H-Y in the absence of CD4 help. C57Bl/6 female mice were primed *in vivo* with an injection of 2 × 10⁶ male spleen cells (*lines with no symbols*) or left unprimed (*squares*). Two weeks later the spleens were harvested, depleted (**b, c**) or not (**a**) of CD4 T cells, and then stimulated *in vitro* with male spleen cells without (**a, b**) or with (**c**) 10% Con A supernatant (CAS) containing IL-2. The cultures were tested for their ability to kill male targets (*solid lines*) and female targets (*dashed lines*) 6 days later.

In this state they are unable to act as efficient APCs for any T cells. The process of isolating and culturing them overnight in IL-4 and granulocyte/macrophage colony-stimulating factor (GM-CSF), however, activates them to upregulate these molecules and become powerful APCs for T-helper cells.

There have been some hints that enriched, activated dendritic cells might be able to stimulate CD8 T-killers under conditions where help is minimal (22). For example, newborn female mice, which have only a minute number of anti-male T cells, and bm12 mice, which carry a mutated MHC-II molecule and are consequently deficient in H-Y-specific T-helpers, cannot be primed against H-Y with an injection of male spleen cells; but both types of mice respond quite well when primed with enriched, activated dendritic cells (22,23). It turns out, however, that minimal help is different from no help at all. Figure 23-2 shows that enriched and activated dendritic cells were unable to stimulate memory CD8 killers when CD4 helper cells were completely removed (Fig. 23-2b) and

that the response was restored if we cultured the dendritic cells overnight with a small number of cells from Marilyn, a CD4⁺, H-Y-specific, T-helper-1 (Th1) cell clone (2c). Thus a small number of helpers can go a long way, but without them the dendritic cells are unable to stimulate CD8 memory cells against H-Y.

Help Delivered Through the APC

Our next step was to search for the mechanism by which T-helper cells deliver help. Specificlly, we asked if the helper cells interacted with the dendritic cells to enhance their ability to stimulate a CD8 killer. Taking a hint from T–B interactions, we looked at MHC-II and CD40 molecules because cross-linking antibodies to CD40 have been shown to stimulate B cells to proliferate (24) and enhance the ability of dendritic cells to present antigen and stimulate T-helper cells (25). We found that antibodies to MHC-I or MHC-II had no effect, whereas antibodies to CD40 were able to subsitute for T-helper

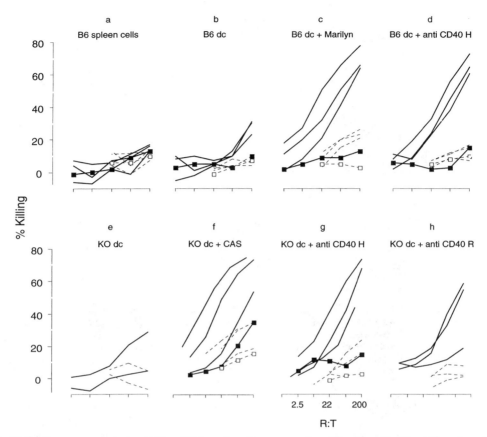

FIG. 23-2. Four ways to help a killer. B6 female mice were primed *in vivo* with 3×10^6 male spleen cells (*lines with no symbols*) or untreated (*squares*). Two weeks later spleens were taken and depleted of CD4 cells, then stimulated with male stimulators of various sorts: B6 spleen cells (**a**); B6 dendritic cells (*dc*) (**b**); B6 dendritic cells incubated with Marilyn, a CD4 Th1 clone specific for H-Y (**c**); B6 dendritic cells treated overnight with the Hamster mAb HM40-3 to crosslink CD40 (**d**); MHC-II KO dc (**e**); KO dc with 10% Con A supernatant (**f**); KO dc crosslinked with the hamster anti-CD40 antibody HM40-3 (**g**); and KO dc crosslinked with the rat anti-CD40 mAb 3/23 (**h**). Six days later these cultures were tested for their ability to kill male (*solid lines*) and female (*dashed lines*) targets. In panels **f–h,** some lines are shifted. The highest R/T is 100:1 rather than 200:1 because of a shortage of responder cells.

cells. Figure 23-2 shows that an enriched population of dendritic cells, stimulated overnight with cross-linking antibodies to CD40, gained the ability to stimulate an anti-H-Y response (Fig. 23-2d).

No CD4-depleting regimen is perfect. Therefore to exclude the possibility that our anti-CD40-treated dendritic cells were simply stimulating IL-2 production from contaminating memory CD4 helper T-cells, we

tested the response using dendritic cells from mutant MHC-II knockout mice (KO), which have no MHC-II and cannot therefore stimulate CD4 helper cells. Figure 23-2e shows that enriched and activated KO dendritic cells, like their unmutated cousins, cannot stimulate killer responses from CD4-depleted memory populations; and that it is not due to the lack of the H-Y antigen because the response can be restored by the addition of an IL-2-containing supernatant (Fig. 23-2f). Nevertheless, though the absence of MHC-II molecules prevents these KO dendritic cells from displaying antigen to any contaminating T-helper cells, they can be activated by overnight treatment with either of two anti-CD40 antibodies to become excellent stimulators of a killing response (Fig. 23-2g,h). We call the DCs that have been driven into this CD40-induced state "superactivated."

Thus the requirement for help can be bypassed in two ways: by adding supernatants containing factors (which may have their effect on the dendritic cells or the CD8 cell) or by superactivating the dendritic cells through CD40, the molecule most likely to be stimulated by CD4$^+$ T-helpers. After such stimulation, the super-activated dendritic cells themselves gain the ability to activate CD8 killers without the need for any further interaction with a helper T cell.

Stimulation by a T-Helper Independent Antigen

There are several viruses known to elicit killer responses in the absence of help. For example, MHC-II KO or CD4-depleted mice make undiminished responses to Sendai virus and diminished but still potent responses to lymphocytic choriomeningitis and influenza virus. We reasoned (7,15) that these viruses might infect dendritic cells and induce a change in differentiation state similar to that induced by T-helper cells. To test this notion, we infected enriched male MHC-II KO dendritic cells with influenza and used them to stimulate an anti-H-Y killing response from primed, CD4-depleted, B6 spleen cells. Figure 23-3 shows that the infected MHC-II KO male dendritic cells (Fig. 23-3e) were nearly as potent as those stimulated with anti-CD40 (Fig. 23-3d) in their ability to stimulate the killers.

Figure 23-4 is a summary of the responses from 102 tests, showing the range of the normal, CD4 depleted, and reconstituted responses. Although there is a certain amount

of variation, it is clear that memory CD8 T-killers can be stimulated *in vitro* by dendritic cells that have been superactivated by stimulation with CD4 T-helpers, treatment with anti-CD40, or virus infection. Thus a rare antigen-specific helper T cell need not communicate directly with the responding killers. It can delegate its function by superactivating a dendritic cell.

The Co-stimulatory Molecules Involved

The superactivated state is not characterized by any obvious surface changes. CD40 modulation of B cells (24) or resting dendritic cells grown *in vitro* from stem cells (26), as well as viral infection of unseparated spleen cells (27), leads to increased expression of the B7 surface molecules involved in co-stimulation of T-helper cells. By fluorescence-activated cell sorter (FACS) analysis, however, our spleen-derived dendritic cells are already activated by the enrichment procedure and express high levels of both B7.1 and B7.2 that do not increase upon CD40 modulation. Although B7.1 and B7.2 levels do not change when dendritic cells move from the activated to the superactivated state, we found that these co-stimulatory molecules were nevertheless important in CTL stimulation. Recombinant mouse CTLA-4-Ig (a soluble form of a receptor for these two molecules) blocked stimulation of unseparated B6 spleen cells by superactivated B6 dendritic cells (Fig. 23-5, top, a culture where both helpers and killers can respond to the dendritic cells) as well as the stimulation of CD4-depleted spleen cells stimulated with modulated MHC-II KO dendritic cells (where the killers are stimulated directly) (Fig. 23-5, bottom). Though the human form of CTLA4-Ig has been shown to block the proliferation of mouse CD4 T cells (28) it did not block the stimulation of mouse CD8 T cells. The nonactivating control antibody Ly5.2 (Rat IgG2a) does not block and, interestingly, neither antibodies to B7.1 or B7.2 were able to block alone, even at very high doses, whereas the two together

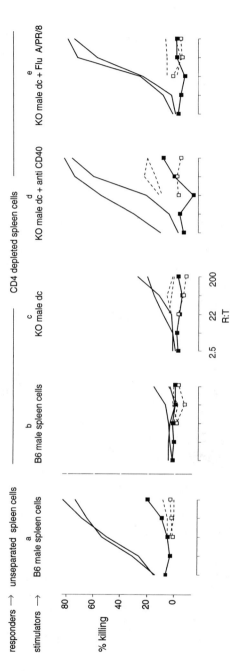

FIG. 23-3. Influenza-infected dendritic cells are superactivated and can stimulate killers in the absence of help. B6 female mice were primed *in vivo* with an injection of male spleen cells or left unprimed (*squares*). Two weeks later their spleens were harvested, depleted (**b–e**); or not (**a**); of CD4 cells, and incubated with irradiated B6 male spleen cells (**a, b**); MHC-II KO dc (**c**); II-KO dc treated with anti-CD40 antibodies (**d**); II-KO dc infected with influenza A/PR/8 (**e**). After 6 days in culture, killing was tested on male (*solid lines*) and female (*dashed lines*) targets.

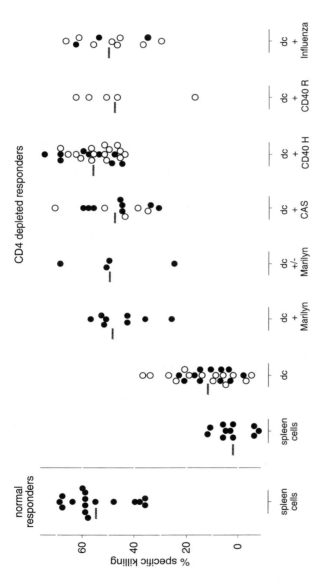

FIG. 23-4. Memory killers can be stimulated *in vitro* by superactivated dendritic cells. Spleen cells from primed female B6 mice were depleted or not of CD4 cells and then stimulated *in vitro* with various normal (*filled circles*) or MHC-II KO (*open circles*) male cell preparations: male spleen or dendritic cells, dendritic cells incubated overnight with Marilyn (a CD4 T cell clone specific for H-Y), dendritic cells + 10% Con A supernatant (as a source of helper factors), dendritic cells crosslinked with the hamster anti-CD40 antibody HM40-3 or the rat anti-CD40 antibody 3/23, dendritic cells infected with influenza A/PR/8. All these cultures were tested for H-Y killing at day 6. Each point represents the activity at a responder/target ratio at which killing from control mice drops off the plateau. Background killing on female targets is subtracted (it was never more than 10% of the killing on male targets). *Horizontal lines* are the group average.

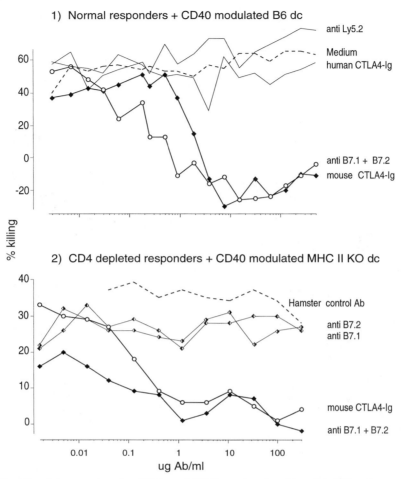

FIG. 23-5. Co-stimulatory molecules B7.1 and B7.2 are involved in stimulation by superactivated dendritic cells. 1×10^5 spleen cells per well from primed B6 (experiment 1) or from CD4 depleted primed B6 responders (experiment 2) were set up in a 96-well format with 5×10^4 superactivated male B6 dendritic cells (treated with anti-CD40 antibody [*Ab*]). Blocking antibodies were titrated into the wells at the concentrations shown, in twofold dilutions starting from 500 (exp. 1) or 300 (exp. 2) μg/ml. After 6 days labeled male targets were added and killing assayed.

blocked very well, suggesting that T-killers may be able to use either of the two co-stimulatory molecules interchangeably. These results show that although, the co-stimulatory molecules involved in the activation of T-helper cells are not sufficient for the stimulation of killers they are nevertheless necessary. They also suggest that human and mouse CTLA-4 may have species-specific components and should not be used interchangeably.

INVESTIGATING THE ABILITY OF CYTOKINES TO CONDITION DENDRITIC CELLS

As stated by Lanzavecchia (29), T-helper cells and inflammatory stimuli induce dendritic cells to produce IL-12 and upregulate the co-stimulatory molecules, which are known to be necessary for the activation of T-helper cells. It has been shown that inflammatory cytokines such as tumor necrosis factor-α (TNF-α), alone or in combination with interferon-α (IFN-α), induce the maturation of immature dendritic cells into mature cells expressing higher levels of co-stimulatory molecules that can functionally activate T cell clones to a greater degree than immature dendritic cells (25). We therefore investigated the effect of these inflammatory cytokines on the MHC-II KO dendritic cells used in our system. By the end of our enrichment procedure the dendritic cells we harvest from the spleens of mice are quite activated and express high levels of the co-stimulatory molecules CD40, B7.1, and B7.2, which do not change significantly after "superactivation" by the crosslinking of CD40

(Fig. 23-6). We therefore asked what effect the overnight incubation of the dendritic cells with inflammatory cytokines would have. We found that the interferons were somewhat able to upregulate CD40, B7.1, and B7.2, whereas the potent cytokine TNF-α had a minor effect only on B7.2. Though the changes in co-stimulatory molecules were small, they nevertheless led us to determine whether a functional change could also be induced by these inflammatory cytokines. In Figure 23-7 we stimulated CD4 T cell-depleted spleen cells from H-Y primed female mice with male spleen cells, or with MHC-II KO male dendritic cells (DCs) that had been treated overnight with anti-CD40, IFN-α, IFN-γ, and TNF-α. The only effective treatment was the crosslinking of CD40 molecules on the cell surface. Hence the slight changes induced by the cytokines did not correlate with the ability to stimulate CD8

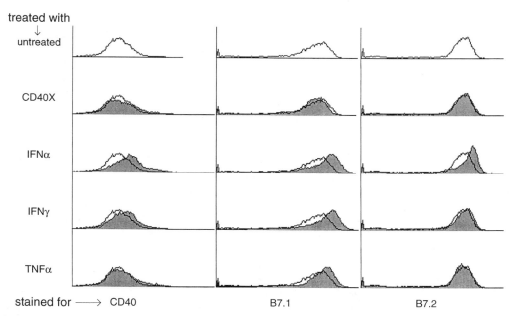

FIG. 23-6. Inflammatory cytokines cause a small amount of upregulation of co-stimulatory molecules. Dendritic cells were prepared and left untreated, CD40 crosslinked, or incubated overnight with 10,000 units of recombinant mouse IFN-α (Gibco/BRL), 120 ng/ml recombinant mouse IFN-γ (Pharmingen), or 10 pg/ml recombinant mouse TNF-α (Pharmingen). Cells were harvested the following morning, and some cells were used as *in vitro* stimulators and the remainder were analyzed by FACS. FACS profiles of the untreated dendritic cells (*top line*). The profiles of treated cells (*filled gray*) are overlaid on those of the untreated cells (*unfilled line*).

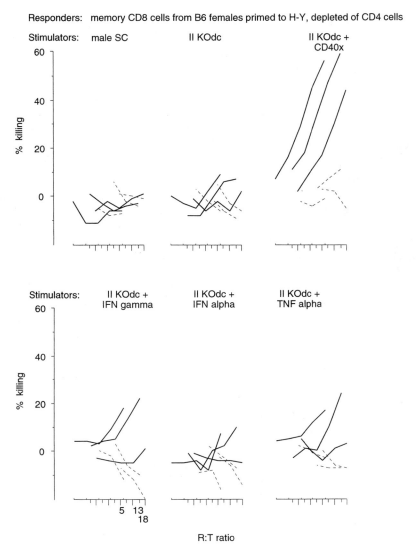

FIG. 23-7. Killing activity on male (*solid lines*) and female (*dashed lines*) targets of CD4-depleted spleen cells from primed female mice after 6 days of culture with the DCs from Fig. 23-6. The R/T ratios shown on the x-axis are different for each mouse because of differences in recovery of the CD4-depleted cells. The titrations begin at 18:1, 13:1, or 5:1 and continue in twofold dilutions.

killers. The conditioning of DCs requires CD40 crosslinking and cannot be substituted by any one of the inflammatory cytokines acting alone. Perhaps in future studies we will find that combinations of inflammatory cytokines have an effect where the individual molecules do not.

One cytokine known to be produced by CD40-crosslinked DCs is IL-12. Because IL-12 is important for the initiation of Th1 immune responses, we asked if it could act directly on the CD8 T cells to bypass help. In experiments where we added IL-12 to MHC-II knockout DCs, we saw little if any produc-

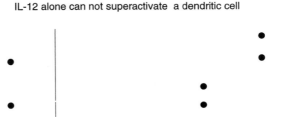

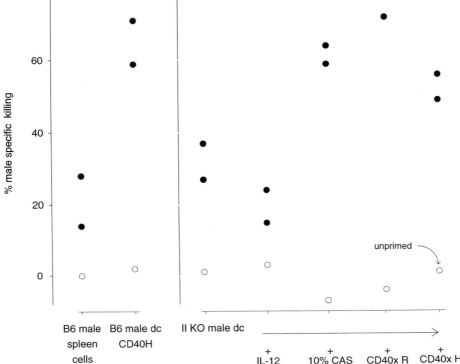

FIG. 23-8. Mouse IL-12 does not substitute for help. Spleen cells from anti H-Y primed or unprimed female B6 mice were depleted of CD4 T cells and were then stimulated with male spleen or dendritic cells from normal male B6 or MHC-II KO mice. Reading left to right: B6 male spleen cells, dendritic cells modulated with hamster anti-mouse CD40, MHC-II KO dc, KO dc with 100 ng/ml recombinant mouse IL-12, KO dc plus 10% Con A supernatant, KO dc modulated with rat or hamster anti-mouse CD40. Each point represents the killing from a single culture at an R/T ratio at which killing shown by cultures from control mice drops off the plateau. Background killing of female targets is subtracted. Killing derived from spleen cells of unprimed control mice treated in the same way as the primed cells is shown as *open circles*.

tion of CTL effectors (Fig. 23-8). Similar results were seen *in vivo* where MHC-II KO female mice were injected intraperitoneally with male MHC-II knockout DCs along with mouse recombinant IL-1 2, 300 ng/day for 3 days. Spleen cells from these mice did not give rise to CTL effectors when restimulated *in vitro* (data not shown). Thus the mechanism by which superactivated DCs turn on CD8 T cells must involve other cytokines or be a more complex process.

DISCUSSION

Combining our results with those of others (30–32), we separate dendritic cells into three activation (or maturation) states.

1. *Resting:* the state of an immature DC, residing quietly in a tissue in which it cannot stimulate any T cell
2. *Activated:* the state in which a DC has become activated and is able to act as an APC for T-helper but not T-killer cells

3. *Superactivated:* the state in which a DC is able to directly stimulate a killer

The signals that move a resting DC to an activated state are not yet fully known, though they include bacterial products such as lipopolysaccharide (LPS) and endogenous molecules such as TNF-α.

The signals that move an activated DC to a superactivated state include CD40 cross-linking and infection by certain viruses. We do not yet know whether the virus induces DC superactivation via a surface receptor or the DC must become productively infected. Preliminary experiments showed that the virally induced superactivation is not due solely to INF-α secretion by infected cells, as the addition of IFN-α alone had no super-activating effect. Experiments with various forms of inactivated virus are now in progress.

We also do not yet know how the superactivated DC differs from a merely activated DC or how it manages to stimulate the killer. There are no obvious consistent surface changes, and tests of IL-12, IL-6, and purified IL-2 also gave no promising results thus far. There is either a new cytokine involved, a new surface marker (perhaps a B7-like co-stimulatory molecule specific for CD8 cells), or an as yet untested combination of surface markers or cytokines that does the job.

We do not know the fate of a killer that recognizes (and is not stimulated by) a normally activated APC. In the absence of the signals offered by superactivated DCs, the killer remains unactivated, but is it unaffected? Studies *in vivo* have shown that CD8 killers become tolerant if they are presented with antigen in the absence of help (4,6–9). If, as we expect, the resulting tolerance is due to the lack of DC superactivation, reagents blocking superactivation should be useful for inducing transplantation tolerance. Recent studies using kidney transplants in primates suggest that a short course of reagents blocking CD40 ligand can lead to effective tolerance and acceptance of the grafts (33).

Finally, we do not know if there is only one superactivated state or many. We know that a DC interaction with a Th1 clone or a virus leads to a Th1-like superactivated state. There may also be superactivated states that drive Th2 or Th3 responses. In this light the DC may resemble a B cell, which can move from the production of IgM to IgG, IgE, and IgA under the influence of different cytokine signals.

APPENDIX: MATERIALS AND METHODS

Mice and Immunizations

C57Bl/6 (B6) mice were purchased from Taconic farms, Germantown, NY. MHC-II KO mice (KO), backcrossed to B6 (N13) or C57Bl/10 (N11), were from the NIAID breeding contract at Taconic. Mice were primed by an intraperitoneal injection of 3×10^6 male spleen cells in 200 μl of sterile phosphate-buffered saline (PBS).

Cells

For CD4 purification; spleen cells, depleted using a Midi MACs (Miltenyi Biotec, Germany) and anti-mouse CD4 monoclonal antibody (mAb), GK1.5, yielded less than 0.2% remaining CD4 cells by FACS analysis with the noncompeting anti-CD4 mAb RM4-4 (Pharmingen, San Diego, CA).

Dendritic cells were isolated as described elsewhere (23).

CD40 crosslinking and cytokine treatments were done as follows: Dendritic cells were incubated on ice for 10 minutes in PBS plus 10% mouse serum, for 20 minutes with hamster (HM40-3, 5 μg/ml) or IgG2a rat (3/23, 3.5 μg/ml; Pharmingen) anti-mouse CD40 mAbs, and then overnight at 37°C with goat anti-hamster or goat anti-rat antibodies (Caltag, Burlingame, CA) in Iscove's medium plus 10% fetal calf serum (IF10) plus GM-CSF 2 ng/ml and IL-4 200 U/ml. To these overnight dendritic cell cultures mouse recombinant IFN-α, IFN-γ, TNF-α, and IL-12 were added at 10,000 U/ml, 120 ng/ml, 10 pg/ml and 100 ng/ml, respectively. The cells were washed after the incubations, irradiated (1,500 rad), and used as *in vitro* stimulators.

The cells were then stimulated with Marilyn. Male B6 dendritic cells 1×10^6 were incubated overnight with 1.5×10^5 Marilyn, a CD4 Th1 clone specific for H-Y/A^b isolated from a B6 × CBA/N female mouse, then irradiated and used as *in vitro* stimulators. In some experiments we removed the Marilyns by FACS sorting with anti-H-2^k before using the dendritic cells as stimulators. We tested for the efficiency of depletion by staining for CD4, Thy1, and T cell receptor (TCR), and by culturing an aliquot of the (nonirradiated) dendritic cell populations and testing for proliferation. In no case did we find evidence of contaminating Marilyn cells.

Infection with influenza: Dendritic cells were infected with influenza virus A/PR/8 as elsewhere described (34), then irradiated and used as *in vitro* stimulators.

In Vitro Cultures

For *standard cultures:* Two weeks to 1 year after *in vivo* immunization, 4×10^6 untreated or CD4-depleted spleen cells were restimulated in 2-ml cultures with 2×10^6 irradiated male spleen cells or 1.5×10^5 dendritic cells, with or without an exogenous source of mouse IL-2, (10% rat Con A supernatant, depleted of ConA; Collaborative Biomedical Products, Bedford, MA). Six days later killing was tested on male and female targets using the JAM Test (35).

For *antibody blocking cultures:* Anti-mouse B7.1 (17A10, hamster), anti-mouse B7.2 (2D10, rat IgG2b), CTLA4-Ig (recombinant human or mouse CTLA4/Ig fusion protein), and control anti-mouse antibodies Ly5.2 (A20.1.7, rat IgG2b), were titrated 1:2 in IF10, starting at 1 mg or 600 μg/ml in 100-μl volumes in 96-well round-bottomed plates. Aliquots of 50 μl containing 1×10^5 primed unseparated or CD4-depleted B6 female spleen cells plus 50 μl containing 5×10^4 conditioned B6 or KO male dendritic

cells were added to give a final volume of 200 μl. Seven days later the medium was removed and replaced with 200 μl medium containing 10^4 target cells for the JAM test (35). We also used hamster antibody UC3-10A6 anti-mouse Vγ2. It did not block and is not reported for clarity.

For *FACS staining:* Dendritic cells were counted, and their Fcγ III/II receptors were blocked with rat anti-mouse anti-CD16/CD32 (24G2) for 10 minutes on ice, then incubated with hamster anti-mouse CD40 clone HM40-3 (fluorescein isothiocyanate), rat IgG2a anti-mouse B7.1 clone 1G10 (phycoerythrin), or rat IgG2a anti-mouse B7.2 clone GL1 (fluorescein isothiocyanate) for 20 minutes on ice. All antibodies were purchased from Pharmingen. The cells were then analyzed on an FACS calibur.

Acknowledgment

Some figures are reproduced by the kind permission of Nature.

REFERENCES

1. Vann DC, Dotson CR. Cellular cooperation and stimulatory factors in antibody responses: limiting dilution analysis in vitro. *J Immunol* 1974; 112:1149–1157.
2. Kennedy JC, Till JE, Siminovitch L, McCulloch, EA. The proliferative capacity of antigen-sensitive precursors of hemolytic plaque-forming cells. *J Immunol* 1966;96:973–980.
3. Tony HP, Parker DC. Major histocompatibility complex-restricted, polyclonal B cell responses resulting from helper T cell recognition of anti-immunoglobulin presented by small B lymphocytes. *J Exp Med* 1985;161:223–241.
4. Keene JA, Forman J. Helper activity is required for the in vivo generation of cytotoxic T lymphocytes. *J Exp Med* 1982;155:768–782.
5. Mitchison NA, O'Malley C. Three-cell-type clusters of T cells with antigen-presenting cells best explain the epitope linkage and noncognate requirements of the in vivo cytolytic response. *Eur J Immunol* 1987;171:579–1583.
6. Bennett SR, Carbone FR, Karamalis F, Miller JF, Heath WR. Induction of a CD8$^+$ cytotoxic T lymphocyte response by cross-priming requires cognate CD4$^+$ T cell help. *J Exp Med* 1997;186:65–70.
7. Guerder S, Matzinger P. A fail-safe mechanism for maintaining self-tolerance. *J Exp Med* 1992;176:553–564.
8. Guerder S, Matzinger P. Activation versus toler-

ance: a decision made by helper T cells. *Cold Spring Harb Symp Quant Biol* 1989;54:799–809.

9. Ress MA, Rosenberg AS, Munitz TI, Singer A. In vivo induction of antigen-specific transplantation tolerance to Qa1a by exposure to alloantigen in the absence of T-cell help. *Proc Natl Acad Sci USA* 1990;87:2765–2769.

10. Tripp RA, Sarawar SR, Doherty PC. Characteristics of the influenza virus-specific CD8⁺ T cell response in mice homozygous for disruption of the H-2lAb gene. *J Immunol* 1995;155:2955–2959.

11. Doherty PC, Topham DJ, Tripp RA. Establishment and persistence of virus-specific CD4⁺ and CD8⁺ T cell memory. *Immunol Rev* 1996;150:23–44.

12. Cardin RD, Brooks JW, Sarawar SR, Doherty PC. Progressive loss of CD8⁺ T cell-mediated control of a gamma-herpesvirus in the absence of CD4⁺ T cells. *J Exp Med* 1996;184:863–871.

13. Hou S, Mo XY, Hyland L, Doherty PC. Host response to Sendai virus in mice lacking class II major histocompatibility complex glycoproteins. *J Virol* 1995;69:1429–1434.

14. Castrucci MR, Hou S, Doherty PC, Kawaoka Y. Protection against lethal lymphocytic choriomeningitis virus (LCMV) infection by immunization of mice with an influenza virus containing an LCMV epitope recognized by cytotoxic T lymphocytes. *J Virol* 1994;68:3486–3490.

15. Gill RG, Lafferty KJ. A quantitative analysis of lymphokine release from activated T cells. *J Immunol* 1989;143:4009–4014.

16. Lassila O, Vainio O, Matzinger P. Can B cells turn on virgin T cells? *Nature* 1988;334:253–255.

17. Steinman RM. The dendritic cell system and its role in immunogenicity. *Annu Rev Immunol* 1991;9:271–296.

18. Roopenian DC, Widmer MB, Orosz CG, Bach FH. Helper cell-independent cytolytic T lymphocytes specific for a minor histocompatibility antigen. *J Immunol* 1983;130:542–545.

19. Simpson E, Gordon RD. Responsiveness to HY antigen Ir gene complementation and target cell specificity. *Immunol Rev* 1977;35:59–75.

20. Gray D, Matzinger P. T cell memory is short-lived in the absence of antigen. *J Exp Med* 1991;174:969–974.

21. Fuchs EJ Matzinger P. B cells turn off virgin but not memory T cells. *Science* 1992;258:1156–1159.

22. Boog CJ, Kast WM, Timmers HT, Boes J, de Waal LP, Melief CJ. Abolition of specific immune response defect by immunization with dendritic cells. *Nature* 1985;318:59–62.

23. Ridge JP, Fuchs EJ, Matzinger P. Neonatal tolerance revisited: turning on newborn T cells with dendritic cells [see comments]. *Science* 1996;271:1723–1726.

24. Saeland S, Duvert V, Moreau I, Banchereau J. Human B cell precursors proliferate and express CD23 after CD40 ligation. *J Exp Med* 1993;178:113–120.

25. Cella M, Scheidegger D, Palmer-Lehmann K, Lane P, Lanzavecchia A, Alber G. Ligation of CD40 on dendritic cells triggers production of high levels of interleukin-12 and enhances T cell stimulatory capacity: T-T help via APC activation. *J Exp Med* 1996;184:747–752.

26. Caux C, Massacrier C, Vanbervliet B, et al. Activation of human dendritic cells through CD40 cross-linking. *J Exp Med* 1994;180:1263–1272.

27. Wu Y, Liu Y. Viral induction of co-stimulatory activity on antigen-presenting cells bypasses the need for CD4⁺ T-cell help in CD8⁺ T-cell responses. *Curr Biol* 1994;4:499–505.

28. Linsley PS, Brady W, Urnes M, Grosmaire LS, Damle NK, Ledbetter JA. CTLA4 is a second receptor for the B cell activation antigen B7. *J Exp Med* 1991;174:561–569.

29. Lanzavecchia A. News and views: licence to kill. *Nature* 1998;393:413–414.

30. Ridge JP, Di Rosa F, Matzinger P. A conditioned dendritic cell can be a temporal bridge between a CD4⁺ T-helper and a T-killer cell [see comments]. *Nature* 1998;393:474–478.

31. Pierre P, Turley SJ, Gatti E, et al. Developmental regulation of MHC class II transport in mouse dendritic cells [see comments]. *Nature* 1997;388:787–792.

32. Cella M, Engering A, Pinet V, Pieters J, Lanzavecchia A. Inflammatory stimuli induce accumulation of MHC class II complexes on dendritic cells [see comments]. *Nature* 1997;388:782–787.

33. Kirk AD, Harlan DM, Armstrong NN, et al. CTLA4-Ig and anti-CD40 ligand prevent renal allograft rejection in primates. *Proc Natl Acad Sci USA* 1997;94:8789–8794.

34. Nonacs R, Humbory C, Tam JP, Steinman RM. Mechanism of mouse spleen dendritic cell function in the generation of influenza specific cytolytic T lympphocytes. *J Exp Med* 1997;176:519–529.

35. Matzinger P. The JAM test: a simple assay for DNA fragmentation and cell death. *J Immunol Methods* 1991;145:185–162.

Cytotoxic Cells: Basic Mechanisms and Medical Applications, edited by Michail V. Sitkovsky and Pierre A. Henkart. Lippincott Williams & Wilkins, Philadelphia © 2000.

Chapter 24
Cytotoxic T Cell Memory

Arno Müllbacher and Robert V. Blanden

Division of Immunology and Cell Biology, John Curtin School of Medical Research, Australian National University, Canberra City, ACT 2601 Australia

Immunologic memory underpins all vaccine strategies and is defined as an altered response of the immune system to a second encounter with the same or a related, cross-reactive antigen. Thus evidence of suppression also fulfills the definition (1). Conventionally, it mainly refers to enhancement, and it is in this sense that it is referred to in this review. Immunologic memory was initially studied predominantly in B cells (2); T cell memory also exists and is one of the defining parameters of the adaptive immune response. It was Medawar's seminal experiments during the 1940s (3) on skin homograft rejection in rabbits and the observation of accelerated rejection (memory) of a second set homograft, the specificity of the reaction, and its systemic nature that allowed him to conclude that skin graft rejection was an immunologic phenomenon. The same experimental procedures are still employed today to probe for the phylogenetic emergence of the T cell response in early vertebrates.

It is surprising to us, that despite the clear demonstration of the existence of T cell memory, we cannot point to a single piece of direct experimental evidence conclusively demonstrating that T cell memory is of crucial importance for a mammalian host to survive an infection. A possible role of persistent cross-reactive memory cytotoxic T cells in immunity to viral infections has been suggested (4). We expect that appropriately designed experiments will eventually demonstrate a survival advantage confered by a T cell memory response, justifying efforts to harness it in preventive or therapeutic vaccine strategies. Such hopes have certainly been raised during the last two decades, especially for tumor therapy (5), human immunodeficiency virus (HIV) infection prevention and therapy (6,7), and other viral and parasitic diseases for which conventional and antibody-based vaccine strategies so far have been suboptimal (e.g., influenza and malaria).

The mechanisms underlying the generation, maintenance, and activation of B cell memory uncovered so far are different from those for T cell memory. Whether there are differences in those parameters between $CD4^+$ and $CD8^+$ T cells is less likely. We review here predominantly data from memory responses of $\alpha\beta$ T cell receptor (TCR) $CD8^+$ cytotoxic T cell (CTL) responses and anticipate that most of these functional properties will be applicable to other T cell subsets.

MEMORY CTL PHENOTYPE

The defining characteristics of immunologic memory is an enhanced response upon encounter with the same or related (cross-reactive) antigen, or as we see later, with a nonantigenic stimulus that can activate resting T cells into effector cells. "Enhanced" generally refers to a response with accelerated kinetics, greater potency, and increased duration than a primary response. For CTL responses this has been most beautifully demonstrated in the influenza A virus model in the mouse (8–10) (Fig. 24-1). All the hallmarks of a memory response are there: early onset and increased and prolonged potency. One of the reasons secondary CTL responses *in vivo* are infrequently observed is due to the effect of persisting antibody responses that neutralize the second viral inoculum (12). Thus one of the prerequisites for the activation of memory CTLs *in vivo* is that the primary and secondary antigen must contain the same or a cross-reactive CTL peptide determinant, and the antibody elicited to the primary antigen should not cross-neutralize the secondary antigen. Strains of influenza A virus fulfill these criteria perfectly in the mouse model. The dominant CTL determinants in the mouse are peptides from the conserved nucleoprotein, whereas antibodies are predominantly made against the hem-

agglutinin and neuraminidase, antigens subject to continuous antigenic drift.

The availability of recombinant virus vectors encoding individual proteins with CTL peptide antigenic determinants of foreign pathogens similarly allows avoidance of interfering antibody responses in memory experiments *in vivo* (13).

The much more common experimental approach demonstrating CTL memory makes use of the fact that lymphocytes from animals previously primed *in vivo* can be activated and expanded in a secondary response *in vitro* when boosted with antigen. It was initially employed to amplify weak responses to minor histocompatibility antigens (14), including H-Y (15). Later, the method was also employed to generate potent viral-immune CTLs by co-culturing splenocytes or lymph node cells from primed animals with virus-infected stimulator cells (16). In certain instances, to generate detectable CTLs immune to viruses such as alphaviruses, *in vitro* secondary responses were obligatory (17). The ability to generate such secondary CTL populations is a long-lived property of previously primed splenocytes and in most cases lasts for the lifetime of the mouse (17,18). This contrasts with the difficulty generating anti-viral CTLs from unprimed lymphocyte populations *in vitro*, which requires special conditions such as enrichment of antigen-presenting cells (APCs) (19–21) or addition of exogenous cytokines (22).

In humans, the ability to obtain effector CTLs from peripheral blood leukocytes after *in vitro* boosting with antigen is accepted as evidence that a past encounter with antigen has occurred and thus is a manifestation of memory (23).

An additional difference between primary and secondary CTLs is that secondary CTLs have a lower requirement for accessory molecules in target cell recognition. Using antibodies to CD8 in CTL killing assays, we (9) and others (24) could show that primary antiviral or alloreactive CTLs were blocked at much lower antibody concentrations than secondary effectors. This was interpreted at

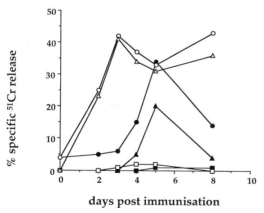

FIG. 24-1. Kinetics of activation of influenza immune CTLs. Percent specific ^{51}Cr release of P815 targets infected with A/JAP (○●), modified with 10^{-4} M influenza virus nucleoprotein-derived peptide with motif for K^d (11) (△▲) or unmodified (□■) by splenocytes from naive (●▲■) or memory (○△□) mice immunized with A/JAP 0 to 8 days previously. All values are taken from a four-fold titration curve at an effector/target (E/T) ratio of 30:1. Duration of assay was 6 hours. (From ref. 10, with permission.)

the time to mean that memory CTLs had higher-affinity TCRs than primary CTLs. High-affinity memory CTLs presumably could be the result of selection by limiting antigen concentration.

The more commonly referred to phenotypic characteristics of memory CTLs concern differences of cell surface markers to naive CTLs (25–31) and their physical properties (32–34). So far none of the identified "memory" markers has proved to be a reliable tag (35) allowing definitive distinction of naive versus memory CTLs. More importantly, there now exists good evidence that memory CTLs are a heterogeneous population consisting of small resting and large activated T cells (36,37). Thus most of the markers originally thought to identify memory T cells turned out to be also expressed on activated primary T cells (35). It has also been of some concern that certain memory markers seem to be mouse strain-specific (24), and markers found in different species such as humans and the mouse are often not related and probably functionally different (35).

INDUCTION OF CTL MEMORY

It is now well documented that upon primary stimulation of the immune system, especially after virus infections, massive proliferation of antigen-specific CD8$^+$ T cells occurs. The functional properties and the precise biologic role of all members of this population of CD8$^+$ T cells are not clear. Most of them are positive in regard to intracellular interferon-γ (INF-γ) synthesis but only a small subset of these cells give rise to cytolytic effector cells *in vitro* (38). It is not known whether this is a limitation of the assay system or it reflects the *in vivo* situation. One approach toward resolving this question would be to analyze perforin and granzyme expression at the single cell level. It is also established that upon antigen elimination, most effector CTLs undergo apoptosis, possibly owing to a lack of interleukins. An expanded antigen-specific pool of CD8$^+$ T cells remains, the so-called memory population,

which as stated above consists of a heterogeneous pool of small resting and large "activated" T cells without detectable cytolytic activity. The developmental pathway and essential signals that lead some but not all antigen-specific CTLs to become memory cells are not understood.

We have advocated a deterministic model of CTL memory formation (13). The model proposes that there is asymmetric cell division of naive T cells following primary recognition of antigen plus co-stimulation, giving rise to effector and memory cell progeny, resulting in an equal number of memory T cells as there were naive T cells activated. The memory T cell enters an antigen-refractory period and develops into a mature memory T cell with all the changed phenotypic characteristics described above and the altered signaling requirements (see below). The increased number of antigen-specific memory T cells observed (38) can be accounted for by the fact that some memory T cells continually divide at low levels due to signal 2-mediated activation (see below). Another option is a stochastic model of T cell memory maturation. In such a model one must postulate that some but not all of the primary effector T cells are selected—for yet unknown reasons—to become long-lived memory precursor T cells.

The role of CD4$^+$ T cells in the generation of memory CTLs was originally investigated in the mouse influenza virus model by adoptive transfer of T subset-depleted splenocytes (39). We could find no evidence for a role of CD4$^+$ T cells in the generation of memory CTLs *in vivo;* this reflected similar findings for the induction of primary antiviral CTLs *in vivo* (40). However, CD4 T cell involvement in the generation of CD8 CTLs immune to ectromelia has been observed when infection was via the intravenous route (Müllbacher, unpublished observation). Thus a role for CD4 T cells in the generation of CTLs may vary depending on physiologic and biochemical parameters, which are at present poorly understood. These findings of the independence of CTL memory formation from CD4$^+$ T cell involvement have been confirmed (41). However, results showing a diminished memory CTL response to lymphocytic choriomeningitis virus (LCMV) in CD4 T cell KO mice has been documented (42) emphasizing the complexity of the immunologic interactions when dealing with viral infections. Additional studies have also shown that B cells are not involved in CTL memory generation, suggesting that they are not involved in antigen processing and presentation for Tc cell responses (41,43). The interpretation of data obtained with CD40-ligand (CD40-L) KO mice, which showed impairment of memory CTL formation in response to LCMV infection (44), is potentially of a more complex nature. In view of the independence of Tc cell memory from B and CD4 T cells, a direct, possibly thymic developmental defect in CD8 T cells as a consequence of the absence of CD40-L cannot be ruled out. Thus most of the maturation pathway that leads from a naive antigen-reactive CD8$^+$ Tc cell to a long-lived memory precursor Tc cell has yet to be uncovered.

MAINTENANCE OF CTL MEMORY

The CTL memory is long-lived in humans and the mouse (17,18,45) even when nonreplicating antigens are used for priming (45,46). Two mechanisms can account for this longevity. First, memory CTLs may be short-lived (48) but are continuously replenished by activation and mitosis for which antigenic stimulation is essential. Activation was thought to be mediated by either of two mechanisms: persistence of the original antigen (49,50) or via cross-reactive stimulation (51). Alternatively, the memory CTLs may be long-lived or be replenished by non-antigen-specific activation (13,52).

The difficulty with the notion of required persistence of original antigen always was how to explain long-lived CTL memory after immunization with non-replicating antigen (46,47). There is also a theoretic problem with the requirement for persisting antigen to drive the maintenance of memory CTLs. It is generally accepted, on the weight of available evidence, that CTL responses evolved to eliminate acute, life-threatening viral infections. They achieve this by lysing all cells that display on their surface complexes of viral peptides with self-major histocompatibility complex (MHC) antigens. It would be a nice trick of evolution to select for CTL responses that somehow stop short of complete elimination of acute infections, a phenomenon that would be neccessary to allow the evolution of a requirement for persisting antigen to maintain CTL memory.

In a recent report (53) a novel proposition to explain continued antigen expression and consequently maintenance of memory was advanced. It was found that after LCMV infection, LCMV RNA was reverse-transcribed into DNA and was present in the nuclei of infected spleen or cell lines. The sequence of the immunodominant CTL peptide determinant was encoded in the cDNA. Whether this surprise finding provides a generalized explanation for the maintenance of memory CTLs remains to be determined. If these virus-derived DNA sequences are indeed transcribed, translated, and give rise to viral peptide–MHC complexes necessary for memory CTL activation, why are these cells not recognized by effector CTLs and eliminated, especially as a single appropriately modified MHC class I (MHC-I) molecule on a target cell is sufficient to trigger CTL-mediated recognition and lysis (54). Furthermore, in every case the cDNA would need to encode the peptide determinants to which the primary CTL response was directed and be capable of cellular transcription and translation. The long-lasting memory response to cellular antigens such as major and minor histocompatibility antigens (including H-Y) requires additional assumptions if a universal explanation of DNA-based persistence of antigen is to apply.

The notion of longevity of memory T cells, for which there exists good evidence, is by itself sufficient to explain most of the experimental findings on long-term Tc cell memory (30,34,55,56). Occasional antigen-independent stimulation of memory precursor CTLs may constitute an additional mechanism to amplify memory T cell numbers periodically (see below).

ACTIVATION OF MEMORY CTLs

As we have mentioned, it became apparent early on that for the induction of anti-viral MHC-restricted CTL responses *in vitro* priming was essential, unless special APC enrichment procedures were undertaken. This differed dramatically from CTL responses generated *in vitro* against allogeneic MHC-I. This discrepancy between primary anti-allo versus primary anti-viral MHC-restricted CTL responses *in vitro* led to the proposition that the strength of the anti-allo response is due to it being in effect a secondary response as a consequence of cross-reactivity after priming with "environmental" antigens (49).

Two mechanisms could potentially account for the difference *in vitro*. First, the strong secondary response could be due simply to an elevated number of precursors; and second, qualitative changes in the stimulation requirements of memory versus naive Tc cell precursors could account for the observed phenomena. An analysis of the two-signal model of T cell activation (57) showed that for the generation of alloreactive CTLs *in vitro* there was a need for both antigen (allo-MHC) and co-stimulatory molecules (CD80) to be expressed on the stimulator cell (58). However, using previously alloantigen-primed splenocytes, no requirement for CD80/CD28-mediated co-stimulation was necessary (59) (Fig. 24-2). Two important conclusions can be gained from these findings. First, memory

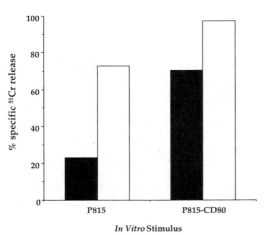

FIG. 24-2. Memory alloreactive CTLs do not require CD28–CD80 interactions for *in vitro* activation. A/J (K^{k}D^d) mice were immunized intraperitoneally with 10^7 pfu of VV (■) or VV encoding the MHC-I, K^d (□). Three weeks later splenocytes were stimulated *in vitro* with mitomycin C-treated P815 (K^{d}D^d) or P815 transfected with CD80 (P815–CD80) cells for 5 days at a responder/stimulator ratio of 5:1. Lysis of D2 (K^{d}D^d) targets at an effector/target ratio of 10:1 is shown. (From ref. 59, with permission.)

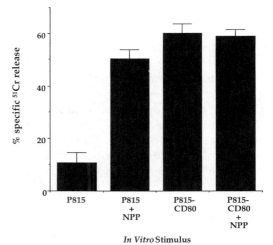

FIG. 24-3. Generation of antiviral cytotoxic activity in the absence of antigen (signal 1). Viral-immune CTLs from influenza A virus-primed BALB/c (K^{d}D^d) animals were stimulated *in vitro* with P815 or P815-CD80 either pulsed with nucleoprotein peptide 147-158 R156$^-$ with high affinity for K^d (60) or left untreated. Following 5 days of culture, effectors were tested for cytotoxicity against influenza virus-infected H-2 matched targets. Lysis of uninfected targets was less than 20%. (From ref. 52, with permission.)

CTL precursors have a less stringent signaling requirement for activation; and second, memory is not the explanation for the strong *in vitro* anti-allo response. Further analysis of anti-influenza-memory CTLs using stimulator cells either pulsed with peptide antigen or co-transfected with CD80 clearly established that biologically relevant memory Tc cells can be activated by either signal 1 (MHC-I plus peptide) or signal 2 (CD80/CD28 interaction) alone (Fig. 24-3). However, there are different requirements for activation of memory cells depending on the presence or absence of antigen. Activation *in vitro* of memory CTLs from influenza-primed mice by co-stimulation in the absence of antigen (MHC–peptide complexes) require exogenous interleukin-2 (IL-2) signaling via the cell surface-expressed IL-2 receptor, which under conditions of IL-2 blockade can be replaced by exogenous IL-7. Activation of memory CTLs by co-stimulation and antigen is independent of IL-2 and IL-7 (Fig. 24-4). Although memory anti-influenza Tc cells do respond to CD80 in the absence of antigen, the additional presence of antigen enables an earlier induction of these CTLs to become cytolytic, and they retain their lytic activity *in vitro* over a longer time period (Fig. 24-5). The capacity of memory CTLs to be activated by CD80/CD28 interaction alone provides a plausible explanation for the observed heterogeneity of phenotype of memory T cells *in vivo* (31,36,37,61) and suggests a mechanism for the stimulation of memory cell division in the absence of persisting antigen (52).

There have been additional reports of other antigen-independent activation mechanisms for memory T cells (62,63), that have been implicated as responsible for the observed bystander effect *in vivo* (38,64–66). It is not clear if bystander activation is an undesirable side effect that must be accommodated in a response to a new pathogenic onslaught, or if bystander activation plays a role in the renewal of the memory response and thus is a part of the

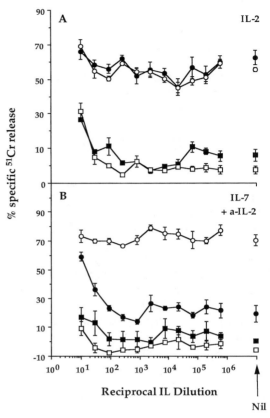

FIG. 24-4. Induction of influenza-immune effector CTLs in the presence of antigen (Ag) and CD80 or CD80 in the absence of Ag. Effect of IL-2 and of IL-7 under conditions of IL-2 blockade. Splenocytes from A/WSN-primed BALB/c mice were cultured as described for Figure 24-1 in the presence of P815-CD80 (●■) or P815-CD80 pulsed with 10^{-4} M NPP (□○). Cultures were supplemented with IL-2 (**A**) or IL-7 in the presence of 50 mg · ml⁻¹ of antibody to IL-2 (**B**). The cytolytic activity of effector CTLs was tested in a 6-hour ^{51}Cr-release assay against uninfected (■□) or A/WSN-infected (●○) D2 target cells. Results are expressed as the mean percent specific lysis ± SE of triplicate cultures. *Nil,* absence of IL-2 (**A**) or IL-7 (**B**). (From ref. 52, with permission.)

strategy of long-term memory maintenance. The report by Selin et al. (67) suggests that the former is the more likely cause, and bystander activation does not confer obvious advantages on the host.

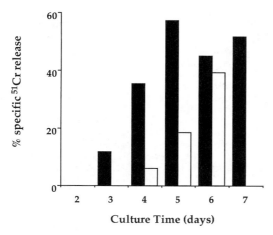

FIG. 24-5. Kinetics of secondary antiviral CTL responses *in vitro* following stimulation of influenza-primed CTLs with Ag in the absence of CD80 or CD80 in the absence of Ag. Spleens were harvested from two A/WSN-primed BALB/c mice per day for 6 consecutive days. Each day, spleen cells from the two animals were pooled and *in vitro* cultures prepared. Responders were stimulated *in vitro* in individual cultures with P815 pulsed with 10^{-4} M NPP (■) or with P815-CD80 (□) at an R/S of 10:1. Cell cultures were harvested on day 7, and effectors were used in a ^{51}Cr-release assay against A/WSN-infected B10.D2 target cells. The result depicts logarithmic regression analysis from a fourfold titration curve at an E/T of 5:1. Lysis of uninfected targets was less than 8%. (From ref. 52, with permission.)

CONCLUSIONS

Although T cell memory was first described more than 50 years ago, much remains to be learned about the biochemical and cellular basis of the phenomenon. We do not have detailed knowledge of the cellular events that lead to the establishment of T cell memory (e.g., the probability of an asymmetric mitosis model). We are not even able to identify a memory CTL phenotype precisely. Most progress has been made in analyzing the general functional properties and activation requirements of memory T cells. The availability of a virus model that allows induction of primary CTL responses but does *not* lead to the generation of long-lasting memory CTLs (68) may prove to be a valu-

able tool in unraveling further aspects of T cell memory.

REFERENCES

1. Celada F. The cellular basis of immunologic memory. *Progr Allergy* 1971;15:223–267.
2. Klinman NR. The mechanism of antigenic stimulation of primary and secondary clonal precursor cells. *J Exp Med* 1972;136:241–260.
3. Medawar PB. The behaviour and fate of skin autografts and skin homografts in rabbits. *J Anat* 1944; 78:176–197.
4. Welsh RM, Lin MY, Lohman BL, Varga SM, Zarozinski CC, Selin SK. Alpha beta and gamma delta T-cell networks and their roles in natural resistance to viral infections. *Immunol Rev* 1997;159:79–93.
5. Melief CJM, Kast WM. T-cell immunotherapy of tumors by adoptive transfer of cytotoxic T lymphocytes and by vaccination with minimal essential epitopes. *Immunol Rev* 1995;146:167–177.
6. Ada GL, Prospects for HIV vaccines. *J AIDS* 1988; 1:259–303.
7. Ada GL, McElrath MJ. HIV type 1 vaccine-induced cytotoxic T cell responses: potential role in vaccine efficacy. *AIDS Res* 1997;13:205–210.
8. Effros RB, Bennink J, Doherty PC. Characteristics of secondary cytotoxic T cell responses in mice infected with influenza virus. *Cell Immunol* 1978; 36:345–353.
9. Hill AB, Blanden RV, Parrish CR, Müllbacher A. Restimulated memory Tc cells have a higher apparent avidity of interaction with targets than primary virus-immune Tc cells as indicated by anti-CD8 blocking. *Immunol Cell Biol* 1992;70:259–265.
10. Müllbacher A, Tha Hla R. In vivo administration of major histocompatibility complex class I-specific peptides from influenza virus induces specific cytotoxic T cell hyporesponsivness. *Eur J Immunol* 1993;23:2526–2531.
11. Rammensee H-G, Friede T, Stevanovic S. MHC ligands and peptide motifs: first listing. *Immunogenetics* 1995;41:178–228.
12. Müllbacher A, Blanden RV. The effect of virus-immune serum on antiviral cytotoxic T cells in vivo and in vitro. *J Gen Virol* 1979;45:73–80.
13. Müllbacher A, Flynn K. Aspects of cytotoxic T cell memory. *Immunol Rev* 1996;150:113–127.
14. Bevan M. Interaction antigens detected by cytotoxic T cells with the major histocompatibility complex as modifier. *Nature* 1975;256:419–422.
15. Simpson E, O'Hopp S, Wunderlich J. Life span and cytotoxic activity and memory activity following allogeneic skin grafting in the mouse. *Transplantation* 1974;18:374–377.
16. Gardner ID, Blanden RV. The cell-mediated immune response to ectromelia virus infection. II. Secondary response in vitro and kinetics of memory T cell production in vivo. *Cell Immunol* 1976; 22:283–296.
17. Müllbacher A, Blanden RV. Murine cytotoxic T-cell response to alphavirus is associated mainly with H-2Dk. *Immunogenetics* 1978;7:551–561.

18. Ashman RB. Persistence of cell-mediated immunity to influenza A virus in mice. *Immunology* 1982; 47:165–168.
19. Blanden RV, Kees U, Dunlop MBC. In vitro primary induction of cytotoxic T cells against virus-infected syngeneic cells. *J Immunol Methods* 1977; 16:73–89.
20. Macatonia SE, Taylor PM, Knight SC, Askonas BA. Primary stimulation by dendritic cells induces antiviral proliferative and cytotoxic T cell responses in vitro. *J Exp Med* 1989;169:1255–1264.
21. Inaba K, Metlay JP, Crowley MT, Steinman RM. Dendritic cells pulsed with protein antigens in vitro can prime antigen-specific, MHC-restricted T cells in situ. *J Exp Med* 1990;172:631–640.
22. Kos FJ, Müllbacher A. Induction of primary antiviral cytotoxic T cells by in vitro stimulation with short synthetic peptide and interleukin-7. *Eur J Immunol* 1992;22:3183–3185.
23. Beverley PCL. Human T-cell memory. *Curr Top Microbiol Immunol* 1990;159:111–122.
24. Shimonkevitz R, Luescher B, Cerottini J-C, MacDonald HR. Clonal analysis of cytolytic T lymphocyte-mediated lysis of target cells with inducible antigen expression: correlation between antigen density and requirement for Lyt-2/3 function. *J Immunol* 1985;135:892–899.
25. MacDonald HR, Budd RC, Cerottini J-C. Pgp-1 (Ly 24) as a marker of murine memory T lymphocytes. *Curr Top Microbiol Immunol* 1990;159:97–109.
26. McFarland HI, Nahill SR, Maciaszek JW, Welsh RM. CD11b (Mac-1): a marker for CD8+ cytotoxic T cell activation and memory in virus infection. *J Immunol* 1992;149:1326–1333.
27. Akbar A, Salmon M, Janossy G. The synergy between naive and memory T cells during activation. *Immunol Today* 1991;12:184–188.
28. Bradley LM, Croft M, Swain SL. T-cell memory: new perspectives. *Immunol Today* 1993;14:197–199.
29. Sanders ME, Makgoba MW, Shaw S. Human naive and memory T cells: reinterpretation of helper-inducer and suppressor-inducer subsets. *Immunol Today* 1988;9:195–199.
30. Tripp RA, Hou S, Doherty PC. Temporal loss of the activated L-selectin-low phenotype for virus-specific CD8+ memory T cells. *J Immunol* 1995; 154:5870–5875.
31. Walunas TL, Bruce DS, Dustin L, Loh DY, Bluestone JA. Ly-6C is a marker of memory CD8+ T cells. *J Immunol* 1995;155:1873–1883.
32. Hall BM, Dorsch SE, Roser BJ. The complex basis of allograft rejection in vivo. II. The nature of memory cell mediating second-set heart graft rejection. *J Exp Med* 1978;148:879–889.
33. Cerottini J-C, Brunner KT. Cell-mediated cytotoxicity, allograft rejection, and tumor immunity. *Adv Immunol* 1974;18:67–132.
34. Bruno L, Kirberg J, von Boehmer H. On the cellular basis of immunological T cell memory. *Immunity* 1995;2:37–43.
35. Dutton RW, Bradley LM, Swain SL. T cell memory. *Annu Rev Immunol* 1998;16:201–223.
36. Razvi ES, Welsh RM, McFarland HI. In vivo state of antiviral CTL precursors: characterization of a

cycling cell population containing CTL precursors in immune mice. *J Immunol* 1995;154:620–632.
37. Tough DF, Sprent J. Turnover of naive- and memory-phenotype T cells. *J Exp Med* 1994;179:1127–1135.
38. Murali Krishna K, Altman JD, Suresh M, et al. Counting antigen-specific CD8 T cells: a reevaluation of bystander activation during viral infection. *Immunity* 1998;8:177–187.
39. Liu Y, Müllbacher A. The generation and activation of memory class I MHC restricted cytotoxic T cell responses to influenza A virus in vivo do not require CD4+ T cells. *Immunol Cell Biol* 1989;67:413–420.
40. Buller RML, Holmes KL, Hügin A, Fredericks TN, Morse HC. III. Induction of cytotoxic T-cell responses in vivo in the absence of CD4 helper cells. *Nature* 1987;328:77–79.
41. Di Rosa F, Matzinger P. Long-lasting CD8 T cell memory in the absence of CD4 T cells or B cells. *J Exp Med* 1996;183:2153–2163.
42. Von Herrath MG, Yokoyama M, Dockter J, Oldstone MB, Whitton JL. CD4-deficient mice have reduced levels of memory cytotoxic T lymphocytes after immunization and show diminished resistance to subsequent virus challenge. *J Virol* 1996;70:1072–1079.
43. Asano MS, Ahmed R. CD8 T cell memory in B cell-deficient mice. *J Exp Med* 1996;183:2165–2174.
44. Borrow P, Tishon A, Lee S, et al. CD40L-deficient mice show deficits in antiviral immunity and have an impaired memory CD8+ CTL response. *J Exp Med* 1996;183:2129–2142.
45. McMichael AJ, Doughworth DW, Gotch FM, Clark A, Potter CW. Declining T-cell immunity to influenza, 1977–1982. *Lancet* 1983;762–764.
46. Müllbacher A, Sheena JH, Fierz W, Brenan M. Specific haplotype preference in congenic F1 hybrid mice in the cytotoxic T cell response to the male specific antigen H-Y. *J Immunol* 1981;127:686–689.
47. Müllbacher A, Ada GL, Hla RT. Gamma-irradiated influenza A virus can prime for a cross-reactive and cross-protective immune response against influenza A viruses. *Immunol Cell Biol* 1988;66:153–157.
48. Gray D, Sprent J. Preface. *Curr Top Microbiol Immunol* 1990;159:V–VII.
49. Matzinger P. Immunology: memories are made of this? *Nature* 1994;369:605–606.
50. Zinkernagel RM. Antiviral T-cell memory. *Curr Top Microbiol Immunol* 1990;159:65–77.
51. Beverley PCL. Is T-cell memory maintained by crossreactive stimulation? *Immunol Today* 1990; 203–205.
52. Flynn K, Müllbacher A. The generation of memory antigen-specific cytotoxic T cell responses by CD28/CD80 interaction in the absence of antigen. *Eur J Immunol* 1997;27:456–462.
53. Klenerman P, Hengartner H, Zinkernagel RM. A non-retroviral RNA virus persists in DNA form. *Nature* 1997;390:298–301.
54. Sykulev Y, Joo M, Vturina I, Tsomides TJ, Eisen HN. Evidence that a single peptide-MHC complex on a target cell can elicit a cytolytic T cell response. *Immunity* 1996;4:565–571.
55. Müllbacher A. The long-term maintenance of cyto-

toxic T cell memory does not require persistence of antigen. *J Exp Med* 1994;179:317–321.

56. Lau LL, Jamieson BD, Somasundaram T, Ahmed R. Cytotoxic T-cell memory without antigen. *Nature* 1994;369:648–652.

57. Schwartz RH, Mueller DL, Jenkins MK, Quill H. T-cell clonal anergy. *Cold Spring Harbor Symp Quant Biol* 1989;54:605–610.

58. Harding FA, Allison JP. CD28-B7 interactions allow the induction of CD8$^+$ cytotoxic T lymphocytes in the absence of exogenous help. *J Exp Med* 1993;177:1791–1796.

59. Flynn K, Müllbacher A. Memory alloreactive cytotoxic T cells do not require costimulation for activation in vitro. *Immunol Cell Biol* 1996;74:413–420.

60. Bodmer HC, Pemberton RM, Rothbard JB, Askonas BA. Enhanced recognition of a modified peptide antigen by cytotoxic T cells specific for influenza nucleoprotein. *Cell* 1988;52:253–258.

61. Kos FJ, Müllbacher A. IL-2-independent activity of IL-7 in the generation of secondary antigen-specific cytotoxic T cell responses in vitro. *J Immunol* 1993;150:387–93.

62. Tough DF, Borrow P, Sprent J. Induction of bystander T cell proliferation by viruses and type I interferon in vivo. *Science* 1996;272:1947–1950.

63. Coppola MA, Blackman MA. Bacterial superantigens reactivate antigen-specific CD8$^+$ memory T cells. *Int Immunol* 1997;9:1393–1403.

64. Ehl S, Hombach J, Aichele P, Hengartner H, Zinkernagel RM. Bystander activation of cytotoxic T cells: studies on the mechanism and evaluation of in vivo significance in a transgenic mouse model. *J Exp Med* 1997;185:1241–1251.

65. Cose SC, Jones CM, Wallace ME, Heath WR, Carbone FR. Antigen-specific CD8$^+$ T cell subset distribution in lymph nodes draining the site of herpes simplex virus infection. *Eur J Immunol* 1997; 27:2310–2316.

66. Zarozinski CC, Welsh RM. Minimal bystander activation of CD8 T cells during the virus-induced polyclonal T cell response. *J Exp Med* 1997;185:1629–1639.

67. Selin LK, Vergilis K, Welsh RM, Nahill SR. Reduction of otherwise remarkably stable virus-specific cytotoxic T lymphocyte memory by heterologous viral infections. *J Exp Med* 1996;183:2489–2499.

68. Lobigs M, Blanden RV, Müllbacher A. Flavivirus-induced up-regulation of MHC class I antigens; implications for the induction of CD8$^+$ T-cell-mediated autoimmunity. *Immunol Rev* 1996;152:5–19.

Cytotoxic Cells: Basic Mechanisms and Medical Applications, edited by Michail V. Sitkovsky and Pierre A. Henkart. Lippincott Williams & Wilkins, Philadelphia © 2000.

Chapter 25

CD8 Memory to Viruses and the T Cell Network

Liisa K. Selin, Meei Y. Lin, Steven M. Varga, and Raymond M. Welsh

Pathology Department, University of Massachusetts Medical Center, Worcester, Massachusetts, 01655, USA

Many viruses are potent inducers of antigen-specific CD8 cytotoxic T lymphocyte (CTL) responses, which are important for the clearance of these viruses and the recovery from infection. This acute CD8 T cell response returns to homeostasis once the virus is cleared, but a portion of the CD8 cells enter the T cell memory pool, where they can be rapidly accessed when the host is rechallenged with the same virus. Two important features of this T cell response are antigen specificity and memory. T cell antigen specificity has been extensively studied and can be clearly defined in biomolecular terms. In contrast, although the concept of T cell memory is easy to comprehend, the molecular characterization of memory T cells has been more difficult.

T cell antigen specificity occurs as a consequence of the rearrangement of T cell receptor (TCR) gene families that give rise to T cell clones with epitope-specific repertoires. T cells recognize virus-infected target cells by virtue of TCR interactions with major histocompatibility complex (MHC) molecules presenting viral peptides (1). Additional molecules have been defined as essential for a successful TCR–antigen interaction. The CD8 molecule, which defines a subset of class I MHC (MHC-I)-restricted T cells mediating cytotoxic function and cytokine production, binds directly to the MHC-I

molecules, whereas the CD4 molecule, which defines class II-restricted T cells involved in regulatory functions via the production of cytokines, binds directly to MHC-II molecules. T cell–target cell conjugation is enhanced by a variety of adhesion molecules, including CD2/LFA3, and LFA-1 (CD11a) or Mac-1 (CD11b)/ICAM-1 (2,3). Initial activation of T cells on contact with antigen-presenting cells (APCs) is further enhanced by signals mediated through CD40L–CD40 interactions (4) and by co-stimulatory signals through CD28 on the T cell and B7 on the APCs (5).

An operational definition for T cell memory, as with B cell memory, is that it provides a faster, stronger immune response to a host upon reexposure to an antigen, resulting in more rapid clearance of the invading pathogen. Memory T cells are effective at providing protective immunity because they can be present at high frequency long after clearance of the primary infection (6–8). Unlike B cells, there is no clear anatomic site where memory T cells develop, no isotype switching of TCR genes, and no somatic mutations selecting for higher affinity T cells. Memory T cells have some functional characteristics different from those of naive cells that make them much easier to activate into effectors. They can respond to a 50-fold lower dose of antigen (9), without stringent requirements

TABLE 25-1. *Expression of cell surface markers on naive and memory T cells*

Marker	Naive cells	Effector cells	Memory cells	References
CD2	Low	High	High	17, 18
CD44	Low	High	High	17, 19
CD45R	High	Low/high	Low	17, 18
CD45RO	Low	Low/high	High	17, 18
CD45RB[a]	High	Low/high	Low	20, 21
CD49d	Low	High	High	22
CD62L	High	Low	Low/high	23–28
CZ-1[a]	Low	High	High	29
ICAM-1	Low	High	High	30, 31
IL-2Rα	Low	High	Low, high on blasts	28, 32, 33
IL-2Rβ	Low	High	High	16, 32, 33
LFA-1	Low	High	High	17, 18
LFA-3	Low	High	High	18, 31
Ly6C[b]	Low	High	High	14, 34
MAC-1[b]	Low	High	High	3

Human naive and memory T cells are generally distinguished using the CD45RA and CD45RO markers.
Mouse naive and memory T cells are generally distinguished by using the CD44 and CD62L markers.
[a] Modulation of these angitens occurs mainly on the CD4[+] T cell subset.
[b] Modulation of these antigens occurs mainly on the CD8[+] T cell subset.

for co-stimulation (10–14) and have been shown to secrete much higher levels of cytokines (12). Upon restimulation they develop effector function more rapidly than naive T cells (15), which could be related to the fact that they constitutively express cytokine receptors such as interleukin-2β (IL-2β) (16). Memory T cells also differ phenotypically from naive cells by expressing different cell surface markers (Table 25-1), but no single marker consistently differentiates between naive, effector, and memory T cells.

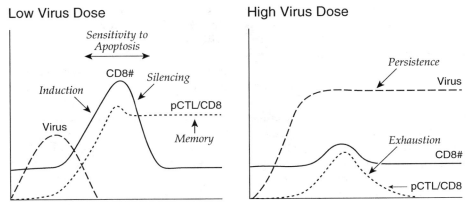

FIG. 25-1. Dynamics of the T cell response to a low dose and a high (disseminating) dose of LCMV in mice. Note the dramatic differences in the immune response to LCMV (*left*), where a modest dose of virus induces a potent CTL response. These T cells enter a state of sensitivity to apoptosis as the virus is cleared, and then the immune response "silences," as the T cell number and activation state decline. However, the CTL precursors per CD8 cells (*pCTL/CD8*) ratio remains high, and stable. In contrast, mice receiving high doses of viral strains (*right*) that can disseminate develop only a modest CTL response, which becomes "clonally exhausted" by mechanisms that might involve activation-induced cell death (AICD) of the T cell population. (From ref. 35, with permission of Munksgaard International Publishers.)

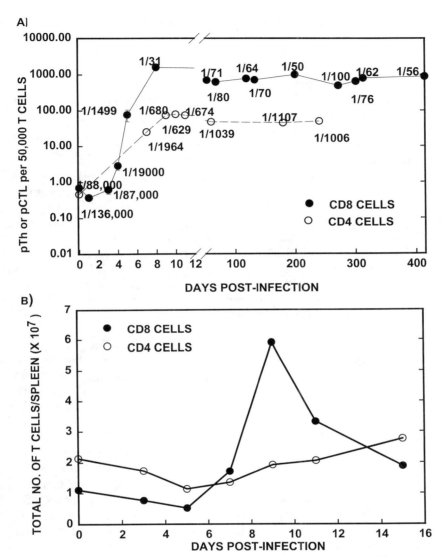

FIG. 25-2. A: LCMV-specific precursors CTLs (*pCTL*) and precursor T-helper cells (*pTh*) frequencies in C57BL/6 mice. Plotted are the frequencies of pCTLs (CD8) and pTh (CD4) cells during the acute and memory stages of the LCMV infection. The numbers were derived from cytotoxic limiting dilution assays (LDAs) for pCTLs and LDAs of purified CD4 cells for IL-2 production. [The data here are based on data from Selin et al. (6) and Varga and Welsh (36).] **B:** Kinetics of CD8 and CD4 T cell number, during the acute T cell response to LCMV infection. Shown here is the dichotomy in CD8 and CD4 total T cell number, during an acute LCMV infection. There is no increase in CD4 total number, whereas CD8 cells increase six-fold by day 8 after infection and then return to homeostasis by day 14. [This figure is based on data from Varga and Welsh (36).]

This chapter focuses on the specificities of T cells that become activated during viral infections, how these T cells are quantitatively and qualitatively modulated throughout the acute infection and into the memory state, and how subsequent infections modulate the preexisting pool of memory cells. The lymphocytic choriomeningitis virus (LCMV) model in mice has been used extensively to demonstrate the role of acute effector and memory CD8 T cells in the clearance of virus and in virus-induced immunopathology. Therefore studies with this virus are the major focus of this chapter, with reference to other viral systems where information is available. Intraperitoneal infection with low to moderate doses of LCMV (Armstrong strain) results in an *induction phase* of CTL activity leading to a five- to tenfold increase in the total CD8 T cell number, an *apoptosis phase* during which the T cells become sensitized to activation-induced cell death (AICD) and when the host enters a stage of transient "immune deficiency," a *silencing phase* during which the T cell number and activation state are reduced, and a *memory phase* associated with the stable preservation of a high frequency of virus-specific memory CTL precursors that have permanently altered the T cell repertoire (Fig. 25-1, low virus dose; Fig. 25-2). In contrast, intravenous infection of mice with high doses of highly disseminating strains of LCMV (clone 13, Docile) results in an initial CTL response that becomes "exhausted" by the overwhelming antigen load, and these mice develop persistent infections in the absence of CTL memory (Fig. 25-1, high virus dose). Each phase of the CD8 T cell response to the low-dose infection is discussed in terms of how it contributes to the generation and maintenance of memory. It is demonstrated that memory cells are not a dormant population of cells but are in continuous dynamic flux, perpetually in cell cycle, and can be cytolytically active in a resting immune host. These CD8 memory cells are part of an immunologic network whereby they are frequently modulated by cross-reactive interactions with new antigens and by apoptotic depletions, both of which may lead to altering the course of subsequent infections.

INDUCTION PHASE OF CTL MEMORY

Specificity of the Virus-Induced CD8 T Cell Population

Because discrete antigen specificity is required for the CTL to recognize virus-infected cells, a great deal of effort has gone into defining immunodominant epitopes, largely in an attempt to develop appropriate vaccine strategies. In C57BL/6 mice four H-2D^b-restricted LCMV-specific immunodominant peptides recognized by CTLs have been defined, three on the LCMV glycoprotein (GP33, GP92, GP276) and one on the nucleoprotein (NP396) (37–40). This chapter discusses research involving predominantly three of these epitopes (GP33, GP276, NP396), as the fourth epitope GP92 was only recently defined. Knowledge of the CD8 T cell epitopes made it possible to investigate if the massive expansion of CD8 T cells during the acute response to viruses was predominantly antigen-specific or was the consequence of a small number of antigen-specific cells causing a substantial bystander proliferation of T cells not specific for the virus. For many years the main techniques available to quantify antigen-specific CTLs have been the seldom used single-cell cytotoxicity assays and the more commonly used limiting dilution assays (LDAs), where replicate wells of various dilutions of responder T cells from the acutely infected spleens are stimulated *in vitro* with virus-infected APCs. A linear curve could be derived by quantifying microwells that gave rise to T cells able to lyse the appropriate virus-infected target; and from this curve could be calculated the precursor frequency of virus-specific CTLs (pCTL). LDA analyses in several virus systems originally showed very low levels of virus-specific CTLs (<1/1,000) (41,42), but as techniques improved, substantially higher levels were observed (6,7,43). For instance, at the peak of LCMV infection (day 8) 1 of 31 of the CD8 splenocytes was shown to be LCMV-specific, representing about 3.3% of the total CD8 pool at that time point (Fig. 25-2A) (6). This frequency was comparable to that reported for single-cell cytotoxicity assays (44). These techniques nevertheless could identify only a small proportion of the CD8 cells as being virus-specific.

New technologies have become available to quantify antigen-specific T cells directly. Altman et al. (45) designed and constructed soluble MHC-I tetramers linked by avidin. These tetramers can be fluorescein-labeled, loaded with an immunodominant T cell peptide, and used to enumerate T cells expressing receptors for that peptide–MHC combination. By another approach, Schneck and colleagues (46) have generated chimeric immunoglobulin G (IgG) molecules in which a truncated heavy chain is fused to a class I α-chain. When this fusion molecule is incubated with β_2-microglobulin, complete MHC-I dimers are produced; and these too can be loaded with peptide and used to enumerate antigen-binding T cells. Techniques based on short term-cytokine production in the presence of interleukin-2 (IL-2) and a stimulating class I peptide have also been newly developed. Intracellular interferon-γ (IFN-γ) or other cytokine production can be quantified by flow cytometry if cells are incubated for several hours in brefeldin A or monensin, which prevents secretion of the cytokine (47–49). Efficient quantification of cytokine-secreting cells has now been efficiently done in Elispot assays using T cells stimulated with peptide and IL-2 (47). Antigen-specific T cell frequencies are similar with each of these techniques, and all have shown that the high percentages of T cells induced during LCMV and other virus infections are indeed virus-specific. Studies showed that in the LCMV infection of mice at least 40% to 60% of the CD8 population was LCMV-specific (47), in influenza A infection of mice 20% of the CD8 population in the bronchoalveolar lavage (BAL) was

influenza NP366 peptide-specific (50), and in human Epstein-Barr virus (EBV) infection up to 40% of the CD8 population was specific to a single EBV epitope (51).

Allo-cross-reactive T Cells Generated During Acute Virus Infections

The LCMV infection, other murine viruses—vaccinia, herpes simplex, pichinde, murine cytomegalovirus—and human viruses such as EBV induce the generation of not only virus-specific CTLs but also CTLs capable of lysing uninfected allogeneic target cells (52–56). These effector cells are typical CD3+, CD8+, $\alpha\beta$ TCR+ T cells recognizing allogeneic MHC-I antigens. Much of the allospecific CTL induction during the LCMV infection can be accounted for by individual T cell clones cross-reacting between allogeneic targets and virus-modified self targets (57). Cross-reactivity of T cells against two different targets is a common event often noted during analyses of defined CTL clones in other systems (58–62). Using an interesting mathematic model, Mason calculated that one T cell has the potential to react productively with approximately 10^6 different MHC-associated minimal peptide epitopes (63). This capacity of individual T cells to recognize several antigens can thus result in an antigen-specific response that is quite degenerate. In the LCMV infection of C57BL/6 (H-2^b) mice, about 10% of the LCMV-specific pCTLs in either the acute infection or the memory state cross react with the H-2^k alloantigens (Fig. 25-3) (57). Thus a history of infection with an immunogenic virus can influence an individual's responsiveness to alloantigens.

This activation of allo-cross-reactive T cells during acute virus infection may underlie the observed clinical association between viral status and graft-versus-host disease and transplant rejection (64–67). These associations have been shown with several types of herpes virus infections, including that of EBV (64–67). Analyses of the B8-restricted response to the immunodominant EBV

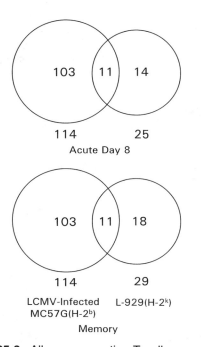

FIG. 25-3. Allo-cross-reactive T cell responses during the LCMV infection. Shown here is the target specificity of LCMV-induced C57BL/6 mouse (H-2^b) short-term T cell clones propagated on LCMV-infected C57BL/6 peritoneal cells. T cells were either isolated from 8-day infected mice or from mice several weeks after clearance of the LCMV infection. H-2^k-specific T cells cross-reactive with LCMV-infected syngeneic targets are elicited during acute infection and remain present in the memory response. [These data were derived from Nahill and Welsh (57).]

EBNA 3A 325 (FLRGRAYGL) epitope showed that a subset of the epitope-specific memory CTL clones also mediated cross-reactive lysis of uninfected target cells expressing the B44.02 alloantigen (52). B8 individuals co-expressing B44.02 generated B8-restricted CTLs to the EBNA 3A 325 epitope, but their CTLs did not lyse uninfected B44.02 targets, presumably because those individuals were tolerant to self-peptide-presenting B44.02 (68). Similar levels of self tolerance were seen in the LCMV system (55–57). EBV-induced CTLs from the B8 individuals have recently been shown also to lyse uninfected targets expressing B14 or

B35.01 alloantigens (69,70). Some evidence suggests that the cross-reactive allospecific response against B35.01 targets was directed against an endogenous peptide derived from liver-specific cytochrome p450 (69,70). This is an interesting example of molecular mimicry with potential relevance to the pathogenesis of autoimmune hepatitis, a liver disease with a suspected EBV association and a strong link to HLA-B8 (71).

Research into the molecular mechanism for alloreactivity has been strongly driven by the significant mortality and morbidity during organ transplantation caused by the high frequency of alloreactive T cells. Two studies examining the biomolecular nature of the interaction between antigen-specific T cell clones recognizing an alloantigen have demonstrated that the mechanism is consistent with true molecular mimicry; that is, the cross-reactive antigen-specific T cell recognizes the allo-MHC molecule and the self-peptide together, but the sites of interaction with the TCR are different from those with the syngeneic MHC and foreign antigen (72,73).

Reactivation of Cross-Reactive Memory CTLs by Heterologous Virus Infection

Memory CTLs specific for one virus can be reactivated and contribute to the primary CTL response to heterologous viruses not considered related to the first virus. Infection of LCMV-immune mice with Pichinde virus (PV), vaccinia virus (VV), or murine cytomegalovirus (MCMV) caused reactivation of LCMV-specific CTLs as measured in bulk cytotoxicity assays (55,74). During the early phase of a PV infection in an LCMV-immune mouse LDAs demonstrated a significant frequency of memory LCMV-specific T cells cross-reactive with PV (35,74). Immunity to either of these viruses normally yields only a few pCTLs specific for the heterologous virus. However, PV infection of LCMV-immune mice induces a much larger population of T cells reactive with both viruses. Splenocytes from an LCMV-immune mouse 5 days after infection with PV and stimulated *in vitro* with PV yielded 1 of 4,068 pCTLs as LCMV-specific and 1 of 1,508 pCTLs as PV-specific. By day 7 of the PV infection the PV-specific pCTL is predominant (1/280 pCTLs per splenocyte) with still 1 of 3,846 pCTLs recognizing LCMV-infected targets.

Of the short-term clones derived from splenocytes in LCMV-immune mice acutely infected for 6 days with PV and grown on PV-infected APCs 21% of the clones that lysed PV-infected targets also lysed LCMV-infected targets (Fig. 25-4) (74). It is noteworthy that 58% of those LCMV-specific clones propagated on PV-infected APCs lysed both LCMV-infected targets and PV-infected targets, the other 42% lysed only the LCMV-infected targets (Fig. 25-4). This phenomenon of preferential lysis against targets different from the stimulating cells was similar to that reported for cross-reactive T cell responses between viral antigens and alloantigens (Fig. 25-3) (57). This observation could be explained by affinity differences or altered TCR signaling depending on

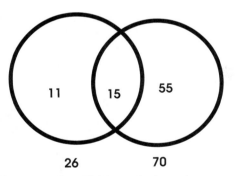

FIG. 25-4. Specificities of the short term, Pichinde virus (PV)-induced CTL clones derived from PV-infected LCMV-immune mice. CD8 clones were generated from LCMV-immune C57BL/6 mice acutely infected with PV for 6 days and grown on PV-infected APCs. The CD8 clones derived this way were tested for what proportion of the clones specifically lysed LCMV-infected targets, PV-infected targets, or both. During an acute PV infection of LCMV-immune mice CD8 clones were generated that were cross-reactive and lysed both types of target. [The data on which this model is based are from Selin et al. (74).]

the antigen, resulting in different functional responses. Anti-CD8 can block low-affinity CTL responses but not high-affinity CTL responses. Nearly all of the LCMV-specific lysis but only some of the PV-specific lysis by T cells propagated on PV-infected APCs is blocked by anti-CD8, suggesting that those LCMV-immune T cells that are stimulated by PV probably have low affinity for LCMV (74).

There are many examples of well defined T cell clones and lines that cross-react between relatively unrelated peptide sequences. An influenza A NP-specific CTL line lysed not only NP peptide-sensitized targets but also targets sensitized with two different influenza A basic polymerase 2 (PB2) peptides (75). An HLA-A2.1-restricted CTL line induced by an influenza A matrix peptide also recognized in a cross-reactive manner a human rotavirus VP4 peptide (76). An H-2K^d-restricted influenza-specific clone recognized two distinct influenza peptides from HA and NS1 (77). Immunization of mice with a VV recombinant of the M2 protein of respiratory syncytial virus (RSV) induced CTLs that lysed in a cross-reactive manner targets sensitized with either of two peptides derived from different nonoverlapping regions of the same M2 protein (78). Some of these cross-reactive peptides have relatively little amino acid homology, with the exception that the peptides complied with the sequence motif for the presenting MHC molecule.

Cross-reactivity at the T cell level obviously is much less dependent on conserved linear sequences of several amino acids and is most likely dependent on the three-dimensional structure of the peptide bound to the MHC peptide-binding groove, such as has been described earlier for allo-cross-reactive responses (72,73). Therefore when thousands of T cell clones are examined by LDA methods, the probability of finding cross-reactive clones between apparently unrelated viruses increases greatly. It is not surprising that the introduction of a second virus into a host with a high frequency of memory T cells from a previous virus infection would result in the activation of cross-reactive memory T cells, especially because memory cells can be stimulated by lower affinity interactions than those with naive cells.

Evaluation of Bystander Stimulation of T Cells During Acute Virus Infections

Some investigators have suggested that non-specific bystander activation of T cells not specific for the virus plays a major role in the acute CD8 T cell proliferative response (14,79–81). This argument has been partially negated by the recent direct quantification studies indicating that most of the activated T cells present during an acute virus infection are virus-specific; but those studies did not completely rule out that there still could be some nonspecific activation of CD8 T cells. In fact, type I interferon and IL-15, cytokines liberated at high levels during viral infections, appear to stimulate DNA synthesis in memory (CD44$^+$) CD8 T cells, suggesting that some bystander events are occurring (14,16). However, experiments specifically designed to address directly whether T cells not specific for a virus increase in number during infection argue that bystander proliferation contributes little to the virus-induced CD8 T cell response (Fig. 25-5) (82). In HY-TCR transgenic C57BL/6 mice, about 30% of the CD8 cells express an HY (male antigen)-specific transgenic TCR that is not cross-reactive with LCMV. In HY-transgenic mice harboring a limited T cell repertoire and in HY-transgenic mice replenished with a complete T cell repertoire by adoptive transfer of normal spleen cells, the acute LCMV infection caused activation and expansion of non-HY-specific T cells, but the HY-specific cells remained small, did not increase in number, and there was no increase in the frequency of blast size HY T cells or of cells expressing the activation phenotype of CD62L^{low} and CD44^{high}. A similar result was observed in mice harboring CD44^{high} memory phenotype HY-specific T cells, resulting as a consequence of *in vivo* stimulation in a male mouse and then parking these cells into

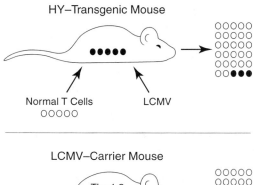

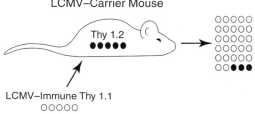

FIG. 25-5. Models for examining the fate of T cells not specific for the virus during a virus-specific T cell response. **Top:** HY-TCR transgenic mice, in which the transgenic T cells are not cross-reactive with the virus, LCMV. Transfer of a normal T cell repertoire into these mice along with an LCMV infection results in expansion of the CD8 T cells but no expansion (in fact, a decrease) in the number of HY-specific T cells. **Bottom:** LCMV-carrier Thy 1.2 mice congenitally and persistently infected and tolerant to LCMV antigens. Into these mice are transferred LCMV-immune Thy 1.1 T cells, which vigorously become activated and expand in number, but the host T cells do not expand and, in fact, decrease in number. [These models are based on that described by Zarozinski and Welsh (82).]

a female $\alpha\beta$ TCR-KO mouse. In each case there was a *decrease* in the total number of HY-positive cells per spleen after virus infection. These results strongly argue that bystander proliferation of nonspecific cells contributes little to the magnitude of the virus-induced CD8 T cell response.

The fact that many T cell clones are cross-reactive between alloantigens and virus-modified self-antigens does not rule out the possibility that some of the allospecific CTL response induced during virus infections is a consequence of bystander stimulation. Evidence against this concept of bystander stimulation of allospecific CTLs was provided by additional experiments using LCMV-infected HY-TCR-transgenic mice (82). T cells from these mice generated comparable levels of anti-H-2^d- and anti-H-2^k-allospecific CTLs in mixed lymphocyte cultures. CTLs to both of those allospecificities are normally elicited by LCMV infection of normal C57BL/6 mice; but in the HY-mice, which have a restricted T cell repertoire, the LCMV infection stimulated the generation of H-2^k- but not H-2^d-specific CTLs. This is an argument against LCMV-induced bystander stimulation of allospecific CTLs, as only one of the two specificities was engendered by the LCMV infection in this limited TCR milieu. These results support the concept that many of the virus-specific CD8 cells induced during an acute virus infection may be cross-reactive and argues against this allospecific CTL activity as being a consequence of bystander activation.

The existence of T cell cross-reactivity between viruses does not rule out that memory T cells could also be nonspecifically activated by cytokines produced during the T cell response to the second infection. It has been shown in an LCMV GP33-epitope specific TCR-transgenic host that VV and *Listeria monocytogenes* infections, as well as high-dose IL-2, could cytolytically activate these LCMV-specific transgenic T cells (81). These experiments must be interpreted with some caution, as there is the possibility that heterologous infectious agents are cross-reactively stimulating the TCRs of the transgenic T cells. In contrast, the experiments using HY-transgenic mice and LCMV persistently infected mice suggest that bystander proliferation of non-cross-reactive T cells is minimal during infection (82).

Differential Stimulation of TCRs

The subject of T cell "specificity" is complex because a "specific" interaction of a TCR with its peptide–MHC ligand does not always result in the same type of response. Peptide–MHC complexes can be classified as: *agonists,* which deliver a rather complete positive signal to the T cell; *partial agonists,* which may stimulate certain (e.g., cytolytic activity) but not other (e.g., IFN-γ production) activities of the T cells; and *antagonists,* which can act dominantly to inhibit T cell function (83–90). Some of the differences between agonists and partial agonists relate to differences in affinities between the TCR and the peptide–MHC complex; and these translate into differences in phosphorylation of signal transduction molecules (89,90). Extremely strong agonists may also have the paradoxical ability to be particularly effective at driving T cells into apoptosis. One must therefore be careful about concluding that a T cell is not specific for a particular antigen or virus. Such issues as cross-reactivity and differential stimulation have relevance when memory CTLs are exposed to heterologous antigens, such as those encoded by another pathogen, as discussed.

APOPTOSIS PHASE AND THE GENERATION OF T CELL MEMORY

General Features of Apoptosis in T Cell Regulation

The vigorous proliferation of lymphocytes during the induction period of immune responses can occur at the rate of three cell divisions a day and therefore must be tightly regulated, as the host otherwise would risk damage from overzealous cytokine production and the potential for developing autoimmunity or leukemia. Of the body's organ systems, the immune system is the only one called on to double or triple in size and then return to a normal homeostatic state, all within a few days. To accomplish this homeostatic regulation, lymphocyte proliferation is tightly regulated by both proliferative and apoptotic signals. T cells are stimulated most efficiently from the resting state, where TCR–ligand events and the interactions of co-stimulatory molecules combine to induce cell proliferation. Among the early molecules expressed during this process is Bcl-X$_L$, an antiapoptotic member of the Bcl-2 family of proteins that regulate the activity of a group of cysteine aspartases (caspases), which act in a cascade to mediate apoptosis (91,92). Bcl-X$_L$ expression therefore protects cells from their innate tendency to undergo apoptosis as they pass through the cell cycle. Proliferating T cells ultimately lose Bcl-X$_L$ expression and instead express CD95 (Fas) and Fas ligand (FasL) (93,94). These highly activated cells become less stable and can be induced into apoptosis on strong TCR signaling by a process known as "activation-induced cell death" (AICD), which is normally a Fas-dependent process (95). The Fas signaling pathway is initiated on crosslinking of Fas with FasL. This stimulates the Fas-activated death domain (FADD), which activates the caspase FLICE (FADD-like IL-1 convertase enzyme) and initiates the caspase cascade (93,94). In some circumstances of AICD, tumor necrosis factor-α (TNF-α)– TNF receptor interactions may substitute for Fas–FasL interactions, particularly in activated CD8 T cells (96). The ligated TNF receptor engages the adaptor molecule TRADD (TNF receptor-associated death domain), which bridges the TNF receptor with FADD (93,94). Apoptosis of activated T cells is not only driven through TCRs; it can also occur through less defined mechanisms, such as by growth factor deprivation due to the removal of IL-2 (97,98). Expression of Bcl-2, which decreases in highly activated cells, can inhibit growth factor deprivation-induced apoptosis (91,92,98). During the complex process of a viral infection, apoptosis may be driven by such processes as AICD, growth factor deprivation, or exposure of activated cells to toxic cytokines, steroids, or other metabolites (99).

Silencing of the Immune Response and Generation of T Cell Memory

Low-dose LCMV infection induces a peak CTL response at 8 to 9 days after infection (Fig. 25-1). At that time there is a five- to tenfold increase in the total number of CD8 T cells per spleen; the CD4/CD8 ratio has changed from 2:1 to 1:2 or 1:3; and the spleen, as a consequence of T cell and B cell hyperplasia, has doubled in size. One week thereafter the CD4 and CD8 T cell numbers and ratios are back to normal, and the spleen has undergone a substantial loss in total splenocyte number (Fig. 25-2B). This loss in cell number is heralded by a peak at day 11 in apoptotic cells, as detected in spleen tissue sections by an *in situ* nucleotidyl transferase (TUNEL) assay, which measures fragmented DNA in cells in tissue sections or as detected in incubated freshly isolated T cell preparations (Fig. 25-6) (98,100). Thus the silencing phase of the immune response to infection is mediated at least in part by apoptotic events. Factors regulating this apoptosis remain unclear. The timing of this apoptotic peak is shortly after the clearance of viral antigens and the decline in the production of IL-2, which is needed to maintain T cell proliferation. Thus apoptosis associated with the silencing phase of the T cell response may be caused by growth factor deprivation, though this does not rule out the effects of inhibitory cytokines or steroids. Apoptosis during this silencing phase occurs relatively normally in mice bearing mutations in Fas (*lpr* mutation), FasL (*gld* mutation), or harboring Bcl-2 transgenes in their T and B cells (98,101–103). In systems of LCMV infections using TCR transgenic LCMV-specific T cells, there is a normal decline in the number of the transgenic T cells, even when they are double transgenic and have enforced expression of Bcl-X$_L$ or Bcl-2 transgenes (103). One might have predicted that these transgenes would protect against a growth-factor-deprivation-induced apoptosis, but the down-regulatory event *in vivo* must supersede any protective effects mediated by those antiapoptotic transgenes.

Although there is much selection of the TCR repertoire during the induction phase of the T cell response, it is less clear whether any selection occurs during the apoptotic phase, nor is it known what determines which T cells survive and which undergo apoptosis. Limiting dilution assays for pCTL CD8 cells

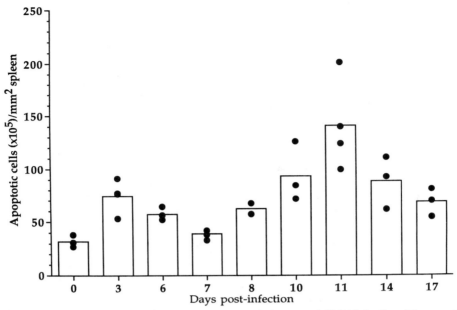

FIG. 25-6. Leukocyte expansion, decline, and apoptosis in acute LCMV infection. The numbers of apoptotic cells in the spleen as assessed by the *in situ* nucleotidyl transferase assay demonstrate an increase in apoptotic splenic lymphocytes initially early in LCMV infection (at day 3) and an even greater increase at day 11 after infection as the acute response downregulates and returns to homeostasis. Each *data point* represents one mouse; *bars* show averages of the individual data points. [This figure is based on data from Razvi et al. (98).]

and for precursor T-helper (pTh) IL-2-producing CD4 cells and the enumeration of implanted LCMV-specific TCR transgenic T cells all reveal about a twofold loss in virus-specific cells per T cell between the peak of the acute infection and the memory state (Fig. 25-2A) (6,26,36). Tetrameric staining data and peptide-specific IFN-γ-producing cell data, however, reveal about a sixfold reduction in the proportion of LCMV-specific T cells between the peak of infection and memory (47,49). The numbers of LCMV-specific T cells detected by tetramer binding or LDA in the memory state are fairly similar. This difference in the techniques between the acute and memory responses may reflect the possibility that some of the tetramer-staining CD8 T cells in the acute infection have not yet differentiated into a form in which they can become memory cells (as detected in LDA), or it could be due to the

enhanced sensitivity of the acute CD8 cells to apoptosis. In either case the efficiency of the LDA, compared to the tetramer staining assay, would be compromised. The use of vital dyes to follow the phenotype of TCR transgenic CD8 cells after exposure to LCMV antigen has shown that CD8 cells change in their expression of cell surface markers with successive cell divisions and are likely to be in different states of differentiation *in vivo* (27). Not all differentiation stages may give rise to precursors during the acute response, but the memory CD8 cells in the immune state may be in a differentiation state that allows them to respond to antigen. Another possible explanation to the dichotomy in techniques is that the higher-affinity cells (i.e., the pCTLs, pTh IL-2-producing cells, and transgenic cells) are preserved with more efficiency into the memory state, but more work needs to be done to determine that this is clearly the case. CDR3 spectratype analyses (see Evolution of CD8 T Cell Repertoire, below) show many LCMV-induced dominant clones at the peak of infection; and virtually all of them remain present as the immune system contracts by apoptosis and enters the memory state (104). This argues against repertoire selection during the apoptosis phase, but it does not exclude the possibility of selective loss of very low affinity cells, as spectratype analyses detect dominant clones that may be of sufficiently high affinity for preservation into the memory state. Neither the Bcl-2 transgene nor the *lpr* or *gld* mutations have much effect on the memory T cell levels after infection (98,101,102).

Stability of T Cell Memory

After the apoptotic phase of the T cell response a portion of the antigen-specific T cells enter the memory pool, and thereafter memory T cells remain remarkably stable at a high level. LCMV-specific memory in C57BL/6 mice is maintained at 1:50 (2%) pCTL per CD8 cells, as measured against LCMV-infected targets (6). Using more sensitive techniques, such as immunodominant peptide-coated targets (Selin et al., in preparation), the total LCMV-specific pCTLs per CD8 is 5%, and by peptide-specific tetramer staining it is 10% (47). The LCMV-encoded immunodominant peptides also each represent a fixed portion of this total LCMV-specific CD8 response, and their relative proportion remains fixed from the peak of the acute response into memory, remaining stable throughout the lifetime of the host (6). When mice exist in a highly controlled environment and do not encounter any other pathogens, the CD8 memory response not only to LCMV but also to other viruses such as PV, VV, influenza virus, and Sendai virus in mice (6,105–107), remain high and remarkably stable. Over a 3-year period influenza memory in humans also remained stable (42,108).

Precursor CD4 T cells, as detected by their ability to secrete IL-2, are at an approximately 10- to 20-fold lower frequency per CD4 cell than pCTL/CD8 cells; but their frequencies are also quite stable between the peak of acute infection (~1/600) and memory (~1/1,200), as with CD8 T cells, and remain stable for the lifetime of the host (29,86). Intracellular IFN-γ assays detect a much higher percentage of antigen-specific CD4 cells during infection, as nearly 10% of the CD4 cells are specific for two of the LCMV-encoded MHC-II peptides. These IFN-γ-producing cell frequencies decline approximately sixfold per CD4 cell between the peak of acute infection and memory (49). It is clear that in a controlled environment after the apoptotic phase the CD4 and CD8 T cell memory becomes heavily biased and remains stable for the lifetime of the host.

T Cell Clonal Exhaustion and Loss of Memory

Virus-specific CTL responses can be ablated under conditions of high antigen load during some viral infections, such as during the late stages of human immunodeficiency virus (HIV) infection, overwhelming hepatitis virus infections, and high-dose infection with rapidly disseminating LCMV strains (109–112). The balance between antigen dose and the T cell response can be tipped such that instead of an infection resolving in antigen clearance and the development of long-term CTL memory the virus becomes persistent and the CTLs are cleared. Such clearance of memory CTLs is most often seen with viral infections that are not overwhelmingly cytopathic, as it is likely that the host would not survive a T cell clonal exhaustion with highly disseminating, highly cytopathic viruses.

Clonal exhaustion under conditions of high-dose LCMV infection has been demonstrated by the loss of memory pCTLs detected in LDAs (101,110), by the disappearance of LCMV-specific TCR transgenic T cells (110), by the loss of CD8 cells enumerated by tetramer staining (113), and by CDR3 spectratype analyses (88). Work with transgenic T cells has suggested that T cells may undergo a period of anergy before they disappear, and that CD8 cells may be driven into clonal exhaustion sooner than CD4 T cells (114).

The mechanism of clonal exhaustion remains unclear, though it is likely to reflect an apoptotic mechanism, as delivery of high doses of an LCMV GP33 peptide into mice directly induces observable apoptosis in GP33-specific transgenic T cells (115). Some work has suggested that the killing of professional APCs by LCMV-specific CTLs during the high-dose infection may result in elimination of survival factors for the CTLs (111,116). Of note is that clonal exhaustion is defective in mice lacking the gene for perforin, which is important for CTL killing (113). Under those perforin-deficient conditions there is a high antigen load, but the APCs, which may be producing survival factors, are not eliminated.

Although it is compelling to speculate that clonal exhaustion is mediated by AICD mechanisms, clonal exhaustion occurs in mice mutant in Fas, FasL, or lacking IFN-γ receptors, even though T cells from such LCMV-infected mutant mice resist AICD *in vitro* (101,102). It should be noted, however, that the TNF/TNF receptor system may provide an alternative pathway for AICD, and experiments have not been done in mice deficient in both the Fas and the TNF pathways (96). An analogous paradox has been observed with antiapoptotic proteins. LCMV GP33-specific double transgenic T cells harboring either the Bcl-2 or Bcl-X$_L$ transgene resisted deletion *in vivo* under conditions of high-dose GP33 peptide treatment, but they still underwent clonal exhaustion during the normal course of the high-dose LCMV infection (103). Thus the mechanism of clonal exhaustion is not resolved.

EVOLUTION OF CD8 T CELL REPERTOIRE

Studies on T cell responses to viral infections have focused on both the specificity of the T cells and the molecular nature of the TCR

used in the response. The initial encounter of a T cell with an APC is probably a stochastic process, presumably leading to a competitive advantage for the first cell encountering antigen. Thereafter it is presumed that cells with TCRs of high affinity to the antigen would have a competitive advantage, assuming that they are not stimulated so strongly they undergo AICD. Only recently has the evolution of the T cell repertoire been systematically studied in response to viruses and other antigens. These analyses strongly suggest that the continued evolution of the CD8 T cell repertoire depends on both the presence of the antigen and the antigen load. In situations where infectious agents are cleared, the T cell repertoire becomes significantly skewed but stops evolving after clearance of the virus (6,104), resulting in a memory CD8 T cell repertoire that reflects the skewed repertoire elicited during the acute infection (6,7,47,104,117,118). In contrast, the T cell repertoire continues to evolve in the presence of antigen, such as during persistent infections (81,104,119,120), or by repeated stimulation of antigen by secondary exposure (121). Persistent infections resulting from high antigen load lead to a loss of memory CD8 T cells due to T cell clonal exhaustion and to conversion of the repertoire to a more naive form (101,104,110,113).

The technologies described earlier in this chapter defined T cells in terms of their specificity but did not evaluate any changes in TCR usage that may develop during the progression of an infection. One way to study the T cell repertoire has been to analyze TCR sequences of peptide-specific T cell lines or clones by polymerase chain reaction (PCR) amplification of the TCR message and DNA sequencing of the cloned PCR products. Another new molecular technique now being widely applied to viral infections is CDR3 length spectratyping, which is based on the fact that TCR VDJ recombination events result in different-length regions of the complementarity-determining region (CDR3) antigen-binding domain of the TCR (122). The size distribution of CDR3 regions in a normal

T cell population is gaussian, but a strong dominant clone can disrupt this distribution and give a characteristic "spectratype." This technique entails amplification of TCR mRNA by reverse transcriptase (RT)-PCR and analysis of Vβ and/or Jβ usage by primer extension reactions across the CDR3. These different-sized products are run on sequencing gels to display the spectratype of sizes, and an increase in the height and area of a particular peak signals expansion of T cell clones. Therefore one can obtain distinct CDR3 profiles to detect changes of TCR repertoire during infection. Spectratype analyses of the T cell response to the low-dose and high-dose LCMV systems support the conclusions on repertoire selection mentioned above.

Evolution of the CD8 T Cell Repertoire When Infectious Agents Are Cleared

Evolution of the CD8 T cell repertoire from acute infection into memory has been well studied in mice infected with low-dose LCMV (6,7,47,104,117) and, to some degree, of mice infected with *Listeria monocytogenes* (102). Several approaches, including LDA (6,7), MHC-I–peptide tetramer staining, intracellular IFN-γ staining, TCR "fingerprint" analyses (47,117), and CDR3 length spectratyping (104,117), have been applied to the LCMV system. The results derived from these approaches invariably show that the diverse TCR repertoire during the acute infection stops evolving after the virus is cleared and is then preserved into memory.

The LDA data showed that the ratios of three immunodominant peptide (GP33, GP276, NP396)-specific pCTLs to total LCMV-specific pCTLs remained unchanged after day 7 of infection, when virus was cleared (6). Analyses of MHC-I–peptide tetramer and Vβ antibody staining showed that the LCMV-specific memory CD8 T cell repertoire was similar to the primary effector CD8 T cell repertoire (117). In addition, functional TCR fingerprinting based on recognition of variant peptides derived from

NP118-126 in BALB/C mice suggested that the finger prints of the LCMV immunodominant peptide-specific CD8 T cells were almost identical in the primary response and in the memory pool (117).

CDR3 length spectratyping showed that the acute LCMV infection expanded a broad spectrum of Vβ8.1 T cells (104) specific for three of the immunodominant peptides (GP33, GP276, NP396). Analyses of the Vβ8.1 T cell repertoire showed that genetically identical mice generated remarkably different T cell responses to the same virus, as reflected by different spectratypes (Fig. 25-7) and different TCR sequences in same-sized bands. However, a conserved motif was detected in the CDR3 region within some same-size bands. This observation of individual variation in TCR repertoire usage but preservation of conserved motifs has also been observed in the CD8 T cell response to a defined peptide derived from a human HLA-CW3 MHC molecule and presented by a mouse MHC (121). This variation of T cell usage between individual animals may be a consequence of a stochastic process, whereby the T cell that randomly encounters a T cell antigen first has a selective advantage over other T cells that have receptors with comparable affinity to the antigen. Alternatively, the starting population may be different as a consequence of prior exposure to environmental antigens or as a consequence of a random generation of the T cell repertoire during thymic selection. Interestingly, recent work from Bousso et al. demonstrated that even in the naive state mice displayed important individual variations in their HLA-A2 peptide-specific repertoire, suggesting that the starting antigen-specific T cell repertoire can be different among mice (123). Some conclusions have been made based on comparisons of spectratypes between different mice (117), but because of the individual variation among mice, meaningful studies on the evolution of the T cell repertoire require longitudinal studies within individual mice.

Longitudinal studies in LCMV-infected mice showed that spectratypes began to

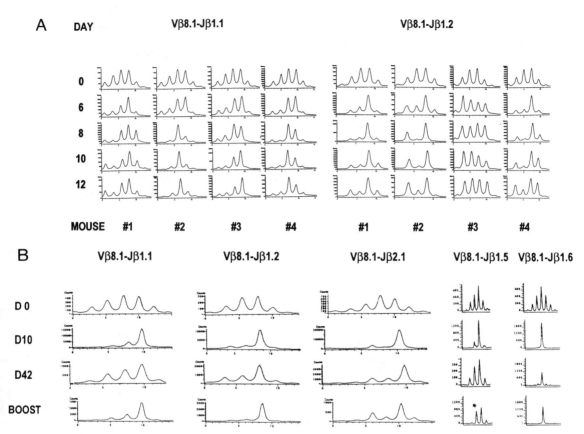

FIG. 25-7. Evolution of the Vβ8.1 spectratypes throughout the acute LCMV infection, into memory and secondary responses. **A:** The Vβ8.1 spectratypes remained stable during the T cell apoptosis phase from days 8 to 12 after LCMV infection. The representative CDR3 profiles from the peripheral blood lymphocytes (PBLs) of four acutely LCMV-infected mice at days 6 to 12 after infection are displayed. Because the naive spectratypes invariably have a normal gaussian distribution, day 0 spectratypes plotted at the top of each columns were from the same two naive control mice. The PCR products were subjected to runoff reactions using [γ-^{33}P]-ATP-labeled Jβ primers. **B:** The Vβ8.1 spectratypes in the immune state resembled those of acute LCMV infection, and most of the spectratypes detected in the primary infection were preserved during secondary infection. The CDR3 profiles were obtained from PBLs of one mouse at days 10 and 42 after primary LCMV infection and at day 5 after secondary infection. Day 0 spectratypes were obtained from a naive control. For a secondary infection, a newly formed peak in Jβ1.5 is marked with an *asterisk*. The runoff reactions were primed with [γ-^{33}P]-ATP-labeled primers (Jβ1.1, Jβ1.2, and Jβ2.1) or with fluorescent Jβ primers (Jβ1.5, Jβ1.6). [These figures are derived from data in Lin and Welsh (104).]

change by day 5, evolved to a distinct spectrum by day 8, and remained stable from days 8 to 12 after LCMV infection, suggesting that there was no further selection of the LCMV-induced T cell repertoire after clearance of the virus and during the apoptosis phase (Fig. 25-7). DNA sequence data obtained from

direct sequencing of dominant singular peaks at days 8 and 12 after infection further supported the finding that the LCMV-induced T cell repertoire remained unchanged during the apoptosis phase (104).

The LDA data originally showed that a high frequency of LCMV-specific pCTLs remained remarkably stable throughout the lifetime of the mouse (6,7), and recent work using MHC-I–peptide tetramer staining, IFN-γ Elispot and intracellular assays, and CDR3 length spectratyping assays has demonstrated that the dominant and subdominant LCMV peptide-specific CD8 T cells were equally well maintained in long-term memory and that the number of LCMV peptide-specific memory CD8 T cells remained at high levels (47,104). MHC tetramer binding analyses have shown that 10% or more of the CD8 T cells in the memory state can be defined as LCMV-specific. Thus a substantial proportion of LCMV-induced T cells can be stably preserved into long-term memory, and the consequence is a significant skewing of the host T cell repertoire.

Evolution of the CD8 T Cell Repertoire During Persistent Infections

In contrast to the stable CD8 T cell repertoires detected after clearance of the infectious agents, the T cell repertoires continue to evolve during persistent infections (104). Persistent infections resulting from high antigen load can lead to a loss of memory CD8 T cells due to T cell clonal exhaustion (Fig. 25-1B). In contrast, oligoclonal memory CD8 T cell repertoires reflecting part of the primary CD8 effector T cell repertoire are detected in persistent infections associated with latent viruses that sporadically become reactivated.

Persistent infections associated with clonal exhaustion due to high antigen load have been described in the high-dose LCMV infections of mice (101,104,110,113), in chronic hepatitis B infection in humans (124), and possibly in HIV patients (112). Analyses of memory CD8 T cells by LDA, by MHC-I–peptide tetramer staining, and by analysis of TCR-transgenic T cells have demonstrated that the virus-specific memory T cells were undetectable under conditions of clonal exhaustion by high-dose LCMV clone 13 or LCMV-Docile infections (101,110,113). Direct ex vivo analysis of the TCR repertoire

by CDR3 length spectratyping showed that, in contrast to the low-dose model where the T cell repertoire became fixed by day 8 after infection, the T cell repertoire continued to evolve from day 7 to day 13 and for several weeks thereafter. Ultimately, however, the spectratypes returned to a naive repertoire-like gaussian distribution, reflective of the clonal exhaustion of the LCMV-specific T cells (104). Studies on hepatitis B virus (HBV) infection used a strategy involving in vitro stimulation of peripheral blood mononuclear cells (PBMCs) with HBV-derived synthetic peptides containing HLA binding motifs to identify epitopes in the HBV nucleoprotein, envelope, and polymerase (124–126). The results demonstrated polyclonal and multispecific CTL responses detectable in PBMCs for more than a year after complete clinical recovery and clearance of virus from the blood. In contrast, CTL responses were not detectable in peripheral blood of patients with chronic HBV infection (124), indicating either clonal exhaustion or an exclusive homing of the CTL to the liver (127). At late stages of the HIV infection, when the CD4 T cell levels have collapsed, the HIV antigen load rises and a selective loss in HIV-specific CD8 pCTLs occurs even though EBV-specific pCTLs are still detected (112). Taken together, these results demonstrate that high antigen load can lead to the disappearance of the virus-specific TCR repertoire.

Many human infections involve latent viruses such as EBV that sporadically reactivate and restimulate the immune system. Analyses of the EBV-specific CD8 T cell lines or clones have demonstrated that only a subset of T cells generated during the acute response are preserved into long-term memory. A longitudinal study on infectious mononucleosis patients of different HLA types showed that differences in the relative frequencies of CTLs to immunodominant versus subdominant epitopes appeared to be much less marked in memory than in primary populations, arguing for continued evolution of the response. In one example, an

EBNA3A peptide-specific pCTL detected during the primary response could not be found in memory (120). Similar continued evolution of CTL responses has been seen in individuals infected with human cytomegalovirus (HCMV) and HIV. A report on memory CTL responses to HCMV has analyzed the clonal composition of the memory CTL response to four epitopes of HCMV tegument protein pp65 by sequencing the TCRs of multiple independently derived CTL clones from healthy virus carriers (128). The results showed a narrow repertoire of CTLs from different donors recognizing similar peptide–MHC complexes, and CTL clones specific to a defined pp65 epitope from any one virus carrier used only one or two different TCR sequences in the TCR α- and β-chain. A limited TCR repertoire has also been described in long-term HIV infections prior to the late stages associated with clonal exhaustion. One report addressed the breadth and duration of the CD8 T cell response to an HIV glycoprotein 41 (gp 41) epitope within an individual by analyzing ten CTL clones isolated at multiple time points over 31 months from an asymptomatic HIV-1-infected individual (129). All ten clones used Vα14 and Vβ4 genes, and nine of the isolated clones shared identical TCR sequences, again indicating a narrow repertoire during a persistent infection. This high degree of clonal focusing was also seen by analysis of TCR Vβ usage in HIV-specific T cells identified by tetramer staining (130). This continued evolution and focusing of memory T cell responses to EBV, CMV, and HIV infections is likely due to the continued stimulation of T cells with persistent antigen.

Evolution of the CD8 T Cell Repertoire Under Conditions of Secondary Stimulation

Individuals may completely clear a virus infection but in the case of ubiquitous viruses may become reexposed to antigens in the environment. As we described above for persistent infections, repeated antigenic stimula-

tion leads to a continued evolution of the TCR repertoire. Basic studies on TCR evolution under conditions of secondary antigen exposure have examined mouse CD8 T cell responses to a human HLA-CW3 peptide presented in the context of H-2K^d in HLA-CW3-transfected P-815 (H-2^d) cells. The HLA-CW3 170-179 epitope-specific T cell repertoire mostly used Vβ10-Jβ1.2 and was analyzed by single-cell PCR analysis (121). For each of the mice analyzed, 40% to 100% of the TCRs amplified during the primary response were found in the secondary infection. In general, most of the T cell clones in the secondary response were similar to those in the primary response, although some additional clones did develop. Similar conclusions were reached after CDR3 spectratype analyses of LCMV-immune mice following a secondary *in vivo* stimulation with LCMV (Fig. 25-7), when it was shown that the relative frequency of NP-specific CTLs increases (Selin et al., in preparation). Most of the dominant spectratype bands present in the acute infection were amplified, and some additional bands appeared (104). These results indicate that some additional evolution of the TCR repertoire occurs during secondary stimulation, but changes in the repertoire are not as dramatic as those seen with persistent infections.

MAINTENANCE OF T CELL MEMORY

Life-Span of Memory T Cells

Memory T cells appear to be a long-lived, complex population of cells. At any given time in an LCMV-immune mouse approximately 10% to 20% of the CD8 pool were found to be blast-sized and in cell cycle (28). By LDA analysis approximately 60% of the polyclonal LCMV-specific pCTLs were present in the CD62L^{high} subset and 40% in the CD62L^{low} subset. The CD62L^{high} group could be further subdivided phenotypically and functionally. One group of these CD62L^{high} memory T cells expressed IL-2α (CD25) receptors was in cell cycle, and did not require exogenous IL-2 during *in vitro* restimulation with antigen to become functional CTLs. A second group of these CD62L[high] memory T cells was noncycling, was small, lacked IL-2Rα, and did require exogenous IL-2 to be activated *in vitro* into functional CTLs. The CD62L[low] T cell subset was small, was noncycling, and did not require exogenous IL-2 for activation *in vitro* into functional CTLs. Other studies using the LCMV TCR transgenic mouse model, which has 80% to 90% GP33-specific CD8 cells, have demonstrated by fluorescent staining that the memory transgenic cells can exist in fairly equal proportions as both CD44[high], CD62L[high] and as CD44[high], CD62L[low] (26,27). These studies did not directly examine the functional characteristics of these two memory subsets.

It is not clear if the resting (80–90%) and cycling (10–20%) memory CD8 cells represent two distinct populations or if over some period of time all the memory cells undergo cell division. As the total number of memory CTLs, under controlled environmental conditions, remains relatively constant, this amount of turnover must be enough to compensate for the rate of cell death. Studies using continuous BrdU labeling of memory GP33-specific CD8 cells in transgenic mice (26) or memory phenotype cells (CD44[high], CD62L[low]) in mice not immunized with a known pathogen (79,80,131) suggested that during a 7- to 8-week period 70% to 80% of the memory T cell population had divided. Because BrdU uptake is a continuous curve and has not reached a plateau in either of these experiments at the time of discontinuation of the experiment, these data strongly suggest that had these mice been followed for a few more weeks perhaps the entire memory populations would have divided. It certainly shows that because the memory cells are cycling slowly many are in a resting state for prolonged periods of time.

Potential mechanisms for driving the cycling of memory cells have not yet been clearly defined. They could include signaling

via the TCRs by cross-reactive environmental antigens or self-antigens (31,132,133), signaling through adhesion molecules known to be upregulated on memory T cells (32,131,134,135), enhanced responsiveness to cytokines because of increased expression of cytokine receptors (16,33), or a biologic clock mechanism, whereby memory T cells automatically divide after a specific length of time.

Cytolytically Active Memory T Cells

The fact that a certain portion of the memory pool is cycling indicates that some memory cells are at least partially activated, and it suggests that they might have effector function. This suggestion has been confirmed by studies indicating that some memory cells are cytotoxic directly *ex vivo* (136). Sorted blast-sized CD8 T cells from LCMV-immune mice lysed sensitive LCMV-specific peptide-coated target cells, even as long as a year after the acute infection had cleared. This lysis was not blocked by cyclosporin, indicating that these cells were already cytolytically active and not simply activated during the 6-hour cytotoxic assay. Cytotoxicity was also observed to be mediated by purified TCR transgenic memory T cells specific for LCMV GP33-coated targets (26). The fact that some memory cells are cytolytically active may enable them to respond to and lyse virus-infected cells rapidly on secondary infection.

Role of CD4 Cells in Maintaining T Cell Memory

Because cytokines may play a role in driving memory T cells to cycle, it has been postulated that CD4 T cells may play a role in maintaining CD8 memory. Female C57BL/6 mice immunized with male splenocytes depleted of CD4 cells with monoclonal antibody (mAb) continuously for 9 months starting 2 months after immunization showed no loss of HY(male-antigen)-specific CD8 T cells. These results suggest that HY-specific CD8 T cell memory persists in the absence of CD4 T cells (137). However, recent work in the LCMV system, where CD4 knockout mice were infected with LCMV and examined for many months did demonstrate a gradual loss of LCMV-specific CD8 memory, suggesting that CD4 T cells may be necessary to maintain virus-specific memory CD8 pCTLs (138). Both experimental designs have their technical deficiencies in that depletion with multiple sequential doses of CD4 mAb may not give a continuous and complete effect. Alternatively, in the LCMV model CD8 memory cells may not differentiate properly into memory CD8 cells in the absence of CD4 cells and therefore are not maintained. There is indirect evidence that LCMV-specific CD8 memory cells generated in the presence of poorly functioning CD4 cells in B-cell-deficient mice are defective. They were unable to clear LCMV, unlike memory LCMV-specific CD8 cells generated in normal mice, when they were transferred into persistently infected mice (139).

It is possible that CD8 T cells require cytokines such as IL-2 to maintain their gradual cycling in memory, as ovalbumin-specific memory CTLs declined when transferred into IL-2 knockout mice (140). CD40L has also been found to be important in the generation of CD8 memory CTLs in the LCMV system. Splenocytes from LCMV-immune CD40L knockout mice, when transferred into LCMV persistently infected mice, were unable to clear LCMV (141). It is possible that some interaction between CD40L on the CD4 cell and CD40 on APCs is required to help CD4 cells generate and maintain CD8 memory (141).

Persistence of Antigen for Maintenance of Memory?

One of the main issues concerning the topic of maintenance of memory T cells is whether memory can remain relatively stable in the absence of specific antigen (7,10,105,137,142) or is it strictly dependent on stimulation by specific antigen (143–146). The common experimental approach to address this issue has been to use adoptively transferred primed T cells into naive recipients and follow their survival in the apparent absence of specific antigen. Data from adoptive transfer studies must be interpreted with caution, though, as the transfer process itself can introduce an element of selective bias. Memory cells appear to be a complex population, and perhaps the various types of memory cell do not survive transfer equally well. Transfer into an empty space, such as nude mice or irradiated hosts, may result in strong activation of the transferred cells as homeostatic mechanisms act to fill in space. In contrast, transfer into normal mice may result in significant loss of the transferred cells as they compete for space with host T cells. Some of these differences in protocols and other technical differences that exist in the following studies addressing this issue may help explain the differing results. These differences as well as others in these studies have also been more closely examined by Dutton et al. (147).

Purified LCMV-specific memory CD8 cells were transferred into uninfected irradiated mice and were shown to persist as demonstrated by LDA and by providing protective immunity for more than 2 years (7), suggesting that CD8 memory is stable without specific antigen. Similar studies with influenza virus came to the same conclusion (105). Studies in which purified T cells from the spleen of female C57BL/6 mice, which had been immunized with male spleen cells 2 months previously, transferred into athymic nude mice showed a decline in memory recall responses to HY-antigen over a 3-month period, suggesting an antigen requirement (132) for maintenance of CD8 memory. This same group of investigators took another experimental approach to this issue that did not involve cell transfer. They showed that C57BL/6 female mice immunized with male splenocytes maintained their HY-specific memory response when depleted of CD4 cells starting 1 month after immunization. They also found that B-cell-deficient female mice immunized with male splenocytes maintained CTL recall responses (137).

These results suggested that CD4 cells were not required to maintain memory nor was antigen retention in the form of immune complexes by follicular dendritic cells (FDCs), if B cells were not required. LCMV-specific CD8 memory is also stable in B-cell-deficient mice (148). Another group of investigators transferred HY-specific TCR-transgenic memory cells into athymic nude female mice and documented that memory persists without specific antigen (142). Zinkernagel and his colleagues have suggested that persistent specific antigen is required (143,145,146) to maintain CD8 memory to LCMV, but in their more recent studies (143,149) they hypothesized that memory cells exist in at least two compartments: as activated effector cycling memory cells, which require persistent antigen for maintenance, or as resting long-lived memory T cells that do not require antigen for maintenance. The issue of whether antigen is required for the persistence of memory is still not completely decided, as the many variations in the study protocols may contribute to difficulty interpreting the results, but the general consensus at present appears to be that most likely immunizing antigen is not required to maintain memory.

Interrelated with whether antigen is needed to maintain T cell memory is the question of whether TCR triggering is required for maintenance of memory and if it is mediated by MHC-I (150–152). Tanchot et al. (151), using a model wherein memory HY-transgenic T cells were adoptively transferred into various environments, suggested that T cell memory can be maintained by multiple signals. Their results suggest that there is a hierarchy of mechanisms that can maintain CD8 memory. MHC-I-presenting specific antigen is better at maintaining memory than MHC-I-containing self-peptides, which is better then allogeneic MHC-I, which is better than nonspecific stimuli such as cytokines. Addressing this issue from another perspective, Markiewicz et al. (152), using a similar system, demonstrated that HY-specific CD8 T cell memory is not main-tained in TAP-1-deficient mice, where the major route of peptide loading of class I molecules is blocked. Alternatively, there have been experiments done in the Sendai virus system (106) where transferred Sendai virus-specific memory CD8 cells are well maintained in a β_2-microglobulin-deficient (MHC-I-deficient) host, suggesting that MHC-I is not needed for maintenance of CD8 memory. At the present time this issue is unresolved. It has also been suggested that some cross-reactive self-peptide presented by MHC-I may play a role in maintaining T cell memory (31,132,137). Interestingly, in the same study adoptive transfer of TCR transgenic CD4 T cells specific for an influenza antigen, continued to cycle in the absence of antigen, whereas transfer of TCR transgenic CD4 T cells specific to pigeon cytochrome C did not continue to cycle in the absence of antigen. This finding suggests that the specificity of the TCR decides whether peripheral T cells cycle in secondary lymphoid tissue in the absence of antigen stimulation (153). Based on these studies it has been postulated that a hypothetical ligand (150,152,153), which may or may not be MHC-I-associated, exists. This ligand does not drive a primary or secondary response but does interact with the TCR in an altered manner, such as a partial agonist signal, which would be enough to keep the cell slowly turning over much as a ligand exists that originally positively selects the T cell in the thymus. At the present time definitive data to support such a hypothesis do not exist.

QUANTITATIVE REDUCTION AND QUALITATIVE ALTERATION OF T CELL MEMORY DURING AND AFTER SUBSEQUENT VIRAL INFECTIONS

Attrition of T Cells Not Specific for the Virus During Viral Infections

Events leading to the vigorous T cell response to viral infections take a toll on T cells not specific for the virus. For example, the number of TCR transgenic T cells with an irrelevant specificity (male antigen-specific HY-transgenic T cells) decline in number during a vigorous T cell response to LCMV (Fig. 25-5) (82). This decline occurs with either naive phenotype or memory phenotype HY-specific T cells and is associated with higher frequencies of cells staining with Annexin V, which detects cells in the early stages of apoptosis (J. McNally and R. Welsh, in preparation). A second model to determine the fate of T cells not specific for the virus has used LCMV-carrier mice infected congenitally with LCMV. These mice have clonally deleted all of their LCMV-specific T cells and are relatively normal, except for the fact that they harbor a persistent infection with the relatively noncytopathic LCMV. Transfer of LCMV-immune Thy 1.1+ T cells into Thy 1.2+ carrier mice results in a vigorous donor T cell response but leads to a substantial loss (30–40%) of the host CD8 T cells, even though the CD8 cells are not LCMV-infected and not susceptible to lysis by LCMV-specific T cells (82). These host cells also display enhanced Annexin V staining under these conditions. Thus it seems that there is a significant apoptosis-mediated attrition of T cells not specific for the virus during viral infections. This may clear room for the virus-specific T cells to expand in number and control the infection. The mechanism for this type of apoptosis is unclear, but work from our laboratory has indicated that apoptosis in CD8 T cell populations can be induced *in vivo* by the interferon inducer polyinosinic:polycytidylic acid (poly I:C) (J. McNally and R. Welsh, in preparation). This reagent also induces a substantial decrease in the number of CD8 T cells per spleen (82). Some of this decrease may be due to cell migration, but Annexin V staining reveals substantially elevated numbers of apoptotic CD8 cells, particularly within the CD44high memory T cell population. LCMV, a good IFN inducer, similarly induces apoptosis and a reduction in the number of CD8 T cells early in infection; at 3 days after

an LCMV infection staining of spleen tissue sections reveals an early peak of apoptosis preceding the later peak that heralds the decline in lymphocyte number associated with the silencing phase of the response (Figs. 25-2B, 25-5).

Transient Immune Deficiency and Impaired Memory T Cell Function During Acute Viral Infections

Many viruses of humans and animals induce a transient period of immune deficiency that occurs during the peak of the T cell response (99,154). This immune deficiency is associated with the failure of T cells isolated from the host to proliferate in response to strong TCR signaling by mitogenic lectins, anti-CD3, or superantigens and by the failure of memory T cells from these individuals to respond to recall antigens. Such patients also have deficiencies in their abilities to mount delayed-type hypersensitivity (DTH) skin reactions, as was first noted in 1908 by von Pirquet, who reported deficient tuberculin-induced skin DTH responses in patients acutely infected with measles virus (155). Although such immune deficiencies may have many mechanisms, one common mechanism is likely to be due to the tendency of highly activated T cells to undergo AICD on strong TCR stimulation. Enhanced AICD has been reported in T cells from patients infected with HIV, EBV, and CMV infections (156–159). In the murine LCMV system AICD was directly correlated with the duration of immunodeficiency, as analyzed by the failure of virus-induced T cells to proliferate in response to anti-CD3 (Fig. 25-1A) (160). With several human and murine viral infections activated T cells have been shown to upregulate Fas and FasL and downregulate Bcl-2 (159). The significance of the Fas/FasL system in AICD during viral infections was illustrated in the LCMV system, where highly activated T cells isolated from *lpr* or *gld* mice resisted apoptosis on TCR stimulation (102). Notably, T cells from LCMV-infected mice lacking receptors for IFN-γ were particularly resistant to AICD and were highly proliferative (101). Earlier work consistent with this result had shown that AICD in cultured T cells could be blocked by antibody to IFN-γ (161). How IFN-γ regulates this process is not known, but it has been shown to upregulate the expression of Fas on T cells (162); also, enforced expression of the IFN-induced enzyme PKR (protein kinase activated by RNA) can lead directly to apoptosis (163). Another factor enhancing the sensitivity of T cells to apoptosis is IL-2, present at high levels during the potent T cell responses to viral infection (160,164). IL-2 can ultimately induce T cells to produce IFN-γ, Fas, and FasL; regulate the levels of NFκB, and induce cells to cycle, all of which are important for apoptotic regulation (165).

From what we know of the sensitivity of highly activated T cells to AICD, it is not surprising that virus-induced T cell populations, which are mostly virus-specific, would undergo apoptosis on strong TCR stimulation; but how would this explain the failure of memory T cells unrelated to the virus to proliferate poorly in response to antigen? Some work has indicated that T cells not specific for the virus become conditioned in the milieu of the virus-specific T cell response to undergo AICD on receptor ligation. Adoptive reconstitution of LCMV-carrier mice with LCMV-immune T cells results in a potent antiviral T cell response (82). Both donor and host T cells isolated from these mice proliferate poorly and undergo AICD on stimulation with anti-CD3 (35). This sensitization of host T cells to AICD does not occur efficiently if the host cells lack IFN-γ receptors or if the donor cells are from FasL-mutant (*gld*) mice (C. Zarozinski and R. Welsh, in preparation). We hypothesize that in the environment of a vigorous T cell response Fas/FasL interactions with IFN-γ-sensitized cells may induce cells to undergo apoptosis on TCR stimulation. Thus it might be expected that initiating new T cell responses or stimulating recall responses of memory cells would be impaired at the peak of the vigorous virus-induced T cell response.

Reduction of CD8 T Cell Memory After Subsequent Viral Infections

Although the mechanisms that maintain stable T cell memory to viral infections under controlled environmental conditions have not been elucidated, the observations concerning attrition of T cells nonspecific for the challenge virus predict that subsequent infections could disrupt this stability. In fact, that is the case. When an immune mouse is infected with another virus, the T cells specific for the second virus are preferentially selected for, and the T cells specific for the first virus are selected against (74). This selection may be a dilutional effect due to the enhanced proliferation of high-affinity T cells specific for the second virus when antigen is present. Alternatively, those T cells not encountering a ligand may be negatively selected by apoptotic events, as described above. After the infection is over the T cells undergo downregulation via apoptotic mechanisms and return to homeostasis. The tetramer technique has indicated that at least 10% of CD8 T cells are LCMV-specific in LCMV-immune mice (47). This is a high proportion of the immune system devoted to one virus, thereby warranting homeostatic mechanisms to clear space for new memory cells as the normal host is exposed to multiple pathogens throughout a lifetime. Analyses of CD8 pCTL frequencies by LDA (6) or by intracellular IFN-γ staining (Selin et al., in preparation) have revealed that each successive systemic heterologous virus infection results in a reduction of the T cells recognizing the earlier viruses (Fig. 25-8). On average, one additional infection reduces pCTL frequencies to an earlier virus by threefold, whereas two additional infections reduce the pCTL frequency by about eightfold, as measured by LDA (6). It appears that T cell memory, in controlled environmental conditions without persistent viral infection, is a stable phenom-

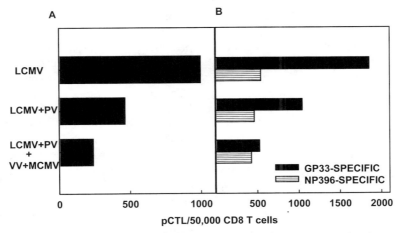

FIG. 25-8. Quantitative reduction and qualitative alteration in CTL memory after heterologous viral infections. **A:** LCMV-specific pCTL frequency of LCMV-specific CTLs, as measured on LCMV-infected KO cells (6,74), from mice immune to LCMV or subsequently infected with other viruses and tested after the response had reached homeostasis after the last infection. There is a gradual loss of LCMV-specific pCTL memory cells as the host is exposed to new viruses. *VV*, vaccinia virus; *MCMV*, murine cytomegalovirus. [This figure is based on data from Selin et al. (6).] **B:** LCMV-specific pCTLs recognizing the immunodominant peptides GP33 and NP396: pCTL frequency of peptide specific CTLs, as measured by peptide-coated KO targets. In this sequence of subsequent viruses, there is a decrease in GP33-specific pCTLs after subsequent virus infections, whereas the NP-specific pCTLs remained stable. [This figure is based data from Welsh et al. (35).]

enon, but it can wane if the host develops strong immune responses to other viruses.

An alternative approach to conserving room in a limited shelf space would be preservation of T cells cross-reactive between two pathogens. Because cross-reactive T cell responses have been defined between heterologous viruses, one might predict that any deletion in T cell memory would not affect all memory cells equally. After an LCMV infection the pCTL frequencies to the three immunodominant LCMV-specific peptides remain fixed in relation to each other from the peak of the T cell response into long-term memory (6). However, when heterologous virus infections disrupt this immune system, the relative numbers of pCTLs responsive to the different peptides become skewed (Fig. 25-8). Similar results are obtained if the memory cell frequencies are measured by intracellular IFN-γ staining. These studies suggested that the memory CD8 cells cross-reactive with the challenging virus are being

maintained whereas the non-cross-reactive memory T cells are lost (Selin et al., in preparation). Therefore not only is there a quantitative reduction in T cell memory after a second infection, there also is a qualitative change in the T cell repertoire, endowing the host with a substantially different memory pool to help control a secondary infection. It thus appears that the immune system uses two strategies to maintain homeostasis: (a) cross-reactivity of T cells between heterologous viruses and (b) deletion of a portion of the memory T cell pool during each newly acquired infection.

In contrast, the memory LCMV-specific CD4[+] pTh frequency is resistant to reduction by subsequent heterologous virus infections, even under conditions that reduce the LCMV-specific CD8 pCTL frequency (Varga et al., in preparation). Several factors may account for this dichotomy in CD8 and CD4 LCMV-specific memory pools. First, there is a large difference in the total number of virus-specific CD8 and CD4 cells generated following these virus infections. It may be that all of the available CD8 T cell memory pool is filled after each infection, and memory cells to earlier infections must therefore be deleted to make room for the newly generated memory cells. Second, it is also possible that CD4 memory T cells are even more commonly cross-reactive than CD8 T cells. If these highly cross-reactive memory CD4 T cells are maintained, it would become difficult to detect any significant reduction in the antigen-specific memory CD4 T cells. Third, it is possible that the CD4 cells are more resistant than CD8 cells to apoptosis signals, though no evidence for this exists. Nevertheless, the waning of the CD8 memory pool under conditions of stability of the CD4 memory pool is an interesting dichotomy that illustrates how the size of the CD8 and CD4 T cell memory pools are regulated differently.

CD8 MEMORY CELLS IN RESISTANCE TO HOMOLOGOUS CHALLENGE AND IN VACCINE DEVELOPMENT

Some virus infections are undoubtedly regulated by CD8 T cells more than others, and one might expect a significant role for CD8 T cells in secondary immune responses against viruses that induce strong CTL responses but weak neutralizing antibody. HIV and LCMV are examples of such viruses. It has been suggested that B cell membrane-bound immunoglobulin specific to the LCMV attachment protein (GP1) facilitates the selective infection of those anti-LCMV antibody-expressing B cells (166). These infected B cells then become lysed by the LCMV-specific CTLs and thus fail to survive and secrete neutralizing antibody. Possibly because of this weak neutralizing antibody, homologous viral challenge of LCMV-immune mice can lead to a rapid increase in the number of LCMV-specific CD8 T cells and elevated CTL memory after the virus has been cleared (6,47). The resistance of HIV to neutral-

izing antibody may be a function of the heavy glycosylation of the HIV gp 120 env protein, as well as the tendency of the virus to rapidly mutate its neutralization epitopes and thereby escape inactivation (167). The need to develop effective vaccines for viruses such as HIV has engendered a focus on developing immunization strategies directed against T cell epitopes. Work in this area is proceeding with many viruses; perhaps the most elegant work has been done in the LCMV system, in which it has clearly been shown that immunization with LCMV-encoded class I epitopes provide protective immunity against homologous challenge.

Different strategies of immunizing mice against internal LCMV proteins (e.g., NP), which have no neutralizing epitopes, or against minimal T cell epitopes have shown that memory virus-specific CTLs can be effective at conferring resistance to infection in the absence of antibody or CD4-dependent immunity. Vaccinia virus recombinants have been used successfully as vectors encoding LCMV genes or "minigenes" encoding LCMV CD8 T cell epitopes (8,37–39,168). Other infectious vaccine approaches have used Mengo virus, influenza virus, and *Listeria monocytogenes* recombinants expressing LCMV T cell epitopes to immunize against LCMV (169–171). Successful immunization against LCMV has also been elicited with DNA vaccines encoding NP CTL epitopes (172–174). Strong, protective CTL memory can also be elicited by immunodominant peptides inoculated alone (175,176), in the presence of complete Freund's adjuvant (177,178), bound to heat shock protein 70 (176), or as a chimeric fusion protein in which the peptide is complexed to a *Bordetella pertussis* adenylate cyclase toxin (179). Each of these strategies elicited memory CTL responses that were rapidly activated on challenge and that provided some degree of protective immunity, clearly illustrating the potent antiviral capacities of memory CTL in at least some viral infections.

Experience with human vaccines has

shown that in some cases incomplete immunity can lead to more severe disease on secondary infection. During the 1960s a vaccine against respiratory syncytial virus (RSV) provided little protective immunity and instead resulted in more severe disease in children who contracted a subsequent infection with RSV (180). CD8 T cells can mediate both protective immunity and immunopathology, and there are potential problems with their pathogenic capacity when vaccines are constructed to provide only T cell immunity and no antibody-dependent immunity. For example, mice immunized with a VV-LCMV NP recombinant, which can elicit no protective antibody response, had accelerated kinetics of a lethal T-cell dependent encephalitis in mice challenged intracranially with LCMV (8). Mice immunized with a VV-LCMV GP recombinant, which does induce an antibody response, were protected from that immunopathology. Similarly, mice receiving an LCMV NP DNA vaccine had accelerated kinetics of encephalitis on challenge (172). This illustrates how a weak or incomplete memory CTL response may do more harm than good. This can become an issue when a host is challenged with heterologous viruses that may, by virtue of cross-reactivity, reactivate CTLs specific to other viruses (see next section).

CROSS-REACTIVE MEMORY T CELLS AND VIRAL PATHOGENESIS

Protective Heterologous Immunity Mediated by Memory T Cells

One of the basic tenets of immunology is that immunity to a virus results in complete protection against that virus. However, if a heterologous virus infection can serve to prime a T cell response against a second unrelated virus by activation of cross-reactive memory cells (Fig. 25-4), one might predict that a history of one virus infection could influence the course of the second infection. In fact, studies with a panel of heterologous viruses, including LCMV, PV, VV, and

MCMV, showed that prior immunity with one of these viruses in many cases enhanced clearance of a second, unrelated virus early in infection (Table 25-2) (181). This protection was not as complete as that seen with a homologous virus challenge but was equivalent to the type of early protection induced by natural killer (NK) cells, with virus titers usually 3- to 20-fold lower than in naive hosts. This type of protective immunity was common, but it was dependent on the virus sequence and was not necessarily reciprocal. For instance, VV, PV, and MCMV did not provide as much protection against LCMV as LCMV did against them. VV showed almost no protective immunity against any of the viruses, but all three viruses resulted in significant protective immunity against VV. A possible explanation for this unidirectionality of the protective immunity depends on whether the immunizing virus has a dominant response against a determinant that can cross-react with the second virus. If the immune repertoire is rich in T cells responsive to this cross-reactive epitope, the second virus may vigorously stimulate the memory T cells, which would then assist in control of

TABLE 25-2. *Decrease in challenge virus following immunity to heterologous viruses*

Immunizing virus	Challenge virus (mean log$_{10}$ decrease)			
	LCMV	PV	MCMV	VV
LCMV	—	0.8	0.4	1.4
PV	0.4	—	0.7	1.9
MCMV	0.8	0.4	—	1.8
VV	0.3	0.1	0	—

Mice were immunized with one virus and more than 6 weeks later were challenged with a second, unrelated virus. At 3 to 5 days after the second infection, the spleen, fat pads, and liver were harvested and plaqued for virus. The numbers in the table demonstrate the mean log$_{10}$ decrease in virus titer in the immunized mice versus the naive mice challenged with these viruses. The mean log$_{10}$ decrease is based on the average decrease of the virus titer in the three organs as measured in two to four experiments.

LCMV, lymphocytic choriomeningitis virus; PV, Pichinde virus; MCMV, murine cytomegalovirus; VV, vaccinia virus.

This table is based on data from Selin et al. (181).

the infection. However, if the immunodominant repertoire to the first virus did not include a cross-reactive epitope with the second virus, this enriched cross-reactive T cell memory pool would be absent, and there would be no additional assistance in clearance of the second virus. This variability and selectivity does, however, suggest that T cell cross-reactivity, instead of nonspecific bystander activation, is important for protective immunity by heterologous memory T cells to occur.

Further studies have addressed the immunologic mechanisms required for heterologous protective immunity (181). Adoptive transfer of LCMV-immune splenocytes depleted of either CD4 or CD8 T cells into naive mice challenged with the heterologous viruses VV or PV demonstrated that both memory cell types were required for protective immunity. IFN-γ played a significant role in protection against VV by LCMV-specific memory T cells. There was enhanced recruitment of memory phenotype IFN-γ-secreting CD4 and CD8 T cells into the peritoneal cavity and increased IFN-γ levels in this initial site of virus replication (Fig. 25-9). Studies with IFN-γ receptor knockout mice and *in vivo* injection of anti-IFN-γ mAb confirmed a role for IFN-γ in the protection by LCMV-immune memory T cells against VV but not against PV, suggesting that memory T cells may utilize different mechanisms depending on the challenging heterologous virus.

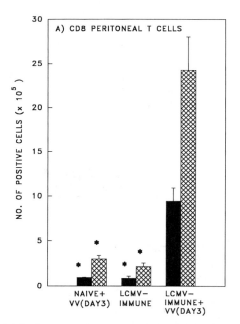
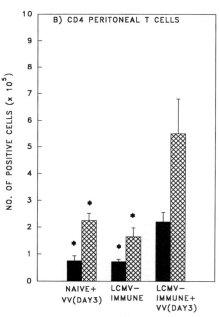

FIG. 25-9. Increased numbers of IFN-γ-secreting **(A)** CD8 and **(B)** CD4 T cells in the peritoneum of LCMV-immune mice challenged with VV (day 3). Peritoneal cells were examined by intracellular IFN-γ staining from age-matched naive and LCMV-immune C57BL/6 mice challenged with purified VV at day 3 of infection or from LCMV-immune mice challenged with control purified cell supernatant (day 3). **A:** There was a tenfold increase in the total number of CD8 (*cross-hatched bars*) and IFN-γ-secreting CD8 (*filled bars*) T cells in LCMV-immune mice versus naive mice challenged with VV. **B:** There was a similar threefold increase in the total number of CD4 cells (*cross-hatched bars*) and IFN-γ-secreting CD4 cells (*solid bars*) in LCMV-immune mice versus naive mice challenged with VV. *Statistically significant difference from the LCMV-immune + VV group ($p < 0.01$). [This figure is reprinted with the permission of The Rockefeller University Press and is based on data from Selin et al. (181).]

Enhanced Immunopathology as a Consequence of Memory T Cell Activation in Response to Heterologous Virus Infections

T cells not only can be mediators of protective immunity they also can induce substantial immunopathology, as discussed above (see CD8 Memory Cells in Resistance to Homologous Challenge). Classic examples are that of LCMV, where the same T cells responsible for viral clearance can mediate a severe leptomeningitis if the virus is replicating in the brain (182,183), and the respiratory viruses, RSV (184,185) and influenza (186), where T cells have been shown to help clear virus but at the same time augment lung pathology.

There is considerable variation in individual responses to infection, ranging from subclinical to severe. It depends on many factors, such as dose, route of infection, and the physiologic state and genetic background of the host. Memory T cells specific to heterologous viruses may also contribute to the host's response to a second infection (Fig. 25-10). As described above, a beneficial effect of these early protective memory T cells is to slow the spread of infection, allowing time for high-affinity antigen-specific T and B cell responses to develop. It is also possible that heterologous memory T cells are detrimental during infections. They may play a role in human infections, such as with EBV or varicella-zoster virus, which lead to more severe disease in young adults than in young children, who presumably have a more restricted memory T cell repertoire (187,188). Dengue hemorrhagic fever (DHF) is the classic example of enhanced disease when the host has complete protection against challenge with the same serotype but only partial protection to the other three serotypes (189). It has been postulated that the T cell responses in secondary infections are predominantly due to reactivation of highly cross-reactive memory T cells from the primary infection and contribute to the severe immunopathology of DHF.

The history of one virus infection can predispose the host to develop more severe im-

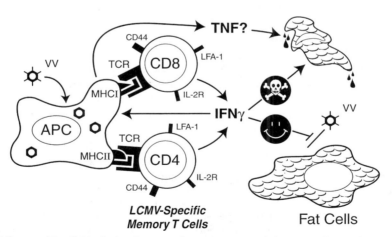

FIG. 25-10. Memory T cells to heterologous viruses can result in protection or immunopathology. This model depicts some of the immunologic events that occur during an acute VV infection of an LCMV-immune mouse that result in either protective immunity or immunopathogenesis. VV infection in an LCMV-immune mouse reactivates LCMV-specific memory T cells early in the VV infection (day 3) in a cross-reactive manner. These cross-reactive memory T cells produce increased amounts of IFN-γ early in infection, which acts to decrease VV titers, but this overactive, partially protective T cell response leads to the occurrence of acute fatty necrosis. [This model is based on data from Selin et al. (181).]

munopathology during a second, unrelated virus infection (181,190). Mice infected intraperitoneally with LCMV developed severe immunopathology in visceral fat pads after challenge with a dose of VV that did not induce severe pathology in nonimmunized mice. This pathology was associated with necrosis of fat tissue and mononuclear infiltrates that contained high levels of CTL activity against both VV and LCMV. This pathology occurred if naive mice were reconstituted with LCMV-immune spleen leukocytes but did not occur in IFN-γ receptor knockout mice, suggesting that IFN-γ was involved in the pathology (Fig. 25-10). Analyses of IFN-γ concentrations in the peritoneal fluid early in infection revealed a fivefold increase in LCMV-immune mice infected with VV compared to control mice infected with VV. Thus the IFN-γ response is greater in immune mice challenged with VV, and this IFN-γ plays a role in protective immunity against VV and in the induction of immunopathology. Memory T cells are known to produce higher levels of cytokines than recently stimulated naive T cells, and this stimulation of cross-reactive memory cells might account for the IFN-γ-dependent effects seen in these systems. Mice immune to both LCMV and PV and then challenged with VV developed even more severe pathology than those immune to either LCMV or PV individually. Recently, we have used the more natural intranasal route of infection (rather than the intraperitoneal route) and

found that mice immune to LCMV develop symptoms of disease more rapidly when challenged with VV, even though VV is cleared more rapidly (Chen et al., unpublished data).

It is possible that reactivation of heterologous memory T cells potentially plays a role in the exacerbation of autoimmune diseases, such as multiple sclerosis or diabetes. Transgenic mice were generated that express the nucleoprotein or glycoprotein of LCMV as a self-antigen in oligodendrocytes (191). An intraperitoneal LCMV infection led to infection of the periphery but not the central nervous system (CNS), although after viral clearance a chronic inflammation of the CNS occurred and resolved over time. A second infection with a heterologous cross-reactive virus (VV or PV) led to disease enhancement. These observations may explain the association of some human autoimmune diseases with several different viruses. These results indicate that how a host responds to an infectious agent is a function of its history of previous infections and their influence on the memory T cell pool.

CONCLUSIONS: CD8 MEMORY AND THE T CELL NETWORK

It has long been known that memory T cells are produced following virus infections and assist in resistance to reinfection. Research has shed light on new ways of viewing CD8 T cell responses (Fig. 25-11). Much higher percentages of T cells are virus-specific in

---

FIG. 25-11. Modulation of the T cell network by viral infections. This model depicts how viral infections modulate the T cell repertoire by stimulating cross-reactive memory T cells and by depleting some portion of the memory pool from previous infections. The *circles* represent T cell clones, with similar specificities depicted horizontally and progressively different specificities depicted vertically. LCMV, shown in darker circles, stimulates the expansion of high-affinity (*dark gray circles*) and lower-affinity (*light gray and black circles*) T cells, which after clearing the virus undergo apoptosis but remain in the immune spleen at high frequency. When PV (*light gray circles*) is introduced into this LCMV-immune animal, it stimulates cross-reactive (*darker gray circles*) T cells. Ultimately, high-affinity (*light gray circles*) PV-specific T cells are driven to proliferate more strongly than the cross-reactive T cells. After this second infection has been silenced, there is a reduction in memory pCTLs to the first virus most likely due to bystander attrition by apoptosis of non-antigen-specific memory T cells to the first virus. This virus model is based on original data presented elsewhere (6,74,82,181), and diagramed in modified forms by others (35,192,193).

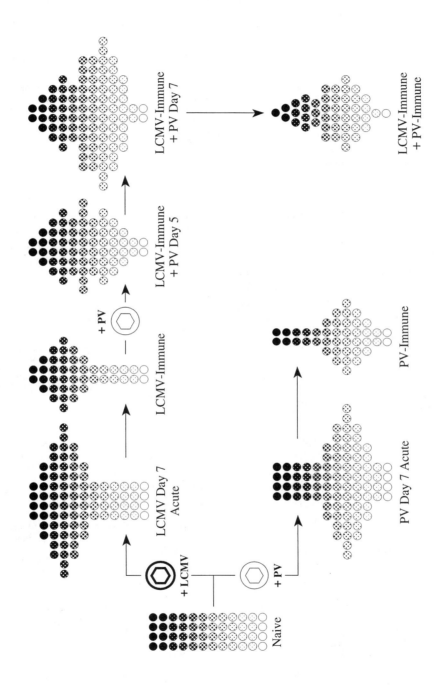

Naive

+ LCMV

+ PV

LCMV Day 7
Acute

LCMV-Immune

+ PV

LCMV-Immune
+ PV Day 5

LCMV-Immune
+ PV Day 7

LCMV-Immune
+ PV-Immune

PV Day 7 Acute

PV-Immune

memory than was previously thought. Memory CD8 T cells are not inert but are continually dividing and capable of cytotoxic function. CD8 memory T cells are much more degenerate in their antigen recognition in that they often have dual specificities, cross-reacting with alloantigens or antigens from unrelated viruses that can influence the host's response to subsequent infections. Apoptosis may be a major modulating mechanism in the generation of memory cells, but the exact molecular pathways involved in generating memory T cells have been difficult to delineate. Memory T cells are found after the acute CD8 response downregulates by apoptosis and returns to homeostasis. Antigen is cleared under conditions of low-dose infection. CTL memory is preserved, and the T cell number declines without a selection based on TCR specificity, at least to the high-affinity immunodominant epitopes. Under conditions of high antigen load, the CTLs undergo an antigen-specific apoptosis and clonal exhaustion, resulting in a persistent infection without memory CTLs. In fact, the immune deficiency observed during many virus infections may be a secondary effect of these TCR-mediated apoptotic effects on memory T cells.

The immune system becomes strongly biased with virus-specific cells capable of cross-reacting with alloantigens and other viruses. They remain stable by mechanisms that are not clearly understood, but this stability can be disrupted with heterologous virus infections. The second infection can result in reactivation of the cross-reactive memory CD8 T cells that are maintained preferentially, whereas there is a bystander apoptotic attrition of the non-cross-reactive memory CD8 cells, leading to loss of a portion of the CD8 memory to the first virus infection. During the heterologous virus infection the cross-reactive memory CD8 cells can play a beneficial role by helping control the infection or a harmful role under some circumstances by enhancing immunopathology. The highly efficient immune system is able to maintain homeostasis by saving space with two mecha-

nisms: (a) deletion of a portion of the memory CD8 pool and (b) salvaging dual-functioning, cross-reactive CD8 memory T cells. Memory T cells are therefore an important component of an immunologic network in which CD8 T cells often cross-react with more than one antigen, and where memory T cell pools are continually being modified as they contribute to the immune responses against unrelated pathogens.

Acknowledgments

This work was made possible by grants AR35506, AI17672, CA34461, and AI01362 from the National Institutes of Health. Its contents are solely the responsibility of the authors and do not necessarily represent the official views of NIH.

REFERENCES

1. Monaco JJ. Pathways of antigen processing: a molecular model of MHC class I-restricted antigen processing. *Immunol Today* 1992;13:173–179.
2. Sanders ME, Makgoba MW, et al. Human memory T lymphocytes express increased levels of three adhesion molecules (LFA-3, CD2, and LFA-1) and three other molecules (UCHL1, CDw29, and Pgp-1) and have enhanced IFN-gamma production. *J Immunol* 1995;140:1401–1407.
3. McFarland HI, Nahill SR, Maciaszek JW, Welsh RM. CD11b (Mac-1). A marker for CD8+ cytotoxic T cell activation and memory in virus infection. *J Immunol* 1992;149:1326–1333.
4. Grewal IS, Flavell RA. CD40 and CD154 in cell-mediated immunity. *Annu Rev Immunol* 1998;16:111–136.
5. Lenschow DJ, Walunas TL, Bluestone JA. CD28/B7 system of T cell costimulation. *Annu Rev Immunol* 1996;14:233–258.
6. Selin LK, Vergilis K, Welsh RM, Nahill SR. Reduction of otherwise remarkably stable virus-specific cytotoxic T lymphocyte memory by heterologous viral infections. *J Exp Med* 1996;183:2489–2499.
7. Lau LL, Jamieson BD, Somasundaram T, Ahmed R. Cytotoxic T-cell memory without antigen. *Nature* 1994;369:648–652.
8. Oehen S, Waldner H, Kundig TM, Hengarter H, Zinkernagel RM. Antivirally protective cytotoxic T cell memory to lymphocytic choriomeningitis virus is governed by persisting antigen. *J Exp Med* 1992;176:1273–1281.
9. Pihlgren M, Dubois PM, Tomkowiak M, Sjogren T, Marvel J. Resting memory CD8+ T cells are hyperactive to antigenic challenge in vitro. *J Exp Med* 1996;184:2141–2151.

10. Swain SL, Croft MC, Dubey C, et al. From naive to memory T cells. *Immunol Rev* 1996;150:143–167.
11. Tabi Z, Lynch F, Ceredig R, Allan JE, Doherty PC. Virus-specific memory T cells are Pgp-1+ and can be selectively activated with phorbol ester and calcium ionophore. *Cell Immunol* 1988; 113:268–277.
12. Bradley LM, Croft M, Swain SL. T-cell memory: new perspectives. *Immunol Today* 1993;14:197–199.
13. Carter LL, Zhang X, Dubey C, Rogers P, Tsui L, Swain SL. Regulation of T cell subsets from naive to memory. *J Immunother* 1998;21:181–187.
14. Tough DL, Borrow P, Sprent J. Induction of bystander T cell proliferation by viruses and type I interferon. *Science* 1996;272:1947–1950.
15. Lalvani A, Brookes R, Hambleton S, Britton WJ, Hill AV, McMichael AJ. Rapid effector function in CD8+ memory T cells. *J Exp Med* 1997; 186:859–865.
16. Zhang X, Sun S, Hwang I, Tough DF, Sprent J. Potent and selective stimulation of memory-phenotype CD8+ T cells in vivo by IL-15. *Immunity* 1998;8:591–599.
17. Cerottini JC, MacDonald HR. The cellular basis of T-cell memory. *Annu Rev Immunol* 1989;7:77–89.
18. Sanders ME, Makgoba MW, Shaw S. Human naive and memory T cell: reinterpretation of helper-inducer and suppressor-inducer subsets. *Immunol Today* 1988;9:195–199.
19. Budd RC, Cerottini JC, Horvath C, et al. Distinction of virgin and memory T lymphocytes: stable acquisition of the Pgp-1 glycoprotein concomitant with antigenic stimulation. *J Immunol* 1987;138: 3120–3129.
20. Lee WT, Yin X-M, Vitetta ES. Functional and ontogenetic analysis of murine CD45Rhi and CD45lo CD4+ T cells. *J Immunol* 1990;144:3288–3295.
21. Gray D. Immunological memory. *Annu Rev Immunol* 1993;11:49–77.
22. Ewing C, Topham DJ, Doherty PC. Prevalence and activation phenotype of Sendai virus-specific CD4+ T cells. *Virology* 1995;210:179–185.
23. Bradley LM, Duncan DD, Tonkonogy S, Swain SL. Characterization of antigen-specific CD4+ effector T cells in vivo: immunization results is a transient population of MEL-14−, CD45RB− helper cells that secretes interleukin 2 (IL-2), IL-3, IL-4, and interferon-gamma. *J Exp Med* 1991;174: 547–559.
24. Bradley LM, Atkins GG, Swain SL. Long-term CD4+ memory T cells from the spleen lack MEL-14, the lymph node homing receptor. *J Immunol* 1992;148:324–331.
25. Tripp RA, Hou S, Doherty PC. Temporal loss of the activated L-selectin-low phenotype for virus-specific CD8+ memory T cells. *J Immunol* 1995; 154:5870–5875.
26. Zimmermann C, Brduscha-Riem K, Blaser C, Zinkernagel RM, Pircher H. Visualization, characterization, and turnover of CD8+ memory T cells in virus-infected hosts. *J Exp Med* 1996;183:1367–1375.
27. Oehen S, Brduscha-Reim K. Differentiation of na-

ive CTL to effector and memory CTL: correlation of effector function with phenotype and cell division. *J Immunol* 1998;161:5538–5346.
28. Razvi ES, Welsh RM, McFarland HI. In vivo state of antiviral CTL precursors: characterization of a cycling population containing CTL precursors in immune mice. *J Immunol* 1995;154:620–632.
29. Varga SM, Welsh RM. The CD45RB-associated epitope defined by monoclonal antibody CZ-1 is an activation and memory marker for mouse CD4 T cells. *Cell Immunol* 1996;167:56–62.
30. Buckle AM, Hogg N. Human memory T cells express intercellular adhesion molecule-1 which can be increased by interleukin 2 and interferon-gamma. *Eur J Immunol* 1990;20:337–341.
31. Beverly PCL. Is T-cell memory maintained by cross-reactive stimulation? *Immunol Today* 1990; 11:203–205.
32. Swain SL, Bradley LM, Croft M, et al. Helper T-cell subsets: phenotype, function and the role of lymphokines in regulating their development. *Immunol Rev* 1991;123:115–144.
33. Unutmaz D, Pileri P, Abrignani S. Antigen-independent activation of naive and memory resting T cells by a cytokine combination. *J Exp Med* 1994;180:1159–1164.
34. Cerwenka A, Carter LL, Reome JB, Swain SL, Dutton RW. In vivo persistence of CD8 polarized T cell subsets producing type 1 or type 2 cytokines. *J Immunol* 1998;161:97–105.
35. Welsh RM, Lin M-Y, Lohman BL, Varga SM, Zarozinski CC, Selin LK. Alpha-beta and gamma-delta T-cell networks and their roles in natural resistance to viral infections. *Immunol Rev* 1997; 159:79–93.
36. Varga SM, Welsh RM. Stability of virus-specific CD4+ T cell frequencies from acute infection into long term memory. *J Immunol* 1998;161:367–374.
37. Whitton JL, Southern PJ, Oldstone MBA. Analyses of the cytotoxic T lymphocyte responses to glycoprotein and nucleoprotein components of lymphocytic choriomeningitis virus. *Virology* 1988; 162:321–327.
38. Whitton JL, Tishon A, Lewicki H, et al. Molecular analyses of a five-amino-acid cytotoxic T-lymphocyte (CTL) epitope: an immunodominant region which induces nonreciprocal CTL cross-reactivity. *J Virol* 1989;63:4303–4310.
39. Whitton JL, Gebhard JR, Lewicki H, Tishon A, Oldstone MBA. Molecular definition of a major cytotoxic T-lymphocyte epitope in the glycoprotein of lymphocytic choriomeningitis virus. *J Virol* 1988;62:687–695.
40. Van der Most RG, Sette A, Oseroff C, et al. Analysis of cytotoxic T cell responses to dominant and subdominant epitopes during acute and chronic lymphocytic choriomeningitis virus infection. *J Immunol* 1996;157:5543–5554.
41. Borysiewicz LK, Graham S, Hickling J, Mason PD, Sissons JGP. Human cytomegalovirus-specific cytotoxic T cells: their precursor frequency and stage specificity. *Eur J Immunol* 1988;18:269–275.
42. Prevost-Blondel A, Lengagne R, Letourneur F, Pannetier C, Gomard E, Guillet J. In vivo longitudinal analysis of a dominant TCR repertoire se-

lected in human response to influenza virus. *Virology* 1997;233:93–104.

43. Moskophidis D, Assmann-Wischer U, Simon MM, Lehmann-Grube F. The immune response of the mouse to lymphocytic choriomeningitis virus V: high numbers of cytotoxic T lymphocytes are generated in the spleen during acute infection. *Eur J Immunol* 1987;17:937–942.

44. Biron CA, Pedersen KF, Welsh RM. Aberrant T cells in beige mutant mice. *J Immunol* 1987; 138:2050–2056.

45. Altman JD, Moss PAH, Goulder PJR, et al. Phenotypic analysis of antigen-specific T-lymphocytes. *Science* 1996;274:94–96.

46. Dal Porto J, Johansen TE, Catipovic B, et al. A soluble divalent class I major histocompatibility complex molecule inhibits alloreactive T cells at nanomolar concentrations. *Proc Natl Acad Sci USA* 1993;90:6671–6675.

47. Murali-Krishna K, Altman JD, Suresh M, et al. Counting antigen-specific CD8 T cells: a re-evaluation of bystander activation during viral infection. *Immunity* 1998;8:177–187.

48. Openshaw P, Murphy EE, Hosken NA, et al. Heterogeneity of intracellular cytokine synthesis at the single-cell level in polarized T helper 1 and T helper 2 populations. *J Exp Med* 1995;182:1357–1367.

49. Varga SM, Welsh RM. Cutting edge: detection of a high frequency of virus-specific CD4+ T cells during acute infection with lymphocytic choriomeningitis virus. *J Immunol* 1998;161:3215–3218.

50. Flynn KJ, Belz GT, Altman JD, Ahmed R, Woodland DL, Doherty PC. Virus-specific CD8+ T cells in primary and secondary influenza pneumonia. *Immunity* 1998;8:683–691.

51. Callan MFC, Tan L, Annels N, et al. Direct visualization of antigen-specific CD8+ T cells during the primary immune response to Epstein-Barr Virus in vivo. *J Exp Med* 1998;187:1395–1402.

52. Burrows SR, Khanna R, Burrows JM, Moss DJ. An alloresponse in humans is dominated by cytotoxic T lymphocytes (CTL) cross-reactive with a single Epstein-Barr virus CTL epitope: implications for graft-versus-host disease. *J Exp Med* 1994;179:1155–1161.

53. Strang G, Rickinson AB. Multiple HLA class I-dependent cytotoxicities constitute the "non-HLA-restricted" response in infectious mononucleosis. *Eur J Immunol* 1987;17:1007–1013.

54. Tomkinson BE, Maziarz R, Sullivan JL. Characterization of the T cell-mediated cellular cytotoxicity during infectious mononucleosis. *J Immunol* 1989;143:660–670.

55. Yang H, Dundon PL, Nahill SR, Welsh RM. Virus-induced polyclonal cytotoxic T lymphocyte stimulation. *J Immunol* 1989;142:1710–1718.

56. Yang H, Welsh RM. Induction of alloreactive cytotoxic T cells by acute virus infection of mice. *J Immunol* 1986;136:1186–1193.

57. Nahill SR, Welsh RM. High frequency of cross-reactive cytotoxic T lymphocytes elicited during the virus-induced polyclonal cytotoxic T lymphocyte response. *J Exp Med* 1993;177:317–327.

58. Russell JH, Dobos CB. Characterization of a "heteroclitic" cytotoxic lymphocyte clone: hetero-

geneity of receptors or signals? *J Immunol* 1983; 130:538–541.

59. Braciale TJ, Andrew ME, Braciale VL. Simultaneous expression of H-2 restricted and alloreactive recognition by a cloned line of influenza virus-specific cytotoxic T lymphocytes. *J Exp Med* 1981; 153:1371–1376.

60. Sheil JM, Bevan MJ, Lefrancois L. Characterization of dual-reactive H-2K^b-restricted anti-vesicular stomatitis virus and alloreactive cytotoxic T cells. *J Immunol* 1987;138:3654–3660.

61. Stukart MJ, Boes J, Melief CJM. Recognition of H-2K^b mutant target cells by Moloney virus-specific cytotoxic T lymphocytes from bm13 (H-2D^b-mutant) mice. *J Immunol* 1984;133:28–32.

62. Jennings SR. Cross-reactive recognition of mouse cells expressing the bm3 and bm11 mutations within H-2K^b by H-2K^b-restricted herpes simplex virus-specific cytotoxic T lymphocytes. *J Immunol* 1985;135:3530–3536.

63. Mason D. A very high level of crossreactivity is an essential feature of the T cell repertoire. *Immunol Today* 1998;19:395–404.

64. Jakel KT, Lonig T. Herpes virus infections, acute rejection, and transplant arteriosclerosis in human cardiac allografts. *Transplant Proc* 1993;25:2029–2030.

65. Pouteil-Noble C, Ecochard R, Landrivon G, et al. Cytomegalovirus infection: an etiological factor for rejection? *Transplantation* 1993;55:851–857.

66. Appleton AL, Sviland L. Pathogenesis of GVHD: role of herpesviruses. *Bone Marrow Transplant* 1993;11:349–355.

67. Van Dorp WT, van Wieringen PAM, Marselis-Jones E, et al. Cytomegalovirus directly enhances MHC class I and intercellular adhesion molecule-1 expression on cultured proximal tubular epithelial cells. *Transplantation* 1993;55:1367–1371.

68. Burrows SR, Silins SL, Moss DJ, Khanna R, Misko IS, Argaet VP. T cell receptor repertoire for a viral epitope in humans is diversified by tolerance to a background major histocompatibility complex antigen. *J Exp Med* 1995;182:1703–1715.

69. Rickinson AB, Moss DJ. Human cytotoxic T lymphocyte responses to Epstein-Barr virus infection. *Annu Rev Immunol* 1997;15:405–431.

70. Burrows SR, Silins SL, Khanna R, et al. Cross-reactive memory T cells for Epstein-Barr virus augment the alloresponse to common human leukocyte antigens: degenerate recognition of major histocompatibility complex-bound peptide by T cells and its role in alloreactivity. *Eur J Immunol* 1997;27:1726–1736.

71. Vento S, Guella L, Mirandola F, et al. Epstein-Barr virus as a trigger for autoimmune hepatitis in susceptible individuals. *Lancet* 1995;346:608–609.

72. Daniel C, Horvath S, Allen PM. A basis for alloreactivity: MHC helical residues broaden peptide recognition by the TCR. *Immunity* 1998;8:543–552.

73. Speir JA, Garcia C, Brunmark A, et al. Structural basis of 2C TCR allorecognition of H-2L^d peptide complexes. *Immunity* 1998;8:553–562.

74. Selin LK, Nahill SR, Welsh RM. Cross-reactivities in memory cytotoxic T lymphocyte recognition of

heterologous viruses. *J Exp Med* 1994;179:1933–1943.

75. Anderson RW, Bennick JR, Yewdell JW, Maloy WL, Coligan JE. Influenza basic polymerase 2 peptides are recognized by influenza nucleoprotein-specific cytotoxic T lymphocytes. *Mol Immunol* 1992;29:1089–1096.

76. Shimojo N, Maloy WL, Anderson RW, Biddison WE, Coligan JE. Specificity of peptide binding by the HLA-A2.1 molecule. *J Immunol* 1989; 143:2939–2947.

77. Kuwano K, Reyes RE, Humphreys RE, Ennis FA. Recognition of disparate HA and NS1 peptides by an H-2k^d-restricted, influenza specific CTL clone. *Mol Immunol* 1991;28:1–7.

78. Kulkarni AB, Morse HC III, Bennink JR, Yewdell JW, Murphy BR. Immunization of mice with vaccinia virus-M2 recombinant induces epitope-specific and cross-reactive K^d-restricted CD8$^+$ cytotoxic T cells. *J Virol* 1993;67:4086–4092.

79. Tough DF, Sprent J. Viruses and T cell turnover: evidence for bystander proliferation. *Immunol Rev* 1996;150:129–142.

80. Tough DF, Sprent J. Turnover of naive- and memory-phenotype T cells. *J Exp Med* 1994;179:1127–1135.

81. Ehl S, Hombach J, Aichele P, Hengartner H, Zinkernagel RM. Bystander activation of cytotoxic T cells: studies on the mechanism and evaluation of in vivo significance in a transgenic mouse model. *J Exp Med* 1997;185:1241–1251.

82. Zarozinski CC, Welsh RM. Minimal bystander activation of CD8 T cells during the virus-induced polyclonal T cell response. *J Exp Med* 1997; 185:1629–1639.

83. Bachmann MF, Sebzda E, Kundig TM, et al. T cell responses are governed by avidity and costimulatory thresholds. *Eur J Immunol* 1996;26:2017–2022.

84. Bertoletti A, Sette A, Chisari FV, et al. Natural variants of cytotoxic epitopes are T-cell receptor antagonists for antiviral cytotoxic T cells. *Nature* 1991;369:407–410.

85. Cao W, Tykodi SS, Esser MT, Braciale VL, Braciale TJ. Partial activation of CD8$^+$ T cells by a self-derived peptide. *Nature* 1995;378:295–298.

86. Corr M, Slaneta AE, Boyd LF, et al. T cell receptor-MHC class I peptide interactions: affinity, kinetics and specificity. *Science* 1994;265:946–949.

87. Evavold BD, Allen PM. Separation of IL-4 production from T cell proliferation by an altered T cell receptor ligand. *Science* 1991;252:1308–1310.

88. Jameson SC, Carbone FR, Bevan MJ. Clone-specific T cell receptor antagonists of major histocompatibility complex class-I-restricted cytotoxic T cells. *J Exp Med* 1993;177:1541–1550.

89. Madrenas J, Chau LA, Smith J, Bluestone JA, Germain RN. The efficiency of CD4 recruitment to ligand-engaged TCR controls the agonist/partial agonist properties of peptide-MHC molecule ligands. *J Exp Med* 1997;185:219–229.

90. Sloan-Lancaster J, Shaw AS, Rothbard JB, Allen PM. Partial T cell signaling: altered phospho- and lack of zap70 recruitment in APL-induced T cell anergy. *Cell* 1994;79:913–922.

91. Gombert W, Borthwick NJ, Wallace DL, et al. Fibroblasts prevent apoptosis of IL-2-deprived T cells without inducing proliferation: a selective effect on Bcl-XL expression. *Immunology* 1996; 89:397–404.

92. Barinaga M. Death by dozens of cuts. *Science* 1998;280:32–34.

93. Gottlieb RA, Babior BM. Regulation of Fas-mediated apoptosis. *Curr Top Cell Regul* 1997; 35:69–105.

94. Chinnaiyan AM, Dixit VM. Portrait of an executioner: the molecular mechanism of Fas/APO-1-induced apoptosis. *Semin Immunol* 1997;9:69–76.

95. Russell JH, White CL, Loh DY, Meleedy-Rey P. Receptor-stimulated death pathway is opened by antigen in mature T cells. *Proc Natl Acad Sci USA* 1991;88:2151–2155.

96. Zheng L, Fisher G, Miller RE, Peschon J, Lynch DH, Lenardo MJ. Induction of apoptosis in mature T cells by tumour necrosis factor. *Nature* 1995; 377:348–351.

97. Crowston JG, Salmon M, Khaw PT, Akbar AN. T-lymphocyte-fibroblast interactions. *Biochem Soc Trans* 1997;25:529–531.

98. Razvi ES, Jiang Z, Woda BA, Welsh RM. Lymphocyte apoptosis during the silencing of the immune response to acute viral infections in normal, lpr and Bcl-2-transgenic mice. *Am J Pathol* 1995; 147:79–91.

99. Razvi ES, Welsh RM. Apoptosis in viral infections. *Adv Virus Res* 1995;45:1–60.

100. Christensen JP, Ropke C, Thomsen AR. Virus-induced polyclonal T cell activation is followed by apoptosis: partitioning of CD8$^+$ T cells based on alpha 4 integrin expression. *Int Immunol* 1996; 8:707–715.

101. Lohman BL, Welsh RM. Apoptotic regulation of T cells and absence of immune deficiency in virus-infected IFN-gamma receptor knock-out mice. *J Virol* 1998;72:7815–7821.

102. Lohman BL, Razvi ES, Welsh RM. T-lymphocyte downregulation after acute viral infection is not dependent on CD95 (Fas) receptor-ligand interactions. *J Virol* 1996;70:8199–8203.

103. Petschner F, Zimmerman C, Strasser A, Grillot D, Nunez G, Pircher H. Constitutive expression of Bcl-xL or Bcl-2 prevents peptide antigen-induced T cell deletion but does not influence T cell homeostasis after a viral infection. *Eur J Immunol* 1998; 28:560–569.

104. Lin MY, Welsh RM. Stability and diversity of T cell receptor (TCR) repertoire usage during lymphocytic choriomeningitis virus infection of mice. *J Exp Med* 1998;188:1993–2005.

105. Mullbacher A. The long-term maintence of cytotoxic T cell memory does not require persistence of antigen. *J Exp Med* 1994;179:317–321.

106. Hou S, Hyland L, Ryan W, Portner A, Doherty PC. Virus-specific CD8$^+$ T-cell memory determined by clonal burst size. *Nature* 1994;369:652–654.

107. Doherty PC, Topham DJ, Tripp RA, Cardin RD, Brooks JW, Stevenson PG. Effector CD4$^+$ and CD8$^+$ T-cell mechanisms in the control of respiratory virus infections. *Immunol Rev* 1997;159: 105–117.

108. Naumov YN, Hogan KT, Naumova EN, Pagel JT, Gorski J. A class I MHC-restricted recall response to a viral peptide is highly polyclonal despite stringent CDR3 selection: implications for establishing memory T cell repertoires in "real-world" conditions. *J Immunol* 1998;160:2842–2852.

109. Ahmed R, Salmi A, Butler LD, Chiller JM, Oldstone MBA. Selection of genetic variants of lymphocytic choriomeningitis virus in spleens of persistently infected mice: role in suppression of cytotoxic T lymphocyte response and viral persistence. *J Exp Med* 1984;160:521–540.

110. Moskophidis D, Lechner F, Pircher H, Zinkernagel RM. Virus persistence in acutely infected immunocompetent mice by exhaustion of antiviral cytotoxic effector T cells. *Nature* 1993;362:758–761.

111. Borrow P, Evans CF, Oldstone MBA. Virus-induced immunosuppression: immune system-mediated destruction of virus-infected dendritic cells results in generalized immune suppression. *J Virol* 1995;69:1059–1070.

112. Carmichael A, Jin X, Sissons P, Borysiewicz L. Quantitative analysis of the human immunodeficiency virus type 1 (HIV-1)-specific cytotoxic T lymphocyte (CTL) response at different stages of HIV-1 infection: differential CTL responses to HIV-1 and Epstein-Barr virus in late disease. *J Exp Med* 1993;177:249–256.

113. Gallimore A, Glithero A, Godkin A, et al. Induction and exhaustion of lymphocytic choriomeningitis virus-specific cytotoxic T lymphocytes visualized using soluble tetrameric major histocompatibility complex class I-peptide complexes. *J Exp Med* 1998;187:1383–1393.

114. Oxenius A, Zinkernagel RM, Hengartner H. Comparison of activation versus induction of unresponsiveness of virus-specific CD4+ and CD8+ T cells upon acute versus persistent viral infection. *Immunity* 1998;9:449–457.

115. Kyburz D, Aichele P, Speiser DE, Hengartner H, Zinkernagel RM, Pircher H. T cell immunity after a viral infection versus T cell tolerance induced by soluble viral peptides. *Eur J Immunol* 1993; 23:1956–1962.

116. Althage A, Odermatt B, Moskophidis D, et al. Immunosuppression by lymphocytic choriomeningitis virus infection: competent effector T and B cells but impaired antigen presentation. *Eur J Immunol* 1992;22:1803–1812.

117. Sourdive DJD, Murali-Krishna K, Altman JD, et al. Conserved T cell receptor repertoire in primary and memory CD8 T cell responses to an acute viral infection. *J Exp Med* 1998;188:71–82.

118. Busch DH, Pilip I, Palmer EG. Evolution of a complex T cell receptor repertoire during primary and recall bacterial infection. *J Exp Med* 1998; 188:61–70.

119. Silins SL, Cross SM, Elliott SL, et al. Development of Epstein-Barr virus-specific memory T cell receptor clonotypes in acute infectious mononucleosis. *J Exp Med* 1996;184:1815–1825.

120. Steven NM, Leese AM, Annels NE, Lee SP, Rickinson AB. Epitope focusing in the primary cytotoxic T cell response to Epstein-Barr Virus and its

121. Maryanski JL, Jongeneel CV, Bucher P, Casanova JL, Walker PR. Single-cell PCR analysis of TCR repertoires selected by antigen in vivo: a high magnitude CD8 response is composed of very few clones. *Immunity* 1996;4:47–55.

122. Pannetier C, Cochet M, Darche S, Casrouge A, Zoller M, Kourilisky P. The sizes of the CDR3 hypervariable regions of the murine T-cell receptor β chains vary as a function of the recombined germline segments. *Proc Natl Acad Sci USA* 1993; 90:4319–4323.

123. Bousso P, Casrouge A, Altman JD, et al. Individual variations in the murine T cell response to a specific peptide reflect variability in naive repertoire. *Immunity* 1998;9:169–178.

124. Rehermann B, Fowler P, Sidney J, et al. The cytotoxic T lymphocyte response to multiple hepatitis B virus polymerase epitopes during and after viral hepatitis. *J Exp Med* 1995;181:1047–1058.

125. Nayersina R, Fowler P, Guilhot S, et al. HLA A2 restricted cytotoxic T lymphocyte response to multiple hepatitis B surface antigen epitopes during hepatitis B virus infection. *J Immunol* 1993; 150:4659–4671.

126. Penna A, Chisari FV, Bertoletti A, et al. Cytotoxic T lymphocytes recognize an HLA-A2-restricted epitope within the hepatitis B virus nucleocapsid antigen. *J Exp Med* 1991;174:1565–1570.

127. Barnaba V, Franco A, Alberti A, Balsano C, Benvenuto R, Balsano F. Recognition of hepatitis B virus envelope protein by liver-infiltrating T lymphocytes in chronic HBV infection. *J Immunol* 1989;143:2650–2655.

128. Weekes MP, Wills MR, Mynard K, Carmichael AJ, Sissons JGP. The memory cytotoxic T-lymphocyte (CTL) response to human cytomegalovirus infection is contains individual peptide-specific CTL clones that have undergone extensive expansion in vivo. *J Virol* 1999;73:2099–2108.

129. Kalams SA, Johnson RP, Trocha AK, et al. Longitudinal analysis of T cell receptor (TCR) gene usage by human immunodeficiency virus 1 envelope-specific cytotoxic T lymphocyte clones reveals a limited TCR repertoire. *J Exp Med* 1994;179:1261–1271.

130. Wilson JDK, Ogg GS, Allen RL, et al. Oligoclonal expansions of CD8+ T cells in chronic HIV infection are antigen specific. *J Exp Med* 1998; 188:785–790.

131. Sprent J, Tough DF. Lymphocyte life-span and memory. *Science* 1996;265:1395–1400.

132. Matzinger P. Memories are made of this? *Nature* 1994;369:605–606.

133. Jameson SC, Hogquist KA, Bevan MJ. Positive selection of thymocytes. *Annu Rev Immunol* 1995;13:93–126.

134. Mackay CR. Immunological memory. *Adv Immunol* 1992;53:217–265.

135. Vitteta ES, Berton MT, Burger C, Kepron M, Lee WT, Yin XM. Memory B and T cells. *Annu Rev Immunol* 1991;9:193–217.

136. Selin LK, Welsh RM. Cytolytically active memory CTL present in lymphocytic choriomeningitis virus

(LCMV)-immune mice after clearance of virus infection. *J Immunol* 1997;158:5366–5373.

137. Di Rosa F, Matzinger P. Long-lasting CD8 T cell memory in the absence of CD4 T cells or B cells. *J Exp Med* 1996;183:2153–2163.

138. Von Herrath MG, Yokoyama M, Dockter J, Oldstone MBA, Whitton JL. CD4-deficient mice have reduced levels of memory cytotoxic T lymphocytes after immunization and show diminished resistance to subsequent virus challenge. *J Virol* 1996;70:1072–1079.

139. Homann D, Tishon A, Berger DP, Weigle WO, von Herrath MG, Oldstone MBA. Evidence for an underlying CD4 helper and CD8 T-cell defect in B-cell-deficient mice: failure to clear persistent virus infection after adoptive immunotherapy with virus-specific memory cells from μMT/μMT mice. *J Virol* 1998;72:9208–9216.

140. Ke Y, Ma H, Kapp JA. Antigen is required for the activation of effector activities, whereas interleukin 2 is required for the maintenance of memory in ovalbumin-specific, CD8$^+$ cytotoxic T lymphocytes. *J Exp Med* 1998;187:49–57.

141. Borrow P, Tishon A, Lee S, et al. CD40L-deficient mice show deficits in antiviral immunity and have an impaired memory CD8$^+$ CTL response. *J Exp Med* 1996;183:2129–2142.

142. Bruno L, Kirberg J, von Boehmer H. On the cellular basis of immunological T cell memory. *Immunity* 1995;2:37–43.

143. Kundig TM, Bachmann MF, Oehen S, et al. On the role of antigen in maintaining cytotoxic T-cell memory. *Proc Natl Acad Sci USA* 1996;93:9716–9723.

144. Gray D, Matzinger P. T cell memory is short-lived in the absence of antigen. *J Exp Med* 1991;174:969–974.

145. Oehen S, Waldner H, Kundig TM, Hengartner H, Zinkernagel RM. Antivirally protective cytotoxic T cell memory to lymphocytic choriomeningitis virus is governed by persisting antigen. *J Exp Med* 1992;176:1273–1281.

146. Bachmann MF, Odermatt B, Hengartner H, Zinkernagel RM. Induction of long-lived germinal centers associated with persisting antigen after viral infection. *J Exp Med* 1996;183:2259–2269.

147. Dutton RW, Bradley LM, Swain SL. T cell memory. *Annu Rev Immunol* 1998;16:201–223.

148. Asano MS, Ahmed R. CD8 T cell memory in B cell-deficient mice. *J Exp Med* 1996;183:2165–2174.

149. Bachmann MF, Kundig TM, Hengartner H, Zinkernagel RM. Protection against immunopathological consequences of a viral infection by activated but not resting cytotoxic T cells: T cell memory without "memory T cells"? *Proc Natl Acad Sci USA* 1997;94:640–645.

150. Kirberg J, Berns A, von Boehmer H. Peripheral T cell survival requires continual ligation of the T cell receptor to major histocompatibility complex-encoded molecules. *J Exp Med* 1997;186:1269–1275.

151. Tanchot C, Lemonnier FA, Perarnau B, Freitas AA, Rocha B. Differential requirements for survival and proliferation of CD8 naive or memory T cells. *Science* 1997;276:2057–2062.

152. Markiewicz MA, Girao C, Opferman JT, et al. Long-term T cell memory requires the surface expression of self-peptide/major histocompatibility complex molecules. *Proc Natl Acad Sci USA* 1998;95:3065–3070.

153. Bruno L, von Boehmer H, Kirberg J. Cell division in the compartment of naive and memory T lymphocytes. *Eur J Immunol* 1996;26:3179–3184.

154. Mims CA, Wainwright S. The immuno depressive action of lymphocytic choriomeningitis virus in mice. *J Immunol* 1968;101:717–724.

155. Von Pirquet C. Das verhalten der kutanen tuberkulin-reaktion wahrend der Masern. *Dtsch Med Wochenschr* 1908;34:1297–1300.

156. Van den Berg AP, Meyaard L, Otto SA, et al. Cytomegalovirus infection associated with a decreased proliferative capacity and increased rate of apoptosis of peripheral blood lymphocytes. *Transplant Proc* 1995;27:936–938.

157. Meyaard L, Otto SA, Jonker RR, Mijnster MJ, Keet RPM, Miedema F. Programmed death of T cells in HIV-1 infection. *Science* 1992;257:217–219.

158. Groux H, Torpier G, Monte D, Mouton Y, Carpon A, Ameisen JC. Activation-induced death by apoptosis in CD4$^+$ T cells from human immunodeficiency virus-infected asymptomatic individuals. *J Exp Med* 1992;175:331–340.

159. Akbar AN, Borthwick N, Salmon M, et al. The significance of low bcl-2 expression by CD45RO T cells in normal individuals and patients with acute viral infections: the role of apoptosis in T cell memory. *J Exp Med* 1993;178:427–438.

160. Razvi ES, Welsh RM. Programmed cell death of T lymphocytes during acute viral infection: a mechanism for virus-induced immune deficiency. *J Virol* 1993;67:5754–5765.

161. Liu Y, Janeway CAJ. Interferon gamma plays a critical role in induced cell death of effector T cell: a possible third mechanism of self-tolerance. *J Exp Med* 1990;172:1735–1739.

162. Oyaizy N, McCloskey TW, Than S, Hu R, Kalyanaraman VS, Pahwa S. Cross-linking of CD4 molecules upregulates Fas antigen expression in lymphocytes by inducing interferon-gamma and tumor necrosis factor-α secretion. *Blood* 1994;84:2622–2631.

163. Lee SB, Esteban M. The interferon-induced double-stranded RNA-activated protein kinase induces apoptosis. *Virology* 1994;199:491–496.

164. Lenardo MJ. Interleukin-2 programs mouse αβ T lymphocytes for apoptosis. *Nature* 1991;353:858–861.

165. Leonard WJ, Shores EW, Love PE. Role of the common cytokine receptor gamma chain in cytokine signalling and lymphoid development. *Immunol Rev* 1995;148:97–114.

166. Planz O, Seiler P, Hengartner H, Zinkernagel RM. Specific cytotoxic T cells eliminate B cells producing virus-neutralizing antibodies. *Nature* 1996;382:726–729.

167. Luciw PA. Human immunodeficiency viruses and their replication. In Fields BN, Knipe DM, Howley PM (eds) *Fields Virology*, vol 2. Philadelphia, Lippincott-Raven, 1995, pp 1881–1952.

168. An LL, Whitton JL. A multivalent minigene vac-

cine, containing B-cell, cytotoxic T-lymphocyte, and Th epitopes from several microbes, induces appropriate responses in vivo and confers protection against more than one pathogen. *J Virol* 1997;71:2292–2302.

169. Slifka MK, Shen H, Matloubian M, Jensen ER, Miller JF, Ahmed R. Antiviral cytotoxic T-cell memory by vaccination with recombinant *Listeria monocytogenes*. *J Virol* 1996;70:2902–2910.

170. Altmeyer R, Girard M, van der Werf S, Mimic V, Seigneur L, Saron MF. Attenuated Mengo virus: a new vector for live recombinant vaccines. *J Virol* 1995;69:3193–3196.

171. Castrucci MR, Hou S, Doherty PC, Kawaoka Y. Protection against lethal lymphocytic choriomeningitis virus (LCMV) infection by immunization of mice with an influenza virus containing an LCMV epitope recognized by cytotoxic T lymphocytes. *J Virol* 1994;68:3486–3490.

172. Zarozinski CC, Fynan EF, Selin LK, Robinson HL, Welsh RM. Protective CTL-dependent immunity and enhanced immunopathology in mice immunized by particle bombardment with DNA encoding an internal virion protein. *J Immunol* 1995; 154:4010–4017.

173. Yokoyama M, Zhang J, Whitton JL. DNA immunization confers protection against lethal lymphocytic choriomeningitis virus infection. *J Virol* 1995;69:2684–2688.

174. Martins LP, Lau LL, Asano MS, Ahmed R. DNA vaccination against persistent viral infection. *J Virol* 1995;69:2574–2582.

175. Aichele P, Brduscha-Riem K, Oehen S, et al. Peptide antigen treatment of naive and virus-immune mice: antigen-specific tolerance versus immunopathology. *Immunity* 1997;6:519–529.

176. Ciupitu A-MT, Petersson M, O'Donnell CL, et al. Immunization with a lymphocytic choriomeningitis virus peptide mixed with heat shock protein 70 results in protective antiviral immunity and specific cytotoxic T lymphocytes. *J Exp Med* 1998; 187:685–691.

177. Schulz M, Zinkernagel RM, Hengartner H. Peptide-induced antiviral protection by cytotoxic T cells. *Proc Natl Acad Sci USA* 1991;88:991–993.

178. Aichele P, Hengartner H, Zinkernagel RM, Schulz M. Antiviral cytotoxic T cell response induced by in vivo priming with a free synthetic peptide. *J Exp Med* 1990;171:1815–1820.

179. Saron MF, Fayolle C, Sebo P, Ladant D, Ullmann A, Leclerc C. Anti-viral protection conferred by recombinant adenylate cyclase toxins from *Bordetella pertussis* carrying a CD8+ T cell epitope from lymphocytic choriomeningitis virus. *Proc Natl Acad Sci USA* 1997;94:3314–3319.

180. Kapikian AZ, Mitchell RH, Chanock RM, Shvedoff RA, Stewart CE. An epidemiological study of altered clinical reactivity to respiratory syncytial (RS) virus infection in children previously vaccinated with an inactivated RS virus vaccine. *Am J Epidemiol* 1969;89:405–421.

181. Selin LK, Varga SM, Wong IC, Welsh RM. Protective heterologous antiviral immunity and enhanced immunopathogenesis mediated by memory T cell populations. *J Exp Med* 1998;188:1705–1715.

182. Doherty PC, Zinkernagel RM. T-cell-mediated immunopathology in viral infections. *Transplant Rev* 1974;19:89–120.

183. Cole GA, Nathanson N, Prendergast RA. Requirement for Φ-bearing cells in lymphocytic choriomeningitis virus-induced central nervous system disease. *Nature* 1972;238:335–337.

184. Cannon MJ, Openshaw PJM, Askonas BA. Cytotoxic T cells clear virus but augment lung pathology in mice infected with respiratory syncytial virus. *J Exp Med* 1988;168:1163–1168.

185. Graham BS, Bunton LA, Wright PF, Karzon DT. Role of T lymphocyte subsets in the pathogenesis of primary infection and rechallenge with respiratory syncytial virus in mice. *J Clin Invest* 1991; 88:1026–1033.

186. Moskophidis D, Kioussis D. Contribution of virus-specific CD8+ cytotoxic T cells to virus clearance or pathologic manifestations of influenza virus infection in a T cell receptor transgenic mouse model. *J Exp Med* 1998;188:223–232.

187. Weinstein L, Meade RH. Respiratory manifestations of chickenpox. *Arch Intern Med* 1956; 98:91–99.

188. Rickinson AB, Kieff E. Epstein-Barr virus. In Fields BN, Knipe DM, Howley PM, et al (eds) *Virology*, vol 2. Philadelphia: Lippincott-Raven, 1996, pp 2397–2446.

189. Matthew A, Kurane I, Green S, et al. Predominance of HLA-restricted cytotoxic T-lymphocyte responses to serotype-cross-reactive epitopes on nonstructural proteins following natural secondary dengue virus infection. *J Virol* 1998;72:3999–4004.

190. Yang H, Joris I, Majno G, Welsh RM. Necrosis of adipose tissue induced by sequential infections with unrelated viruses. *Am J Pathol* 1985; 120:173–177.

191. Evans CF, Horwitz MS, Hobbs MV, Oldstone MB. Viral infection of transgenic mice expressing a viral protein in oligodendrocytes leads to chronic central nervous system autoimmune disease. *J Exp Med* 1996;184:2371–2384.

192. Janeway CA. Innate immunity acknowledged. *Immunologist* 1995;3:198–200.

193. Welsh RM, Tay C, Varga SM, O'Donnell CL, Vergilis KL, Selin LK. Lymphocyte-dependent "natural" immunity to virus infections mediated by both natural killer cells and memory T cells. *Semin Virol* 1996;7:95–102.

Cytotoxic Cells: Basic Mechanisms and Medical Applications, edited by Michail V. Sitkovsky and Pierre A. Henkart. Lippincott Williams & Wilkins, Philadelphia © 2000.

Chapter 26

Tumor Antigens Recognized by Cytotoxic Lymphocytes

Paul F. Robbins, Rong-Fu Wang, and Steven A. Rosenberg

Surgery Branch, National Cancer Institute, Bethesda, Maryland 20815, USA

Studies carried out during the 1980s indicated that tumor-reactive T cells could be isolated from tumor-bearing mice and human cancer patients. Tumor-infiltrating lymphocytes (TILs) cultured *in vitro* with interleukin-2 (IL-2), and cultures derived by *in vitro* stimulation of peripheral blood mononuclear cells (PBMCs) with tumor cells from melanoma patients, were found to contain CD8$^+$ T cells that lysed tumor cells but not a variety of normal cells in a major histocompatibility complex class I (MHC-I)-restricted manner. In addition, these cells were found specifically to release a variety of cytokines including interferon-γ (IFN-γ), granulocyte/macrophage colony-stimulating factor (GM-CSF), and tumor necrosis factor-α (TNF-α) in response to tumor stimulation. Studies demonstrating the efficacy of TILs in mouse tumor models led to clinical trials in melanoma patients. In comparison with previous trials carried out with IL-2 treatment, treatment with TILs appeared to enhance clinical responses, but most patients still failed to respond to immunotherapy.

To gain a better understanding of the nature of antitumor immune responses and thereby hopefully improve anticancer treatment, studies have been carried out by a number of investigators using a variety of techniques to identify the antigens recognized by tumor-reactive T cells. Initially, cells that expressed the appropriate MHC-I haplotype but that did not express the tumor antigen were stably transfected with plasmid constructs containing genomic or cDNA libraries derived from tumor cells. Tumor-reactive T cells were then assayed for their ability specifically to release cytokines in response to transfectant clones. In subsequent studies, cDNA pools were transiently transfected into targets expressing the appropriate class I restriction element and assayed for their ability to stimulate cytokine release from T cell lines or clones. The peptides recognized by tumor-reactive T cells have also been directly identified by fractionating peptides isolated from tumor cell surface MHC-I molecules.

Gene products that are expressed in a limited number of normal tissues or overexpressed in tumors have been identified by independent means and represent potential or candidate antigens. Peptides that bind to particular MHC-I alleles have been identified from candidate antigens and have been examined for their ability either to be recognized by or induce tumor-reactive T cells. Screening of cDNA expression libraries using antisera derived from cancer patients (SEREX) has resulted in the cloning of several genes that are recognized by CD8$^+$ T cells and the identification of potentially important T cell targets.

These studies have demonstrated that tumor-reactive T cells recognize a wide variety

TABLE 26-1. *Cancer/testis antigens*

Gene	HLA allele	Peptide epitope	Reference
MAGE-1	A1	EADPTGHSY	1
MAGE-1	Cw16	SAYGEPRKL	2
MAGE-3	A1	EADPIGHLY	3
MAGE-3	A2	FLWGPRALV	4
MAGE-3	B44	MEVDPIGHLY	5
GAGE-1/2	Cw6	YRPRPRRY	6
BAGE	Cw16	AARAVFLAL	7
RAGE	B7	SPSSNRIRNT	8
NY-ESO-1	A2	SLLMWITQCFL	9
NY-ESO-1	A2	SLLMWITQC	9
NY-ESO-1	A2	QLSLLMWIT	9

of antigens. These antigens can be grouped into a number of categories based on their expression patterns in tumor and normal tissues (Tables 26-1 through 26-4). Identification of the T cell epitopes has revealed that several novel mechanisms are involved in generating the T cell epitopes in these molecules. In some cases, posttranslational modification of the amino acid side chains has been observed. Peptide epitopes have been shown to be encoded by intronic sequences, presumably resulting from incomplete splicing of mRNA transcripts, and from the translation of alternative open reading frames.

A number of these antigens are now being tested in clinical trials for their ability to cause tumor regression and to stimulate antitumor immune responses. A better understanding of the nature of these molecules should hopefully allow the development of more effective anticancer vaccines.

CANCER-TESTIS ANTIGENS

The first cloned human tumor antigen recognized by T cells was isolated following the screening of a genomic library from the melanoma patient MZ2 with an autologous, melanoma-reactive T cell clone (10). This gene, termed MAGE-1, was found to belong to a relatively large multigene family containing at least 12 genes that had not been previously described. These genes do not appear to be expressed in most normal adult tissues; however, several members of this gene family are expressed in either testicular germ cells or placental trophoblasts, two tissues that do not express MHC-I molecules (11,12). Members of the MAGE gene family have been shown to be expressed in tumors derived from a variety of additional tissue types including prostate, mammary, ovarian, colorectal, and esophageal carcinomas. Multiple members of the MAGE gene family have been found to be expressed in these tumors, with MAGE-3 expressed in the highest percentage of tumors (13). The BAGE (7) and GAGE (6) genes, which appear to be representatives of multigene families with expression patterns similar to those of the genes of the MAGE family, were isolated by screening a cDNA library from patient MZ2 with autologous T cell clones.

To identify the peptide epitopes in these molecules, fragments of these genes have been generated using the polymerase chain reaction (PCR) and exonuclease digestion. Epitopes that are recognized in the context of HLA-A1 and Cw16 were identified in MAGE-1 by synthesizing peptides from truncated constructs that fit the appropriate class I binding motif (1,2). An epitope of MAGE-3 recognized in the context of HLA-A1 was found to be encoded by the same region that encoded the MAGE-1 HLA-A1 epitope, differing at two of the nine amino acid residues within the epitope (3). Both of the peptides conformed to the consensus for binding to HLA-A1 (D or E at position 3, Y at position 9).

The identification of additional T cell epitopes from the MAGE-3 gene has been carried out by identifying potential epitopes using previously described HLA binding motifs, followed by screening those peptides for their binding to the appropriate class I allele. Following *in vitro* sensitization with peptides, peripheral blood lymphocytes (PBLs) were then tested for reactivity with class I binding peptide pulsed and tumor targets. Using this approach, T cells have been generated using peptide from MAGE-3 that are recognized in the context of HLA-A2 (4), HLA-B44 (14), and HLA-A24 (15). It will be crucial to demonstrate that T cells generated using these peptides can recognize a variety of tumor cells that express MAGE-3. Studies carried out with MAGE-1-reactive cytotoxic T lymphocytes (CTLs) indicated that many tumor cell lines express insufficient levels of this gene product to allow recognition by the CTLs (16).

Transgenic mice expressing the human HLA-A2 class I molecule have also been immunized with candidate peptides from the human MAGE-2 gene. Three HLA-A2-binding MAGE-2 peptides were found to be immunogenic in HLA-A2 transgenic mice, and two of these peptides appeared to elicit T cells that recognized peptide pulsed targets and tumor cells expressing HLA-A2 and MAGE-3 (17). Future studies demonstrating that these peptides can induce immune responses in human cancer patients are needed, as these peptides may be more immunogenic in mice, where they represent foreign epitopes, than in humans.

Screening of a melanoma cDNA expression library with serum from a patient with squamous cell carcinoma of the esophagus resulted in isolation of a previously unidentified gene that was termed NY-ESO-1 (18). Expression of this gene in normal tissues appeared to be limited to testis and ovary, but a wide variety of tumors including melanomas and carcinomas of the breast, prostate, ovaries, and bladder appeared to express this gene product. A survey carried out using serum from patients with melanoma and ovarian, lung, breast, and colon cancer demonstrated that approximately 10% of patients developed high-titered antibody against NY-ESO-1 protein (19). Subsequently, an HLA-A2-restricted CTL line derived from a melanoma patient with a high titer of antibodies to NY-ESO-1 was found to react with this antigen (9). Twenty-six peptides from the NY-ESO-1 coding sequence that conformed to the HLA-A2-binding motif were then synthesized and tested for recognition by the NY-ESO-1-reactive CTL line. Three par-

tially overlapping peptides (SLLMWITQC, SLLMWITQCFL, QLSLLMWIT) appeared to be recognized when pulsed on HLA-A2-expressing target cells. Although peptides containing cysteine and threonine at anchor residue positions were not identified in the original analysis of HLA-A2-binding peptides, peptide epitopes derived from tumor antigens containing these amino acids at the anchor residue positions have recently been described, as discussed later in this chapter.

The NY-ESO-1 gene was also isolated independently following the screening of a cDNA library with HLA-A31-restricted CTL clones (20). When a number of T cell clones were analyzed, two were found to recognize a peptide derived from the normal NY-ESO-1 open reading frame (ORF), whereas two additional CTL clones were found to recognize a peptide derived from an alternative ORF of NY-ESO-1. This alternative ORF, which initiated at an AUG codon that was 40 nucleotides downstream from the putative start codon, encoded a short 58-amino-acid polypeptide. Both of these products appear to be processed and presented naturally in melanoma and breast cancer cells, as all four of the T cell clones recognized melanomas and breast tumor cells expressing HLA-A31 and NY-ESO-1 (20).

Studies have suggested that class I-restricted T cells can recognize peptides derived from alternative ORFs of the α-tubulin (21), and influenza (22,23) nucleoprotein genes. Alternative splicing of the *p16* gene has also been shown to result in two products that are translated in different ORFs (24). These results, taken together with the results discussed below demonstrating that T cells recognize the product of alternative ORFs of the human melanoma antigen TRP-1 (25), indicate that similar cryptic products are expressed from a variety of genes. These transcripts appear generally to be expressed at relatively low levels in cells; however, antigen-specific T cells appear to be capable of responding to fewer than five peptide–MHC complexes on the cell surface (26,27).

DIFFERENTIATION ANTIGENS

Analysis of the specificity of a number of T cell lines and clones derived from melanomas has indicated that many of these cells recognized differentiation antigens that are expressed in normal cultured melanocytes. Screening of melanoma cDNA libraries carried out with an HLA-A2-restricted, melanoma-reactive TIL line (28) and a T cell clone derived from a mixed lymphocyte-tumor culture (MLTC) (29) resulted in isolation of a previously unknown gene termed MART-1 or Melan-A. Expression of this gene product appeared to be limited in normal tissues to the retina, which contains large numbers of melanocytes, and cultured skin melanocytes. MART-1 also appears to be expressed in skin *in vivo,* although the small percentage of melanocytes present in this tissue prevents precise quantitation of the level of expression of this gene product in skin. This gene encodes a 108-amino-acid protein

of unknown function that does not appear to be homologous to other known proteins. A hydrophobic region between amino acids 27 and 47 of the MART-1 protein may represent a transmembrane region, and preliminary studies indicate that MART-1 is expressed in melanosomes (30).

To identify the MART-1 peptide epitope, 23 peptides within this sequence that fit the HLA-A2 binding motif were synthesized and tested for reactivity with MART-1-reactive TILs (31). The results demonstrated that 10 of 10 MART-1 reactive TILs and a MART-1-reactive T cell clone reacted with a single nanomer peptide, AAGIGILTV (MART-1:27–35) (Table 26-2). Decamer peptides that contain one amino acid on the amino-terminus (EAAGIGILTV) and carboxy-terminus (AAGIGILTVI) of MART-1:27–35 were also recognized by these TILs at similar concentrations similar to that of the nanomer peptide. Additional testing has revealed that 22 of 30 HLA-A2-restricted TILs recognized MART-1 and the MART-1:27–35 peptide, indicating that it represented a dominant T cell epitope in patients expressing this

TABLE 26-2. *Melanocyte differentiation antigens*

Gene	HLA allele	Peptide epitope	Reference
MART-1	A2	AAGIGILTV	31
MART-1	A2	EAAGIGILTV	31
MART-1	A2	AAGIGILTVA	31
MART-1	B45	AEEAAGIGILT	32
MART-1	B45	AEEAAGIGIL	32
Gp100	A2	KTWGQYWQV	33
Gp100	A2	ITDQVPFSV	33
Gp100	A2	YLEPGPVTA	33
Gp100	A2	LLDGTATLRL	33
Gp100	A2	VLYRYGFSV	33
Gp100	A2	RLMKQDFSV	33
Gp100	A2	RLPRIFCSC	34
Gp100	A3	SLIYRRRLMK	34
Gp100	A3	ALLAVGATK	35
Gp100	A24	VYFFLPDHL(intron)	36
Tyrosinase	A2	MLLAVLYCL	37
Tyrosinase	A2	YMDGTMSQV	37
Tyrosinase	A24	AFLPWHRLF	38
Tyrosinase	A1	KCDICTDEY	39
Tyrosinase	A1	SSDYVIPIGTY	34
TRP-1	A31	MSLQRQFLR	25
TRP-2	A31	LLPGGRPYR	40
TRP-2	A2	SVYDFFVWL	41
TRP-2	A68	EVISCKLIKR(intron)	42

MHC-I haplotype (43). Studies have suggested that some HLA-A2-restricted, MART-1-reactive T cells recognize the peptide ILTVILGVL, which partially overlaps with MART-1:27–35 (44), but most MART-1-reactive T cells do not appear to react with this peptide (45; Y. Kawakami, unpublished observations).

The ability of peptides such as MART-1 to elicit T cell responses has been examined in patients expressing a number of HLA-A2 subtypes. The results indicated that MART-1:27–35 responses could be elicited in HLA-A*0201 individuals but not individuals of closely related subtypes including HLA-A*0202, 0205, 0206, and 0226 (46).

Recently, an HLA-B45 restricted melanoma-reactive T cell was found to recognize MART-1 (32). Mapping of the epitope through the use of exonuclease III deletions revealed that the region encoding the HLA-A2 epitope also encoded the HLA-B45 epitope. The peptides AEEAAGIGILT and AEEAAGIGIL appeared to represent the optimal epitopes recognized by two T cell clones isolated from melanoma patient SK29. It is not clear if there is any significance to the overlap between these peptides and the HLA-A2 epitope, but it could indicate that there is some bias in the processing of peptides from MART-1.

It is not clear what is responsible for the immune dominance of the response to the MART-1. One explanation put forth is that the MART-1 epitope represents an epitope mimic (47). In this study, evidence was presented indicating that MART-1-reactive T cells also reacted with a number of peptides derived from viral proteins. Thus T cells that recognize a common infectious agent could potentially cross-react with the MART-1 peptide, providing an explanation for the apparently high precursor frequency of T cells reactive with this tumor antigen.

Expression cloning carried out with an additional TIL line resulted in the identification of gp100 as a melanoma tumor antigen (48). This gene, which had previously been isolated, encoded a 661-amino-acid glycopro-

tein that was recognized by a number of monoclonal anti-melanoma antibodies (49). The gp100 protein is expressed in the melanosomal matrix and has been shown to represent an enzyme that is involved in melanin synthesis (50). In addition, a mutation in the murine gp100 gene has been shown to result in the mouse silver coat color phenotype (51). Studies carried out using reverse transcriptase PCR (RT-PCR) techniques have suggested that essentially all normal tissues and a variety of tumors of different histologies express low levels of gp100 (52,53). Nevertheless, expression of the protein product of this gene appears to be undetectable in nonmelanocyte lineage cells.

In contrast to MART-1, a large number of gp100 peptide epitopes have been identified. Screening carried out with TILs from four patients resulted in the identification of three nanomer peptides (gp100:154–162, 209–217, and 280–288) and two decamer peptides (gp100:457–466 and 476–485) (33). In another study, peptides were eluted from HLA-A2 molecules isolated from the surface of melanoma cells, fractionated by reverse-phase high performance liquid chromatography (HPLC) columns, and tested for recognition by HLA-A2-restricted melanoma-reactive MLTC lines (54). Two of the lines recognized multiple HPLC fractions, two of which appeared to contain shared epitopes. Peptides from one of these fractions were rechromatographed, and screening of the peptides identified following the second separation indicated that the gp100:280–288 peptide represented the active peptide in this fraction. Three additional CTL lines that were tested also reacted with this peptide, indicating that it represents an immunodominant epitope. Additional studies have indicated that about 20% of TILs react with each of the peptide epitopes gp100:154–162, 209–217, and 280–288 (43).

Several additional HLA-A2-restricted gp100 epitopes have been identified. Candidate peptides from gp100 were initially identified based on their binding to HLA-A2 and then tested for their ability to stimulate *in vitro* responses (55). Three of six additional gp100 peptides that had been identified on the basis of their high to moderate affinity for HLA-A2 appeared capable of stimulating melanoma-reactive CTLs *in vitro*. Stimulation with two of the six peptides resulted in generation of peptide-reactive T cells that failed to recognize tumor targets. Subsequent studies have demonstrated that the gp100:619–627 peptide was recognized by CTL clones isolated from a melanoma patient (34). In the study cited above (55), the gp100:619–627 peptide appeared to induce peptide-reactive T cells, but clear tumor reactivity could not be demonstrated with these T cells. Thus stimulation with peptide pulsed targets expressing relatively high levels of MHC-I complexes appears in some cases to result in stimulation of low-affinity T cells that cannot recognize targets expressing relatively low levels of endogenously processed antigens. T cells that result from *in vitro* or *in vivo* stimulation with tumor, such as TILs, generally contain T cells with relatively high-affinity receptors that are capable of recognizing processed antigens. T cell tolerance may also play a role in skewing the T cell repertoire toward low-affinity T cells in the case of self antigens such as gp100.

An additional HLA-A2-restricted, gp100 epitope, gp100:639–647 (RLPRIFCSC), was found to be recognized by the bulk TIL 1200 cell line (34). Previous results indicated that this TIL line recognized two gp100 epitopes, gp100:154–162 and 457–465 (33). This peptide contained two cysteine residues, one at position 7 and one at position 9 at the C-terminal anchor residue position. Peptides were then synthesized in which the cysteine residues were substituted with α-aminobutyric acid, an amino acid that cannot be oxidized but that contains a side chain similar in size to the cysteine side chain. Replacement of the cysteines at either position individually or at both of these positions with α-aminobutyric acid significantly enhanced T cell recognition. This finding indicates that formation of disulfide bonds, with a second

cysteine residue or another sulfhydryl compound, may inhibit binding of the peptide to class I. Interactions with amino acids in the HLA-A2 binding pocket may prevent further modification of the cysteine residue side chains in the naturally processed epitope.

Epitopes of gp100 that are recognized in the context of additional class I restriction elements have also been described. Screening of a melanoma cDNA library with an HLA-A24-restricted T cell cloid resulted in the isolation of a cDNA clone that encoded the first 158 amino acids of gp100 (36). Following nucleotide 469 of the normal gp100 coding region, the sequence of the cDNA clone corresponded to the fourth intron of gp100, indicating that it represented an aberrantly spliced product of the gp100 gene. A peptide epitope that conformed to the HLA-A24 binding motif was found to be encoded within the intronic region of this transcript. In addition, the T cell cloid also appeared to recognize normal cultured melanocytes, and RT-PCR analysis indicated that this transcript appeared to be expressed at relatively similar levels in melanomas and melanocytes. This transcript was not, however, detected by Northern blot analysis, indicating that it is expressed at relatively low levels in these cells.

Tyrosinase, a critical enzyme involved in the first steps of melanin synthesis, has also been shown to be recognized by melanoma-reactive T cells. The gene encoding tyrosinase was first isolated in 1987 (56). Two HLA-A2-restricted, melanoma-reactive T cell clones were found to recognize distinct epitopes of tyrosinase, one beginning at the amino-terminal methionine of the tyrosinase signal sequence (MLLAVLYCL, tyr:1–9) and a second beginning with amino acid residue 368 (YMNGTMSQV, tyr:368–376) (57). Subsequent studies demonstrated that tyrosinase-specific CTLs could be elicited by stimulating T cells from cancer patients or healthy donors with the tyr:368–376 peptide (58).

A peptide with a sequence similar to the tyr:368–376 peptide but containing a substitution at the third position of aspartic acid for asparagine was identified by the analysis of peptides that had been eluted from MHC-I molecules isolated from melanoma cells (54). Subsequent studies indicated that it represented the natural peptide recognized by HLA-A2-restricted tyrosine-reactive T cells (59). The asparagine residue at position 3 of this peptide is part of an N-linked glycosylation site, and a mammalian enzyme has been isolated that removes N-linked oligosaccharide side chains from glycopeptides and converts the asparagine residue at this position to aspartic acid (60). Presentation of the tyr:368–376 peptide appeared to involve processing in the cytosol, and was TAP- and proteosome-dependent, indicating that conversion of the asparagine to aspartic acid in this peptide may take place in this compartment (61). Peptide-specific T cells from HLA-A2 transgenic mice that had been immunized with the aspartic acid-containing peptide recognized human melanomas but failed to recognize targets pulsed with the asparagine-containing peptide (61). Conversely, T cells isolated from mice that had been immunized with the asparagine-containing peptide reacted with targets that had been pulsed with the asparagine-containing but not the aspartic acid-containing peptide; however, these T cells failed to recognize human HLA-A2$^+$ melanoma cells. In addition, only the aspartic acid-containing peptide could be eluted from HLA-A2 molecules isolated from the melanoma cell surface, indicating that it represents the naturally processed epitope recognized by T cells.

Further studies have resulted in identification of additional tyrosinase epitopes. Two HLA-A24-restricted TILs were found to recognize tyrosinase. The peptide epitope recognized by one of the TILs, AFLPWHRLF, conformed to the normal HLA-A24-binding motif (38); and the second HLA-A24-restricted TIL failed to recognize this epitope and recognizes an as yet unidentified epitope (62). Additional tyrosinase epitopes have been found to be recognized in the context of HLA-B44 (63). Autologous cells that had

been infected with a recombinant vaccinia virus construct encoding tyrosinase have also been used to stimulate *in vitro* responses of PBLs from melanoma patients (64). T cells clones that recognized tyrosinase in the context of a variety of MHC-I alleles were isolated from five of the eight patients' PBLs examined.

Recent studies have resulted in identification of a tyrosinase epitope that is recognized in the context of HLA-A1 (39). Melanoma-reactive CTLs that were isolated from five of six HLA-A1 patients were all found to recognize the nanomer KCDICTDEY and the overlapping dodecamer DAEKCDICTDEY. Relatively high concentrations of peptide, on the order of 1 μM, were required to sensitize targets for T cell recognition. Serine or alanine residues, two amino acids containing side chains similar in size to the cysteine side chain, were then substituted for cysteine at either position 2 or 5 of the nanomer peptide. Peptides containing either a serine or alanine residue at position 2 of the nanomer and the corresponding residue in the dodecamer were recognized at concentrations that were 100- to 1,000-fold lower than the natural peptide. The effects of modification of the cysteine at position 5 were less clear, as recognition of the nanomer did not appear to be affected significantly, whereas recognition of the dodecamer was abolished by this change. These results indicate that the cysteine residue near the N-terminus of the natural epitope may reside in the HLA-A1-binding groove and therefore be protected from modification. The cysteine residue that is nearer to the C-terminus would be predicted to possess an exposed side chain and may be linked either to cysteine or another sulfhydryl compound.

Screening a melanoma cDNA library using TIL586 resulted in isolation of the gene encoding TRP-1 (gp75) (65), a molecule that had previously been shown to be recognized by immunoglobulin G (IgG) antibodies in the serum of a patient with melanoma (66). The gp75 protein is one of the most abundant intracellular glycoproteins in melanocyte-lineage cells but is not expressed in nonmelanocytic cell types (67). The gp75 molecule has been shown to have DHI-2-carboxylic acid oxidase activity involved in the synthesis of melanin (68).

To identify a T cell epitope from gp75, a number of peptides were synthesized based on the predicted amino acid sequence of gp75 from a small region known to confer T cell recognition when co-transfected with an HLA-A31 cDNA into COS-7 cells. None of the peptides tested were found to stimulate cytokine release from TIL586 when pulsed onto HLA-A31$^+$ Epstein-Barr virus (EBV)-transformed B cells (25). To explore the possibility that T cell epitopes are derived from gene products of alternative ORFs, three peptides derived from ORF2 and two peptides from ORF3 were selected and synthesized on the basis of the HLA-A31-binding motif. Surprisingly, the peptide that was derived from ORF3, MSLQRQFLR, was capable of stimulating cytokine release from TIL586 when pulsed onto HLA-A31$^+$ EBV-transformed B cells.

Additional HLA-A31-restricted, melanoma-reactive CTL clones isolated from TIL586 failed to recognize TRP-1 but still recognized HLA-A31$^+$ melanocytes. Screening of an autologous cDNA library with one of these clones resulted in the isolation of TRP-2 (40). TRP-2 is a member of the tyrosinase-related family of proteins and is 40% to 45% identical at the amino acid sequence level to both tyrosinase and TRP-1/gp75. The antigenic peptide recognized by the CTL clone was encoded by the normal ORF of TRP-2. Another study demonstrated that CTLs reactive with the murine B16 melanoma recognized a distinct peptide encoded by the mouse TRP-2 gene (69).

To broaden the clinical utility of tumor antigens such as TRP-1 and TRP-2, both of which are recognized in the context of HLA-A31, an attempt was made to identify T cell epitopes from these proteins that are restricted by additional MHC-I alleles. Studies of the structural similarities of a group of HLA alleles and peptide binding motifs has led to the grouping of HLA alleles into "supertypes" (70). The HLA-A31 molecule belongs to a member of the HLA-A3-like supertype that encompasses 45% to 50% of all ethnic populations. In a recent study, the TRP-1 and TRP-2 peptides were found to bind to HLA-A3, -A11, -A31, -A33, and -A68. Furthermore, the TRP-2 peptide was recognized by T cells in the context of HLA-A31 and HLA-A33 (71). These studies indicate that it may be possible to immunize patients expressing one of the HLA-A3 superfamily members with the TRP-1 and TRP-2 peptides that have already been identified.

Recent studies have also focused on the identification of peptide epitopes from these antigens that are recognized in the context of more widely expressed class I alleles, such as HLA-A2. Peptides from TRP-2 that fit the HLA-A2-binding motif were initially tested for their affinity for this class I allele using a standard competitive inhibition assay (72). Twenty-one peptides that inhibited the binding of a standard peptide at a concentration of 2 μM or less were then used to generate CTLs *in vitro* using PBLs from HLA-A2 melanoma patients. Repetitive *in vitro* stimulations with one of these peptides, SVYDFFVWL (TRP2:180–188), was found to generate CTLs from patient PBLs that recognized T2 cells pulsed with this peptide as well as HLA-A2$^+$, TRP-2$^+$ melanomas (41). This peptide is identical to the TRP-2 peptide previously found to be recognized by B16-reactive CTLs in the context of H-2K^b (69). Use of the TRP-2 antigen and peptide epitopes identified from this antigen may allow the development of immunotherapeutic protocols in cancer patients, and parallel with studies in mouse model systems may allow further evaluation of these strategies.

WIDELY EXPRESSED PROTEINS

Several tumor antigens that appear to be expressed in a variety of normal tissues have been isolated (Table 26-3). A tumor derived from melanoma patient LB33, termed

TABLE 26-3. *Widely expressed antigens*

Gene	HLA allele	Peptide epitope	Reference
SART-1	A26	KGSGKMKTE	73
PRAME	A24	LYVDSLFFL	74
P15	A24	AYGLDFYIL	75

LB33.MEL.A, was initially shown to express at least five distinct tumor antigens that were recognized by autologous CTLs in the context of the HLA-A28, -B13, -B44, and -Cw6 class I genes (76). This CTL failed to recognize a tumor cell line, termed MEL.B, that was derived from a recurrent tumor isolated from the same patient 3 years after resection of the original tumor. Analysis of this tumor indicated that it had lost the expression of all HLA class I alleles with the exception of HLA-A24. Stimulation of PBLs from patient LB33 with the MEL.B cell line resulted in stimulation of CTLs that recognized MEL.B tumor; however, these CTLs failed to recognize the MEL.A tumor. The cloning of this antigen, which was carried out using a conventional cDNA library approach, demonstrated that these CTLs recognized a novel antigen in the context of HLA-A24. This antigen, termed PRAME, appeared to be expressed at relative high levels in the testis and endometrium. The level of expression of this product in other normal tissues, such as the ovary, adrenals, kidney, brain, and skin, was estimated using a semiquantitative PCR to be only a small percentage of that found in melanoma cells. The PRAME-reactive T cell line was found to express a natural killer (NK) cell inhibitory receptor that bound to the HLA-Cw7 class I molecule expressed by the MEL.A but not the MEL.B tumor.

A screening assay carried out using an HLA-A24-restricted, melanoma-reactive T cell line resulted in isolation of a previously undescribed gene that was termed p15 and that appeared to be expressed in a number of normal tissues as well (75). It is not clear at the present time how these T cells discriminate tumor from normal cells. One caveat

must be raised, however: Gene products that are overexpressed as a result of transfection might be recognized even if they do not represent the normal target antigen due to the degeneracy of T cell recognition.

Expression cloning techniques were also used to isolate a novel antigen recognized by a CTL line that was derived by stimulation with an autologous squamous cell carcinoma (73). This antigen was encoded by a previously undescribed gene, termed SART-1, which seemed to be expressed in lung adenocarcinomas as well as lung and esophageal squamous cell carcinomas. In addition, this product appeared to be expressed in normal proliferating cell lines but not in normal tissues with the exception of fetal liver and testis. A second protein product of this gene that was derived by initiation from an internal AUG codon appeared to be expressed in the cytoplasm of tumor cells but not normal cells, which may account for the tumor specificity of this response.

TUMOR-SPECIFIC ANTIGENS

Most of the antigens that have been isolated appear to be expressed in at least some normal tissues, although tumor antigens with a more limited expression pattern have been observed (Table 26-4). A number of the antigens in this category arise from somatically mutated gene products. In some cases these mutations have been observed in only a single tumor isolate, whereas in other cases mutations have been found in multiple tumors. Nonmutated transcripts that appear to be expressed only in tumor cells have also been observed.

TABLE 26-4. *Tumor-specific antigens*

Gene	HLA	Peptide epitope	Reference
CDK-4	A2	ACDPHSGHFV	77
MUM-1	B44	EEKLIVVLF	29
β-Catenin	A24	SYLDSGIHF	78
Caspase-8	B35	FPSDSWCYF	79
KIAA0205	B44	AEPINIQTV	80
HPV E7	A2	YMLDLQPETT	81

Screening a cDNA library with a T cell clone isolated from melanoma patient LB33 resulted in isolation of a previously undescribed gene whose product was recognized in the context of HLA-B44 (82). This cDNA clone contained a sequence that appeared to represent an intron that was removed inefficiently from the primary RNA transcript, and the T cell epitope was found to be encoded by the region that spanned the intron/exon boundary. In addition, a single basepair change altered an amino acid that seemed to affect a T cell contact residue, as both the normal and mutated peptides appeared to bind equivalently to HLA-B44.

Expression cloning carried out with an HLA-A2-restricted, melanoma-reactive T cell resulted in isolation of a mutated product of the cyclin-dependent kinase 4 (CDK4) gene (77). The CDK4 protein plays an important role in cell cycle progression. A single basepair change in the region encoding the minimal T cell epitope, ACDPHSGHFV, resulted in substitution of cysteine for arginine at the second position in this peptide. T cell clones could recognize targets pulsed with approximately 100-fold lower concentrations of the mutant than the normal peptide, but antigen processing may also be affected by this mutation. Binding of the normal CDK4 inhibitor, p16^{INK4a}, to CDK4 appeared to be partially disrupted by the CDK4 mutation. The p16^{INK4a} gene appears to be frequently mutated in a variety of cancers including melanomas, and genetic susceptibility to melanoma is associated with mutations of the p16^{INK4a} locus (83). Unregulated cell growth may result from inactivation of the p16 gene product or mutation of key residues in the CDK4 gene product. The identical CDK4 mutation was also observed in 1 of 28 additional melanomas examined, providing further support for the role of this mutation in carcinogenesis.

Expression cloning carried out using T cells reactive with a squamous cell carcinoma resulted in isolation of a cDNA encoding caspase-8 (CASP-8) (79), a protein that appears to play a critical role in apoptosis mediated by Fas and TNFR1. This gene was found to contain a point mutation in the normal CASP-8 stop codon that resulted in a carboxy-terminal extension of the normal ORF by 88 amino acids. This appears to be a relatively rare mutation, as it was not found in 150 additional tumors that were analyzed. The peptide epitope, which was recognized in the context of HLA-B*3503, was encoded by sequences within the extended region. The CASP-8 mutation appeared to interfere with the apoptotic activity of this protein; thus it is possible that this product plays some role in tumorigenesis.

Screening of a cDNA library using an HLA-A24-restricted tumor reactive CTL line resulted in isolation of a β-catenin cDNA clone (84). The peptide epitope that was identified, SYLDSGIHF, corresponded to amino acids 29 to 37 of the β-catenin molecule. A single point mutation found in the codon 37 resulted in a change from serine to phenylalanine at this position. This alteration appeared to create an optimal HLA-A24-binding peptide, and binding studies indicated that the mutated peptide had a significantly higher binding affinity than the normal peptide for HLA-A24. Mutations at the same site, as well as positions 41 or 45 of β-catenin, were found in melanomas isolated from different patients, and these mutations appeared to enhance the stability of this molecule (78). Additional studies have demonstrated the presence of β-catenin mutations in colon (85,86) and hepatocellular (87) carcinomas. These mutations stabilize the β-catenin molecule, allowing it to form complexes with members of the Tcf family of DNA-binding proteins. The activation of as yet unidentified target genes by these complexes could potentially play some role in tumorigenesis.

A previously unidentified gene was recently isolated after screening a bladder cancer cDNA library with autologous tumor-reactive T cells in the context of HLA-B*4403 (80). This product, which appeared to be expressed in a wide variety of normal tissues and cell lines, contained a single point mutation in the region of the transcript encoding the T cell epitope. This mutation resulted in substitution of an asparagine for an aspartic acid residue at position 5 of the peptide, which appears to represent a T cell contact residue, as binding of this peptide to HLA-B*4403 was unaffected by this alteration. This mutation was expressed only in the tumor cell line and a fresh tumor sample that was isolated from the autologous patient, but it was not found in more than 100 additional tumors that were examined, indicating that this represented a relatively rare event.

A product of the *N*-acetylglucosaminyltransferase V (GnT-V) gene appears to represent a shared tumor-specific antigen (88). The transcript isolated using conventional expression cloning techniques initiated from a cryptic promoter present within one of the introns of the normal GnT-V gene. The intronic region present within this transcript encoded a 74-amino-acid polypeptide that included the T cell epitope. Approximately half of the melanomas tested expressed significant levels of this product, whereas other tumor types generally did not express the GnT-V intronic transcript. Normal tissues including skin did not appear to express this transcript, although *in vitro* cultured melanocytes expressed this product. Expression of the GnT-V product may have been induced as a result of proliferation induced by *in vitro* culture, and thus it is possible that tissue melanocytes may either not express this gene product or express it at relatively low levels.

Screening assays carried out using T cells that recognize a renal carcinoma resulted in isolation of a mutated HLA-A2 molecule (89). This mutation was present in the α helix region of the HLA-A2 α2 domain, effectively resulting in generation of an allogeneic MHC molecule in this tumor. Somatic mutations that alter the amino acid sequence of an MHC molecule have not previously been observed and thus appear to represent relatively rare events.

A tumor-specific epitope encoded by a retained intronic sequence has been identified using an HLA-A*6801-restricted, melanoma-reactive CTL clone (42). The cDNA clone that was isolated appeared to contain the second intron of the TRP-2 gene and a portion of the fourth intron of this gene. Read through of the normal TRP-2 ORF into the second intron would result in the production of a 227-amino-acid protein, 39 of which would be derived from the intronic sequence. The peptide epitope EVIS CKLIKR, which was encoded by sequences within the second intron, conformed to the HLA-A*68 binding motif (90). The CTL clone used in this study failed to recognize melanocytes expressing HLA-A*68, and data obtained using PCR demonstrated that transcripts containing the second intron were either not detected or expressed at low levels in melanocytes. This transcript was, however, readily detected in all melanomas that expressed the normal TRP-2 gene product.

Viral antigens such as those derived from the human papillomavirus (HPV), which has been shown to be present in more than 90% of cervical carcinomas and is implicated in the etiology of this disease, represents a tumor-specific target for immunotherapy. *In vitro* stimulations carried out with three HLA-A2-binding peptides from the HPV E6 protein appeared to result in the generation of T cells reactive with cervical carcinoma (91). Additional studies carried out with two of these peptides have indicated that peptide and tumor-reactive T cells can be generated from only a minority of cervical carcinoma patients (81,92). Nevertheless, these results support additional efforts to identify immunogenic HPV epitopes.

IDENTIFICATION OF EPITOPES ON CANDIDATE ANTIGENS

A number of approaches have been used to identify new tumor antigen peptide epitopes, including *in vitro* sensitization with synthetic peptides that have been found to bind to particular MHC alleles and immunization of transgenic mice expressing human MHC alleles. In a recent study the gp100 gene was scanned for peptides that bind to HLA-A2, and a number of peptides were synthesized and used to stimulate *in vitro* responses (55). Five peptides that bound to HLA-A2 with high-affinity peptides were identified, and three of them were found to elicit T cells that recognized tumor cells. As described above, one of these peptides, gp100:619–627, was subsequently found to be recognized by melanoma-reactive T cell clones (34).

A recent attempt has been made to identify peptide epitopes derived from the melanocortin 1 receptor (MC1R) (93). This protein, which is a member of a family of G-protein-coupled receptors that bind melanocyte-stimulating hormone (MSH), appears to be primarily expressed in cells of the melanocyte lineage. The MC1R sequence was initially scanned for peptides that fit the HLA-A2-binding motif, followed by testing these peptides for their ability to bind to purified HLA-A2. The 12 highest MHC binding peptides were then tested for their ability to elicit peptide-reactive CTLs. Three peptides with either high or intermediate affinity for HLA-A2 were found to elicit peptide-specific T cells in most normal donors tested. CTL lines generated with each of the three peptides appeared to recognize HLA-A2$^+$, M1CR$^+$ melanomas but did not recognize melanomas expressing only HLA-A2 or M1CR.

A number of attempts have also been made to identify T cell epitopes from the HER-2/neu protein. This protein, a member of the tyrosinase kinase family of receptors, is frequently amplified and overexpressed in a variety of tumors including breast, ovarian, and colorectal tumors (94). Studies have indicated that overexpression of HER-2/neu may influence the tumorigenicity of cancer cells (95,96), making it an attractive target for the development of anticancer therapies. Several HLA-A2-binding peptides were found to be recognized by tumor-associated lymphocytes (TALs) that had been isolated from malignant ascites and cultured in the presence of IL-2 (97). A single peptide, HER-2/neu:369–377, appeared to represent the immunodominant peptide, as all of four

TAL lines appeared to recognize this peptide. It has also been reported that the HER-2/neu:654–662 peptide was recognized by breast and ovarian cancer TILs (98). Additional HER-2/neu peptides have been identified by immunizing double transgenic mice expressing the human HLA-A2 and CD8 molecules (99) and by stimulating normal PBLs with peptide-pulsed dendritic cells (100).

These findings, indicating that the HER-2/neu:369–377 peptide represents an immunodominant epitope of this protein, served as the basis for a clinical trial involving immunization with this peptide in incomplete Freund's adjuvant that was recently carried out in the Surgery Branch, National Cancer Institute. The CTL response of PBMCs obtained before or after peptide immunization was examined following a single *in vitro* stimulation with peptide for 7 to 10 days. In three of the four patients examined, a vigorous peptide-specific T cell response was elicited by *in vitro* stimulation of postimmunization PBMCs. The *in vitro* stimulation of preimmunization PBMCs resulted in generation of peptide-reactive T cells from only one of four patients (101). These peptide-reactive CTLs failed to react with HLA-A2$^+$ breast and ovarian tumor cell lines that naturally overexpressed HER-2/neu, however, and did not react with transfected cell lines expressing both of these gene products.

It is not clear how to reconcile these observations with previous results. Peptide immunization may have resulted in stimulation of T cells with only a low affinity for this antigen; however, targets pulsed with as little as 1 ng/ml of the HER-2/neu:654–662 peptide could be recognized by these CTLs (101). In one study, PBMCs from normal donors were stimulated with autologous dendritic cells that had been pulsed with the HER-2/neu:369–377 peptide (100). When replicate wells containing peptide-reactive cells were assayed, only 2 of 29 of the cultures appeared to recognize tumors that overexpressed this gene product. Thus stimulation with this peptide may generally elicit T cells that can recognize only the relatively high amounts of peptide present on the cell surface following exogenous peptide pulsing. The tumor cell lines used in this study were also treated with interferon-γ (IFN-γ), and it is not clear how well these T cells would recognize unmanipulated targets. Thus cells that endogenously express the HER-2/neu antigen may not generally process and present detectable levels of this peptide on the cell surface.

As another approach to the screening of candidate antigens, antigen-presenting cells (APCs) have been either directly transfected with constructs encoding target molecules or infected with recombinant viral constructs. As mentioned above, tyrosinase-reactive T cells could be elicited by stimulation with autologous adherent cells from peripheral blood that had been infected with a recombinant vaccinia virus encoding tyrosinase (64). In addition, dendritic cells that had been transfected with genes encoding MART-1 and gp100 were shown to stimulate responses against these antigens (102).

A number of molecules that represent potential T cell targets have been identified through the use of the SEREX technique (103,104). Genetic techniques that rely on differences in the expression in various tissues have also been used to isolate a new member of the MAGE gene family (105) as well as LAGE (106), a gene that is highly homologous to NY-ESO-1. The development of efficient methods for stimulating T cell responses against processed epitopes of these molecules should allow generation of therapeutic reagents that can be used for the treatment of a large number of tumor types.

INFLUENCE OF EXPRESSION LEVEL AND AFFINITY ON IMMUNE RESPONSE

A number of factors may influence antigenicity and immunogenicity of a particular epitope, including the endogenous level of expression of a particular gene product, the affinity of the peptide for the MHC-I molecule, and the affinity of the T cell receptor

(TCR) for the peptide–MHC complex. Analysis of the expression of MAGE-1 using a quantitative PCR technique indicated that at least 10% of the level found in a reference melanoma was required for recognition by specific CTLs (16). Studies of tumor variants raised *in vitro* by cloning (107) or the selection of resistant tumor lines (108) have indicated that the level of HLA class I gene expression on tumor cells can influence T cell recognition.

A number of the HLA-A2 epitopes appear to have a relatively low binding affinity for MHC-I molecules, which may affect the immunogenicity of these antigens. Modifications of T cell epitopes that increase MHC-I binding affinities have been shown to enhance peptide immunogenicity, as discussed below. In addition, the recognition of a target antigen is dependent on the levels of class I and antigen expression as well as the TCR affinity for that complex, which has implications for the use of these products as immunogens. Peptide epitopes that have been predicted to bind to MHC-I molecules when used as immunogens have been found in some cases to lead to the stimulation of T cells that react with peptide-pulsed targets but that fail to recognize cells expressing the antigen endogenously. Endogenous protein expression may result in either no expression or relatively low levels of expression of processed peptides on MHC-I molecules. T cell tolerance may also influence responses to self antigens, resulting in the deletion of T cells with high-affinity TCRs and leaving only T cells with low-affinity receptors that may not respond to the relatively low levels of expression resulting from endogenous processing. Clearly, a combination of factors may influence the ability of T cells to recognize a particular epitope, helping to explain some of the discrepancies between results reported by different investigators.

Several studies have suggested that the equilibrium binding affinity (109) and the stability of peptide–MHC complexes (110) are important determinants of peptide immunogenicity. A number of the tumor antigen peptides that have been identified do not fit the optimal HLA-A2 binding motif, which consists of a leucine or methionine residue at position 2 and a valine or leucine residue at the last position, and appear to bind to HLA-A2 with relatively low or intermediate affinities. The gp100:209–217 peptide contains a threonine residue at position 2; however, substitutions of either leucine or methionine for threonine at this position enhanced the HLA-A2-binding affinity of this peptide by a factor of 52 and 9, respectively (111). Analysis of the T cells elicited following multiple *in vitro* stimulations demonstrated that the tumor-reactive T cells could be elicited more reliably and after fewer stimulations with the modified peptides than with the native gp100:209–217 peptide. As discussed below, use of the modified peptide in clinical trials has been shown to result in stimulation of enhanced T cell responses (112).

Attempts have also been made to enhance the immunogenicity of the HLA-A2 MART-1 peptide. Results suggest that certain peptide-reactive T cells recognize the decamer EAAGIGILTV (MART-1;26–35) at significantly lower concentrations than the nanomer peptide (32,113). Varying recognition patterns were observed when 5 MART-1 reactive T cell clones were tested for their ability to respond to peptides containing modifications at different positions (45). Measurement of the binding and the dissociation of this complex indicated that the MART-1;26–35 peptide that contained a leucine or methionine substitution at position 2 was significantly more stable than the unmodified decamer and nanomer. Substitution of tyrosine or phenylalanine for glutamic acid at position 1 of the decamer also enhanced the binding and stability of the peptide; however, only the decamer containing leucine at position 2 was recognized by all of the T cell clones. The relative ability of this peptide to be recognized by these clones was enhanced by 100- to 20,000-fold in comparison to the native nanomer, suggesting that it might represent a more potent immunogen *in vitro* and *in vivo*.

Initially it was reported that tumor-reactive T cells could be generated using targets that had been pulsed with an HLA-A2-binding peptide from MAGE-3 (4). In a second study, however, T cells stimulated with targets that had been pulsed with an HLA-A2-binding MAGE-3 peptide recognized peptide-pulsed targets and cells that had been transfected with the MAGE-3 cDNA, but failed to recognize tumor cells expressing normal endogenous levels of this protein (114). The influence of tumor antigen expression on CTL recognition has also been demonstrated in an analysis of tumor cell lines with varied levels of expression of the MART-1 and gp100 proteins (115). The levels of expression of adhesion molecules has also been shown to affect tumor cell recognition (116).

Studies of peptides derived from the p53 tumor-suppressor protein have demonstrated that the induction of tolerance by peptides expressed on normal tissues plays an important role in influencing the T cell repertoire. A number of peptides from the human and mouse p53 sequence were tested for their ability to stimulate T cell responses in normal or p53 knockout mice expressing the HLA-A2 class I transgene (117). For a number of peptides, immune responses could be generated only in knockout mice, indicating that T cells may be tolerized in normal mice owing to the expression of these peptides on normal cells. Immunization of p53 knockout mice with a tumor expressing p53 resulted in tumor regression, which was shown to result from recognition of a p53 peptide (118). A single nonmutated p53 peptide (amino acids 261–269) was capable of generating a response in normal and knockout mice; however, the avidity of T cells stimulated with this peptide appeared to be significantly lower in the normal mice than in knockout mice. The CTLs generated in normal mice appeared to recognize peptide-pulsed targets but failed to recognize tumor cells that overexpressed p53. Two studies using human PBLs have indicated, however, that it is possible to generate T cells that recognize tumor cells by stimulating with the human p53:264–272 peptide, which is identical to the mouse p53:261–269 peptide. In one study, a CTL clone generated against this peptide appeared to recognize two squamous carcinoma cell lines (119). There did not appear to be a correlation between recognition and overexpression of p53, as one of the cell lines that was recognized did not appear to overexpress p53, whereas an HLA-A2$^+$ squamous carcinoma cell line that overexpressed p53 was not recognized. Thus, additional factors may influence the recognition of tumor cells by p53-reactive T cells. In a second study, two CTL lines generated from a single healthy donor appeared to recognize peptide-pulsed targets as well as one melanoma and two breast cancer cell lines (120). Immunohistochemical data indicated that the tumor cell lines that were recognized overexpressed p53, although one of the breast cancer cell lines that was recognized did not express a mutated p53 gene product.

Cross-reactive T cell responses have also been elicited using a natural peptide variant that possesses a higher affinity for MHC-I molecules than the parental peptide. Stimulation of mice with a peptide from the human gp100 molecule was found to result in generation of T cells that can recognize the homologous mouse peptide (121). Binding studies indicated that the human peptide, which differs from the mouse sequence at the first three positions, had a significantly higher affinity for the H-2D^b molecule involved in presenting this epitope than the homologous mouse peptide. Presumably the higher affinity of the human peptide facilitated the induction of CTLs that cross-reacted with the mouse peptide.

Tolerance mechanisms may influence the nature of immune responses to melanocyte antigens. In this report patients with vitiligo were examined for their ability to recognize the MART-1 antigen using an MHC-I tetramer containing an optimized MART-1 peptide (122). These results indicated that T cells from HLA-A2$^+$ vitiligo patients reacted with the MART-1 peptide, and that these T cells in addition expressed high levels of the skin homing receptor cutaneous lymphocyte-associated antigen (CLA), a form of the P selectin-binding glycoprotein 1 (123).

T CELL RECEPTOR ANALYSIS

Initial studies indicated that there may be some restriction in the repertoire of TCRs expressed in response to a particular peptide epitope (124), but subsequent studies have shown that a wide array of TCRs can be expressed in response to a single antigenic epitope (125). Recent studies have suggested that T cells expressing particular TCRs may be enriched in populations of TILs isolated from untreated melanoma patients (126) and from patients immunized with either dinitrophenyl-modified tumor cells or the HLA-A1 MAGE-3 peptide epitope (127). In addition, expansion of the T cells using specific antibodies directed against these receptors can result in generation of cell lines that specifically recognize tumors. Thus although the repertoire of TCRs present on tumor-reactive T cells may be quite varied in the peripheral blood of patients, a restricted set of tumor-reactive T cell clonotypes may be expanded at the tumor site.

CLINICAL STUDIES

Previous studies suggested that recognition of gp100 correlated with response to TIL therapy (33). In a recent study, 13 of 30 HLA-A2-restricted TILs were found to recognize gp100, and there appeared to be a significant correlation between patient response to TIL therapy and the ability of TILs to recognize gp100 (34). Of the same 30 TILs, 22 recognized MART-1 transfectants as well as and all of them recognized the MART-1:27–35 peptide; however, there was no significant correlation between patient response and recognition of MART-1. These observations indicate that gp100 might represent a significant tumor rejection antigen.

In a clinical trial using immunization with the soluble HLA-A1-binding MAGE-3 peptide, there was no evidence of generation of CTLs in the peripheral blood of treated patients, but partial tumor regression was observed in 2 of the 12 patients who completed the study (128). In a second study, six patients with evaluable metastatic melanoma were immunized with HLA-A2-restricted peptides from the MART-1, tyrosinase, and gp100 antigens (129). Modest enhancement of *in vitro* antipeptide responses were reported against the MART-1 and gp100 but not the tyrosinase peptides, and no clinical antitumor responses were seen.

Peptide immunization trials carried out in the Surgery Branch, National Cancer Institute (NCI) with the MART-1 and gp100: 209–217 peptides demonstrated evidence for modest enhancement in the induction of antipeptide immunity following injection of the native peptide in incomplete Freund's adjuvant (130,131). No significant clinical responses were seen in these trials. Immunization with the MAGE-1 peptide that had been pulsed on autologous APCs also demonstrated evidence for a low level of immunization; but again no significant clinical responses were seen (132). In another study, immunization with the MAGE-1 HLA-A1-binding peptide appeared to increase the precursor frequency of peptide and tumor-reactive T cells at the tumor sites (133).

Clinical trials carried out in the Surgery Branch (NCI) have utilized immunization with the modified peptide antigen gp100: 209–217 (2M) in combination with IL-2 (112). Preliminary results indicate that 42% of 31 patients exhibited objective tumor regression to the peptide–IL-2 combination, a significantly higher percentage than was seen in previous clinical trials using IL-2 alone. Long-term studies and randomized phase 3 clinical trials are needed at this point to confirm these observations.

The extent of tumor antigen expression represents an important variable that may influence clinical responses to therapy. One study has suggested that tumors can express relatively homogeneous levels of tyrosinase, but that the expression of gp100 and TRP-1 was more variable (134). Expression of the MAGE-1 protein was found to be variable in tumors by RT-PCR analysis, and this appeared to correlate with recognition by MAGE-1 reactive T cells (16). In addition, IFN-γ treatment of small cell lung cancer cells was able to induce expression of class I and restore recognition by MAGE-3-reactive T cells (135).

Some studies have provided indirect evidence that antitumor responses result in the selection of tumor variants *in vivo*. As described above, autologous CTLs appeared to recognize a melanoma cell line derived from patient LB33 in 1988 in the context of HLA-A28, -B13, -B44, and -Cw6. A subsequent metastasis isolated from this patient was found to have lost all of the class I alleles with the exception of HLA-A24 (76). Studies of sequential biopsy specimens from patients revealed loss of melanoma antigens as well as HLA class I (136). Results of a study analyzing responses to peptides derived from melanoma antigens also suggest that CTL may be involved in the selection of tumor antigen loss variants *in vitro* (137).

These findings suggest that the most effective immunization strategy employs immunization with a number of antigens to prevent the outgrowth of tumor antigen loss variants. Coordinate expression of the MAGE, BAGE, GAGE, tyrosinase, and Melan-A/MART-1 antigens in tumors suggests that therapy could be directed against these antigens in a high percentage of melanoma patients (138). In a clinical trial recently initiated in the Surgery Branch (NCI), melanoma patients are being immunized simultaneously with peptides from the MART-1 and tyrosinase antigens, as well as two peptides from gp100, gp100:209–27, and gp100:280–280, that contain modifications that enhance HLA-A2 binding. Ongoing studies to evaluate methods to enhance the immunogenicity of these antigens should hopefully lead to the generation of more effective tumor vaccines.

REFERENCES

1. Traversari C, van der Bruggen P, Luescher IF, et al. A nonapeptide encoded by human gene MAGE-1

is recognized on HLA-A1 by cytolytic T lymphocytes directed against tumor antigen MZ2-E. *J Exp Med* 1992;176:1453–1457.

2. Van der Bruggen P, Szikora JP, Boel P, et al. Autologous cytolytic T lymphocytes recognize a MAGE-1 nonapeptide on melanomas expressing HLA-Cw* 1601. *Eur J Immunol* 1994;24:2134–2140.

3. Gaugler B, Van den Eynde B, van der Bruggen P, et al. Human gene MAGE-3 codes for an antigen recognized on a melanoma by autologous cytolytic T lymphocytes. *J Exp Med* 1994;179:921–930.

4. van der Bruggen P, Bastin J, Gajewski T, et al. A peptide encoded by human gene MAGE-3 and presented by HLA-A2 induces cytolytic T lymphocytes that recognize tumor cells expressing MAGE-3. *Eur J Immunol* 1994;24:3038–3043.

5. Herman J, van der Bruggen P, Luescher IF, et al. A peptide encoded by the human MAGE3 gene and presented by HLA-B44 induces cytolytic T lymphocytes that recognize tumor cells expressing MAGE3. *Immunogenetics* 1996;43:377–383.

6. Van den Eynde B, Peeters O, De Backer O, et al. A new family of genes coding for an antigen recognized by autologous cytolytic T lymphocytes on a human melanoma. *J Exp Med* 1995; 182:689–698.

7. Boel P, Wildmann C, Sensi ML, et al. BAGE: a new gene encoding an antigen recognized on human melanomas by cytolytic T lymphocytes. *Immunity* 1995;2:167–175.

8. Gaugler B, Brouwenstijn N, Vantomme V, et al. A new gene coding for an antigen recognized by autologous cytolytic T lymphocytes on a human renal carcinoma. *Immunogenetics* 1996;44:323–330.

9. Jager E, Chen YT, Drijfhout JW, et al. Simultaneous humoral and cellular immune response against cancer-testis antigen NY-ESO-1: definition of human histocompatibility leukocyte antigen (HLA)-A2-binding peptide epitopes. *J Exp Med* 1998;187:265–270.

10. Van der Bruggen P, Traversari C, Chomez P, et al. A gene encoding an antigen recognized by cytolytic T lymphocytes on a human melanoma. *Science* 1991;254:1643–1647.

11. De Plaen E, Arden K, Traversari C, et al. Structure, chromosomal localization, and expression of 12 genes of the MAGE family. *Immunogenetics* 1994;40:360–396.

12. Takahashi K, Shichijo S, Noguchi M, et al. Identification of MAGE-1 and MAGE-4 proteins in spermatogonia and primary spermatocytes of testis. *Cancer Res* 1995;55:3478–3482.

13. Van den Eynde B, van der Bruggen P. T cell defined tumor antigens. *Curr Opin Immunol* 1997;9:684–693.

14. Fleischhauer K, Fruci D, Van Endert P, et al. Characterization of antigenic peptides presented by HLA-B44 molecules on tumor cells expressing the gene MAGE-3. *Int J Cancer* 1996;68:622–628.

15. Tanaka F, Fujie T, Tahara K, et al. Induction of antitumor cytotoxic T lymphocytes with a MAGE-3-encoded synthetic peptide presented by human leukocytes antigen-A24. *Cancer Res* 1997;57:4465–4468.

16. Lethe B, van der Bruggen P, Brasseur F, et al. MAGE-1 expression threshold for the lysis of melanoma cell lines by a specific cytotoxic T lymphocyte. *Melanoma Res* 1997;7(suppl 2):S83–88.

17. Visseren MJ, van der Burg SH, van der Voort EI, et al. Identification of HLA-A*0201-restricted CTL epitopes encoded by the tumor-specific MAGE-2 gene product. *Int J Cancer* 1997; 73:125–130.

18. Chen YT, Scanlan MJ, Sahin U, et al. A testicular antigen aberrantly expressed in human cancers detected by autologous antibody screening. *Proc Natl Acad Sci USA* 1997;94:1914–1918.

19. Stockert E, Jager E, Chen YT, et al. A survey of the humoral immune response of cancer patients to a panel of human tumor antigens [see comments]. *J Exp Med* 1998;187:1349–1354.

20. Wang R-F, Johnston SL, Zeng G, Topalian SL, Schwartzentruber DJ, Rosenberg SA. A breast and melanoma-shared tumor antigen: T cell responses to antigenic peptides translated from different open reading frames. *J Immunol* 1998;161:3596-3606.

21. Malarkannan S, Afkarian M, Shastri N. A rare cryptic translation product is presented by Kb major histocompatibility complex class I molecule to alloreactive T cells. *J Exp Med* 1995;182:1739–1750.

22. Elliott T, Bodmer H, Townsend A. Recognition of out-of-frame major histocompatibilty complex class I-restricted epitopes in vivo. *Eur J Immunol* 1996;26:1175–1179.

23. Bullock TN, Patterson AE, Franlin LL, et al. Initiation codon scan through versus termination codon readthrough demonstrates strong potential for major histocompatibility complex class I-restricted cryptic epitope expression. *J Exp Med* 1997; 186:1051–1058.

24. Quelle DE, Zindy F, Ashmun RA, et al. Alternative reading frames of the INK4a tumor suppressor gene encode two unrelated proteins capable of inducing cell cycle arrest. *Cell* 1995;83:993–1000.

25. Wang RF, Parkhurst MR, Kawakami Y, et al. Utilization of an alternative open reading frame of a normal gene in generating a novel human cancer antigen. *J Exp Med* 1996;183:1131–1140.

26. Brower RC, England R, Takeshita T, et al. Minimal requirements for peptide mediated activation of CD8+ CTL. *Mol Immunol* 1994;31:1285–1293.

27. Sykulev Y, Joo M, Vturina I, et al. Evidence that a single peptide-MHC complex on a target cell can elicit a cytolytic T cell response. *Immunity* 1996;4:565–571.

28. Kawakami Y, Eliyahu S, Delgado CH, et al. Cloning of the gene coding for a shared human melanoma antigen recognized by autologous T cells infiltrating into tumor. *Proc Natl Acad Sci USA* 1994;91:3515–3519.

29. Coulie PG, Brichard V, Van Pel A, et al. A new gene coding for a differentiation antigen recognized by autologous cytolytic T lymphocytes on HLA-A2 melanomas [see comments]. *J Exp Med* 1994;180:35–42.

30. Kawakami Y, Battles JK, Kobayashi T, et al. Production of recombinant MART-1 proteins and spe-

cific antiMART-1 polyclonal and monoclonal anti-bodies: use in the characterization of the human melanoma antigen MART-1. *J Immunol Methods* 1997;202:13–25.

31. Kawakami Y, Eliyahu S, Sakaguchi K, et al. Identification of the immunodominant peptides of the MART-1 human melanoma antigen recognized by the majority of HLA-A2 restricted tumor infiltrating lymphocytes. *J Exp Med* 1994;180:347–352.

32. Schneider J, Brichard V, Boon T, et al. Overlapping peptides of melanocyte differentiation antigen Melan-A/MART-1 recognized by autologous cytolytic T lymphocytes in association with HLA-B45.1 and HLA-A2.1. *Int J Cancer* 1998;75:451–458.

33. Kawakami Y, Eliyahu S, Jennings C, et al. Recognition of multiple epitopes in the human melanoma antigen gp100 associated with in vivo tumor regression. *J Immunol* 1995;154:3961–3968.

34. Kawakami Y, Robbins PF, Wang X, et al. Identification of new melanoma epitopes on melanosomal proteins recognized by tumor infiltrating lymphocytes restricted by HLA-A1, -A2 and -A3 alleles. *J Immunol* 1998;6985–6992.

35. Skipper JC, Kittlesen DJ, Hendrickson RC, et al. Shared epitopes for HLA-A3-restricted melanoma-reactive human CTL include a naturally processed epitope from Pmel-17/gp 100. *J Immunol* 1996;157:5027–5033.

36. Robbins PF, El-Gamil M, Li YF, et al. The intronic region of an incompletely spliced gp100 gene transcript encodes an epitope recognized by melanoma-reactive tumor-infiltrating lymphocytes. *J Immunol* 1997;159:303–308.

37. Wolfel T, Van Pel A, Brichard V, et al. Two tyrosinase nonapeptides recognized on HLA-A2 melanomas by autologous cytolytic T lymphocytes. *Eur J Immunol* 1994;24:759–764.

38. Kang X-Q, Kawakami Y, Sakaguchi K, et al. Identification of a tyrosinase epitope recognized by HLA-A24 restricted tumor-infiltrating lymphocytes. *J Immunol* 1995;155:1343–1348.

39. Kittlesen DJ, Thompson LW, Gulden PH, et al. Human melanoma patients recognize an HLA-A1-restricted CTL epitope from tyrosinase containing two cysteine residues: implications for tumor vaccine development. *J Immunol* 1998;160:2099–2106.

40. Wang RF, Appella E, Kawakami Y, et al. Identification of TRP-2 as a human tumor antigen recognized by cytotoxic T lymphocytes. *J Exp Med* 1996;184:2207–2216.

41. Parkhurst MR, Fitzgerald, EB, Southwood S, Sette A, Rosenberg SA, Kawakami Y. Identification of a shared HLA-A*0201 restricted T cell epitope from the melanoma antigen tyrosinase related protein 2 (TRP-2). *Cancer Res* 1998;58:4895–4901.

42. Lupetti R, Pisarra P, Verrecchia A, et al. Translation of a retained intron in tyrosinase-related protein (TRP) 2 mRNA generates a new cytotoxic T lymphocyte (CTL)-defined and shared human melanoma antigen not expressed in normal cells of the melanocytic lineage. *J Exp Med* 1998;188:1005–1016.

43. Kawakami Y, Dang N, Wang X, et al. Recognition of shared melanoma antigens in association with

major HLA-A alleles by tumor infiltrating lymphocytes from 123 patients with melanoma. *J Immunother* (in press).

44. Castelli C, Storkus WJ, Maeurer MJ, et al. Mass spectrometric identification of a naturally processed melanoma peptide recognized by CD8$^+$ cytotoxic T lymphocytes. *J Exp Med* 1995;181:363–368.

45. Valmori D, Fonteneau JF, Lizana CM, et al. Enhanced generation of specific tumor-reactive CTL in vitro by selected Melan-A/MART-1 immunodominant peptide analogues. *J Immunol* 1998;160:1750–1758.

46. Bettinotti MP, Kim CJ, Lee KH, et al. Stringent allele/epitope requirements for MART-1/Melan A immunodominance: implications for peptide-based immunotherapy. *J Immunol* 1998;161:877–889.

47. Loftus DJ, Castelli C, Clay TM, et al. Identification of epitope mimics recognized by CTL reactive to the melanoma/melanocyte-derived peptide MART-1 27–35. *J Exp Med* 1996;184:647–657.

48. Kawakami Y, Eliyahu S, Delgado CH, et al. Identification of a human melanoma antigen recognized by tumor infiltrating lymphocytes associated with in vivo tumor rejection. *Proc Natl Acad Sci USA* 1994;91:6458–6462.

49. Adema GJ, de Boer AJ, van't Hullenaar R, et al. Melanocyte lineage-specific antigens recognized by monoclonal antibodies NKI-beteb, HMB-50, and HMB-45 are encoded by a single cDNA. *Am J Pathol* 1993;143:1579–1585.

50. Lee ZH, Hou L, Moellmann G, et al. Characterization and subcellular localization of human Pmel 17/silver, a 110-kDa (pre)melanosomal membrane protein associated with 5,6,-dihydroxyindole-2-carboxylic acid (DHICA) converting activity. *J Invest Dermatol* 1996;106:605–610.

51. Kwon BS, Halaban R, Ponnazhagan S, et al. Mouse silver mutation is caused by a single base insertion in the putative cytoplasmic domain of Pmel 17. *Nucleic Acids Res* 1995;23:154–158.

52. Schreurs MW, de Boer AJ, Schmidt A, et al. Cloning, expression and tissue distribution of the murine homologue of the melanocyte lineage-specific antigen gp100. *Melanoma Res* 1997;7:463–470.

53. Brouwenstijn N, Slager EH, Bakker AB, et al. Transcription of the gene encoding melanoma-associated antigen gp100 in tissues and cell lines other than those of the melanocytic lineage. *Br J Cancer* 1997;76:1562–1566.

54. Cox AL, Skipper J, Chen Y, et al. Identification of a peptide recognized by five melanoma-specific human cytotoxic T cell lines. *Science* 1994;264:716–719.

55. Tsai V, Southwood S, Sidney J, et al. Identification of subdominant CTL epitopes of the GP100 melanoma-associated tumor antigen by primary in vitro immunization with peptide-pulsed dendritic cells. *J Immunol* 1997;158:1796–1802.

56. Kwon BS, Haq AK, Pomerantz SH, et al. Isolation and sequence of a cDNA clone for human tyrosinase that maps at the mouse c-albino locus. *Proc Natl Acad Sci USA* 1987;84:7473–7477.

57. Brichard V, Van Pel A, Wolfel T, et al. The tyrosi-

nase gene codes for an antigen recognized by autologous cytolytic T lymphocytes on HLA-A2 melanomas. *J Exp Med* 1993;178:489–495.

58. Visseren MJW, van Elsas A, van der Voort EIH, et al. CTL specific for the tyrosinase autoantigen can be induced from healthy donor blood to lyse melanoma cells. *J Immunol* 1995;154:3991–3998.

59. Skipper JC, Hendrickson RC, Gulden PH, et al. An HLA-A2-restricted tyrosinase antigen on melanoma cells results from posttranslational modification and suggests a novel pathway for processing of membrane proteins. *J Exp Med* 1996;183: 527–534.

60. Suzuki T, Seko A, Kitajima K, et al. Identification of peptide: N-glycanase activity in mammalian-derived cultured cells. *Biochem Biophys Res Commun* 1993;194:1124–1130.

61. Mosse CA, Meadows L, Luckey CJ, et al. The class I antigen-processing pathway for the membrane protein tyrosinase involves translation in the endoplasmic reticulum and processing in the cytosol. *J Exp Med* 1998;187:37–48.

62. Robbins PF, El-Gamil M, Kawakami Y, et al. Recognition of tyrosinase by tumor infiltrating lymphocytes from a patient responding to immunotherapy. *Cancer Res* 1994;54:3124–3126.

63. Brichard VG, Herman J, Van Pel A, et al. A tyrosinase nonapeptide presented by HLA-B44 is recognized on a human melanoma by autologous cytolytic T lymphocytes. *Eur J Immunol* 1996; 26:224–230.

64. Yee C, Gilbert MJ, Riddell SR, et al. Isolation of tyrosinase-specific CD8$^+$ and CD4$^+$ T cell clones from the peripheral blood of melanoma patients following in vitro stimulation with recombinant vaccinia virus. *J Immunol* 1996;157:4079–4086.

65. Wang R-F, Robbins PF, Kawakami Y, et al. Identification of a gene encoding a melanoma tumor antigen recognized by HLA-A31-restricted tumor-infiltrating lymphocytes. *J Exp Med* 1995; 181:799–804.

66. Mattes MJ, Thomson TM, Old LJ, et al. A pigmentation-associated, differentiation antigen of human melanoma defined by a precipitating antibody in human serum. *Int J Cancer* 1983;32:717–721.

67. Vijayasyradhi S, Bouchard BB, Houghton AN. The melanoma antigen gp75 is the human homologue of mouse b (brown) locus gene. *J Exp Med* 1990;171:1375–1380.

68. Jimenez-Cervantes C, Solano F, Kobayashi T, et al. A new enzymatic function in the melanogenic pathway. *J Biol Chem* 1994;269:17993–18001.

69. Bloom MB, Perry-Lalley D, Robbins PF, et al. Identification of tyrosinase-related protein 2 as a tumor rejection antigen for the B16 melanoma. *J Exp Med* 1997;185:453–459.

70. Sidney J, Grey HM, Southwood S, et al. Definition of an HLA-A3-like supermotif demonstrates the overlapping peptide-binding repertoires of common HLA molecules. *Hum Immunol* 1996; 45:79–93.

71. Wang RF, Johnston, SL, Southwood S, Sette A, Rosenberg SA. Recognition of an antigenic peptide derived from tyrosinase-related protein-2 by

CTL in the context of HLA-A31 and -A33. *J Immunol* 1998;160:890–897.

72. Sette A, Sidney J, del Guercio M-F, et al. Peptide binding to the most frequent HLA-A class I alleles measured by quantitative molecular binding assays. *Mol Immunol* 1994;31:813–822.

73. Shichijo S, Nakao M, Imai Y, et al. A gene encoding antigenic peptides of human squamous cell carcinoma recognized by cytotoxic T lymphocytes. *J Exp Med* 1998;187:277–288.

74. Ikeda H, Lethe B, Lehmann F, et al. Characterization of an antigen that is recognized on a melanoma showing partial HLA loss by CTL expressing an NK inhibitory receptor. *Immunity* 1997;6:199–208.

75. Robbins PF, El-Gamil M, Li YF, et al. Cloning of a new gene encoding an antigen recognized by melanoma-specific HLA-A24 restricted tumor-infiltrating lymphocytes. *J Immunol* 1995;154:5944–5950.

76. Lehmann F, Marchand M, Hainaut P, et al. Differences in the antigens recognized by cytolytic T cells on two successive metastases of a melanoma patient are consistent with immune selection. *Eur J Immunol* 1995;25:340–347.

77. Wolfel T, Hauer M, Schneider J, et al. A p16INK4a-insensitive CDK4 mutant targeted by cytolytic T lymphocytes in a human melanoma. *Science* 1995;269:1281–1284.

78. Rubinfeld B, Robbins P, El-Gamil M, et al. Stabilization of beta-catenin by genetic defects in melanoma cell lines [see comments]. *Science* 1997;275:1790–1792.

79. Mandruzzato S, Brasseur F, Andry G, et al. A CASP-8 mutation recognized by cytolytic T lymphocytes on a human head and neck carcinoma. *J Exp Med* 1997;186:785–793.

80. Gueguen M, Patard JJ, Gaugler B, et al. An antigen recognized by autologous CTLs on a human bladder carcinoma. *J Immunol* 1998;160:6188–6194.

81. Ressing ME, van Driel WJ, Celis E, et al. Occasional memory cytotoxic T-cell responses of patients with human papillomavirus type 16-positive cervical lesions against a human leukocyte antigen-A*0201-restricted E7-encoded epitope. *Cancer Res* 1996;56:582–588.

82. Coulie PG, Lehmann F, Lethe B, et al. A mutated intron sequence codes for an antigenic peptide recognized by cytolytic T lymphocytes on a human melanoma. *Proc Natl Acad Sci USA* 1995;92:7976–7980.

83. Sherr CJ. Cancer cell cycles. *Science* 1996;274: 1672–1677.

84. Robbins PF, El-Gamil M, Li YF, et al. A mutated β-catenin gene encodes a melanoma-specific antigen recognized by tumor infiltrating lymphocytes. *J Exp Med* 1996;183:1185–1192.

85. Korinek V, Barker N, Morin PJ, et al. Constitutive transcriptional activation by a beta-catenin-Tcf complex in APC$^{-/-}$ colon carcinoma. *Science* 1997;275:1784–1787.

86. Morin PJ, Sparks AB, Korinek V, et al. Activation of beta-catenin-Tcf signaling in colon cancer by mutations in beta-catenin or APC. *Science* 1997;275:1787–1790.

87. De La Coste A, Romagnolo B, Billuart P, et al.

Somatic mutations of the beta-catenin gene are frequent in mouse and human hepatocellular carcinomas. *Proc Natl Acad Sci USA* 1998;80:95:8847–8851.

88. Guilloux Y, Lucas S, Brichard VG, et al. A peptide recognized by human cytolytic T lymphocytes on HLA-A2 melanomas is encoded by an intron sequence of the N-acetylglucosaminyltransferase V gene. *J Exp Med* 1996;183:1173–1183.

89. Brandle D, Brasseur F, Weynants P, et al. A mutated HLA-A2 molecule recognized by autologous cytotoxic T lymphocytes on a human renal cell carcinoma. *J Exp Med* 1996;183:2501–2508.

90. Rammensee HG, Friede T, Stevanoviic S. MHC ligands and peptide motifs: first listing. *Immunogenetics* 1995;41:178–228.

91. Ressing ME, Sette A, Brandt RM, et al. Human CTL epitopes encoded by human papillomavirus type 16 E6 and E7 identified through in vivo and in vitro immunogenicity studies of HLA-A*0201-binding peptides. *J Immunol* 1995;154:5934–5943.

92. Alexander M, Salgaller ML, Celis E, et al. Generation of tumor-specific cytolytic T lymphocytes from peripheral blood of cervical cancer patients by in vitro stimulation with a synthetic human papillomavirus type 16 E7 epitope. *Am J Obstet Gynecol* 1996;175:1586–1593.

93. Salazar-Onfray F, Nakazawa T, Chhajlani V, et al. Synthetic peptides derived from the melanocyte-stimulating hormone receptor MC1R can stimulate HLA-A2-restricted cytotoxic T lymphocytes that recognize naturally processed peptides on human melanoma cells. *Cancer Res* 1997;57:4348–4355.

94. Slamon DJ, Clark GM, Wong SG, Levin WJ, Ulrich A, McGuire WL. Human breast cancer: correlation of relapse and survival with amplification of the HER-2/neu oncogene. *Science* 1987;235:177–182.

95. Katsumata M, Okudaira T, Samanta A, et al. Prevention of breast tumor development in vivo by downregulation of the p185neu receptor. *Nat Med* 1995;1:644–648.

96. Schlegel J, Trenkle T, Stumm G, Kiessling, M. Growth inhibition by dominant-negative mutations of the neu-encoded oncoprotein. *Int J Cancer* 1997;70:78–83.

97. Fisk B, Blevins TL, Wharton JT, et al. Identification of an immunodominant peptide of HER-2/neu protooncogene recognized by ovarian tumor-specific cytotoxic T lymphocyte lines. *J Exp Med* 1995;181:2109–2117.

98. Peoples GE, Goedegebuure PS, Smith R, et al. Breast and ovarian cancer-specific cytotoxic T lymphocytes recognize the same HER2/neu-derived peptide. *Proc Natl Acad Sci USA* 1995;92:432–436.

99. Lustgarten J, Theobald M, Labadie C, et al. Identification of Her-2/Neu CTL epitopes using double transgenic mice expressing HLA-A2.1 and human CD.8. *Hum Immunol* 1997;52:109–118.

100. Kawashima I, Hudson SJ, Tsai V, et al. The multiepitope approach for immunotherapy for cancer: identification of several CTL epitopes from various tumor-associated antigens expressed on solid epithelial tumors. *Hum Immunol* 1998;59:1–14.

101. Zaks TZ, Rosenberg SA. Immunization with a peptide epitope (p369–377) from HER-2/neu leads to peptide specific cytotoxic T lymphocytes which fail to recognize HER-2/neu+ tumors. *Cancer Res* 1998;58:4902–4908.

102. Tuting T, Wilson CC, Martin DM, et al. Autologous human monocyte-derived dendritic cells genetically modified to express melanoma antigens elicit primary cytotoxic T cell responses in vitro: enhancement by cotransfection of genes encoding the Th1-biasing cytokines IL-12 and IFN-alpha. *J Immunol* 1998;160:1139–1147.

103. Tureci O, Chen YT, Sahin U, et al. Expression of SSX genes in human tumors. *Int J Cancer* 1998;77:19–23.

104. Chen YT, Gure AO, Tsang S, et al. Identification of multiple cancer/testis antigens by allogeneic antibody screening of a melanoma cell line library. *Proc Natl Acad Sci USA* 1998;95:6919–6923.

105. Lucas S, De Smet C, Arden KC, et al. Identification of a new MAGE gene with tumor-specific expression by reprsentational difference analysis. *Cancer Res* 1998;58:743–752.

106. Lethe B, Lucas S, Michaux L, et al. LAGE-1, a new gene with tumor specificity. *Int J Cancer* 1998;76:903–908.

107. Rivoltini L, Barracchini KC, Viggiano V, et al. Quantitative correlation between HLA class I allele expression and recognition of melanoma cells by antigen-specific cytotoxic T lymphocytes. *Cancer Res* 1995;55:3149–3157.

108. Kono K, Halapi E, Hising C, et al. Mechanisms of escape from CD8+ T-cell clones specific for the HER-2/neu proto-oncogene expressed in ovarian carcinoma: related and unrelated to decreased MHC class 1 expression. *Int J Cancer* 1997;70:112–119.

109. Sette A, Vitiello A, Reherman B, et al. The relationship between class I binding affinity and immunogenicity of potential cytotoxic T cell epitopes. *J Immunol* 1994;153:5586–5592.

110. Van der Burg SH, Visseren MJW, Brandt RMP, et al. Immunogenicity of peptides bound to MHC class I molecules depends on the MHC-peptide complex stability. *J Immunol* 1996;156:3308–3314.

111. Parkhurst MR, Salgaller M, Southwood S, et al. Improved induction of melanoma reactive CTL with peptides from the melanoma antigen gp 100 modified at HLA-A0201 binding residues. *J Immunol* 1996;157:2539–2548.

112. Rosenberg SA, Yang JC, Schwartzentruber DJ, et al. Immunologic and therapeutic evaluation of a synthetic peptide vaccine for the treatment of patients with metastatic melanoma [see comments]. *Nat Med* 1998;4:321–327.

113. Romero P, Gervois N, Schneider J, et al. Cytolytic T lymphocyte recognition of the immunodominant HLA-A*0201-restricted Melan-A/MART-1 antigenic peptide in melanoma. *J Immunol* 1997;159:2366–2374.

114. Valmori D, Lienard D, Waanders G, et al. Analysis of MAGE-3-specific cytolytic T lymphocytes in human leukocyte antigen-A2 melanoma patients. *Cancer Res* 1997;57:735–741.

115. Cormier JN, Panelli M, Hackett JA, et al. Natural variation of the expression of HLA and endoge-

nous antigen modulates CTL recognition in an in vitro melanoma model. *Int J Cancer* 1999;80:781–790.

116. Mortarini R, Belli F, Parmiani G, et al. Cytokine-mediated modulation of HLA-class II, ICAM-1, LFA-3 and tumor-associated antigen profile of melanoma cells: comparison with antiproliferative activity by rIL1-beta, rTNF-alpha, rIFN-gamma, rIL4 and their combinations. *Int J Cancer* 1990;45:334–341.

117. Theobald M, Biggs J, Dittmer D, et al. Targeting p53 as a general tumor antigen. *Proc Natl Acad Sci USA* 1995;92:11993–11997.

118. Vierboom MP, Nijman HW, Offringa R, et al. Tumor eradication by wild-type p53-specific cytotoxic T lymphocytes. *J Exp Med* 1997;186:695–704.

119. Ropke M, Hald J, Guldberg P, et al. Spontaneous human squamous cell carcinomas are killed by a human cytotoxic T lymphocyte clone recognizing a wild-type p53-derived peptide. *Proc Natl Acad Sci USA* 1996;93:14704–14707.

120. Gnjatic S, Cai Z, Viguier M, et al. Accumulation of the p53 protein allows recognition by human CTL of a wild-type p53 epitope presented by breast carcinomas and melanomas. *J Immunol* 1998; 160:328–333.

121. Overwijk WW, Tsung A, Irvine KR, et al. gp100/pmel 17 is a murine tumor rejection antigen: induction of "self"-reactive, tumoricidal T cells using high-affinity, altered peptide ligand. *J Exp Med* 1998;188:277–286.

122. Ogg GS, Rod Dunbar P, Romero P, et al. High frequency of skin-homing melanocyte-specific cytotoxic T lymphocytes in autoimmune vitiligo. *J Exp Med* 1998;188:1203–1208.

123. Fuhlbrigge RC, Kieffer JD, Armerding D, et al. Cutaneous lymphocyte antigen is a specialized from of PSGL-1 expressed on skin-homing T cells. *Nature* 1997;389:978–981.

124. Sensi M, Traversari C, Radrizzani M, et al. Cytotoxic T lymphocyte clones from different patients display limited T-cell receptors variable gene usage in HLA-A2 restricted recognition of Melan/Mart-1 melanoma antigen. *Proc Natl Acad Sci USA* 1995;92:5674–5678.

125. Cole DJ, Wilson MC, Rivoltini L, Custer M, Nishimura MI. T-cell receptor repertoire in matched MART-1 peptide-stimulated peripheral blood lymphocytes and tumor-infiltrating lymphocytes. *Cancer Res* 1997;57:5320–5327.

126. Clemente C, Rao S, Lupetti R, et al. Immunohistochemical analysis of the T-cell receptor beta-chain variable regions expressed by T lymphocytes infiltrating primary human melanoma. *Lab Invest* 1998;78:619–627.

127. Sensi M, Farina C, Maccalli C, et al. Intralesional selection of T cell clonotypes in the immune response to melanoma antigens occurring during vaccination. *J Immunother* 1998;21:198–204.

128. Marchand M, Weynants P, Rankin E, et al. Tumor regression responses in melanoma patients treated with a peptide encoded by gene MAGE-3 [letter]. *Int J Cancer* 1995;63:883–885.

129. Jaeger E, Bernhard H, Romero P, et al. Generation of cytotoxic T-cell responses with synthetic melanoma-associated peptides in vivo: implications for tumor vaccines with melanoma-associated antigens. *Int J Cancer* 1996;66:162–169.

130. Salgaller ML, Marincola FM, Cormier JN, et al. Immunization against epitopes in the human melanoma antigen gp100 following patient immunization with synthetic peptides. *Cancer Res* 1996; 56:4749–4757.

131. Cormier JN, Salgaller ML, Prevette T, et al. Enhancement of cellular immunity in melanoma patients immunized with a peptide from MART-1/Melan A [see comments]. *Cancer J Sci Am* 1997; 3:37–44.

132. Hu X, Chakraborty NG, Sporn JR, et al. Enhancement of cytolytic T lymphocyte precursor frequency in melanoma patients following immunization with the MAGE-1 peptide loaded antigen presenting cell-based vaccine. *Cancer Res* 1996; 56:2479–2483.

133. Mukherji B, Chakraborty NG, Yamasaki S, et al. Induction of antigen-specific cytolytic T cells in situ in human melanoma by immunization with synthetic peptide-pulsed autologous antigen presenting cells. *Proc Natl Acad Sci USA* 1995;92: 8078–8082.

134. Chen YT, Stockert E, Tsang S, et al. Immunophenotyping of melanomas for tyrosinase: implications for vaccine development. *Proc Natl Acad Sci USA* 1995;92:8125–8129.

135. Traversari C, Meazza R, Coppolecchia M, et al. IFN-gamma gene transfer restores HLA-class I expression and MAGE-3 antigen presentation to CTL in HLA-deficient small cell lung cancer. *Gene Ther* 1997;4:1029–1035.

136. Jager E, Ringhoffer M, Altmannsberger M, et al. Immunoselection in vivo: independent loss of MHC class I and melanocyte differentiation antigen expression in metastatic melanoma. *Int J Cancer* 1997;71:142–147.

137. Jager E, Ringhoffer M, Karbach J, et al. Inverse relationship of melanocyte differentiation antigen expression in melanoma tissues and CD8[+] cytotoxic-T-cell responses: evidence for immunoselection of antigen-loss variants in vivo. *Int J Cancer* 1996;66:470–476.

138. Dalerba P, Ricci A, Russo V, et al. High homogeneity of MAGE, BAGE, GAGE, tyrosinase and Melan-A/MART-1 gene expression in clusters of multiple simultaneous metastases of human melanoma: implications for protocol design of therapeutic antigen-specific vaccination strategies. *Int J Cancer* 1998;77:200–204.

Cytotoxic Cells: Basic Mechanisms and Medical Applications, edited by Michail V. Sitkovsky and Pierre A. Henkart. Lippincott Williams & Wilkins, Philadelphia © 2000.

Chapter 27

Manipulation of T Cell Activation to Generate Antitumor CTLs

Arthur A. Hurwitz,* Andrea van Elsas, Dana R. Leach, Jennifer Ziskin, Jennifer Villasenor, Tan Truong, and James P. Allison

*Department of Microbiology and Immunology, State University of New York Health Sciences Center, Syracuse, New York 13210, USA; and Cancer Research Laboratory, Howard Hughes Medical Institute, University of California, Berkeley, California 94720, USA

Advances in the understanding of T cell activation have led to the development of immunotherapeutic strategies for treating cancer. The idea that T cells require two distinct signals for complete activation has provided many approaches to modulate the antitumor immune response. In this review, we present a historical perspective of tumor immunotherapy and strategies exploiting the current paradigm for T cell activation used to generate a successful tumor vaccine.

IDENTIFICATION OF T CELL EPITOPES ON TUMORS

Until recently it was believed that most, if not all, spontaneously arising tumors do not carry tumor antigens that could be targeted by the immune system. In fact, the immune surveillance hypothesis as postulated by Thomas and Burnet assumed that the organism was capable of recognizing foreign antigens on intruding pathogens but was tolerant to self antigens. As such, the immune system could handle virally induced tumors but not spontaneously arising tumors that lacked a non-self antigen (1). Murine tumors induced with carcinogens were found to contain neoantigens that could be targeted (2). However, these antigens were unique to each tumor and not shared with other variants.

The realization that T cells can recognize tumors has led to a strong effort to identify tumor-associated antigens. During the early 1990s pioneering work by Boon and colleagues has led to identification of tumor antigens that serve as targets for cytotoxic lymphocytes (CTLs) (3). Most of these studies were done on human melanoma for practical reasons: (a) it was relatively easy to grow tumor cell lines from melanoma material (that could easily be accessed); and (b) it was known for quite some time that a small but definite fraction of melanoma patients underwent spontaneous remissions, suggestive of a potent immune (T cell) response. Through expression cloning using CTL clones generated from patients characterized as long-term survivors, three major categories of antigens were discovered (3,4).

The first group is represented by the MAGE family of genes and also contains BAGE, GAGE, and RAGE genes, as well as NY-ESO-1 and relatives. These genes are expressed in early embryonic development and in the testis by HLA class I-negative cells (5). Expression of the MAGE-like antigens is shared between a large portion of human melanomas and unrelated cancers. Therefore these proteins represent good candidate targets for immune intervention; the first immunization trials for melanoma patients were based on CTL epitopes derived from MAGE-1 and MAGE-3 (5).

The second category consists of mutated antigens uniquely expressed in the tumor, and such neoantigens hypothetically represent the ideal candidate targets for immunotherapy. One such antigen is the cell cycle regulatory protein p16/INK4, for which an ultraviolet light (UV)-induced mutation is described that leads to unscheduled entry into the cell cycle and is involved in maintaining the malignant character of the tumor (6). One T cell epitope binds to HLA-A2 as a result of the mutation. The mutated p16/INK4 antigen and a few others described thus far represent the ideal tumor-specific immune targets (6,7). Other tumor-specific epitopes were found to arise from aberrant transcription or splicing events (8). In addition, prediction of potential CTL targets in mutated oncogenes or in p53 was applied to stimulate tumor-specific CTL immunity. In most cases, however, such tumor-specific antigens were found to be unique or poorly antigenic, and are therefore less suitable on which to base immunotherapeutic strategies.

The third category is made up of normal nonmutated self antigens, such as tissue-specific proteins, to which immunologic tolerance is nonexistent or can be broken. These include melanocyte differentiation antigens such as tyrosinase, Melan-A/Mart-1, gp100/Pmel-17, TRP-1/gp75, and TRP-2 (4,5). Within this class, the gp100/Pmel-17 antigen contains multiple CTL epitopes, presented by HLA-A2 or HLA-A3, and appears to be a target for CTLs in many patients (9,10). The tyrosinase gene also contains several epitopes for CTLs, and helper epitopes (11,12). Multiple patients were found to contain CTLs directed against an immunodominant epitope from MelanA/Mart-1 (10,13). Finally, in a few well documented cases, TRP-1 or TRP-2 were targeted by autologous CTLs (14,15). Because most melanoma lesions express such shared antigens, they represent good candidate targets for immunotherapy, despite the obvious risk of developing unwanted autoimmunity. In support of this strategy, objective tumor regressions were documented in melanoma patients after reinfusion of autologous tumor-infiltrating lymphocytes (TILs) that recognize melanocyte differentiation antigens such as gp100/Pmel-17, tyrosinase, and TRP-1 (15,16). The identification of differentiation antigens as targets for CTLs in melanoma patients may explain the interesting association that was noted between the development of skin depigmentation and a favorable clinical response (17). Thus autoreactivity against melanocyte-associated antigens may be an indicator of successful anti-tumor response (spontaneous or treatment-associated). Several of the more commonly recognized epitopes from MelanA/Mart-1, gp100, and tyrosinase are immunogenic *in vitro*, when autologous peripheral blood mononuclear cells (PBMCs) from normal donors are stimulated with peptide pulsed on dendritic cells (18,19). Thus there is a strong case for assuming a role for melanocyte antigen-specific CTLs in the immune control of melanoma. Despite the obvious risk of developing autoimmune depigmentation or vitiligo, tissue-specific antigens are being targeted in new protocols for immunotherapy (20,21) and represent a promising approach to generating antitumor immuntiy.

MODULATION OF CO-STIMULATORY SIGNALS

Identification of antigen receptors for both T and B cells confirmed the idea of the clonality of the adaptive immune response and laid the groundwork for the idea that the immune system could identify antigens on tumors. We now know that one of the signals required for T cell activation involves the interaction of the T cell antigen receptor (TCR) with an antigenic peptide bound to the polymorphic major histocompatibility complex antigens (MHC) (22). This trimolecular interaction alone is not sufficient to activate T cells; an antigen-independent signal is also required. In combination with TCR ligation, this second, co-stimulatory interaction is sufficient to drive cell-cycle progression, clonal expansion, and effector generation (23). Interaction between CD28 on the T cell surface and B7 (CD80 and CD86) on the antigen-presenting cell (APC) can provide this antigen-independent signal. Unlike "professional" APCs (dendritic cells, macrophages, B cells), most tumors do not express B7 and are therefore considered to be poor initiators of an antitumor response (24). During the early 1990s, several laboratories demonstrated that genetically modifying tumors to express B7 could lead to tumor rejection and immunity to rechallenge in a T cell-dependent mechanism (25) (Table 27-1). It was initially reported that this approach rendered the tumor a more potent APC, but a subsequent report suggested that host, bone marrow-derived APCs may initially prime T cells (26). Although this approach was reported to work in tumors of various tissue origins with some inherent immunogenicity (27), few studies demonstrated that this approach could be used to treat more established primary tumors (28–30). Interestingly, in tumor models where conferring B7 was not effective, combination with proinflammatory cytokines could be used to provide more successful treatment (31–35).

Although CD28 is considered to be the principal co-stimulatory receptor expressed by resting T cells, other molecules expressed by T cells can provide co-stimulatory signals. Two such molecules, 4-1BB (36) and OX-40 (37), are members of the tumor necrosis factor (TNF) receptor family and are expressed on the surface of recently activated T cells. The 4-1BB molecule was identified by differential screening of T cells (38). Functionally, ligation of 4-1BB can provide a co-stimulatory signal to purified $CD4^+$ and $CD8^+$ T cells at suboptimal levels of TCR stimulation. It was recently suggested that 4-1BB ligation can support T cell proliferation and effector differentiation in mice deficient in CD28 (39). However, blockade of B7-mediated co-stimulatory pathways has a greater effect on T cell proliferative responses than does blockade of 4-1BB-mediated signals (40). Unlike 4-1BB, OX-40 appears to be exclusively expressed on $CD4^+$ cells. OX-40 ligation can also provide co-stimulatory signals to naive and effector T cells (37,41). Like 4-1BB, OX-40 is also thought to synergize with B7-mediated signals to produce optimal T cell activation (41).

Some studies have implicated both 4-1BB and OX-40 as suitable targets for modulation of the anti-tumor immune response. Two reports by Chen and colleagues (42,43) suggested that ligation of 4-1BB can promote regression of both immunogenic and poorly immunogenic tumors in a T cell- and natural killer (NK) cell-dependent mechanism. Administration of an anti-4-1BB antibody resulted in regression of previously established P815 and Ag104A tumors. Using a different approach, the authors transduced the same

TABLE 27-1. *Modulation of co-stimulation to enhance anti-tumor immunity*

Tumor model	Tumor type/ tisuse origin	Rejection		
		B7	αCTLA-4	Combination[a]
EL4	Lymphoid	+	+/−	NT
SAI/N	Fibrosarcoma	+	+	NT
51BLim 10	Colorectal	+	+	NT
RENCA	Renal carcinoma	+/−	+	NT
K1735	Melanoma	+	+/−	NT
TRAMPC	Prostatic epithelium	+	+	NT
SM1	Mammary epithelium	−	−	+
B16/BL6	Melanocyte	−	−	+
TRAMP	Primary prostate Ca	−	−	+

NT, not tested; +, full rejection (> 80%); +/−, partial rejection (40–80%); −, low rejection (< 40%).
[a] Combination of α-CTLA-4 and GM-CSF-expressing vaccine.

tumors to express the 4-1BB ligand (4-1BBL) and tested their immunogenicity. Although 4-1BBL expression by P815 resulted in rejection, it had no appreciable effect on Ag104A. However, co-expression of 4-1BBL and B7 was sufficient to promote Ag104A regression, thereby demonstrating synergy between the two co-stimulatory pathways. The observation that OX-40 expression is detected on the surface of tumor-infiltrating lymphocytes and T cells from draining lymph nodes (44) from patients with squamous cell carcinoma and melanoma suggested that this pathway may be exploited to enhance tumor immunogenicity. Accordingly, administration of a soluble OX-40 agonist reduced tumor incidence and enhanced survival of mice challenged with a weakly immunogenic mammary carcinoma (37; A. Weinberg, personal communication). Taken together, these findings suggest that modulation of co-stimulatory pathways is an effective way to augment tumor immunity, but that an approach that exploits multiple co-stimulatory receptors may be necessary.

An alternative approach taken to enhance the antitumor response was to bypass the need for direct priming of CTLs by the tumor by providing alternative paracrine signals. By conferring cytokine expression to tumors, autocrine effects on MHC expression or paracrine effects on APCs or T cells may sufficiently enhance the immune response to promote tumor immunity. Interleukin-2 (IL-2) (45) and IL-4 (46), both important for providing help during T cell activation, were demonstrated to augment T cell immunity to tumors of various tissue origins. Interferon-γ (IFN-γ), a T cell-derived cytokine that can modulate T cell activation by directly activating the effector T cell or upregulating MHC expression on APCs, was also capable of enhancing tumor immunity (47) in a T cell-dependent mechanism. In addition to promoting the growth and differentiation of myeloid cells, granulocyte/macrophage colony-stimulating factor (GM-CSF) has pleiotropic effects that can result in APC activation by modulating MHC and co-stimulatory molecule expression. Immunization with irradiated, GM-CSF-expressing melanoma cells was the most effective regimen compared to ten cytokines and adhesion proteins (48); protection was dependent on both T cells and NK cells (49). The demonstration that GM-CSF was the most effective cytokine of those tested suggests that recruitment of professional APCs could enhance the potency of tumor cell vaccines.

MODULATION OF INHIBITORY SIGNALS THAT REGULATE T CELL ACTIVATION

CTLA-4 is a CD28 homolog that is expressed on the surface of T cells soon after activation but has a much higher avidity interaction with CD80 and CD86 than does CD28. Most importantly, unlike CD28, CTLA-4 appears to deliver an inhibitory signal to T cells. In support of this idea, mice deficient in *ctla-4* suffer a severe, lymphoproliferative disorder (50–52). Ligation of CTLA-4 by antibodies blocks cell-cycle progression, decreases cytokine elaboration, and reduces proliferative responses (53,54). *In vivo*, antibodies that block CTLA-4 interactions with B7 appear to enhance T cell activation, as demonstrated using animal models of autoimmune disease, superantigen response, and nominal antigen (55–59).

These findings led us and others to test whether blockade of CTLA-4–B7 interaction might be sufficient to promote tumor regression (60,61) (Table 27-1). When used alone, administration of anti-CTLA-4 antibodies was sufficient to accelerate rejection of tumors modified to express B7 (61). More strikingly, treatment with anti-CTLA-4 antibodies could promote regression of a variety of tumors of different tissue origins. In fact, therapy of some tumors could be delayed until tumor size reached nearly 10 mm in diameter (D. R. Leach, unpublished observation). Rejection of these tumors was accompanied by immunity to rechallenge. Lymphocyte depletion studies indicated that both CD4$^+$ and CD8$^+$ T cells are required for rejection. Because the tumors tested did not express class II MHC (MHC-II), these findings also suggested that anti-CTLA-4 therapy acts by blocking B7 signals derived from class II$^+$, host-derived APCs (D. R. Leach, unpublished observation). Interestingly, for most murine tumor models in which conferring B7 expression was successful, CTLA-4 blockade was also effective (Table 27-1). This supports the idea that the efficacy was reflective of the inherent immunogenicity of the tumor. However, it also implies that CTLA-4 blockade would not be effective for many, if not most, clinically relevant tumors, where immunogenicity is considered to be low.

To overcome this obstacle, we hypothesized that combination of anti-CTLA-4 with another therapy that boosts host-derived tumor antigen presentation might provide a more effective treatment regimen. Given the results of cytokine vaccine studies discussed above, we tested GM-CSF as a candidate cell-based vaccine to combine with anti-CTLA-4 therapy. We initially examined the poorly immunogenic, MHC-II$^-$ mammary carcinoma SM1 (62). Treatment of mice implanted with SM1 using anti-CTLA-4 alone only marginally slowed its growth; there was no effect on tumor incidence. Similarly, treatment with an irradiated, cell-based vaccine transduced to express GM-CSF had no effect on SM1 growth. However, the combination of the GM-CSF-expressing vaccine and anti-CTLA-4 resulted in successful treatment of recently established, unmodified SM1 tumors. Not surprisingly, rejection was dependent on both CD4$^+$ and CD8$^+$ cells and resulted in immunity to rechallenge with SM1. Results of this study demonstrated that in poorly immunogenic tumors, where CTLA-4 blockade alone is not sufficient to enhance anti-tumor immunity, provision of signals to enhance host-derived priming of T cells could overcome the threshold needed to generate a more potent antitumor response.

More recently, we have extended these findings to two murine tumor models. Combination therapy using GM-CSF-producing vaccines and anti-CTLA-4 was also successfully applied to treatment of the poorly immunogenic, C57BL/6-derived melanoma, B16-BL6. Similar to SM1, neither treatment alone produced a significant reduction in tumor incidence, but combination of the two treatments cured up to 80% of the mice from early-stage tumors. Mice that rejected the primary challenge with B16 were immune to rechallenge. The mechanism of immune rejection differed from that found with the SM1 mammary carcinoma in that CD4$^+$ T cells proved to be dispensable during initiation of the antitumor response. Moreover, combination treatment led to complete eradication of B16-F10 lung metastases and long-term survival, whereas each treatment by itself produced little effect. In addition, only the combination therapy induced a strong infiltration of mononuclear cells in the F10 pulmonary lesions when tissues were harvested 4 weeks after tumor challenge.

Most interesting, a large fraction of the surviving mice developed depigmentation of skin and hair, starting at the site of vaccination and challenge and, in some cases, spreading to distant sites. Again, it was found that CD4$^+$ T cells were not required during initiation of the immune response to pigment-containing cells, suggesting that T cell immunity had developed against a tissue-specific antigen involved in pigmentation. Interestingly, we have also detected antibody deposition at the sites of depigmentation, suggesting a role for B cells as well. The findings in this model are reminiscent of the clinical correlation described for vitiligo and improved response in melanoma patients (as described above). Altogether, blockade of CTLA-4 allows recruitment of CTLs directed against a normal self antigen that might otherwise remain tolerant or ignorant.

We have also used this approach to treat primary prostate tumors using the *t*ransgenic *a*denocarcinoma of the *m*ouse *p*rostate (TRAMP) model (63). TRAMP mice carry the SV40 T antigen under the transcriptional regulation of the rat probasin promoter that delivers expression to the prostatic epithelium. Mice exhibit disease pathogenesis similar to that in humans: progression from hyperplasia to neoplasia to invasive adenocarcinoma and ultimately metastasis. Tumor lines derived from TRAMP mice (TRAMPC) transduced to express B7 were rejected by syngeneic, nontransgenic mice (64). In addition, TRAMPC cells were rejected by nontransgenic hosts following anti-CTLA-4 treatment. To test our ability to treat primary tumors, TRAMP mice were treated with anti-CTLA-4 and an irradiated vaccine comprised of TRAMPC cells transduced to express GM-CSF at 15 weeks of age (when prostate pathology is at an early stage of neoplasia). Our results demonstrated that there was a significant reduction in the incidence of primary tumor development in mice given the combination treatment. Moreover, the histologic severity of prostatic lesions in mice treated with the GM-CSF-expressing vaccine and anti-CTLA-4 was significantly lower than in mice given either treatment alone (or given no treatment at all). These findings indicate that immunotherapy of primary tumors is not only feasible but obtainable with relatively modest therapies. The fact that TRAMP tumors are susceptible to this approach is encouraging given that the entire prostate is transformed as a result of the unrelenting expression of the transgene. Generation of tumor-based vaccines could be replaced with defined antigens known to be expressed on individual tumors and containing T cell epitopes presented by the host MHC. Identification of these antigens may render blockade of CTLA-4 a more translatable approach to both primary and metastatic disease in humans.

COMBINATION OF CTLA-4 BLOCKADE WITH TRADITIONAL THERAPIES

Given the success of CTLA-4 blockade both alone and in combination with cell-based vaccines, we have recently undertaken studies to combine this approach with more traditional therapies. In the first set of studies, mice implanted with SM1 mammary tumors were treated with anti-CTLA-4 in combination with cisplatin, a common chemotherapeutic agent. The rationale for this approach was that cisplatin may attack a portion of SM1 tumor cells that could result in tumor cell death and an inflammatory response followed by host APC priming of T cells. Subsequent administration of anti-CTLA-4 might serve to lower the threshold for priming anti-SM1 T cells and facilitate more effective priming. In fact, it has been our observation that whereas either treatment alone has negligible effects on SM1 growth, the combination of cisplatin and anti-CTLA-4 appears to slow tumor growth significantly and induce complete tumor regression in about 20% of mice tested (9 of 50 mice). Further studies using additional tumor models will help determine whether this combinatorial approach can be applied to tumors of multiple tissue specificities. In addition, application of this approach to transgenic models of tumorigenesis will permit assessment of its efficacy on primary tumors.

One other combinatorial approach is underway in our laboratory. One of the most common approaches to treat prostate cancer is androgen ablation therapy. This approach is aimed at eliminating hormone-responsive cancer. Unfortunately, androgen-insensitive disease frequently recurs and is highly aggressive. One common feature of androgen ablation therapy is an inflammatory response in the prostate prior to tissue remodeling. During this response, priming of prostate antigen-specific T cells may take place if additional inhibitory signals are blocked by administration of anti-CTLA-4. Therefore we hypothesized that immunotherapy may be an important adjunctive therapy to androgen ablation for treating prostate cancer. To test this idea, castration of TRAMP mice (a procedure previously demonstrated to alter disease progression in this model) (65) will be combined with immunotherapy as previously described. Mice will be monitored for tumor incidence and histologic disease progression. The outcome of these studies will be directly applicable to ongoing clinical trials.

CONCLUSIONS

The approaches discussed herein suggest that by modulating the process of T cell activation during tumor immunotherapy a more successful outcome can be achieved. Early studies manipulating the role of B7 in T cell priming served to invigorate research in the field. The more recent findings of additional co-stimulatory receptors on T cells can certainly provide another avenue for preclinical studies. The identification of CTLA-4 as an inhibitory receptor on T cells and its manipulation in generating a potent antitumor response represent another turning point in tumor immunology. CTLA-4 may act at two levels that are not mutually exclusive: it may function to terminate ongoing T cell responses, or it may function to set a threshold for the initiation of T cell activation. Our data support the latter in that CTLA-4 blockade may permit priming of T cells under what would normally be an unfavorable condition or insurmountable threshold, regulated by tolerance to self antigens. The ability to combine CTLA-4-based therapy with other antigen-specific vaccination approaches and more traditional cancer therapies could make this an even more powerful tool. Ongoing research aimed at understanding the mechanism of T cell activation can make cancer immunotherapy a more realistic and effective option.

REFERENCES

1. Klein G, Klein E. Immune surveillance against virus-induced tumors and nonrejectability of spontaneous tumors: contrasting consequences of host versus tumor evolution. *Proc Natl Acad Sci USA* 1977;74:2121–2125.
2. Prehn RT. Tumor-specific antigens of putatively nonviral tumors. *Cancer Res* 1968;28:1326–1330.
3. Boon T, Cerottini J-C, Van den Eynde B, van der Bruggen P, Van Pel A. Tumor antigens recognized by T lymphocytes. *Annu Rev Immunol* 1994; 12:337–365.
4. Rosenberg SA. Cancer vaccines based on the identi-

fication of genes encoding cancer regression antigens. *Immunol Today* 1997;18:175–182.
5. Van den Eynde BJ, van der Bruggen P. T cell defined tumor antigens. *Curr Opin Immunol* 1997; 9:684–693.
6. Wölfel T, Hauer M, Schneider J, et al. A p16INK4a-insensitive CDK4 mutant targeted by cytolytic T lymphocytes in a human melanoma. *Science* 1995;269:1281–1284.
7. Robbins PF, El-Gamil M, Li YF, et al. A mutated beta-catenin gene encodes a melanoma-specific antigen recognized by tumor infiltrating lymphocytes. *J Exp Med* 1996;183:1185–1192.
8. Coulie PG, Lehmann F, Lethé B, et al. A mutated intron sequence codes for an antigenic peptide recognized by cytolytic T lymphocytes on a human melanoma. *Proc Natl Acad Sci USA* 1995;92:7976–7980.
9. Cox AL, Skipper J, Chen Y, et al. Identification of a peptide recognized by five melanoma-specific human cytotoxic T cell lines. *Science* 1994;264: 716–719.
10. Kawakami Y, Eliyahu S, Delgado CH, et al. Identification of a human melanoma antigen recognized by tumor-infiltrating lymphocytes associated with in vivo tumor rejection. *Proc Natl Acad Sci USA* 1994;91:6458–6462.
11. Skipper JC, Hendrickson RC, Gulden PH, et al. An HLA-A2-restricted tyrosinase antigen on melanoma cells results from posttranslational modification and suggests a novel pathway for processing of membrane proteins. *J Exp Med* 1996;183:527–534.
12. Topalian SL, Rivoltini L, Mancini M, et al. Human CD4+ T cells specifically recognize a shared melanoma-associated antigen encoded by the tyrosinase gene. *Proc Natl Acad Sci USA* 1994;91:9461–9465.
13. Kawakami Y, Eliyahu S, Delgado CH, et al. Cloning of the gene coding for a shared human melanoma antigen recognized by autologous T cells infiltrating into tumor. *Proc Natl Acad Sci USA* 1994;91:3515–3519.
14. Wang RF, Appella E, Kawakami Y, Kang X, Rosenberg SA. Identification of TRP-2 as a human tumor antigen recognized by cytotoxic T lymphocytes. *J Exp Med* 1996;184:2207–2216.
15. Wang RF, Parkhurst MR, Kawakami Y, Robbins PF, Rosenberg SA. Utilization of an alternative open reading frame of a normal gene in generating a novel human cancer antigen. *J Exp Med* 1996;183:1131–1140.
16. Robbins PF, el-Gamil M, Li YF, et al. Cloning of a new gene encoding an antigen recognized by melanoma-specific HLA-A24-restricted tumor-infiltrating lymphocytes. *J Immunol* 1995;154:5944–5950.
17. Richards JM, Mehta N, Ramming K, Skosey P. Sequential chemoimmunotherapy in the treatment of metastatic melanoma. *J Clin Oncol* 1992;10:1338–1343.
18. Visseren MJ, van Elsas A, van der Voort EI, et al. CTL specific for the tyrosinase autoantigen can be induced from healthy donor blood to lyse melanoma cells. *J Immunol* 1995;154:3991–3998.
19. Bakker AB, Marland G, de Boer AJ, et al. Generation of antimelanoma cytotoxic T lymphocytes from healthy donors after presentation of melanoma-as-

sociated antigen-derived epitopes by dendritic cells in vitro. *Cancer Res* 1995;55:5330–5334.

20. Nestle FO, Alijagic S, Gilliet M, et al. Vaccination of melanoma patients with peptide- or tumor lysate-pulsed dendritic cells. *Nat Med* 1998;4:328–332.

21. Rosenberg SA, Yang JC, Schwartzentruber DJ, et al. Immunologic and therapeutic evaluation of a synthetic peptide vaccine for the treatment of patients with metastatic melanoma. *Nat Med* 1998;4:321–327.

22. Davis MM, Bjorkman PJ. T-cell antigen receptor genes and T-cell recognition. *Nature* 1988;334:395–402.

23. Lenschow DJ, Walunas TL, Bluestone JA. CD28/B7 system of T cell costimulation. *Annu Rev Immunol* 1996;14:233–258.

24. Denfeld RW, Dietrich A, Wuttig C, et al. In situ expression of B7 and CD28 receptor families in human malignant melanoma: relevance for T-cell-mediated anti-tumor immunity. *Int J Cancer* 1995;62:259–265.

25. Allison JP, Hurwitz AA, Leach DR. Manipulation of costimulatory signals to enhance antitumor T cell responses. *Curr Opin Immunol* 1995;7:682–686.

26. Huang AY, Bruce AT, Pardoll DM, Levitsky HI. Does B7-1 expression confer antigen-presenting cell capacity to tumors in vivo? *J Exp Med* 1996;183:769–776.

27. Chen L, McGowan P, Ashe S, et al. Tumor immunogenicity determines the effect of B7 costimulation on T cells-mediated tumor immunity. *J Exp Med* 1994;179:523–532.

28. Baskar S, Glimcher L, Nabavi N, Jones RT, Ostrand-Rosenberg S. Major histocompatibility complex class II+B7-1+ tumor cells are potent vaccines for stimulating tumor rejection in tumor-bearing mice. *J Exp Med* 1995;181:619–629.

29. Li Y, McGowan P, Hellstrom I, Hellstrom KE, Chen L. Costimulation of tumor-reactive CD4+ and CD8+ T lymphocytes by B7, a natural ligand for CD28, can be used to treat established mouse melanoma. *J Immunol* 1994;153:421–428.

30. Townsend SE, Su FW, Atherton JM, Allison JP. Specificity and longevity of anti-tumor immune responses induced by B7-transfected tumors. *Cancer Res* 1994;54:6477–6483.

31. Coughlin CM, Wysocka M, Kurzawa HL, Lee WM, Trinchieri G, Eck SL. B7-1 and interleukin 12 synergistically induce effective antitumor immunity. *Cancer Res* 1995;55:4980–4987.

32. Hurwitz AA, Townsend SE, Yu TF-Y, Atherton J, Allison JP. Enhancement of the anti-tumor immune response using a combination of interferon-γ and B7 expression in an experimental mammary carcinoma. *Int J Cancer* 1998;77:107–113.

33. Katsanis E, Bausero MA, Panoskaltsis-Mortari A, et al. Irradiation of singly and doubly transduced murine neuroblastoma cells expressing B7-1 and producing interferon-gamma reduces their capacity to induce systemic immunity. *Cancer Gene Ther* 1996;3:75–82.

34. Sumimoto H, Tani K, Nakazaki Y, et al. GM-CSF and B7-1 (CD80) co-stimulatory signals co-operate in the induction of effective anti-tumor immunity in syngeneic mice. *Int J Cancer* 1997;73:556–561.

35. Zitvogel L, Robbins PD, Storkus WJ, et al. Interleukin-12 and B7.1 co-stimulation cooperate in the induction of effective antitumor immunity and therapy of established tumors. *Eur J Immunol* 1996;26:1335–1341.

36. Vinay DS, Kwon BS. Role of 4-1BB in immune responses. *Semin Immunol* 1998;10:481–489.

37. Weinberg AD, Vella AT, Croft M. OX-40: life beyond the effector T cell stage. *Semin Immunol* 1998;10:471–480.

38. Kwon BS, Weissman SM. cDNA sequences of two inducible T-cell genes. *Proc Natl Acad Sci USA* 1989;86:1963–1967.

39. DeBenedette MA, Shahinian A, Mak TW, Watts TH. Costimulation of CD28-T lymphocytes by 4-1BB ligand. *J Immunol* 1997;158:551–559.

40. Hurtado JC, Kim SH, Pollok KE, Lee ZH, Kwon BS. Potential role of 4-1BB in T cell activation. comparison with the costimulatory molecule CD28. *J Immunol* 1995;155:3360–3367.

41. Gramaglia I, Weinberg AD, Lemon M, Croft M. Ox-40 ligand: a potent costimulatory molecule for sustaining primary CD4 T cell responses. *J Immunol* 1998;161:6510–6517.

42. Melero I, Bach N, Hellstrom KE, Aruffo A, Mittler RS, Chen L. Amplification of tumor immunity by gene transfer of the co-stimulatory 4-1BB ligand: synergy with the CD28 co-stimulatory pathway. *Eur J Immunol* 1998;28:1116–1121.

43. Melero I, Shuford WW, Newby SA, et al. Monoclonal antibodies against the 4-1BB T-cell activation molecule eradicate established tumors. *Nat Med* 1997;3:682–685.

44. Vetto JT, Lum S, Morris A, et al. Presence of the T-cell activation marker OX-40 on tumor infiltrating lymphocytes and draining lymph node cells from patients with melanoma and head and neck cancers. *Am J Surg* 1997;174:258–265.

45. Fearon E, Pardoll D, Itaya T, et al. Interleukin-2 production by tumor cells bypasses T helper function in the generation of an antitumor response. *Cell* 1990;60:397–403.

46. Golumbek P, Lazanby H, Levitsky H, et al. Treatment of established renal cancer by tumor cells engineered to secrete interleukin-4. *Science* 1991;254:713–716.

47. Gansbacher B, Bannerji R, Daniels B, Zier K, Cronin K, Gilboa E. Retroviral vector-mediated gamma-interferon gene transfer into tumor cells generates potent and long lasting antitumor immunity. *Cancer Res* 1990;50:7820–7825.

48. Dranoff G, Jaffee E, Lazenby A, et al. Vaccination with irradiated tumor cells engineered to secrete murine granulocyte-macrophage colony-stimulating factor stimulates potent, specific, long-lasting anti-tumor immunity. *Proc Natl Acad Sci USA* 1993;90:3539–3543.

49. Levitsky H, Lazenby A, Hayashi RJ, Pardoll DM. In vivo priming of two distinct anti-tumor effector populations: the role of MHC class I expression. *J Exp Med* 1994;179:1215–1224.

50. Waterhouse P, Penninger JM, Timms E, et al. Lymphoproliferative disorders with early lethality in mice deficient in CTLA-4. *Science* 1995;270:985–988.

51. Tivol EA, Borriello F, Schweitzer AN, Lynch WP, Bluestone JA, Sharpe AH. Loss of CTLA-4 leads to massive lymphoproliferation and fatal multiorgan tissue destruction, revealing a critical negative regulatory role of CTLA-4. *Immunity* 1995;3:541–547.

52. Chambers CA, Cado D, Truong T, Allison JP. Thymocyte development is normal in CTLA-4-deficient mice. *Proc Natl Acad Sci USA* 1997;94:9296–9301.

53. Krummel MF, Allison JP. CTLA-4 engagement inhibits IL-2 accumulation and cell cycle progression upon activation of resting T cells. *J Exp Med* 1996;183:2533–2540.

54. Walunas TL, Bakker CY, Bluestone JA. CTLA-4 ligation blocks CD28-dependent T cell activation. *J Exp Med* 1996;183:2541–2550.

55. Hurwitz AA, Sullivan TJ, Krummel MF, Sobel RA, Allison JP. Specific blockade of CTLA-4/B7 interactions results in exacerbated clinical and histologic disease in an actively-induced model of experimental allergic encephalomyelitis. *J Neuroimmunol* 1997;73:57–62.

56. Karandikar NJ, Vanderlugt CL, Walunas TL, Miler SD, Bluestone JA. CTLA-4: A negative regulator of autoimmune disease. *J Exp Med* 1996;184:783–788.

57. Krummel MF, Sullivan TJ, Allison JP. Superantigen responses and co-stimulation: CD28 and CTLA-4 have opposing effects on T cell expansion in vitro and in vivo. *Int Immunol* 1996;8:519–523.

58. Luhder F, Hoglund P, Allison JP, Benoist C, Mathis D. Cytotoxic T lymphocyte-associated antigen 4 (CTLA-4) regulates the unfolding of autoimmune diabetes. *J Exp Med* 1998;187:427–432.

59. Kearney ER, Walunas TL, Karr RW, et al. Antigen-dependent clonal expansion of a trace population of antigen-specific CD4+ T cells in vivo is dependent on CD28 costimulation and inhibited by CTLA-4. *J Immunol* 1995;155:1032–1036.

60. Yang G, Hellstrom KE, Hellstrom I, Chen L. Antitumor immunity elicited by tumor cells transfected with B7-2, a second ligand for CD28/CTLA-4 costimulatory molecules. *J Immunol* 1995;154:2794–2800.

61. Leach DR, Krummel MF, Allison JP. Enhancement of antitumor immunity by CTLA-4 blockade. *Science* 1996;271:1734–1736.

62. Hurwitz AA, Yu TF-Y, Leach DR, Allison JP. CTLA-4 blockade synergizes with tumor-derived granulocyte-macrophage colony-stimulating factor for treatment of an experimental mammary carcinoma. *Proc Natl Acad Sci USA* 1998;95:10067–10071.

63. Greenberg NM, DeMayo F, Finegold MJ, et al. Prostate cancer in a transgenic mouse. *Proc Natl Acad Sci USA* 1995;92:3439–3443.

64. Kwon ED, Hurwitz AA, Foster BA, et al. Manipulation of T cell costimulatory and inhibitory signals for immunotherapy of prostate cancer. *Proc Natl Acad Sci USA* 1997;94:8099–8103.

65. Gingrich JR, Barrios RJ, Kattan MW, Nahm HS, Finegold MJ, Greenberg NM. Androgen-independent prostate cancer progression in the TRAMP model. *Cancer Res* 1997;57:4687–4691.

Cytotoxic Cells: Basic Mechanisms and Medical Applications, edited by Michail V. Sitkovsky and Pierre A. Henkart. Lippincott Williams & Wilkins, Philadelphia © 2000.

Chapter 28

Use of Bacterial DNA in Vaccines for CTL Generation

Grayson B. Lipford and Hermann Wagner

Institute of Medical Microbiology, Immunology, and Hygiene, 81675 Munich, Germany

Bacterial DNA was considered immunologically inert for decades. To the contrary, however, it has been demonstrated that the immune system through pattern recognition discrimination senses prokaryotic DNA and signals infectious danger. Structural and sequence usage differences between pathogen versus host DNA have allowed immune cells to evolve detection systems that key on unmethylated CpG dinucleotides in particular base context. As a result, the presence of bacterial DNA, including vector DNA or mimicking synthetic oligodeoxynucleotide (ODN), activates both innate and adaptive immune cells, such as dendritic cells and macrophages (antigen-presenting cells) or natural killer (NK) cells, B cells, and T cells (lymphocytes). Bacterial DNA can thus serve as an adjuvant for the induction of cytolytic cells or humoral responses to antigen. Responses to antigen or infectious challenge are primarily T-helper (Th1) cell dominated implying a major role for antigen-presenting cell (APC)-derived interleukin-12 (IL-12). Animal models have revealed that CpG ODN could have a major therapeutic impact as a vaccine adjuvant or immunomodulator in cancer, allergic, or infectious disease treatments.

BACTERIAL DNA AS AN IMMUNOSTIMULANT

Freund et al., without recognition of the fact, more than 50 years ago first used DNA as an adjuvant in their description of complete Freund's adjuvant, a mixture of whole mycobacterial extract in oil (1). During the 1960s it was first postulated that foreign DNA can induce interferon (IFN) release (2,3), although this observation was later questioned (4). Subsequently, Yamamoto, Tokunaga, and colleagues pioneered the field by a series of studies originally aimed at analyzing *Mycobacterium bovis*-bacille Calmette-Guérin (BCG)-mediated tumor resistance in mice. A fraction extracted from BCG (designated MY-1) exhibited antitumor activity *in vivo,* augmented NK cell activity, and triggered *in vitro* type I and type II IFN release from murine spleen cells or human peripheral blood lymphocytes (PBLs) (5–7). These activities could be destroyed by DNase pretreatment of MY-1 but not by RNase. Pisetsky and associates independently observed that normal mice and humans respond to bacterial DNA but not vertebrate DNA by producing anti-DNA antibodies (8). They first realized that bacterial DNA was mitogenic for murine B cells and postulated that the activity was due to "nonconserved structural determinants." The differential stimulative capacity of bacterial DNA versus vertebrate DNA was also demonstrated for induction of NK cell activity by Yamamoto et al. (9).

The MY-1 fraction was determined by high performance liquid chromatography (HPLC) analysis to be composed of a broad size range of DNA fragments with a peak at 45 bases. Synthetic single-stranded 45mer ODNs derived from BCG cDNA sequences were analyzed for their IFN-inducing capacity and augmentation of NK cytotoxicity (10). It was concluded that synthetic ODNs containing palindromic sequences could induce these activities; critical, however, was the sequence of the palindrome. Sequences with a central CpG were most active, but an explanation for this phenomenon was not apparent (9,11).

Several investigators using antisense ODNs began to observe sequence-specific immune stimulatory effects. Working from a similar observation, Krieg et al. affected this area of research by formulating a hypothetic framework to understand the pattern recognition of bacterial or synthetic DNA (12). Monitoring B cell proliferation induced by ODNs, they iteratively isolated mitogenicity to specific sequences containing CpG dinucleotides with selective flanking bases. They concluded that DNA motifs displaying a 5'-Pu-Pu-CpG-Pyr-Pyr-3' base sequences were biologically active. It was therefore tempting to speculate that immune cells sense unique base sequences of pathogen-associated DNA.

Bacterial DNA, some viral DNA, and DNA of invertebrates apparently differ structurally from vertebrate DNA. The usage of the dinucleotide motif 5'-CpG-3' in bacterial DNA has the expected statistical frequency of 1:16. In contrast, mammalian DNA exhibits CpG suppression; that is, there is only about one-fourth as many CpG as predicted by random base usage (13). The usage of the 5'-Pu-Pu-CpG-Pyr-Pyr-3' motif is even further suppressed in mammals compared to a normal distribution in the genome of *Escherichia coli* (12). Furthermore, eukaryotic CpG motifs are preferentially methylated, and sequence-specific methylation of CpG abolishes their stimulatory potential (12,13). The realization that CpG sequences are underrepresented in vertebrate DNA provides a theory to explain a number of biologic observations in the context of non-self pattern recognition by the immune system.

Concurrent with these developments, the field of immunization with "naked" vector DNA was developing. The initial observations were that vector DNA, encoding an antigen and unassociated with delivery vehicles, induced cell-mediated and humoral immune responses to the encoded antigen after inoculation [reviewed by Tighe et al. (14)]. Subsequently, it was discovered that the noncoding sequences of the vector influenced the immune response. Sato et al. realized that a β-gal encoding vector containing the ampicillin-resistance gene (ampR) rather than the kanamycin-resistance gene resulted in a stronger immune response to β-gal (15). This phenomenon was correlated with the presence of CpG motifs in the ampR sequence. Thus the immune system senses and responds to DNA by virtue of CpG motifs within extracted bacterial DNA, vector DNA, or synthetic ODNs; and its recognition can influence *in vivo* immune responses.

PATTERN RECOGNITION MOBILIZES THE INNATE IMMUNE RESPONSE

The immune system is based on two distinct pathogen recognition systems: innate (non-clonal host defense) and adaptive (clonal host defense). The innate immune system receptors recognize conserved molecular structures shared by a large group of pathogens, termed pattern recognition receptors (PRRs) (16,17). The adaptive immune system receptors recognize unique pathogen structures and are selected from a pool of T and B clones expressing unique randomly recombined conserved and nonconserved receptor gene domains. The main difference between PRRs and clonally distributed antigen receptors of the adaptive system is that PRR specificities are germline-encoded.

Thus a parameter imposed on PRRs is the recognition of non-self structural patterns. Although T and B cell receptors, through their specificity and diversity, represent the crowning achievement of the vertebrate adaptive immune system, they do not distinguish self from non-self. Thus the innate system senses non-self pathogen invasion and through its activation controls the initiation of the adaptive immune response. Initiation and control of the adaptive response is accomplished by regulating the expression of cell surface co-stimulatory molecules on APCs and instructing the adaptive immune system to develop a particular effector response through the release of effector cytokines.

The APCs (e.g., dendritic cells and macrophages) represent a decisive interface between the innate and adaptive immune system (18). By virtue of their surveillance and phagocytic/endocytic properties, these cells engage pathogens through PRRs at an early stage of the infectious challenge. Signals induced by pattern recognition can be grouped into three categories: (a) inflammatory responses including IL-1, tumor necrosis factor (TNF), IL-6, type I IFN, and chemokines; (b) co-stimulators of T cell activation, including B7.1 (CD80), B7.2 (CD86), and CD40; and (c) effector cytokines, including IL-10, IL-12, transforming growth factor-α (TGF-α), and IFN-γ. Before a productive response can ensue, APCs must be activated, thus acquiring the ability to instigate productive T and B cell activation through the above-mentioned mediators.

CpG MOTIFS INDEPENDENTLY ACTIVATE APC BY PRRs

Macrophages utilizing PRRs recognize non-self DNA through CpG motifs and initiate inflammatory responses. In early work by Yamamoto et al. it was concluded that IFN-α/β produced by ODN-stimulated spleen cells possibly came from an adherent cell

population (6). We and others discovered that extracted DNA from gram-negative or gram-positive bacteria, vector DNA, or synthetic CpG ODN trigger macrophages to activate the stress kinase pathways and various transcription factors, transcribe cytokine mRNAs, and secrete cytokines such as TNF-α, IL-1, IL-6, and IL-12 (15,19–25). Acute release of toxic amounts of TNF-α can follow bacterial DNA challenge *in vivo,* leading to lethal toxic shock in mouse models (20,21). These attributes are similar to previously described PRR signaling induced by the bacterial product lipopolysaccharide (LPS). Bacterial DNA can also sensitize mice for the action of LPS; and more important, bacterial DNA or CpG ODNs synergize with LPS, inducing macrophage cytokine release *in vitro* and toxic amounts of TNF-α *in vivo* (21,26). Unquestionably the worst scenario for bacterial infections is acute systemic stimulation, resulting in overproduction of proinflammatory cytokines that cause toxic shock. Integration of multiple PRR signals by APCs resulting in amplified immune cell mobilization for combating infectious danger, however, appears adaptive.

Dendritic cells (DCs) are considered the premier APC and a pivotal link to productive immune responses. They are ubiquitously distributed but most frequently located as immature DCs at strategically important sites (e.g., epidermis, lung, lymph nodes) (18). Immature DCs phagocytize, pinocytize, and process exogenous antigen; yet they perform poorly as APCs because expression of major histocompatibility complex (MHC) and costimulatory molecules is low. To become effective APCs, the DCs must mature; an activation process leading to enhanced expression of antigen-presentation molecules and cell surface co-stimulatory molecules. After antigen engagement, DCs mature and translocate to T cell areas within draining lymph nodes. DC maturation can be mediated via CD40/CD40L interactions between DCs and antigen-reactive T cells, a situation requiring prior activation of T cells (27). On the other hand, PRR signaling causes direct DC maturation (see below) in a CD40/CD40L-independent fashion (28), allowing activated APCs to engage and stimulate naive T cells (29). The need for adjuvants, which are typically PRR stimuli, for the induction of immune responses to purified protein antigens, might be explained by PRR signals resulting in direct DC maturation.

We analyzed the effects of bacterial DNA or CpG ODN on immature DCs grown in granulyocyte/macrophage colony-stimulating factor (GM-CSF)-conditioned medium from bone marrow cells (BMDDCs) (30). Bacterial DNA displayed three major effects. First, it caused upregulation within hours of the molecules of MHC class II

(MHC-II) and the co-stimulatory molecules CD40 and B7.2 (Fig. 28-1). Second, and in parallel, the phenotypically matured DCs produced large amounts of IL-12, TNF-α, IL-6, and to a lesser extent IL-10 (Figure 28-2 shows representative IL-12 release). Third, matured and activated DCs displayed professional APC function during primary activation of T cells (not shown). These data defined bacterial DNA and CpG ODN as inducers of DC maturation and activation. There is now a need to analyze whether CpG DNA also drives DC maturation *in vivo*, thereby causing translocation to T cell areas within lymph nodes. If so, CpG-mediated maturation/activation of immature DCs might explain aspects of their remarkable adjuvant capacity (see below).

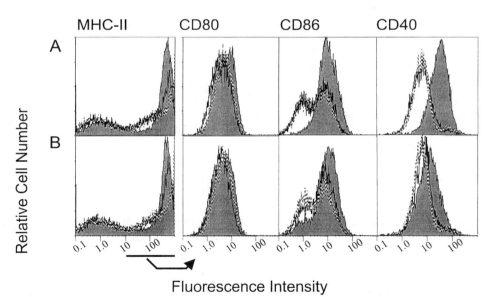

FIG. 28-1. Bacterial DNA and CpG oligodeoxynucleotide (ODN) trigger upregulation of co-stimulatory molecules in bone marrow-derived dendritic cells (BMDDCs). MHC class II (MHC-II)-positive cells (*black bar*) (mean > 10) were gated, and the expression of CD80, CD86, and CD40 are depicted. Synthetic CpG ODN and bacterial DNA induce upregulation of MHC-II, CD86, and CD40. **A:** The CpG containing ODN 1668 (TCCATGA*CG*TTCCTGATGCT) (*solid histograms*), control GpC containing ODN 1720 (TCCATGA*GC*TTCCTGATGCT) (*black lines*), or solvent-only control (*dotted lines*) were used to stimulate nonadherent BMDDCs 1 × 10[6]/ml in LowTox Medium without GM-CSF for 20 hours. **B:** *Escherichia coli* DNA (*solid histograms*), DNase-treated *E. coli* DNA as a control (*black lines*), or solvent-only control (*dotted lines*) were also used to stimulate nonadherent BMDDCs 1 × 10[6]/ml in LowTox Medium without GM-CSF for 20 hours.

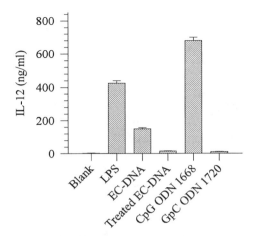

FIG. 28-2. Bacterial DNA and CpG ODN trigger IL-12 release from BMDDCs. BMDDCs (1 × 10⁶/ml) were stimulated with lipopolysaccharide (*LPS*) 0.1 µg/ml, *E. coli* DNA (*EC-DNA*) 1.0 µg/ml, DNase-treated *E. coli* DNA as a control 1.0 µg/ml, CpG ODN 1668 (1.0 µM), or control GpC 1.0 µM containing ODN 1720 for overnight. IL-12 released into the supernatant was measured by ELISA. Bacterial DNA and CpG ODN induced IL-12 release for dendritic cells, whereas DNase-treated bacterial DNA or the GpC ODN 1720 induced the release of only relatively low amounts of IL-12.

CpG ADJUVANT EFFECTS

Fearon and Locksley postulated that innate immune responses could create an immune milieu conducive to the development of antigen-specific immunity (16). Protection against pathogens requires broad-spectrum subunit vaccines that activate both humoral and cell-mediated immune responses. Unfortunately, first-generation killed virus vaccines, although phagocytosed by professional APCs, often lead to nonprotective Th2-dominated humoral immunity with no significant cytotoxic T cell (CTL) responses. To confer protective, (i.e., Th1-oriented) immunogenicity to soluble subunit proteins, the use of adjuvants is often required. Adjuvants are thought to act primarily by activating APCs to express a full complement of costimulatory molecules and effector cytokines. Efficient APC activation can be trig-

gered by a number of environmental stimuli ranging from plant extracts to bacterial components. Because of the intense APC activation that takes place due to CpG motif stimulation it seems logical to assume strong adjuvant activity.

To determine the potential adjuvant qualities of CpG-containing oligonucleotides we synthesized and tested the proven immunostimulatory sequence 1668 (TCCAT GACGTT CCTGATGCT) (31). This sequence contains the motif CpG flanked by two 5' purines and two 3' pyrimidines, which has been previously postulated to be the initiator of B cell mitogenicity, releasing IL-6 from B cells and releasing of IFN-γ from NK1.1 cells (10–12,25,26,32,33). The 1668 ODN was injected into mice with either free ovalbumin or liposome-encapsulated ovalbumin. The mice were boosted at day 14; and after 1 week ovalbumin-specific endpoint antibody titers were determined in an isotype specific enzyme-linked immunosorbent assay (ELISA). Figure 28-3 shows that 1668 strongly potentiated the antibody response and induced class switching toward immunoglobulin G2a (IgG2a) and IgG2b. The mean specific titer was greatest when CpG ODN was used as adjuvant, being a 272-fold increase for IgG2a and 189-fold increase for IgG2b. The adjuvant effect was negligible for IgM, IgG1, or IgG3. Specific titers for IgA and IgE were tested but were not measurable. These data imply that CpG ODN can serve as adjuvant for the induction of specific antibodies to protein antigens. The biasing of CpG ODN-enhanced responses to the IgG2 isotypes may indicate a Th1-dependent, cytokine-induced class switching (34). Results confirming these observations have been reported by others (24,35–37).

Previously, we described the use of liposomes in combination with Quil A or QS-21 to induce CTLs to either protein or MHC-I binding peptides (38). Antigen entrapped in liposomes without adjuvant was an ineffective inducer of CTL activity, but the inoculums became effective with the addition of

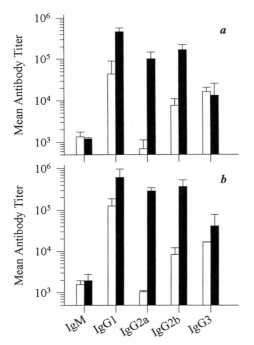

FIG. 28-3. Mean endpoint antibody titers of C57Bl/6 mice injected in the hindfoot pads with 10 nmol CpG ODN and 300 μg free OVA (**a**) or liposome-entrapped OVA (**b**), final volume 100 μl. Three mice per condition were given injections and boosted with inoculums after 2 weeks. One week later blood was taken for ovalbumin specific serum antibody titering through ELISA. The *bars* represent the mean and SD of isotype-specific antibody titers; IgA and IgE titers were not measurable. *Open bars,* inoculums with antigen only; *solid bars,* inoculums including 10 nmol 1668 as adjuvant. Two- to three-log increases in ovalbumin-specific antibody titers can be seen for IgG2a and IgG2b when comparing inoculums plus or minus the adjuvant.

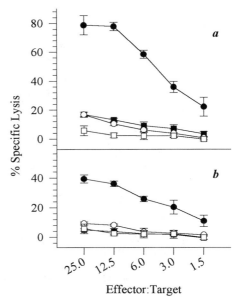

FIG. 28-4. Primary CTL response after injection with oligomers as the adjuvant plus liposome entrapped ovalbumin (**a**) or liposome-entrapped SIINFEKL (**b**), the immunodominant peptide epitope from ovalbumin. C57/B6 mice were injected with antigen only (*squares*) or antigen plus 1668 (*circles*). Draining lymph nodes were harvested at day 4, and lymph node cells were cultured for an additional 4 days in the presence of IL-2 (10 U/ml) but absence of antigen. Specific lysis was measure by a standard ^{51}Cr release assay. The targets were EL-4 cells (*open symbols*) or EL-4 cells pulsed with the SIINFEKL peptide (*closed symbols*). CpG ODN 1668 served as an adjuvant to induce ovalbumin specific CTLs when either whole protein or synthetic peptide was used as the immunogen.

immunostimulatory adjuvant. To test the *in vivo* T cell immunomodulatory potential of CpG ODN we utilized an inoculum of ODN plus liposome-entrapped ovalbumin to demonstrate primary activation of CTLs. The results in Figure 28-4a show a substantial primary CTL response induced by these inoculums. The lytic unit (LU) value at the 30% kill level interpolated from these curves was approximately 500 LU compared to less than 20 LU for ovalbumin liposomes alone. Other non-CpG-containing oligomers did not induce CTLs (data not shown). Addi-

tionally, when the inoculum was formulated with the immunodominant K^b-restricted ovalbumin peptide SIINFEKL (39), the CpG ODN induced a specific primary CTL response (Fig. 28-4b). CTL memory could also be demonstrated with these inoculums. If mice were rested for 2 weeks after the first injection and reinjected with the same inoculum, CpG ODN recalled CTLs displaying lytic units measured at approximately 1,500 LU (data not shown). Thus CpG ODNs serve as a strong *in vivo* stimulus resulting in T cell activation and the proliferation of antigen-specific CTL effectors.

Confirming our initial result, the ability of

CpG DNA to serve as an adjuvant for productive CTL responses to various antigens has subsequently been shown. Similar data were reported for CTL responses to recombinant hepatitis B protein, hen egg lysozyme, and other proteins (24,35,37,40). CpG ODNs thus are a powerful new class of synthetic adjuvants promoting CTL responses and Th1-type responses to proteinaceous antigens.

SOLUBLE PROTEIN PLUS CpG ODN INDUCE CTL *IN VIVO*

It is widely accepted that fully soluble native antigen unassociated with delivery vehicles such as lipids or detergents does not induce CTLs *in vivo* (41). This belief is supported by the dichotomy of antigen processing and routing for peptides that load MHC-I or MHC-II. Active MHC peptide loading is compartmentalized within the cell. Endoplasmic reticulum (ER)-localized MHC-I is supplied with proteosome-degraded, TAP-transported peptide fragments originating from cytosolic proteins. Endosomally localized MHC-II is supplied with enzymatically degraded peptide fragments from exogenously engulfed proteins. CTLs recognize peptides in the context of MHC-I and thus are restricted to peptides processed from cytosolic antigens. Several techniques have been developed to deliver vaccine subunit proteins to the cytosol of APCs, including osmotic shock, cationic lipid carriers, toxin carriers, bacterial or virus carriers, and naked DNA antigen-encoding carriers.

Several investigators have demonstrated that particulate antigen could induce CTLs (42). It was hypothesized that these antigens, which are phagocytosed from the extracellular environment, either enter the cytosol by some form of endosomal leakage or that an alternative processing pathway for MHC-I exists. Brossart and Bevan have subsequently shown that *in vitro* cultured dendritic cells use macropinocytosis to capture soluble antigens and present them in the context of MHC-I (43). The classic presentation pathway was operative, as TAP deficiency, proteosome blockade, or MHC-I ER egress

blockade eliminated presentation. An additional relevant observation was that exogenously added IFN-γ enhanced this form of processing and presentation.

Because of the strong influence CpG ODNs exert on dendritic cells and the ability of CpG DNA to induce IFN-γ, it became imperative to determine if fully soluble native antigen in the context of a natural adjuvant such as CpG DNA would induce CTLs. Figure 28-5 shows that mice injected with soluble ovalbumin plus CpG ODN in phosphate-buffered saline (PBS) generate a primary CTL response specific for ovalbumin. Taken together these observations imply that during infection DCs take up soluble antigen and through concurrent PRR activa-

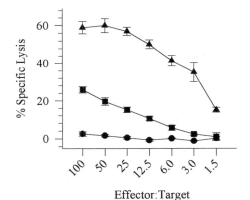

FIG. 28-5. Primary CTL response after injection with soluble ovalbumin in combination with DNA as the adjuvant. Ovalbumin (grade VI; Sigma, Germany) was solubilized in PBS and centrifuged at 25,000 *g* for 30 minutes. The supernatant was harvested, and the protein was measured and termed "soluble ovalbumin." C57/B6 mice were injected with 100 μg soluble ovalbumin plus 50 μg CpG ODN (*triangles*), 100 μg of empty vector DNA that contained the ampicillin-resistance gene (*squares*), or solvent only (*circles*). Draining lymph nodes were harvested at day 4, and lymph node cells were cultured for an additional 4 days in the presence of IL-2 (10 U/ml) but absence of antigen. Specific lysis was measure by a standard ⁵¹Cr release assay. The target cells were EG-7 cells, which are EL-4 cells transfected with the ovalbumin gene (generous gift from M. Bevan). It can be seen that both CpG ODN and vector DNA serve as adjuvant, contributing to the induction of CTLs to fully soluble ovalbumin.

tion mature and recruit precursor CTLs for antigen-specific activation. This observation simplifies what has been a complex immunologic question: How do the most relevant professional APCs induce CTL responses without being infected? Given the proper activation stimulus, DCs apparently ingest and process soluble antigen resulting in antigen activation of primary CTLs.

CpG ODN BIAS ADAPTIVE IMMUNE RESPONSES TO Th1

The Th1-promoting adjuvant effects of CpG ODNs may be useful for the redirection to protective or even curative Th1 responses in Th2-driven disorders. A particular impressive disease model is the modulation of Th2-driven airway inflammation by CpG ODNs in a murine model of asthma (44). CpG ODNs prevented airway eosinophilia, Th2 cytokine induction, IgE production, and bronchial hyperreactivity. Whether CpG ODNs effect Th1-driven protection against exposure to extrinsic allergens (atopic disorders) still needs to be analyzed. A model for redirection of Th2 responses to protective Th1 responses is our demonstration that CpG ODNs protected BALB/c mice against lethal *Leishmania major* (*L.m*) infections (45). In this system of Th2-driven infectious disorder, administration of CpG ODNs cured *L.m*-infected Balb/c mice when applied as late as 15 days after infection. Although we realize that CpG ODNs trigger sustained IL-12 production by DCs and may induce inducible nitric oxide synthase (iNos) activity in *L.m*-infected DCs and macrophages, the cellular and molecular mechanism of the curative effects are yet poorly understood.

DEPENDENT SIGNALING AND CO-RECEPTOR DRIVEN CpG EFFECTS

It has long been claimed that CpG ODNs stimulate the release of IFN-γ from NK cells. Chace et al. determined that NK activation was macrophage-dependent (23). Purified NK cells in the absence of APCs did not respond to bacterial DNA. NK cells could be primed to respond to CpG DNA by co-culture with IL-12. These data demonstrate that NK cells respond to bacterial DNA, although a co-receptor must be engaged, implying dependence in the signal transduction pathways.

The CpG ODNs independently activate resting B cells, immature DCs, and macrophages but apparently not T cells (31). Given the lineage relation between B and T cells, this cell selectivity is surprising. Because T cell activation is tightly controlled, in that T cell receptor (TCR) ligation (signal 1) induces sensitivity to co-stimulation (signal 2), we analyzed *in vitro* the effects of CpG ODNs on purified T cells subjected to TCR ligation (by plastic-bound anti-CD3 monoclonal antibody). It is of note that the culture system used was essentially free of APCs. In this system CpG ODN but not ODN with rearranged CpG-motifs (CpG to GpC) mediated T cell co-stimulation in that T cells upregulated IL-2R, produced IL-2, and thus initiated IL-2-driven growth and differentiation (S. Bendigs et al., submitted) (46). CpG ODN co-stimulation was sufficient to bypass the need for CD28 crosslinking and was operative in CD28$^{-/-}$ knockout mice. We also found that CpG ODN mediated co-stimulation operated more effectively in the CD8$^+$ T cell subset than in CD4$^+$ T cells.

Co-stimulation of T cells by CpG-ODN opens the possibility of promoting cell activation in the apparent absence of APCs and thus circumvents the need for APC-mediated co-stimulation. Obviously, we now have to analyze whether CpG ODN-mediated T cell co-stimulation allows induction of CTLs against tumor cells expressing tumor antigen but lacking co-stimulatory molecules. By the same token, one needs to study whether co-stimulatory active ODNs promote induction of autoimmune responses.

CONCLUSIONS

The immune system senses bacterial DNA and CpG ODNs, probably because of their unique base sequences and methylation status. The ability to detect DNA may be an important signal for infection and results in activation of DCs and macrophages, inducing proinflammatory cytokine secretion. Under physiologic conditions, bacterial DNA promotes professional APC function by causing autonomous maturation/activation of DCs. Although CpG ODNs stimulate DCs and macrophages, they co-stimulate T cells, NK cells, and perhaps also B cells in the apparent absence of APCs. By promoting professional APC function and by co-stimulating lymphocytes, CpG ODNs function as a natural adjuvant. A characteristic of their adjuvant effect is the induction of Th1-type humoral and cell-mediated responses to proteinaceous antigens and to plasmid DNA vaccines. Collectively, these data suggest that bacterial DNA represents a hitherto underestimated pathogen-associated molecular pattern recognized by PRR, which influences early decisions of the immune system. It appears that this discovery along with the realization that synthetic DNA can mimic naturally occurring bacterial DNA will lead to a wealth of therapeutic applications. Translation of the information obtained in mouse models thus far to primates and humans will be challenging and, hopefully, rewarding.

Acknowledgments

This work was supported by SFB 391, BMBF, Deutsche Krebhilfe, and Wilhelm-Sander-Foundation.

REFERENCES

1. Freund J, Casals J, Hismer EP. Sensitization and antibody formation after injection of tubercle bacilli and paraffin oil. *Proc Soc Exp Biol Med* 1937; 37:509–515.
2. Rotem Z, Cox RA, Isaacs A. Inhibition of virus multiplication by foreign nucleic acids. *Nature* 1963;197:564–566.
3. Jensen KE, Neal AL, Owens RE, Warren J. Interferon responses of chick embryo fibroblasts to nucleic acids and related compounds. *Nature* 1963;200:433–434.
4. Isaacs A. Studies on interferon. *Aust J Biol Med Sci* 1965;43:405–412.
5. Tokunaga T, Yamamoto H, Shimada S, et al. Antitumor activity of deoxyribonucleic acid fraction from *Mycobacterium bovis* BCG. I. Isolation, physicochemical characterization, and antitumor activity. *J Natl Cancer Inst* 1984;72:955–962.
6. Yamamoto S, Kuramoto E, Shimada S, Tokunaga T. In vitro augmentation of natural killer cell activity and production of interferon-alpha/beta and -gamma with deoxyribonucleic acid fraction from *Mycobacterium bovis* BCG. *Jpn J Cancer Res* 1988;79:866–873.
7. Mashiba H, Matsunaga K, Tomoda H, Furusawa M, Jimi S, Tokunaga T. In vitro augmentation of natural killer activity of peripheral blood cells from cancer patients by a DNA fraction from *Mycobacterium bovis* BCG. *Jpn J Med Sci Biol* 1988; 41:197–202.
8. Messina JP, Gilkeson GS, Pisetsky DS. Stimulation of in vitro murine lymphocyte proliferation by bacterial DNA. *J Immunol* 1991;147:1759–1764.
9. Yamamoto S, Yamamoto T, Shimada S, et al. DNA from bacteria, but not from vertebrates, induces interferons, activates natural killer cells and inhibits tumor growth. *Microbiol Immunol* 1992;36:983–997.
10. Tokunaga T, Yano O, Kuramoto E, et al. Synthetic oligonucleotides with particular base sequences from the cDNA encoding proteins of *Mycobacterium bovis* BCG induce interferons and activate natural killer cells. *Microbiol Immunol* 1992; 36:55–66.
11. Yamamoto S, Yamamoto T, Kataoka T, Kuramoto E, Yano O, Tokunaga T. Unique palindromic sequences in synthetic oligonucleotides are required to induce IFN and augment IFN-mediated natural killer activity. *J Immunol* 1992;148:4072–4076.
12. Krieg AM, Yi AK, Matson S, et al. CpG motifs in bacterial DNA trigger direct B-cell activation. *Nature* 1995;374:546–549.
13. Bird AP. CpG-rich islands and the function of DNA methylation. *Nature* 1986;321:209–213.
14. Tighe H, Corr M, Roman M, Raz E. Gene vaccination: plasmid DNA is more than just a blueprint. *Immunol Today* 1998;19:89–97.
15. Sato Y, Roman M, Tighe H, et al. Immunostimulatory DNA sequences necessary for effective intradermal gene immunization. *Science* 1996;273: 352–354.
16. Fearon DT, Locksley RM. The instructive role of innate immunity in the acquired immune response. *Science* 1996;272:50–53.
17. Medzhitov R, Janeway CA Jr. Innate immunity: impact on the adaptive immune response. *Curr Opin Immunol* 1997;9:4–9.
18. Banchereau J, Steinman RM. Dendritic cells and the control of immunity. *Nature* 1998;392:245–252.
19. Stacey KJ, Sweet MJ, Hume DA. Macrophages ingest and are activated by bacterial DNA. *J Immunol* 1996;157:2116–2122.
20. Sparwasser T, Miethke T, Lipford G, et al. Bacterial DNA causes septic shock. *Nature* 1997;386:336–337.
21. Sparwasser T, Miethke T, Lipford G, et al. Macrophages sense pathogens via DNA motifs: induction of tumor necrosis factor-alpha-mediated shock. *Eur J Immunol* 1997;27:1671–1679.
22. Lipford GB, Sparwasser T, Bauer M, et al. Immuno-

stimulatory DNA: sequence-dependent production of potentially harmful or useful cytokines. *Eur J Immunol* 1997;27:3420–3426.

23. Chace JH, Hooker NA, Mildenstein KL, Krieg AM, Cowdery JS. Bacterial DNA-induced NK cell IFN-gamma production is dependent on macrophage secretion of IL-12. *Clin Immunol Immunopathol* 1997;84:185–193.

24. Roman M, Martin-Orozco E, Goodman JS, et al. Immunostimulatory DNA sequences function as T helper-1-promoting adjuvants. *Nat Med* 1997;3: 849–854.

25. Halpern MD, Kurlander RJ, Pisetsky DS. Bacterial DNA induces murine interferon-gamma production by stimulation of interleukin-12 and tumor necrosis factor-alpha. *Cell Immunol* 1996;167:72–78.

26. Cowdery JS, Chace JH, Yi AK, Krieg AM. Bacterial DNA induces NK cells to produce IFN-gamma in vivo and increases the toxicity of lipopolysaccharides. *J Immunol* 1996;156:4570–4575.

27. Cella M, Scheidegger D, Palmer-Lehmann K, Lane P, Lanzavecchia A, Alber G. Ligation of CD40 on dendritic cells triggers production of high levels of interleukin-12 and enhances T cell stimulatory capacity: T-T help via APC activation. *J Exp Med* 1996;184:747–752.

28. Verhasselt V, Buelens C, Willems F, et al. Bacterial lipopolysaccharide stimulates the production of cytokines and the expression of costimulatory molecules by human peripheral blood dendritic cells: evidence for a soluble CD14-dependent pathway. *J Immunol* 1997;158:2919–2925.

29. Ridge JP, Di Rosa F, Matzinger P. A conditioned dendritic cell can be a temporal bridge between a CD4+ T-helper and a T-killer cell. *Nature* 1998; 393:474–478.

30. Sparwasser T, Koch ES, Vabulas RM, et al. Bacterial DNA and immunostimulatory CpG oligonucleotides trigger maturation and activation of murine dendritic cells. *Eur J Immunol* 1998;28:2045–2054.

31. Lipford GB, Bauer M, Blank C, Reiter R, Wagner H, Heeg K. CpG-containing synthetic oligonucleotides promote B and cytotoxic T cell responses to protein antigen: a new class of vaccine adjuvants. *Eur J Immunol* 1997;27:2340–2344.

32. Yi AK, Chace JH, Cowdery JS, Krieg AM. IFN-gamma promotes IL-6 and IgM secretion in response to CpG motifs in bacterial DNA and oligodeoxynucleotides. *J Immunol* 1996;156:558–564.

33. Klinman DM, Yi AK, Beaucage SL, Conover J, Krieg AM. CpG motifs present in bacteria DNA rapidly induce lymphocytes to secrete interleukin 6, interleukin 12, and interferon gamma. *Proc Natl Acad Sci USA* 1996;93:2879–2883.

34. Snapper CM, Paul WE. Interferon-gamma and B cell stimulatory factor-1 reciprocally regulate Ig isotype production. *Science* 1987;236:944–947.

35. Chu RS, Targoni OS, Krieg AM, Lehmann PV, Harding CV. CpG oligodeoxynucleotides act as adjuvants that switch on T helper 1 (Th1) immunity. *J Exp Med* 1997;186:1623–1631.

36. Carson DA, Raz E. Oligonucleotide adjuvants for T helper 1 (Th1)-specific vaccination. *J Exp Med* 1997;186:1621–1622.

37. Davis HL, Weeranta R, Waldschmidt TJ, Tygrett L, Schorr J, Krieg AM. CpG DNA is a potent enhancer of specific immunity in mice immunized with recombinant hepatitis B surface antigen. *J Immunol* 1998;160:870–876.

38. Lipford GB, Wagner H, Heeg K. Vaccination with immunodominant peptides encapsulated in Quil A-containing liposomes induces peptide-specific primary CD8+ cytotoxic T cells. *Vaccine* 1994;12:73–80.

39. Lipford GB, Hoffman M, Wagner H, Heeg K. Primary in vivo responses to ovalbumin: probing the predictive value of the Kb binding motif. *J Immunol* 1993;150:1212–1222.

40. Sun S, Kishimoto H, Sprent J. DNA as an adjuvant: capacity of insect DNA and synthetic oligodeoxynucleotides to augment T cell responses to specific antigen. *J Exp Med* 1998;187:1145–1150.

41. Wijburg OL, van den Dobbelsteen GP, Vadolas J, Sanders A, Strugnell RA, van Rooijen N. The role of macrophages in the induction and regulation of immunity elicited by exogenous antigens. *Eur J Immunol* 1998;28:479–487.

42. Speidel K, Osen W, Faath S, et al. Priming of cytotoxic T lymphocytes by five heat-aggregated antigens in vivo: conditions, efficiency, and relation to antibody responses. *Eur J Immunol* 1997;27:2391–2399.

43. Brossart P, Bevan MJ. Presentation of exogenous protein antigens on major histocompatibility complex class I molecules by dendritic cells: pathway of presentation and regulation by cytokines. *Blood* 1997;90:1594–1599.

44. Kline JN, Waldschmidt TJ, Businga TR, et al. Modulation of airway inflammation by CpG oligodeoxynucleotides in a murine model of asthma. *J Immunol* 1998;160:2555–2559.

45. Zimmermann S, Egeter O, Hausmann S, et al. CpG oligodeoxynucleotides trigger protective and curative Th1 responses in lethal murine leishmaniasis. *J Immunol* 1998;160:3627–3630.

46. Bendigs S, Salzer U, Lipford GB, Wagner H, Heeg K. CpG-oligonucleotides costimulate primary T cells in the absence of APC. *Eur J Immunol* 1999;29;1209–1218.

Cytotoxic Cells: Basic Mechanisms and Medical Applications, edited by Michail V. Sitkovsky and Pierre A. Henkart. Lippincott Williams & Wilkins, Philadelphia © 2000.

Chapter 29

Redirected Cellular Cytotoxicity

David M. Segal, Stuart W. Hicks, Alessandra Mazzoni, and Alberto Visintin

Immune Targeting Section, Experimental Immunology Branch, National Cancer Institute, National Institutes of Health, Bethesda, Maryland 20892-1360, USA

The prototypic pathway of cell-mediated cytolysis begins with the formation of bicellular conjugates between effector and target cells, followed by the triggering of a cytotoxic response in the effector cell that results in target cell death (Fig. 29-1). Cytotoxic cells express several types of receptor that bind target cells, but only a limited number of them trigger cytotoxic responses. Several years ago it was shown that antibodies (Abs) against cytotoxic triggering molecules could substitute for the natural ligand and "redirect" effector cells to kill cells they would otherwise ignore (1–6). To mediate redirected lysis, the Ab must not only bind to a triggering molecule on the effector cell but must promote conjugate formation with the target cell. Experimentally, this has been achieved in three ways: (a) By using as targets hybridoma cells that produce monoclonal antibodies (mAbs) against cytotoxic triggering molecules. Hybridoma lines often express a surface form of their mAb, and mAbs against triggering molecules provoke lytic responses from effector cells (3,4,7). This form of redirected lysis (Fig. 29-2, top panel) has provided a convenient means for identifying hybridoma cells that make mAbs specific for cytotoxic triggering molecules. (b) By using immunoglobulin G (IgG) mAbs to redirect the lysis of FcγR$^+$ target cells (8) (Fig. 29-2, middle panel). This process, known as "reverse antibody-dependent cell-mediated toxicity" (ADCC), is especially

convenient for detecting triggering function when only small amounts of mAb are available. (c) By using bispecific antibodies (bsAbs), molecules generated by chemical, biologic, or genetic methods that have two different binding specificities (Fig. 29-2, bottom panel). Depending on their reactivities, bsAbs can redirect the lysis of nearly any type of target cell by a broad selection of cytotoxic cells (1,5,6,9); in particular, their capacity to redirect cellular effectors against tumors and virally infected cells has drawn attention to their possible use in clinical settings.

In this chapter we review the types of cells mediating redirected lysis and their triggering molecules. We then focus on the molecular structures of bsAbs and recent advances in the production of genetically engineered bispecific molecules. Finally, we cover the current state of bsAb-based preclinical and clinical studies. Other recent publications dealing with bsAbs include a book (10) and a report on the 5th World Conference on Bispecific Antibodies (11).

CYTOTOXIC TRIGGERING MOLECULES

Immunotherapy based on redirected cellular cytotoxicity offers numerous choices of triggering molecules and effector cells that can be directed against a tumor or other unwanted cell. The nature of the redirected re-

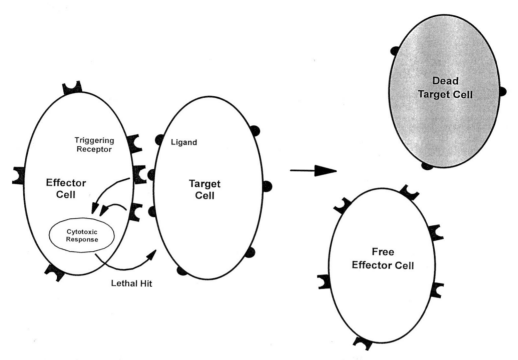

FIG. 29-1. Mechanism of cell mediated lysis. Triggering receptors on an effector cell specifically bind ligands on a target cell, leading to multivalent interactions between the two cells. Stable effector/target conjugates are formed (often aided by adhesion molecules), and ligation of the triggering molecule initiates a response that results in delivery of a lethal hit to the target cell. The two cells detach, leaving a dying target cell and an effector cell that is free to lyse another target.

sponse depends on the triggering molecule recognized by the bsAb; and in this section we briefly discuss the known triggering molecules and the cells that express them.

T Cell Receptors and Fc Receptors

The two classic cytotoxic triggering cell surface structures are the T cell receptor (TCR) and Fcγ receptors (FcγR). The ligand binding components of these receptors are type I integral membrane glycoproteins that consist of extracellular portions containing Ig-like domains, short intracytoplasmic domains, and transmembrane portions that often contain one or two positively charged residues. The TCRs and most FcγRs are noncovalently associated with signal transducing molecules that contain negatively charged residues in their transmembrane portions.

The TCR is constitutively expressed by both CD4⁺ and CD8⁺ T lymphocytes. It is a multiprotein complex comprised of either an α/β or a γ/δ clone-specific binding structure and several invariant signal transducing elements, including CD3 γ/ε and δ/ε heterodimers and ζ/ζ homodimers (12). Their capacity to signal relies on the presence of intracytoplasmic immunoreceptor tyrosine-based activation motifs (ITAMs). It has been demonstrated that both constant and variable portions of the TCR induce cytotoxic responses when engaged by Abs in redirected lysis experiments (5,13–15). Both CD4⁺ and CD8⁺ cytotoxic T lymphocyte (CTL) clones mediate redirected lysis (5,16); but in freshly isolated peripheral blood lymphocytes (PBLs) or PBLs stimulated with interleukin-2 (IL-2) only the small CD8/CD56 double positive subset of T cells mediates this func-

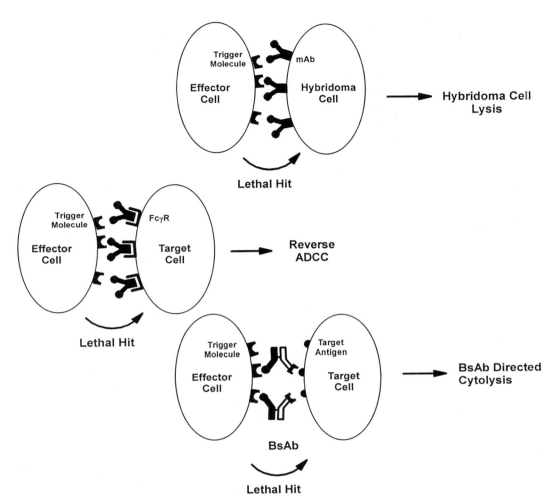

FIG. 29-2. Redirected lysis. **Top:** Hybridoma cell lysis, in which a surface form of the secreted monoclonal antibody (mAb) binds a triggering molecule on a cytotoxic cell, promotes conjugate formation, and induces lysis. **Middle:** Reverse antibody-dependent cell-mediated cytotoxicity (ADCC), where an immunoglobulin G (IgG) mAb simultaneously binds a triggering molecule on a killer cell by its antibody binding site and an FcγR⁺ target via its Fc portion, thereby inducing conjugate formation and target cell lysis. **Bottom:** Bispecific antibody (BsAb)-mediated lysis. Here the BsAb redirects lysis by binding to both effector and target cells by its two antigen-binding sites.

tion (17,18). Most T cells (i.e., CD56⁻ cells) require both IL-2 stimulation and TCR crosslinking to gain cytotoxic function.

The FcγR consists of a number of broadly expressed proteins that bind to the Fc portion of IgG molecules. These proteins are characterized by the presence of an extracellular Fc binding region and one or more intracellular transducing elements that are able to elicit a signaling cascade similar to those used by T and B cell antigen receptors (19,20). In the immune system FcγRs are primarily expressed by cellular mediators of innate immunity, natural killer (NK) cells, monocytes, macrophages, and granulocytes; and they provide a means for these cells to gain the specificities of IgG Abs once the acquired responses have developed. In the human, mAbs have been produced against the three major classes of FcγR—FcγRI (CD64), FcγRII (CD32), and FcγRIIIA/B (CD16)—and all have proven effective at mediating redirected lysis (21). Why should anti-FcγR-containing bsAbs be used when normal ADCC can be induced simply by using an mAb against the target cell? The rationale is that *in vivo* the high concentration of IgG in blood competes with antibodies bound to target cells for FcγR on killer cells, thus serving as a negative regulator of ADCC (22). This competition could be overcome by using a bsAb that binds FcγR either with much higher affinity than the normal ligand or at an epitope outside the Fc binding site; thus bsAbs could induce much more potent responses against target cells than conventional mAbs (1,21).

FcγRI/CD64, the high affinity FcγR expressed predominantly on monocytes, macrophages, and activated neutrophils, is a 72-kDa type I transmembrane glycoprotein (21,23,24). It is normally expressed at low levels but is upregulated by granulocyte colony-stimulating factor (G-CSF), interferon-γ (IFN-γ), IL-10, and IL-13 and downregulated by IL-4. Its engagement leads to cytokine release, ADCC, and phagocytosis. FcγRI/CD64 is currently being used as the triggering molecule in several bsAb-based clinical trials (see below). FcγRII/CD32 is a family of low-affinity 40-kDa isoforms expressed on monocytes, macrophages, B cells, granulocytes, platelets, Langerhans cells, and placental endothelial cells. Its expression on cytotoxic cells (monocytes and granulocytes) is weakly modulated by cytokines, but in neutrophils and eosinophils (but not in monocytes) G-CSF and IFN-γ treatment are required for FcγRII/CD32-triggered cytotoxic activity (25–27). FcγRIII/CD16, a low-affinity receptor for IgG, is encoded by two genes, FcγRIII/CD16 A and B. The B isoform, expressed on polymorphonuclear neutrophils (PMNs), is a 50-kDa GPI-anchored protein that does not serve as a cytotoxic triggering molecule. NK cells and differentiated mononuclear phagocytes express FcγRIII/CD16 A, an 80-kDa transmembrane protein that is a powerful inducer of cytotoxic responses (24,28,29). FcγRI/CD64 and FcγRIII/CD16 A contain no ITAMs but bind to γ-γ or ζ-ζ signal transducing molecules. In the human, FcγRII/CD32 A and FcγRII/CD32 C each contain an ITAM on their cytoplasmic domains and deliver signals in the absence of other molecules (20). Finally, it was recently demonstrated that FcαRI/CD89, a receptor for the Fc portion of IgA that is expressed on most myeloid cells, can also trigger cytotoxic responses. In that study, anti-FcαRI × anti-HER2/neu bsAbs induced neutrophils, monocytes, or whole blood effector cells specifically to kill HER2/neu-bearing tumor cells (30).

Adhesion Molecules and Other Cell Surface Proteins

A number of adhesion molecules can serve as positive triggers for cytotoxic responses. They differ from the TCRs and FcRs in that they do not rely on rearranged V regions for ligand recognition. Early redirected lysis experiments demonstrated that CD2, an adhesion molecule that interacts with CD58 on endothelial and hematopoietic cells, is a cytotoxic triggering molecule in T and NK cells; and later studies revealed that triggering through CD2 requires the presence of either a functional TCR or FcγRIII/CD16 (31–35). CD44, a homing receptor that binds hyaluronic acid and several other components of the extracellular matrix, is ubiquitously expressed on hematopoietic cells and is a cytotoxic triggering molecule in some T cell clones (36–38), PMNs (39), IL-2 activated NK cells, and CD56⁺ T cells (40). In NK cells CD44-directed lysis requires IL-2 activation, and CD44 crosslinking induces the tyrosine phosphorylation of several proteins (41,42). The activation marker CD69 is rapidly expressed on T and NK cells following stimulation with cytokines (43). It serves as a cytotoxic triggering molecule on NK and γ/δ (but not α/β) T cell clones (44,45) and on monocytes (46). Recently, CD38, a type II integral membrane receptor that binds CD31 (PECAM-1) and has ADP-ribosyl cyclase ectoenzymatic activity (47–50), was shown to activate cytolysis in major histocompatibility complex (MHC) nonrestricted CTLs (51). Finally, NK cells express several other cytotoxic triggers, including NKRP-1 (52), NK-TR (53), and activatory forms of killer inhibitory receptors (KIRs) (54). An interesting feature of the cytotoxic triggering function of adhesion molecules is that these same molecules can be expressed on cells, even some cytotoxic cells, where they do not serve as triggers. Unfortunately, from a practical point of view, the widespread expression of many of these adhesion molecules in a non-triggering form may limit their usefulness in clinical applications.

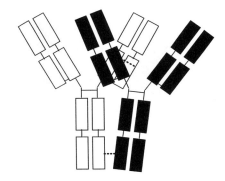

FIG. 29-3. Randomly crosslinked IgG heterodimer. Chemical crosslinkers typically form a covalent bond between any lysine residue on one molecule with a lysine on the other. Two possible crosslinks are indicated as *dotted lines.*

TYPES OF BISPECIFIC ANTIBODY

With the proliferation of chemical, biologic, and genetic methods for creating and modifying proteins, the term "bispecific antibody" has come to mean any single molecule containing two different Ab-based binding specificities, including proteins that vary greatly in homogeneity, size, and ease of production. A major obstacle to clinical development of bsAbs has been the high cost of producing material suitable for use in patients, but recent advances using genetic engineering approaches may provide the large amounts of clinical grade material needed for these studies. In this section, the molecular structures and methods of production of bsAbs are reviewed.

Chemical Crosslinking

The fastest way to produce bsAbs is to randomly crosslink two mAbs, affinity-purified polyclonal Abs, or their proteolytic fragments using bifunctional chemical crosslinking reagents (55) (Fig. 29-3). Most crosslinking reagents form covalent bridges between lysine residues on different Ab molecules; and crosslinkers that prevent the formation of homoconjugates, usually by employing di-

sulfide exchange reactions or thioether formation, are preferred for bsAb production. Such reagents produce a mixture of heterocrosslinked antibodies that differ in size and in the numbers and positions of crosslinks. After purification by gel filtration, randomly crosslinked heteroconjugates work well for most *in vitro* applications, for example, mediating redirected lysis (1), targeting an antigen to an antigen-presenting cell APC (56), or redirecting viral transduction (57,58).

In vivo, however, where size and composition greatly affect biodistribution and stability, heteroconjugates do not give consistent results. One way of overcoming this problem is to make homogeneous hetero-F(ab')$_2$ molecules by crosslinking two F(ab') fragments at their hinge cysteine residues (Fig. 29-4). F(ab')$_2$ fragments, generated from mAbs by proteolytic digestion, are selectively reduced, yielding F(ab') fragments with hinge sulfhydryls in the reduced state. One F(ab') ("donor") is left in the reduced state, and the other ("acceptor") is either oxidized at its hinge sulfhydryl using a dithiol compound such as Ellman's reagent (59) or alkylated with a bis-maleimide compound (60). When the donor and acceptor F(ab') molecules are mixed, a bispecific hetero-F(ab')$_2$, specifically joined at its hinge sulfhydryls and uncontaminated by parental F(ab')$_2$, is formed.

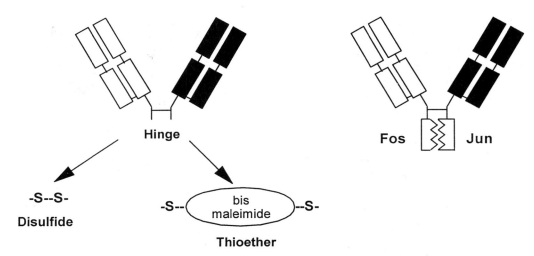

FIG. 29-4. Bispecific hetero-F(ab')$_2$ prepared by chemical (**left**) or genetic (**right**) methods. **Left:** This molecule is produced from F(ab') molecules obtained from intact mAbs by proteolytic degradation and reduction. F(ab') molecules are heterocrosslinked by their hinge cysteines using reagents that give either reducible disulfide bonds or non-reducible thioether linkages. **Right:** In this molecule genetically engineered F(ab')s are produced in prokaryotic or eukaryotic cells and are then linked chemically at their hinge cysteines. One version, shown here, uses a Fos leucine zipper peptide fused to the C-terminus of one F(ab') and a Jun leucine zipper fused to the other to favor heterodimerization.

The oxidized acceptor is linked to the donor through a reducible disulfide bridge, whereas the alkylated acceptor is linked through a nonreducible thioether bond. Thioether linked hetero-F(ab')$_2$s have been prepared in large amounts under GMP conditions and are being used in several clinical trials (61,62). Although hetero-F(ab')$_2$ bsAbs are well defined with respect to size and composition, their preparation requires laborious, multistep procedures, each of which is accompanied by loss of protein.

Hybrid-Hybridomas

Immunoglobulin heavy (H) and light (L) chains associate promiscuously with H and L chains from other Abs. Therefore when two hybridomas that produce different mAbs are fused, a stable "hybrid-hybridoma" or "quadroma" line is generated that secretes as one of its products a bsAb, H_1L_1-H_2L_2 (63,64) (Fig. 29-5). Hybrid-hybridoma lines provide a stable source of bsAb, but unfortunately the bsAb is not the only se-creted product. Random combination of the two heavy and two light chains synthesized by the hybrid hybridoma generates ten different Ig species, only one of which has both Ab activities (Fig. 29-5). Mispairing of heavy and light chains leads to reduced yields of bsAb and may necessitate complicated purification protocols.

Several procedures have been described for producing hybrid-hybridomas (55,65–71). In most, two hybridoma lines are fused using polyethylene glycol, and the resulting hybrid-hybridoma lines are selected from the unfused parental lines using selectable drug markers or electronic cell sorting. Once stable hybrid-hybridoma lines have been established, they are screened for bsAb production. The amount of bsAb secreted is highly variable between lines and depends on the relative rates of synthesis of the four Ig chains and on preferential associations between H and L chains. When synthesis of the four chains is equal and they associate randomly, 12.5% of the total Ig is bsAb (72). When both parental mAbs are of the same

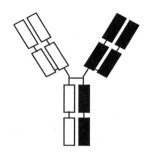

Bispecific Antibody

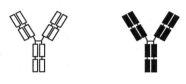

Parental Antibodies

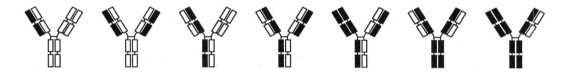

Light Chain Mispaired Species

FIG. 29-5. Hybrid-hybridoma bsAbs. The fusion of two hybridomas produces a hybrid-hybridoma line that secretes two heavy chains (*open and filled symbols*) and two light chains (*open and filled symbols*). Random pairing of these chains generates a bsAb (**top**), the two parental antibodies (**middle**), and seven species with mispaired light chains (**bottom**).

or structurally related IgG isotype, H-H pairings are usually random. By contrast, H-L pairings, which are stabilized in part by interactions between variable (V) residues (73), often show preferences; in some cases homologous H-L chain pairing is favored (74,75), whereas in other cases random or even heterologous pairings predominate (76). Thus depending on the nature of the H-L interaction, the yield of bsAb can vary between 0% and 50%. If the H chains from the parental antibodies are of different IgG isotype, the yield of mixed H-H chain combinations may decrease (64); and if two different classes of H chain are used, association between the heterologous H chains may not occur at all (70). The lower yield of mixed-isotype bsAbs may, however, be offset by an increase in efficiency of purification (55, 64,74); for example, IgG molecules consisting of two different H-chain isotypes may be purified by protein A chromatography by eluting at different pH values (77). Mixed-isotype bsAbs are often incapable of mediating ADCC, which may be advantageous in cases where effector cells bind the bsAb (67,78). Despite their difficulty in production and isolation, clinical grade F(ab')₂ fragments of hybrid-hybridoma antibodies have been prepared in gram amounts and have been tested in patients in two different phase I–II trials (79,80).

Genetically Engineered bsAbs

Genetically engineered bsAb constructs have been designed to aid in the large scale production of homogeneous protein that would be suitable for use in patients. F(ab') constructs, which eliminate the need for proteolytic digestion of intact mAbs, have been expressed in bacteria (81,82) and mammalian cells (83–85). For the preparation of bsAbs, two different F(ab') molecules were expressed and isolated separately; then they were linked via their hinge sulfhydryl groups to give the hetero-F(ab')$_2$. In one study F(ab')s were crosslinked chemically using a bis-maleimide reagent (81), but this step was removed in the other study by inclusion of Fos or Jun leucine zippers at the C-terminal ends of the F(ab') heavy chains (83) (Fig. 29-4). Fos and Jun leucine zippers have a strong tendency to form heterodimers; and when F(ab')s with Fos and Jun zippers are mixed under mildly oxidizing conditions, bispecific hetero-F(ab')$_2$ molecules are obtained in high yields. Animal studies have shown that these bsAbs are stable in serum and are cleared at about the same rate as conventional F(ab')$_2$ fragments (84,86).

Bispecific constructs have also been produced using only the V domains of the H and L chains of antibodies (87–99). The V domains of antibodies associate noncovalently to form the Fv fragment, a 26-kDa heterodimer that is the smallest fragment to bear the antigen-binding site (100) (Fig. 29-6). Unlike Fabs, Fvs are frequently unstable in solution due to weak interactions between V_L and V_H domains. The interface between V_L and V_H contains both framework and CDR residues (73), leading to large differences in stability between Fvs from different antibodies (101). Two structural modifications have been introduced to stabilize Fvs: A polypeptide linker of 15 to 20 residues joining the C-terminus of V_L to the N-terminus of V_H, or vice versa, produces the "single-chain Fv" (scFv) (Fig. 29-6) (102–104); cysteine residues introduced into V_H and V_L result in a "disulfide-stabilized Fv" (101,105,106). Further stabilization of scFvs has been achieved using filamentous phage display libraries that express large numbers of different scFvs as fusions with the phage gene 3 protein (107,108). By employing various selection stategies, stable sFvs, even some lacking intrachain disulfides, have been isolated from scFv phage display libraries (109–112).

Joining two scFvs produces bsAbs having the minimal molecular mass; several ap-

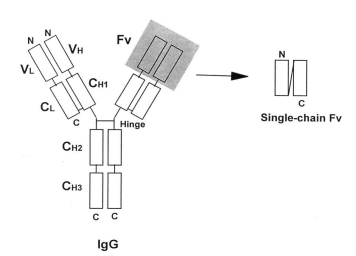

FIG. 29-6. Intact IgG antibody highlighting the Fv portion (**left**) and an scFv (**right**) produced genetically by connecting the C-terminus of one V domain to the N-terminus of the other with a polypeptide linker. The Fv is the smallest fragment of an antibody that has binding activity.

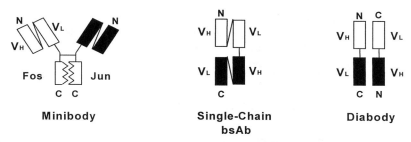

FIG. 29-7. Three Fv-based bispecific antibody (*bsAb*) constructs.

proaches have been described (96) (Fig 29-7). "Miniantibodies" consist of two scFvs that heterodimerize noncovalently due to oligimerization domains (amphipathic helices) (88,113,114) and Ig constant domains (115) fused to the C-termini of the scFvs. A bivalent miniantibody produced in high cell density bacteria culture gave yields of 3 g/L of culture supernatant (116). The inclusion of short interdomain linkers in sFvs prevents proper V_L–V_H pairing within a single chain. Instead, two chains tend to associate laterally, producing a bivalent homodimer known as a "diabody" (89). Co-expression in bacteria periplasm of two separate polypeptide chains with structures V_{HA}–V_{LB} and V_{HB}–V_{LA} (where A and B refer to the parental sFvs) generates protein that is totally heterodimeric and bispecific (89). The crystal structure of one diabody reveals a back-to-back association of V_H domains, with the two Ab binding sites located at opposite ends of the molecule and separated by about 6.5 nM (117). Diabodies, like scFvs, have been selected by phage display (118), stabilized by interchain disulfide bonds (119), and produced in high amounts by bacteria (120). Several bispecific diabodies capable of redirecting lysis have been described (98,99,119–123).

BsAbs in which both binding activities reside in a single polypeptide chain have been produced by concatenating two different sFvs with a polypeptide linker (91–95,97,124). Single-chain bsAbs, when expressed in mammalian cells (92,95) or bacteria (91,93,94,97), bind both antigens, usually with an affinity similar to that of the parental Fab. Those with anti-CD3 activity redirect lysis, often in the nanogram per milliliter range. Diabodies, with their short interdomain linkers, are probably more rigid structures than single-chain bsAbs, which are typically connected by long flexible linkers (117, 123). Diabodies have been found to be more efficient than single-chain bsAbs in redirecting lysis (97,123) and binding to tumor (125), which may be related to their lack of internal segmental flexibility. When tested *in vitro* for stability at 37°C, one single-chain bsAbs was totally active after 4 hours but only 25% active after 24 hours in mouse serum (97), whereas another retained most of its activity after 16 hours in 10% fetal calf serum (FCS) (95). Because of their small size, single-chain constructs have much higher rates of tumor penetration, but much lower rates of serum retention, than intact antibodies (97,114, 126,127). It remains to be seen which factor will prove more advantageous for treating solid tumors, but it has been demonstrated that anti-CD3 × antitumor single-chain bsAbs can cure mice of leukemia, particularly when given with T cell activators (97).

ANIMAL STUDIES

Because bsAbs have the potential of targeting a wide variety of effector responses to tumors in cancer patients, much effort has been expended to learn how bsAbs function in preclinical experimental animal models. Indeed, initial studies demonstrated that the bsAb-based approach was effective when treatment was given locally at the tumor site. Early xenograft studies showed that targeted T (128) and NK (9) cells could mount a potent antitumor response in a Winn-type assay in which effector cells, tumor cells, and bsAbs were mixed and injected subcutaneously into nude mice. Growth of bystander cancer cells was blocked as well, indicating that release of cytokines by lymphocytes played an important role in blocking tumor growth in the subcutaneous environment (129). BsAb treatment to redirect T lymphocytes against tumor cells in a syngeneic rat colon carcinoma model also proved to be effective, provided IL-2 was given along with the bsAb (130).

In subsequent investigations, solid tumors were allowed to become established before local treatment was administered. In one such study nude mice were injected intraperitoneally with human ovarian carcinoma cells; by day 4 the number of cells in ascites had more than doubled, and solid tumor had begun to metastasize to the pancreas and mesenteric lymph nodes (131). Intraperitoneal injection of *in vitro* preactivated human T cells targeted with an anti-CD3 × antitumor bsAb were initiated on day 4 and resulted in a dramatic increase of the mean survival time in comparison to untreated controls (132). In a more recent study, SCID mice bearing intraperitoneal human melanoma cells were treated with intraperitoneal injections of IL-2-activated PBLs retargeted against melanoma cells with an anti-CD3 containing bsAb; again an increase in the survival time together with a reduced incidence of metastases were observed (133). However, in both of the above studies most of the animals eventually died of tumor, indicating that treatment did not destroy all of the tumor cells. On the other hand, retargeting of human NK cells against established human ovarian tumor in SCID mice by means of an anti-FcγRIII/CD16 × antitumor bsAb resulted in an increase in the mean survival time from 80 to 131 days, with up to 70% of mice still tumor-free after 150 days. IL-2

proved to be essential for the effectiveness of the treatment (134).

A more demanding model is one in which established tumor is treated by injections of bsAb and/or cells and cytokine at sites distant from the tumor, thus requiring activated, targeted cells to home to the tumor site. Solid tumors are often refractory to this type of treatment. For example, in a totally syngeneic mouse model, systemic treatment with an anti-CD3 × antitumor bsAb, with or without IL-2, was unable to block the growth of established subcutaneous mammary tumor but did delay the growth of lung metastases (86). By contrast, hematologic malignancies are much more responsive to systemic bsAb therapy, and encouraging results have been obtained in a number of animal studies. Two totally syngeneic mouse models, in which bsAbs target host T cells against the idiotypes of the surface immunoglobulin on BCL_1 (97,135–139) and 38C13 (84,140–144) B lymphoma cells, have demonstrated the efficacy of bsAb treatment. In the case of the BCL_1 lymphoma, most mice treated with intravenous injections of anti-CD3 × anti-idiotype bsAb 9 days after receiving tumor were free of the tumor 150 days later, whereas all mice were dead by 80 days in the untreated control (135). Similar results were obtained using a genetically engineered single-chain bsAb (97). Both $CD4^+$ and $CD8^+$ T cells infiltrated the tumor in bsAb-treated mice, and blockage of tumor growth was at least in part mediated by cytokines such as IFN-γ and tumor necrosis factor-α (TNF-α) that were secreted by the targeted T cells (138). In mice bearing the highly aggressive 38C13 B cell lymphoma, up to 80% of mice treated with a single intravenous injection of the anti-CD3 × anti-idiotype bsAb were cured (140). Intraperitoneal injection was also effective, resulting in a significantly higher mean survival time of treated mice (141); in this case tumor eventually developed, but it was a variant lymphoma that did not express the idiotype recognized by the bsAb. Finally, two studies using SCID mice have shown that systemically administered human T (145) or

NK (146) cells targeted with an appropriate bsAb prolong survival or cure mice from Hodgkin's lymphoma xenografts.

Most T cells, *in vivo,* are in the resting state and must be activated to become competent cytotoxic cells. In general, proper T cell activation is not achieved following bsAb-mediated interactions between T cells and tumor cells, as CD3 crosslinking per se is usually not sufficient; additional co-stimulatory signals are required. From a clinical perspective, it would be desirable to achieve activation of the effector cells directly in the host, thereby avoiding the need for *ex vivo* stimulation. To this purpose, co-administration of bsAb and cytokines such as IL-2 (97,130,147) or superantigens (97,148,149) has been shown to be an effective method of stimulating T cells *in vivo.* Moreover, approaches have been tried that rely on the delivery of co-stimulatory signals via the CD28/B7 pathway. In one study a combination of two bsAbs (anti-CD3 × antitumor and anti-CD28 × antitumor) was used to cure SCID mice of subcutaneously growing Hodgkin's lymphoma. Tumor-bearing mice were given intravenous injections of bsAbs followed by injections of human PBLs. Biodistribution studies and histologic examination established that each bsAb individually reached the tumor and promoted the infiltration of both CD4$^+$ and CD8$^+$ cells (145). In this system, *ex vivo* activation was unnecessary because tumor-bearing mice could be cured with freshly isolated resting human PBLs together with the two bsAbs (150). A number of other studies have also proved the effectiveness of using anti-CD28 mAb as a co-stimulator (139,151–153). Alternatively, tumor cells have been induced to express co-stimulatory signals by giving soluble CD40 along with the anti-CD3 × antitumor bsAb, leading to prolonged mean survival times in lymphoma-bearing mice (144).

CLINICAL STUDIES

The generation of antitumor immune responses in cancer patients remains a fundamental goal of cancer therapy, and bsAbs with specificity for tumor-associated antigens (TAAs) and cytotoxic triggering molecules on immune effector cells could provide a powerful tool for directing immune effector cells against a tumor. Most TAAs are molecules that are overexpressed on tumor cells but that also appear to a lesser extent on some normal cells. Presumably the usefulness of a TAA as a target molecule depends on how infrequently normal cells trigger targeted effector cells and prevent them from acting locally at tumor sites, and whether essential cells that express TAAs can survive bsAb therapy. Indeed, cross reaction of antitumor bsAbs on normal cells might be responsible for some side effects, usually small and manageable, observed in patients following administration of bsAbs (see below). The clinical trials discussed in this section have been designed to direct T cells, NK cells, neutrophils, and monocytes/macrophages against TAAs on tumor cells using FcγRI/CD64, FcγRIII/CD16, and the TCRs as triggering molecules.

Retargeting of T Cells by bsAbs

Results from the first bsAb-based clinical trials agreed with findings from the animal studies demonstrating that local bsAb treatments could be effective. In one study, a F(ab')$_2$ bsAb with anti-CD3 and antiglioma specificities was reported to inhibit tumor growth in 20 patients with advanced malignant glioma (154). Although the initial results were encouraging, these findings have not been confirmed in later studies. More recently, in a phase I–II clinical trial, ovarian cancer patients were treated with repeated intraperitoneal infusions of *ex vivo* activated autologous T lymphocytes retargeted by an anti-CD3 × antiovarian tumor bsAb (that used folate-binding protein as the TAA) (79). Of 26 patients evaluated, 27% responded to therapy, with a mean survival time of more than 22 months. Nineteen patients were evaluated by surgery and histology: Three patients achieved complete responses, one showed a complete intraperitoneal response with progressive disease in retroperitoneal lymph nodes, three gave partial responses, seven had stable disease, and five had progressive disease. This study clearly established that locoregional treatment of at least one type of solid tumor with bsAb-retargeted autologous T cells could lead to the eradication of tumors. However, tumors that were inaccessible to treatment showed progressive growth. Thus another phase I–II clinical study has been initiated in which the activated, retargeted peripheral blood mononuclear cells (PBMCs) are given simultaneously intraperitoneally and intravenously to the patients (155). The data obtained so far indicate mild toxicity of the treatment and confirm its efficacy in about 25% of the cases. It is noteworthy that intravenous infusion of the bsAb alone (i.e., not bound to *ex vivo* activated T cells) resulted in severe toxicity (156). Similar effects were observed in renal cancer patients following infusion of an anti-CD3 × antirenal tumor bsAb (157); in both cases, dramatic increases in the serum levels of TNF-α and IFN-γ were held responsible. Presumably, the bsAbs [both of which were F(ab′)$_2$] induced cytokine release from circulating T cells, probably by crosslinking TCRs after binding to TAAs on normal or tumor cells.

The success in treating B cell lymphomas with TCR-based bsAbs in experimental animals makes this type of malignancy a good candidate for therapy in patients. In preliminary studies (152,158,159) a bsAb redirecting T cells against CD19 on malignant B cells was studied for treatment of non-Hodgkin lymphoma patients. In this case, systemic administration of bsAbs in three patients produced only mild side effects, accompanied by modest activation of CD8$^+$ T cells. In an attempt to increase the effector cell activation, IL-2 or an anti-CD28 mAb was given intravenously in conjunction with the bsAb, but no clear clinic effects have been achieved so far (152,159).

Targeting Through Fcγ Receptors

To date, two FcγRs have been used as triggering molecules in bsAb-based clinical trials. FcγRIII/CD16 is a potent triggering molecule on NK cells and IFN-γ-activated monocytes/macrophages but not PMNs (21,160). FcγRI/CD64, on the other hand, triggers activated PMNs, monocytes, and macrophages but is not expressed on NK cells (21).

In a phase I clinical study (62) 15 patients suffering from advanced breast and ovarian cancers were treated with a single infusion of a F(ab′)$_2$ bsAb with specificities for FcγRI/CD64 and the HER-2/neu oncogene product (the latter being overexpressed in those tumors). The treatment was well tolerated, without severe toxicity. Among ten patients assessed for clinical responses, two showed some antitumor effects: In a breast cancer patient subcutaneous nodules resolved, and an ovarian cancer patient showed a substantial decrease in cervical adenopathy. In attempts to improve the efficacy of this treatment, the bsAb is currently being given in conjunction with subcutaneous injection of G-CSF (161,162). G-CSF induces increases in neutrophil numbers and in the expression levels of FcγRI/CD64 on neutrophils. The rationale for this protocol is that G-CSF together with the bsAb increases the cytotoxic capacity of targeted neutrophils. Early results show that the treatment is well tolerated, and substantial antitumor responses have been obtained in a significant number of renal and prostate cancer patients, thus validating the bsAb plus cytokine combination therapy approach (162).

Two studies have used anti-FcγRIII/CD16-based bsAbs to target patients' effector cells against tumors. In a phase I trial 15 patients with advanced HER-2/neu$^+$ tumors were treated with repeated infusions of an anti-FcγRIII/CD16 × anti-HER2 bsAb

(80). The treatment induced increases in serum levels of a number of cytokines, including IL-6 and TNF-α, and was accompanied by several minor clinical responses, such as reductions in tumor mass and resolution of pleural effusions and ascites. In a second study (163) a bsAb was used to direct FcγRIII/CD16+ effector cells against CD30 on Hodgkin's lymphoma cells. Treatment of 15 patients with repeated infusions of the bsAb gave encouraging clinical responses with only rare side effects consisting of fever and pain in the lymph nodes. Interestingly, most of the Hodgkin's patients exhibited pronounced NK deficiencies before treatment.

Current State of bsAb-Based Therapies

To date, the goals of clinical studies involving bsAb therapy have been to establish maximum tolerated doses, to follow pharmacokinetics, and to look for early signs of biologic or clinical effects of bsAbs. Indeed, several phase I and phase II trials have shown limited toxicities of the various bsAbs and some efficacy in terms of responses in patients with advanced disease. Moreover, bsAb-based treatment of cancer is likely to be even more effective in situations of minimal residual disease (i.e., after initial tumor reduction by conventional treatment modalities). However, there are still many obstacles to overcome and many questions to address before bsAbs can be used effectively.

First, obtaining sufficient quantities of bsAbs suitable for clinical trials remains a major problem, and it is still unclear which type of bsAb would be most effective—a small construct that would have improved tumor penetration or a large construct that would have a prolonged serum half-life? One serious drawback encountered in most of the clinical trials has been the development of an anti-bsAb response, which limits the efficacy of the treatment to a short period of time. Would a totally "humanized" construct allow more prolonged treatments? In addi-

tion, activation of effector cells is required to achieve an optimal antitumor response. This has often been accomplished *ex vivo* using cumbersome procedures that would not be possible on a large scale. Thus development of combination therapies is warranted in which bsAbs are administered together with cytokines, hormones, superantigens, or co-stimulatory signals to directly activate the effector cells *in situ*. Finally, it remains to be established which routes and schedules of administration of bsAbs would be best for getting the largest numbers of effector cells and bsAbs to the tumor sites. The answers to these and other questions require extensive experimentation, but the mere fact that so many options exist gives one hope that ways will be found to improve the effectiveness of bsAb therapy in treating cancers.

REFERENCES

1. Karpovsky B, Titus JA, Stephany DA, Segal DM. Production of target-specific effector cells using hetero-cross-linked aggregates containing anti-target cell and anti-Fc gamma receptor antibodies. *J Exp Med* 1984;160:1686–1701.
2. Kranz DM, Tonegawa S, Eisen HN. Attachment of an anti-receptor antibody to non-target cells renders them susceptible to lysis by a clone of cytotoxic T lymphocytes. *Proc Natl Acad Sci USA* 1984;81:7922–7926.
3. Lancki DW, Ma DI, Havran WL, Fitch FW. Cell surface structures involved in T cell activation. *Immunol Rev* 1984;81:65–94.
4. Hoffman RW, Bluestone JA, Leo O, Shaw S. Lysis of anti-T3-bearing murine hybridoma cells by human allospecific cytotoxic T cell clones and inhibition of that lysis by anti-T3 and anti-LFA-1 antibodies. *J Immunol* 1985;135:5–8.
5. Perez P, Hoffman RW, Shaw S, Bluestone JA, Segal DM. Specific targeting of cytotoxic T cells by anti-T3 linked to anti-target cell antibody. *Nature* 1985;316:354–356.
6. Staerz UD, Kanagawa O, Bevan MJ. Hybrid antibodies can target sites for attack by T cells. *Nature* 1985;314:628–631.
7. Graziano RF, Fanger MW. Human monocyte-mediated cytotoxicity: the use of Ig-bearing hybridomas as target cells to detect trigger molecules on the monocyte cell surface. *J Immunol* 1987;138:945–950.
8. Leeuwenberg JTM, Spits H, Tax WJM, Capel PJA. Induction of nonspecific cytotoxicity by mono-

clonal anti-T3 antibodies. *J Immunol* 1985; 134:3770–3775.

9. Titus JA, Perez P, Kaubisch A, Garrido MA, Segal DM. Human K/NK cells targeted with hetero-crosslinked antibodies specifically lyse tumor cells in vitro and prevent tumor growth in vivo. *J Immunol* 1987;139:3153–3158.

10. Fanger MW. *Bispecific Antibodies.* Austin, R. G. Landes, 1995.

11. Van de Winkel JG, Bast B, De Gast GC. Immuno-therapeutic potential of bispecific antibodies. *Immunol Today* 1997;18:562–564.

12. Cambier JC. Antigen and Fc receptor signaling: the awesome power of the immunoreceptor tyrosine-based activation motif (ITAM). *J Immunol* 1995;155:3281–3285.

13. Staerz UD, Bevan MJ. Cytotoxic T lymphocyte-mediated lysis via the Fc receptor of target cells. *Eur J Immunol* 1985;15:1172–1177.

14. Borst J, van Dongen JJM, Bolhuis RLH, et al. Distinct molecular forms of human T cell receptor gamma/delta detected on viable T cells by a mono-clonal antibody. *J Exp Med* 1988;167:1625–1644.

15. Leo O, Foo M, Sachs DH, Samelson LE, Bluestone JA. Identification of a monoclonal antibody spe-cific for a murine T3 polypeptide. *Proc Natl Acad Sci USA* 1987;84:1374–1378.

16. Liu MA, Kranz DM, Kurnick JT, Boyle LA, Levy R, Eisen HN. Heteroantibody duplexes target cells for lysis by cytotoxic T lymphocytes. *Proc Natl Acad Sci USA* 1985;82:8648–8652.

17. Garrido MA, Perez P, Titus JA, et al. Targeted cytotoxic cells in human peripheral blood lympho-cytes. *J Immunol* 1990;144:2891–2898.

18. Lanier LL, Le AM, Civin CI, Loken MR, Phillips JH. The relationship of CD16 (Leu-11) and Leu-19 (NKH-1) antigen expression on human peripheral blood NK cells and cytotoxic T lymphocytes. *J Immunol* 1986;136:4480–4486.

19. Sanchez-Mejorada G, Rosales C. Signal transduc-tion by immunoglobulin Fc receptors. *J Leukoc Biol* 1998;63:521–533.

20. Daeron M. Fc receptor biology. *Annu Rev Immu-nol* 1997;15:203–234.

21. Wallace PK, Valone FH, Fanger MW. Myeloid cell-targeted cytotoxicity of tumor cells. In Fanger MW (ed) *Bispecific Antibodies.* Austin, R. G. Landes, 1995, pp 43–76.

22. Segal DM, Dower SK, Titus JA. The role of non-immune IgG in controlling IgG-mediated effector functions. *Mol Immunol* 1983;20:1177–1189.

23. Looney RJ, Abraham GN, Anderson CL. Human monocytes and U937 cells bear two distinct Fc receptors for IgG. *J Immunol* 1986;136:1641–1647.

24. Ravetch JV, Anderson CL. Fc gamma R family: proteins, transcripts, and genes. In Metzger H (ed) *Fc Receptors and the Action of Antibodies.* Wash-ington, DC, American Society for Microbiology, 1990, pp 211–235.

25. Fanger MW, Graziano RF, Shen L, Guyre PM. Fc gamma R cytotoxicity exerted by mononuclear cells. *Chem Immunol* 1989;47:214–253.

26. Van de Winkel JG, Anderson CL. Biology of hu-man immunoglobulin G Fc receptors. *J Leukoc Biol* 1991;49:511–524.

27. Heijnen IA, Van de Winkel JG. Human IgG Fc receptors. *Int Rev Immunol* 1997;16:29–55.

28. Lanier LL, Cwirla S, Yu G, Testi R, Phillips JH. Membrane anchoring of a human IgG Fc receptor (CD16) determined by a single amino acid. *Science* 1989;246:1611–1613.

29. Leibson PJ. Signal transduction during natural killer cell activation: inside the mind of a killer. *Immunity* 1997;6:655–661.

30. Deo YM, Sundarapandiyan K, Kelleher K, Wal-lace PK, Graziano RF. Bispecific molecules di-rected to the Fc receptor for IgA (Fc alpha RI, CD89) and tumor antigens efficiently promote cell-mediated cytotoxicity of tumor targets in whole blood. *J Immunol* 1998;160:1677–1686.

31. Siliciano RF, Pratt JC, Schmidt RE, Ritz J, Rein-herz EL. Activation of cytotoxic T lymphocyte and natural killer cell function through the T11 sheep erythrocyte binding protein. *Nature* 1985;317: 428–429.

32. Scott CFJ, Lambert JM, Kalish RS, Morimoto C, Schlossman SF. Human T cells can be directed to lyse tumor targets through the alternative activation/T11-E rosette receptor pathway. *J Im-munol* 1988;140:8–14.

33. Spruyt LL, Glennie MJ, Beyers AD, Williams AF. Signal transduction by the CD2 antigen in T cells and natural killer cells: requirement for expression of a functional T cell receptor or binding of anti-body Fc to the Fc receptor, Fc gamma RIIIA (CD16). *J Exp Med* 1991;174:1407–1415.

34. Howard FD, Moingeon P, Moebius U, et al. The CD3zeta cytoplasmic domain mediates CD2-in-duced T cell activation. *J Exp Med* 1992; 176:139–145.

35. Tutt A, Stevenson GT, Glennie MJ. Trispecific F(ab')₃ derivatives that use cooperative signaling via the TCR/CD3 complex and CD2 to activate and redirect resting cytotoxic T cells. *J Immunol* 1991;147:60–69.

36. Galandrini R, Albi N, Tripodi G, et al. Antibodies to CD44 trigger effector functions of human T cell clones. *J Immunol* 1993;150:4225–4235.

37. Seth A, Gote L, Nagarkatti M, Nagarkatti PS. T-cell-receptor-independent activation of cytolytic activity of cytotoxic T lymphocytes mediated through CD44 and gp90^MEL-14. *Proc Natl Acad Sci USA* 1991;88:7877–7881.

38. Hammond DM, Nagarkatti PS, Gote LR, Seth A, Hassuneh MR, Nagarkatti M. Double-negative T cells from MRL-lpr/lpr mice mediate cytolytic ac-tivity when triggered through adhesion molecules and constitutively express perforin gene. *J Exp Med* 1993;178:2225–2230.

39. Pericle F, Sconocchia G, Titus JA, Segal DM. CD44 is a cytotoxic triggering molecule on human polymorphonuclear cells. *J Immunol* 1996;157: 4657–4663.

40. Sconocchia G, Titus JA, Segal DM. CD44 is a cytotoxic triggering molecule in human peripheral blood NK cells. *J Immunol* 1994;153:5473–5481.

41. Galandrini R, Piccoli M, Frati L, Santoni A. Tyro-sine kinase-dependent activation of human NK cell functions upon triggering through CD44 receptor. *Eur J Immunol* 1996;2807–2811.

42. Sconocchia G, Titus JA, Segal DM. Signaling pathways regulating CD44-dependent cytolysis in NK cells. *Blood* 1997;90:716–725.

43. Testi R, D'Ambrosio D, De Maria R, Santoni A. The CD69 receptor: a multipurpose cell-surface trigger for hematopoietic cells. *Immunol Today* 1994;15:479–483.

44. Moretta A, Poggi A, Pende D, et al. CD69-mediated pathway of lymphocyte activation: anti-CD69 monoclonal antibodies trigger the cytolytic activity of different lymphoid effector cells with the exception of cytolytic T lymphocytes expressing T cell receptor α/β. *J Exp Med* 1991;174:1393–1398.

45. Risso A, Smilovich D, Capra MC, et al. CD69 in resting and activated T lymphocytes: its association with a GTP binding protein and biochemical requirements for its expression. *J Immunol* 1991; 146:4105–4114.

46. De Maria R, Cifone MG, Trotta R, et al. Triggering of human monocyte activation through CD69, a member of the natural killer cell gene complex family of signal transducing receptors. *J Exp Med* 1994;180:1999–2004.

47. Deaglio S, Dianzani U, Horenstein AL, et al. Human CD38 ligand: a 120-kDa protein predominantly expressed on endothelial cells. *J Immunol* 1996;156:727–734.

48. Mehta K, Shahid U, Malavasi F. Human CD38, a cell-surface protein with multiple functions. *FASEB J* 1996;10:1408–1417.

49. Deaglio S, Morra M, Horenstein A, et al. Human CD38 (ADP-ribosyl cyclase) is a ligand of CD31, an Ig superfamily member. *J Immunol* 1998; 160:395–402.

50. Shubinsky G, Schlesinger M. The CD38 lymphocyte differentiation marker: new insight into its ectoenzymatic activity and its role as a signal transducer. *Immunity* 1997;7:315–324.

51. Cesano A, Visonneau S, Deaglio S, Malavasi F, Santoli D. Role of CD38 and its ligand in the regulation of MHC-nonrestricted cytotoxic T cells. *J Immunol* 1998;160:1106–1115.

52. Giorda R, Rudert WA, Vavassori C, Chambers WH, Hiserodt JC, Trucco M. NKR-P1, a signal transduction molecule on natural killer cells. *Science* 1990;249:1298–1300.

53. Frey JL, Bino T, Kantor RR, et al. Mechanism of target cell recognition by natural killer cells: characterization of a novel triggering molecule restricted to CD3-large granular lymphocytes. *J Exp Med* 1991;174:1527–1536.

54. Moretta A, Sivori S, Vitale M, et al. Existence of both inhibitory (p58) and activatory (p50) receptors for HLA-C molecules in human natural killer cells. *J Exp Med* 1995;182:875–884.

55. Segal DM, Bast BJEG. Production of bispecific antibodies. In Coligan JE, Kruisbeek AM, Margulies DH, Shevach EM, Strober W (eds). *Current Protocols in Immunology.* New York, John Wiley & Sons, 1995, pp 2.13.1–2.13.16.

56. Snider DP, Segal DM. Targeted antigen presentation using crosslinked antibody heteroaggregates. *J Immunol* 1987;139:1609–1616.

57. Wickham TJ, Segal DM, Roelvink PW, et al. Targeted adenovirus gene transfer to endothelial and smooth muscle cells by using bispecific antibodies. *J Virol* 1996;70:6831–6838.

58. Wickham TJ, Lee GM, Titus JA, et al. Targeted adenovirus-mediated gene delivery to T cells via CD3. *J Virol* 1997;71:7663–7669.

59. Brennan M, Davison PF, Paulus H. Preparation of bispecific antibodies by chemical recombination of monoclonal immunoglobulin G1 fragments. *Science* 1985;229:81–83.

60. Glennie MJ, McBride HM, Worth AT, Stevenson GT. Preparation and performance of bispecific F(ab)$'_2$ antibody containing thioether-linked Fab$'$ gamma fragments. *J Immunol* 1987;139:2367–2375.

61. Curnow RT. Clinical experience with CD64-directed immunotherapy: an overview. *Cancer Immunol Immunother* 1997;45:210–215.

62. Valone FH, Kaufman PA, Guyre PM, et al. Phase Ia/Ib trial of bispecific antibody MDX-210 in patients with advanced breast or ovarian cancer that overexpresses the proto-oncogene HER-2/neu. *J Clin Oncol* 1995;13:2281–2292.

63. Milstein C, Cuello AC. Hybrid hybridomas and their use in immunohistochemistry. *Nature* 1983;305:537–540.

64. Milstein C, Cuello AC. Hybrid-hybridomas and production of bi-specific monoclonal antibodies. *Immunol Today* 1984;5:299–304.

65. Lanzavecchia A, Scheidegger D. The use of hybrid hybridomas to target human cytotoxic T lymphocytes. *Eur J Immunol* 1987;17:105–111.

66. Karawajew L, Micheel B, Behrsing O, Gaestel M. Bispecific antibody-producing hybrid hybridomas selected by a fluorescence activated cell sorter. *J Immunol Methods* 1987;96:265–270.

67. Clark M, Gilliland L, Waldmann H. Hybrid antibodies for therapy. *Prog Allergy* 1988;45:31–49.

68. Karawajew L, Rudchenko S, Wlasik T, Trakht I, Rakitskaya V. Flow sorting of hybrid hybridomas using the DNA stain Hoechst 33342. *J Immunol Methods* 1990;129:277–282.

69. Wong JT, Colvin RB. Bi-specific monoclonal antibodies: selective binding and complement fixation to cells that express two different surface antigens. *J Immunol* 1987;139:1369–1374.

70. Urnovitz HB, Chang Y, Scott M, Fleischman J, Lynch RG. IgA:IgM and IgA:IgA hybrid hybridomas secrete heteropolymeric immunoglobulins that are polyvalent and bispecific. *J Immunol* 1988;140:558–563.

71. Cao Y, Vinayagamoorthy T, Noujaim AA, Suresh MR. A rapid non-selective method to generate quadromas by microelectrofusion. *J Immunol Methods* 1995;187:1–7.

72. Staerz UD, Bevan MJ. Hybrid hybridoma producing a bispecific monoclonal antibody that can focus effector T-cell activity. *Proc Natl Acad Sci USA* 1986;83:1453–1457.

73. Padlan EA. Anatomy of the antibody molecule. *Mol Immunol* 1994;31:169–217.

74. Lindhofer H, Mocikat R, Steipe B, Thierfelder S. Preferential species-restricted heavy/light chain pairing in rat/mouse quadromas: implications for a single-step purification of bispecific antibodies. *J Immunol* 1995;155:219–225.

75. Massino YS, Dergunova NN, Kizim EA, et al.

Quantitative analysis of the products of IgG chain recombination in hybrid hybridomas based on affinity chromatography and radioimmunoassay. *J Immunol Methods* 1997;201:57–66.

76. De Lau WBM, Heije K, Neefjes JJ, Oosterwegel M, Rozemuller E, Bast BJEG. Absence of preferential homologous H/L chain association in hybrid hybridomas. *J Immunol* 1991;146:906–914.

77. Koolwijk P, Spierenburg GT, Frasa H, Boot JH, Van de Winkel JG, Bast BJ. Interaction between hybrid mouse monoclonal antibodies and the human high-affinity IgG FcR, huFc gamma RI, on U937: involvement of only one of the mIgG heavy chains in receptor binding. *J Immunol* 1989; 143:1656–1662.

78. Clark MR, Waldmann H. T-cell killing of target cells induced by hybrid antibodies: comparison of two bispecific monoclonal antibodies. *J Natl Cancer Inst* 1987;79:1393–1401.

79. Canevari S, Stoter G, Arienti F, et al. Regression of advanced ovarian carcinoma by intraperitoneal treatment with autologous T lymphocytes retargeted by a bispecific monoclonal antibody. *J Natl Cancer Inst* 1995;87:1463–1469.

80. Weiner LM, Clark JI, Davey M, et al. Phase I trial of 2B1, a bispecific monoclonal antibody targeting c-erbB-2 and Fc gamma RIII. *Cancer Res* 1995; 55:4586–4593.

81. Shalaby MR, Shepard HM, Presta L, et al. Development of humanized bispecific antibodies reactive with cytotoxic lymphocytes and tumor cells overexpressing the HER2 protooncogene. *J Exp Med* 1992;175:217–225.

82. Carter P, Kelley RF, Rodrigues ML, et al. High level *Escherichia coli* expression and production of a bivalent humanized antibody fragment. *Biotechnology* 1992;10:163–167.

83. Kostelny SA, Cole MS, Tso JY. Formation of a bispecific antibody by the use of leucine zippers. *J Immunol* 1992;148:1547–1553.

84. Weiner GJ, Kostelny SA, Hillstrom JR, et al. The role of T cell activation in anti-CD3 X antitumor bispecific antibody therapy. *J Immunol* 1994; 152:2385–2392.

85. Link BK, Kostelny SA, Cole MS, Fusselman WP, Tso JY, Weiner GJ. Anti-CD3-based bispecific antibody designed for therapy of human B-cell malignancy can induce T-cell activation by antigen-dependent and antigen-independent mechanisms. *Int J Cancer* 1998;77:251–256.

86. Bakacs T, Lee J, Moreno MB, et al. A bispecific antibody prolongs survival in mice bearing lung metastases of syngeneic mammary adenocarcinoma. *Int Immunol* 1995;7:947–955.

87. Winter G, Milstein C. Man-made antibodies. *Nature* 1991;349:293–299.

88. Pack P, Pluckthun A. Miniantibodies: use of amphipathic helices to produce functional, flexibly linked dimeric FV fragments with high avidity in *Escherichia coli. Biochemistry* 1992;31:1579–1584.

89. Holliger P, Prospero T, Winter G. "Diabodies": small bivalent and bispecific antibody fragments. *Proc Natl Acad Sci USA* 1993;90:6444–6448.

90. Dorai H, McCartney JE, Hudziak RM, et al. Mammalian cell expression of single-chain Fv (sFv) anti-

body proteins and their C-terminal fusions with interleukin-2 and other effector domains. *Biotechnology* 1994;12:890–897.

91. Gruber M, Schodin BA, Wilson ER, Kranz DM. Efficient tumor cell lysis mediated by a bispecific single-chain antibody expressed in *Escherichia coli. J Immunol* 1994;152:5368–5374.

92. Hayden MS, Linsley PS, Gayle MA, et al. Single-chain mono- and bispecific antibody derivatives with novel biological properties and antitumour activity from a COS cell transient expression system. *Ther Immunol* 1994;1:3–15.

93. Mallender WD, Voss EW, Jr. Construction, expression, and activity of a bivalent bispecific single-chain antibody. *J Biol Chem* 1994;269:199–206.

94. Kurucz I, Titus JA, Jost CR, Jacobus CM, Segal DM. Retargeting of CTL by an efficiently refolded bispecific single-chain Fv dimer produced in bacteria. *J Immunol* 1995;154:4576–4582.

95. Jost CR, Titus JA, Kurucz I, Segal DM. A single-chain bispecific Fv2 molecule produced in mammalian cells redirects lysis by activated CTL. *Mol Immunol* 1996;33:211–219.

96. Pluckthun A, Pack P. New protein engineering approaches to multivalent and bispecific antibody fragments. *Immunotechnology* 1997;3:83–105.

97. De Jonge J, Heirman C, De Veerman M, et al. In vivo retargeting of T cell effector function by recombinant bispecific single-chain Fv (anti-CD3 × anti-idiotype) induces long-term survival in the murine BCL1 lymphoma model. *J Immunol* 1998;161:1454–1461.

98. Helfrich W, Kroesen BJ, Roovers RC, et al. Construction and characterization of a bispecific diabody for retargeting T cells to human carcinomas. *Int J Cancer* 1998;76:232–239.

99. Kipriyanov SM, Moldenhauer G, Strauss G, Little M. Bispecific CD3 × CD19 diabody for T cell-mediated lysis of malignant human B cells. *Int J Cancer* 1998;77:763–772.

100. Hochman J, Inbar D, Givol D. An active antibody fragment (Fv) composed of the variable portions of heavy and light chains. *Biochemistry* 1973; 12:1130–1135.

101. Glockshuber R, Malia M, Pfitzinger I, Pluckthun A. A comparison of strategies to stabilize immunoglobulin Fv-fragments. *Biochemistry* 1990;29: 1362–1367.

102. Bird RE, Hardman KD, Jacobson JW, et al. Single-chain antigen-binding proteins. *Science* 1988;242: 423–426.

103. Huston JS, Levinson D, Mudgett-Hunter M, et al. Protein engineering of antibody binding sites: recovery of specific activity in an anti-digoxin single-chain Fv analogue produced in *Escherichia coli. Proc Natl Acad Sci USA* 1988;85:5879–5883.

104. Huston JS, Mudgett-Hunter M, Tai M-S, et al. Protein engineering of single-chain Fv analogs and fusion proteins. *Methods Enzymol* 1991;203:46–78.

105. Almog O, Benhar I, Vasmatzis G, et al. Crystal structure of the disulfide-stabilized Fv fragment of anticancer antibody B1: conformational influence of an engineered disulfide bond. *Proteins* 1998; 31:128–138.

106. Brinkmann U, Di Carlo A, Vasmatzis G, et al.

Stabilization of a recombinant Fv fragment by base-loop interconnection and V(H)-V(L) permutation. *J Mol Biol* 1997;268:107–117.

107. Clackson T, Hoogenboom HR, Griffiths AD, Winter G. Making antibody fragments using phage display libraries. *Nature* 1991;352:624–627.

108. Marks JD, Hoogenboom HR, Bonnert TP, McCafferty J, Griffiths AD, Winter G. By-passing immunization: human antibodies from V-gene libraries displayed on phage. *J Mol Biol* 1991;222:581–597.

109. Jung S, Pluckthun A. Improving in vivo folding and stability of a single-chain Fv antibody fragment by loop grafting. *Protein Eng* 1997;10:959–966.

110. Proba K, Worn A, Honegger A, Pluckthun A. Antibody scFv fragments without disulfide bonds made by molecular evolution. *J Mol Biol* 1998;275:245–253.

111. Martineau P, Jones P, Winter G. Expression of an antibody fragment at high levels in the bacterial cytoplasm. *J Mol Biol* 1998;280:117–127.

112. Worn A, Pluckthun A. An intrinsically stable antibody scFv fragment can tolerate the loss of both disulfide bonds and fold correctly. *FEBS Lett* 1998;427:357–361.

113. Pack P, Muller K, Zahn R, Pluckthun A. Tetravalent miniantibodies with high avidity assembling in *Escherichia coli*. *J Mol Biol* 1995;246:28–34.

114. Kalinke U, Krebber A, Krebber C, et al. Monovalent single-chain Fv fragments and bivalent miniantibodies bound to vesicular stomatitis virus protect against lethal infection. *Eur J Immunol* 1996; 26:2801–2806.

115. Muller KM, Arndt KM, Strittmatter W, Pluckthun A. The first constant domain (C(H)1 and C(L)) of an antibody used as heterodimerization domain for bispecific miniantibodies. *FEBS Lett* 1998; 422:259–264.

116. Horn U, Strittmatter W, Krebber A, et al. High volumetric yields of functional dimeric miniantibodies in *Escherichia coli*, using an optimized expression vector and high-cell-density fermentation under non-limited growth conditions. *Appl Microbiol Biotechnol* 1996;46:524–532.

117. Perisic O, Webb PA, Holliger P, Winter G, Williams RL. Crystal structure of a diabody, a bivalent antibody fragment. *Structure* 1994;2:1217–1226.

118. McGuinness BT, Walter G, FitzGerald K, et al. Phage diabody repertoires for selection of large numbers of bispecific antibody fragments. *Nat Biotechnol* 1996;14:1149–1154.

119. FitzGerald K, Holliger P, Winter G. Improved tumour targeting by disulphide stabilized diabodies expressed in *Pichia pastoris*. *Protein Eng* 1997; 10:1221–1225.

120. Zhu Z, Zapata G, Shalaby R, Snedecor B, Chen H, Carter P. High level secretion of a humanized bispecific diabody from *Escherichia coli*. *Biotechnology* 1996;14:192–196.

121. Krebs B, Griffin H, Winter G, Rose-John S. Recombinant human single-chain Fv antibodies recognizing human interleukin-6: specific targeting of cytokine-secreting cells. *J Biol Chem* 1998;273: 2858–2865.

122. Holliger P, Wing M, Pound JD, Bohlen H, Winter G. Retargeting serum immunoglobulin with

bispecific diabodies. *Nat Biotechnol* 1997;15: 632–636.

123. Holliger P, Brissinck J, Williams RL, Thielemans K, Winter G. Specific killing of lymphoma cells by cytotoxic T-cells mediated by a bispecific diabody. *Protein Eng* 1996;9:299–305.

124. De Jonge J, Brissinck J, Heirman C, et al. Production and characterization of bispecific single-chain antibody fragments. *Mol Immunol* 1995;32:1405–1412.

125. Adams GP, Schier R, McCall AM, et al. Prolonged in vivo tumour retention of a human diabody targeting the extracellular domain of human HER2/ neu. *Br J Cancer* 1998;77:1405–1412.

126. Colcher D, Bird R, Roselli M, et al. In vivo tumor targeting of a recombinant single-chain antigen-binding protein. *J Natl Cancer Inst* 1990;82:1191–1197.

127. Huston JS, McCartney J, Tai M-S, et al. Medical applications of single-chain antibodies. *Int Rev Immunol* 1993;10:195–217.

128. Titus JA, Garrido MA, Hecht TT, Winkler DF, Wunderlich JR, Segal DM. Human T cells targeted with anti-T3 crosslinked to anti-tumor antibody prevent tumor growth in nude mice. *J Immunol* 1987;138:4018–4022.

129. Qian J, Titus JA, Andrew SM, et al. Human PBL targeted with bispecific antibodies release cytokines that are essential for inhibiting tumor growth. *J Immunol* 1991;146:3250–3256.

130. Beun GD, van de Velde CJ, Fleuren GJ, Eggermont AM. T-cell retargeting using bispecific monoclonal antibodies in a rat colon carcinoma model. IV. Tumor neutralization in Winn type assays. *J Immunother* 1993;14:11–15.

131. Garrido MA, Valdayo MJ, Winkler DF, et al. Targeting human T lymphocytes with bispecific antibodies to react against human ovarian carcinoma cells in nu/nu mice. *Cancer Res* 1990;50:4227–4232.

132. Mezzanzanica D, Garrido MA, Neblock DS, et al. Human T-lymphocytes targeted against an established ovarian carcinoma with bispecific F(ab')$_2$ antibody prolong host survival in a murine xenograft model. *Cancer Res* 1991;51:5716–5721.

133. Riedle S, Rosel M, Zoller M. In vivo activation and expansion of T cells by a bi-specific antibody abolishes metastasis formation of human melanoma cells in SCID mice. *Int J Cancer* 1998; 75:908–918.

134. Weiner LM, Holmes M, Adams GP, LaCreta F, Watts P, Garcia de Palazzo I. A human tumor xenograft model of therapy with a bispecific monoclonal antibody targeting c-erbB-2 and CD16. *Cancer Res* 1993;53:94–100.

135. Brissinck J, Demanet C, Moser M, Leo O, Thielemans K. Treatment of mice bearing BCL$_1$ lymphoma with bispecific antibodies. *J Immunol* 1991;147:4019–4026.

136. Demanet C, Brissinck J, Moser M, Leo O, Thielemans K. Bispecific antibody therapy of two murine B-cell lymphomas. *Int J Cancer Suppl* 1992;7: 67–68.

137. Brissinck J, Demanet C, Moser M, Leo O, Thielemans K. Bispecific antibodies in lymphoma. *Int Rev Immunol* 1993;10:187–194.

138. Demanet C, Brissinck J, Leo O, Moser M, Thiele-mans K. Role of T-cell subsets in the bispecific antibody (anti-idiotype × anti-CD3) treatment of the BCL$_1$ lymphoma. *Cancer Res* 1994;54:2973–2978.

139. Demanet C, Brissinck J, De Jonge J, Thielemans K. Bispecific antibody-mediated immunotherapy of the BCL$_1$ lymphoma: increased efficacy with multiple injections and CD28-induced costimulation. *Blood* 1996;87:4390–4398.

140. Demanet C, Brissinck J, Van Mechelen M, Leo O, Thielemans K. Treatment of murine B cell lymphoma with bispecific monoclonal antibodies (anti-idiotype × anti-CD3). *J Immunol* 1991;147:1091–1097.

141. Weiner GJ, Hillstrom JR. Bispecific anti-idiotype/anti-CD3 antibody therapy of murine B cell lymphoma. *J Immunol* 1991;147:4035–4044.

142. Weiner GJ. Bispecific IgG and IL-2 therapy of a syngeneic B-cell lymphoma in immunocompetent mice. *Int J Cancer Suppl* 1992;7:63–66.

143. Link BK, Weiner GJ. Production and characterization of a bispecific IgG capable of inducing T-cell-mediated lysis of malignant B cells. *Blood* 1993;81:3343–3349.

144. Wooldridge JE, Dahle CE, Weiner GJ. T-cell activation induced by anti-CD3 × anti-B-cell lymphoma monoclonal antibody is enhanced by pretreatment of lymphoma cells with soluble CD40 ligand. *Cancer Immunol Immunother* 1997;45:174–179.

145. Renner C, Jung W, Sahin U, et al. Cure of xeno-grafted human tumors by bispecific monoclonal antibodies and human T cells. *Science* 1994;264:833–835.

146. Hombach A, Jung W, Pohl C, et al. A CD16/CD30 bispecific monoclonal antibody induces lysis of Hodgkin's cells by unstimulated natural killer cells in vitro and in vivo. *Int J Cancer* 1993;55:830–836.

147. Kroesen BJ, Helfrich W, Bakker A, et al. Reduction of EGP-2-positive pulmonary metastases by bispecific-antibody-redirected T cells in an immunocompetent rat model. *Int J Cancer* 1995;61:812–818.

148. Penna C, Dean PA, Nelson H. Antitumor × anti-CD3 bifunctional antibodies redirect T-cells activated in vivo with staphylococcal enterotoxin B to neutralize pulmonary metastases. *Cancer Res* 1994;54:2738–2743.

149. Porter LE, Nelson H, Ethem Gecim I, Rice DC, Thibault C, Chapoval AI. T cell activation and retargeting using staphylococcal enterotoxin B and bispecific antibody: an effective in vivo antitumor strategy. *Cancer Immunol Immunother* 1997;45:180–183.

150. Renner C, Bauer S, Sahin U, et al. Cure of dissem-inated xenografted human Hodgkin's tumors by bispecific monoclonal antibodies and human T cells: the role of human T-cell subsets in a preclini-cal model. *Blood* 1996;87:2930–2937.

151. Bohlen H, Manzke O, Titzer S, et al. Prevention

of Epstein-Barr virus-induced human B-cell lymphoma in severe combined immunodeficient mice treated with CD3 × CD19 bispecific antibod-ies, CD28 monospecific antibodies, and autologous T cells. *Cancer Res* 1997;57:1704–1709.

152. Manzke O, Titzer S, Tesch H, Diehl V, Bohlen H. CD3 × CD19 bispecific antibodies and CD28 costimulation for locoregional treatment of low-malignancy non-Hodgkin's lymphoma. *Cancer Immunol Immunother* 1997;45:198–202.

153. Katayose Y, Kudo T, Suzuki M, et al. MUC1-specific targeting immunotherapy with bispecific antibodies: inhibition of xenografted human bile duct carcinoma growth. *Cancer Res* 1996;56:4205–4212.

154. Nitta T, Sato K, Yagita H, Okumura K, Ishii S. Preliminary trial of specific targeting therapy against malignant glioma. *Lancet* 1990;335:368–371.

155. Canevari S, Mezzanzanica D, Mazzoni A, et al. Approaches to implement bispecific antibody treatment of ovarian carcinoma. *Cancer Immunol Immunother* 1997;45:187–189.

156. Tibben JG, Boerman OC, Claessens RAMJ, et al. Cytokine release in an ovarian cancer patient following intravenous administration of bispecific antibody OC/TR F(ab')2. *J Natl Cancer Inst* 1993;85:1003–1004.

157. Kroesen BJ, Buter J, Sleijfer DT, et al. Phase I study of intravenously applied bispecific antibody in renal cell cancer patients receiving subcutaneous interleukin 2. *Br J Cancer* 1994;70:652–661.

158. De Gast GC, Haagen I-A, Van Houten AA, et al. CD8 T cell activation after intravenous administra-tion of CD3 × CD19 bispecific antibody in patients with non-Hodgkin lymphoma. *Cancer Immunol Immunother* 1995;40:390–396.

159. De Gast GC, Van Houten AA, Haagen IA, et al. Clinical experience with CD3 × CD19 bispecific antibodies in patients with B cell malignancies. *J Hematother* 1995;4:433–437.

160. Clark JI, Alpaugh RK, Weiner LM. Natural killer cell-directed bispecific antibodies. In Fanger MW (ed) *Bispecific Antibodies.* Austin, R. G. Landes, 1995, pp 77–87.

161. Van Ojik HH, Repp R, Groenewegen G, Valerius T, Van de Winkel JG. Clinical evaluation of the bispecific antibody MDX-H210 (anti-Fc gamma RI × anti-HER-2/neu) in combination with granu-locyte-colony-stimulating factor (filgrastim) for treatment of advanced breast cancer. *Cancer Immunol Immunother* 1997;45:207–209.

162. James N, Atherton P, Koletsky A, Tchekmedyian N, Curnow RT. Phase II trial of the bispecific anti-body MDX-H210 (anti-Her2/Neu × anti-CD64) combined with GM-CSF in patients with advanced prostate and renal cell carcinomas that express Her2/Neu. *Br J Cancer* 1998;78:19.

163. Hartmann F, Renner C, Jung W, et al. Treatment of refractory Hodgkin's disease with an anti-CD16/CD30 bispecific antibody. *Blood* 1997;89:2042–2047.

Cytotoxic Cells: Basic Mechanisms and Medical Applications, edited by Michail V. Sitkovsky and Pierre A. Henkart. Lippincott Williams & Wilkins, Philadelphia © 2000.

Chapter 30

Clinical Applications of Redirected Cytotoxicity

Reinder L. H. Bolhuis, Ralph A. Willemsen, and Jan W. Gratama

Clinical and Tumor Immunologies, University Hospital Rotterdam, Daniel Den Hoed Cancer Center, P.O. Box 5021, 3000 CA Rotterdam, The Netherlands

Throughout history researchers and clinicians have collaborated and aimed to translate the advances in basic science for medical purposes, in particular to design innovative treatment modalities. For immunotherapy the advent of diverse technologies to (a) produce monoclonal antibodies (mAbs) by somatic hybridization or by establishing phage display libraries; (b) tissue-culture cells for large-scale expansion; (c) clone, isolate, and characterize individual representatives of all kind of somatic cells, including stem cells, and lymphoid cells; (d) clone genes encoding for all possible functional structures, including immune cell receptors; and (e) develop gene transfer vehicles to introduce "genes of choice" to "targets of choice" has created new prospects for immunologically based therapeutic strategies for cancer, autoimmunity, infections, and genetic disorders. Examples of such developments are regularly highlighted in the preclinical and clinical literature, and it is fair to state that the "new" strategies for treatment of patients in essence are a natural phenomenon representing a recurrent theme. No matter what type of new technologic expertise and advance in biology were underlying the development of "new" therapeutic strategies, it always required in-depth knowledge of the biological mechanisms and the technologic skill to take it "from the page to the stage."

Whereas in the past advances in basic sciences were made by academic research, and new drugs and technologies were discovered by industry, today this distinction has largely become blurred. Both sectors now occupy themselves with biology and technology, alone or in collaboration.

The phenomena of cell–cell interactions are studied in many disciplines of biology, ranging from cell differentiation, embryology, organ formation, and function to neuroendocrinology and immunology. A major focus in these studies is how cells of these systems communicate between each other within the organism: through the production and acceptance of soluble factors and through cell–cell contact. The immunologist is faced with the fascinating challenge to dissect these intra- and intercellular relationships of the innate and cognate cellular and humoral members of the immune system on the one hand and their soluble and major histocompatibility complex (MHC)-presented antigens on the other. One member, the natural killer (NK) cell, is unique in the sense that it functions by continuously scanning the cellular environment of the organism and comes to immediate action the moment imbalances occur in the organism. An imbalance may be the consequence of pathologic changes in the internal milieu or the cell membrane makeup, or it may be due to intrusion by infectious or other foreign particles. Other members of the immune system, the B and T cells, require a unique challenge and stimulus before they come into action: T and B cell activation is the result of specific antigen recognition and binding followed by cell differentiation and proliferation. The B and T cell responses also involve many other cell types, including eosinophils, basophils, macrophages, and dendritic cells and the responses are elicited through cell–cell interaction or through production and acceptance of soluble messengers, the lymphokines. The "key" entry point for any cellular component of the immune system is the antigen-recognizing receptor, which has a signaling capacity that can trigger a cascade of immune functions.

IMMUNE RECOGNITION

The hallmark of immunologically based therapeutic strategies is its specificity by virtue of the presence of specific receptors on the immune cells. Foreign antigens comprise viruses, bacteria, MHC antigens on partially or fully mismatched organ grafts, or antigens on malignantly transformed cells. All these "foreign" antigens are distinct from "self" antigens, and even "self" antigens that are expressed in an "aberrant" way may serve as a target structure. When antigens are present in the host in soluble form, they will primarily be neutralized by antibodies (Abs) and by immune cells when presented by MHC [e.g., on antigen-presenting cells, or APCs]. As a consequence, the immune attack leaves normal and noninfected tissues (self) intact and eliminates "non-self." This idea goes back to the beginning of the twentieth century when Paul Ehrlich put forward his hypothesis of "magic bullets" (1), and studies were initiated aimed at active immunization of cancer patients against their own cancerous tissue. During the subsequent six decades cancer patients were nonspecifically immune-stimulated with relatively crude leukocyte extracts such as transfer factor, immune RNA, bacterial extracts such as bacillus Calmette-Guérin (BCG) or Coley's toxin, or levamisol. Little was known, however, about the various components of the immune system that could react against cancer, and even less was known about tumor-associated antigen structures. Nevertheless, the first wave of immunotherapy had started.

In 1970 Burnett revisited the immune-surveillance theory and highlighted the issue that cell-mediated immunity played a critical role in the control of cancer and infectious diseases (2). The study of "self" versus "non-self" recognition by immune cells became the central focus in basic and applied immunology, and it was postulated that T cells learned during ontogeny to distinguish between the two: "Self" should be left intact, and "non-self" should be eliminated. Ridge et al. proposed that discrimination between "self" and "non-self" is an active, lifelong process in which foreign molecules activate immune cells through T cell immune specific receptors only when co-activation together with a "danger" signal is delivered but tolerate T cells in the absence of a danger signal (3). Therefore one of the major tasks of the host immune system was and is to continuously scan whether in the host "self" becomes "non-self" due to viral infections, neoplastic transformation, or aberrant "self" expression. Today it is believed that NK cells are the sentinels in the immune system, vigilantly monitoring the intactness of the interior milieu and always ready to act whenever an alteration in "self" occurs.

During the 1980s NK and T cells became the logical choice to be adoptively transferred to cancer patients for "nonspecific" and "immune-specific immunotherapy of cancer," respectively. Hence the second wave of immunotherapy had started. Large numbers of clinical studies were performed, and adoptive transfer of immune cells was combined with mAbs and cytokines. The ultimate goal of all these efforts was and is to generate a target cell-specific, long-lasting immune response that not only eradicates or controls the growth of tumor cells but provides protection for future encounters: protection through immunologic memory. With this concept immune intervention is thought to trigger *in vivo* a cascade of immune effector functions to involve macrophages, APCs, eosinophils, and the full range of NK, B, and T cells. They are triggered to operate in an orchestrated fashion through cell–cell contact and cytokine production.

NK, B, AND T CELLS

Important members of the cognate immune system are the antigen-specific CD3[+] T lymphocytes and immunoglobulin-positive (Ig[+]) B lymphocytes. Both immune cells demonstrate exquisite antigen specificity. T cells recognize MHC-presented antigens through the T cell receptor (TCR), whereas B cells recognize antigens in a MHC-unrestricted fashion through membrane-anchored immunoglobulins. The T cell population comprises CD8[+] cytotoxic T lymphocytes (CTLs), which kill their target cells, and T-helper (Th) cells, which produce lymphokines and regulate Ig synthesis. APCs such as macrophages, dendritic cells, and others are important initiators of the immune response against foreign invaders. At any rate, all immune cells communicate with each other through membrane-anchored receptors that mediate cell–cell contact, followed by intracellular and intercellular transduction of regulatory signals and through lymphokine production.

T LYMPHOCYTES

The TCRs specifically recognize and bind to antigens presented by MHC class I (MHC-I) or MHC-II molecules. As such, T cells, like NK cells, scan the surface of body cells of the organism for the presence of peptides derived from degraded pathogens. The TCR is a multichain complex consisting of an Ig-like antigen-binding portion (polymorphic $\alpha\beta$ or $\gamma\delta$ TCRs) that are noncovalently linked to nonpolymorphic signal transducing elements (CD3/$\delta\varepsilon$, CD3/$\gamma\varepsilon$, ζ, and η chains). The $\alpha\beta$ and $\gamma\delta$ chains are disulfide-linked heterodimers or tetramers, and both contain an invariant constant (C) region and an antigen-binding variable (V) region (4). The exquisite antigen specificity and diversity of TCRs is the hallmark of the T cell response

and is created through gene rearrangements. These gene rearrangements comprise the V, diversity (D), and joining (J) gene segments, which are combined to form the antigen-binding $\alpha\beta$ and $\gamma\delta$ domains. The C region of the TCR contains a transmembrane structure and has a signaling function to the T cell cytoplasm via the CD3 complex, which is anchored to the T cell membrane. The fashion and form in which TCRs fold intracellularly are critical for their intracellular transport to the T cell membrane, subsequent membrane expression, and capacity to recognize and bind MHC-presented antigens. T lymphocyte immune functions comprise lymphokine production by Th1 and Th2 cells and lytic functions by CTLs to preserve the integrity of the interior milieu of the individual. When T lymphocytes recognize antigens in the absence of co-stimulatory and danger signal(s) they become tolerant or anergic (4). Although the intrinsic binding affinities of TCRs for antigen are low in comparison to Abs, low numbers of MHC–peptide complexes per target cell can trigger T lymphocytes. This is possible because the same antigens can serially bind to TCRs after TCR disengagement from antigen following signal transduction (5,6).

The previously antigen-engaged TCRs become inactivated after signal transduction owing to TCR–CD3 complex degradation. T cells can accumulate the signals individually generated via TCRs until an activation threshold is reached. We proposed that this serial use of sets of TCRs represent the mechanism by which CTLs can lyse multiple target cells (7). Therefore different T lymphocyte responses by the same T cell differ in the required signaling thresholds via TCRs. The signal strength is co-determined by the antigen density and potency on the one hand and the TCR affinity and occupancy on the other.

ADHESION AND CO-ACTIVATION MOLECULES

The TCR-mediated T cell activation requires both T cell adhesion molecules that interact with target cell ligands (e.g., CD11a/ CD18-CD54) and the CD2-CD58 adhesion pathways. The adhesion pathways become more critical in circumstances where only a low density of MHC-presented antigens is expressed on the target cell. A second group of accessory molecules are the very late antigens (VLA), a subfamily of integrins (VLAs 3, 4, 5, and 6). This group of VLAs recognize the collagen, fibronectin, and lamenin present in the intracellular matrix of target cells. CD44, a third category of molecules, recognizes extracellular matrix proteins such as glycosaminoglycans (4). Together, these structures: (a) secure a stable effector cell–target cell interaction; (b) guide lymphocyte trafficking through the dynamic expression of varying combinations of these extracellular matrix proteins; and (c) are thought to govern the maturation process of immune cells (8). In addition to adhesion functions, the CD2, CD8, and CD11a/CD18 receptors play important roles as co-stimulatory molecules in T lymphocyte activation. Indeed, when combinations of mAbs against CD2, CD3, CD16, and other co-activation molecules are used for crosslinking the T lymphocyte (co-)activating receptors, the activation kinetics and levels are critically enhanced. Other molecules that can serve in signaling are CD44 and CD69 (9–11).

The CD8 and CD4 molecules on T lymphocytes specifically associate with the same MHC-I or MHC-II molecules that present antigens and thereby (a) contribute to stabilization of T cell–target cell interactions and (b) amplify the T cell activation signal strength. The important message is that crosslinking of multiple TCRs on individual T cells with multiple antigens on the individual target cells, the additional bond formations between CD4 or CD8 in the T cell membrane with MHC-presented antigens on target cells, and the crosslinking between T lymphocyte adhesion molecules and target cell ligands all act together to establish firm conjugate formation between effector cell and target cell to elicit an effective immune response. All receptor–antigen interactions

function in an organized fashion. During these complex interactions these receptors and their ligands move toward the contact region of the effector cell and target cell, a process that can be visualized under the microscope using fluorochrome labeled Abs specific for these structures (7,12).

NK CELLS

Initially, NK cells were defined by their ability to lyse tumor cells and virus-infected cells without the need for prior sensitization. Indeed, NK cells lack specific receptors, such as TCRs on T cells, that can recognize MHC-presented antigen in a cognate manner. NK cell interaction with target cells therefore appeared to be MHC-unrestricted; and because they were shown to lyse a wide range of histogenetically distinct target cells, even across species, the recognition mechanism was termed "nonspecific," or "innate." Later it was found that they also lyse certain normal cells, particularly hematopoietic blast cells displaying a mismatch at the MHC locus. However, NK cells never lyse normal cells from the same host (self). Hersey and Bolhuis hypothesized that CD3⁻ NK cells demonstrate target cell selectivity through the simultaneous use of varying combinations of distinct receptors. This proposed mechanism of specificity has been backed by extensive research and is widely accepted (13).

Despite these fundamental distinctions in target cell recognition mechanisms between innate and adaptive immune cells, NK and T cells share important characteristics: They have a common progenitor, and the representatives of the NK and T cell lineages express surface markers on their membrane that are important for cell–cell interactions and delivery of co-activation signals (e.g., CD2, CD8, CD16). These common features point to the close relationship between NK and T cells (13–15). The mechanism by which NK and T cells lyse their target cells also share important characteristics: The cells kill via perforin or via induction of apoptosis (16–18). The typical NK or T lineage commitment occurs at an early stage, illustrated by the fact that NK cells do not rearrange TCR-like genes.

The NK cells show a wide variety of functions, such as (a) instant eradication of target cells infected by microorganisms by direct lysis through the release of perforins from cytotoxic granules in the NK cells and (b) immune response regulation through the production of cytokines that mediate inflammatory immune responses. It is noteworthy that NK cells are one of the first immune type cells to respond to interleukin-12 (IL-12) release by macrophages: The cells are active during the early stages of viral infections through the production of interferon-γ (INF-γ). NK cells therefore play a central role within the cytokine network: After all, INF-γ not only, exerts direct antiviral activity, it enhances and regulates immune responses by increasing MHC-I expression in target cell membranes. This upregulated MHC expression in turn allows more efficient target antigen presentation to T lymphocytes to induce Th cell and cytolytic activities. Interestingly, NK cells also directly identify and destroy normal, MHC-mismatched hematopoietic or lymphoid cells as shown by their capacity to reject transplants of mismatched bone marrow cells in hybrid systems *in vivo* (19–22). Rather than being "nonspecific," NK cells demonstrate specificity through the coordinated and selective use of distinct multiple receptors in varying combinations (13). The technique of cell cloning allowed identification of distinct NK clones, which permitted identification of a whole new range of NK receptors, each showing selective expression of different combinations of killer inhibitory receptors (KIRs) and killer activation receptors (KARs). These KIRs and KARs have been shown to be specific for distinct MHC-I molecules (23). To explain the lack of "self" attack by NK cells, Ljunggren and Kärre formulated the "missing-self" hypothesis, which in essence states that NK cells are prevented from responding to "self" through

the specific recognition of "self" MHC-I antigens: "self" MHC triggers the KIRs so they are "signaled off" (24). The "multiple receptor" hypothesis together with the "missing self" hypothesis provide the mechanistic explanation how NK cells (a) demonstrate target cell specificity and (b) can interact with a range of normal, "non-self" target cells such as lymphocytes or bone marrow cells, tumor cells, and virus-infected cells without prior sensitization.

The inhibition of NK activities by "self" MHC-I through KIRs may therefore serve as a security mechanism to prevent highly activated immune cells to overreact against "self" tissues to prevent autoimmunity. The sequences and localizations of the genes encoding the KIRs and KARs have in part been identified and their specific binding patterns to MHC-I are well documented, albeit not fully (25). The NK cell signaling pathways that either prevent or trigger NK cell activities have also been partially unraveled. KIRs belong to a polymorphic group of several receptors that vary in size and structure, but, like TCRs, they all belong to the Ig superfamily (26–31). It is noteworthy that some human KIRs are also expressed in subpopulations of T cells, such as memory T cells (32), on dendritic APCs (33), and on a human CTL clone with specificity for melanoma cells (34).

It has become clear that the specificity of NK cells indeed depends on the interaction between the members of the NK receptor family with MHC specificity. The "multireceptor" and "missing self" hypotheses have thus found a solid molecular basis.

The Fc receptor for IgG (CD16) mediates Ab-dependent cell-mediated cytotoxicity (ADCC) and therefore can also activate NK cells. Hence, in ADCC the NK immune specificity is dictated by the Fab part of the Ig that binds with its Fc part to the Fc receptor. The Fc receptor, however, is not required for NK receptor-mediated target cell recognition and lysis (35). The ultimate lack of susceptibility of a particular target cell to lysis by NK cells, and for that matter by T cells, most likely co-depends on the density and activation level of "co-receptor" molecules anchored in the membrane of the effector cells on the one hand and the density and spatial arrangement of their relevant ligands on the target cells on the other hand. This implies that even changes in the physiologic spatial arrangements of "self" antigens in target cell membrane may make them susceptible to immune cell attack because their cytoskeletal mosaic has become aberrant.

IMMUNOTHERAPY OF DISEASE WITH THE ADOPTIVE TRANSFER OF IMMUNE CELLS

Tumor-Infiltrating Lymphocytes

As mentioned earlier, immune system-based therapies employing tumor-reactive T cells have been developed for patients with, for example, metastatic melanoma, and have resulted in clinically significant tumor reduction and cure. Especially, tumor-infiltrating lymphocytes (TILs) grown from many murine and human tumors were effective in preclinical and clinical studies. In mice, the CD8+ or CD4 TILs were shown to recognize unique antigens on murine transplantable tumor, and the adoptive transfer of TILs mediated rejection of established lung and liver metastasis. Clinical studies were triggered by these observations and yielded the establishment of CD8+ TILs able to recognize unique tumor antigens on human melanoma, breast cancer, colon cancer, ovarian cancer, and lymphomas and allowed the identification, cloning, isolation, and synthesis of these tumor rejection antigens. The antitumor responses in patients were significant, with an objective regression of cancer in 34% of melanoma patients irrespective of whether they had earlier responded to interleukin-2 (IL-2) treatment. These TILs were able to: (a) specifically move to tumor sites; (b) lyse the relevant tumor cells; and (c) produce cytokines following interaction with the tumor targets (36). Unfortunately, TILs could be established only at low frequencies in cancer

patients, with the exception of melanoma where a success rate of 50% was reached. Moreover, many of these TILs recognized only unique tumor rejection antigens; only a few recognized shared tumor rejection antigens, restricted by a variety of MHC-I molecules. At this point the TIL approach therefore does not provide a clinically practical or reliable approach for immunotherapy of cancer patients.

Targeting of CTLs with Bispecific mAbs

In contrast to the lack of success of reliably generating T lymphocytes with tumor-rejection antigen-specific TCRs in patients, a plethora of mAbs were already available with specificity for tumor-associated antigens that are common to a wide range of cancers. To combine the ability of these mAbs to recognize and bind selectively to tumors with the potent antitumor functions of T lymphocytes, we and others designed bispecific (bs)-mAbs with the aim of retargeting the immune specificity of T lymphocytes to tumor-associated antigens by sensitizing them with bs-mAbs. Such bs-mAbs can be produced by chemically coupling two types of mouse mAb with defined specificities against a CTL receptor on the one hand and a tumor-associated antigen on the other. Later, the hybridoma technology became more sophisticated and reliable for the production of bs-mAbs. In principle, bs-mAbs act like to a two-component "glue," bridging the immune effector cell to the tumor target cell. The multiple bonds created by bs-mAbs between tumor-associated antigen and, for example, the CD3 complex on T cells result in crosslinking of receptors and activation of the T lymphocyte machinery for lymphokine production, proliferation, and cytolysis. It should also be noted that all CTLs of an individual can be retargeted using bs-mAbs, provided one of the Fab-binding parts of the bs-mAb recognizes a nonpolymorphic lymphocyte activation site, such as CD3, which is present on all T cells. The induction of human anti-mouse bs-mAb (HAMA) responses observed in the patients could be dramatically reduced or even avoided entirely when gene encoding Ab fragments of human origin were used. Such human origin bs-mAbs are now readily available owing to the advances made in phage display technology.

Phage Display

Phage display involves the expression of proteins on the surface of phage as fusion proteins attach to normal phage code proteins. It is the physical link between the protein on the phage surface and the gene encoding it within the phage that allows the rapid evolution of protein properties on the basis of binding by a series of repetitive cycles of phage binding, elution, and regrowth to amplify the phage population of choice. The phage display technology also allows derivation of mAbs by use of large phage Ab libraries for subsequent improvement of the affinity of selected Abs by mutation and further selection. Phage can be selected from libraries of randomly paired combinations of V domains of heavy and light chains, structurally formatted as single-chain Abs or diabody fragments displayed on the surface of filamentous bacteria. Human mAbs can also be generated when the libraries are constructed from "naive" human B cells or from cloned human gene segments. Indeed large collections have now been made with more than 10 billion different mAbs. Thus Abs to any "chosen" antigen and with an affinity ranging from moderate to high can now be isolated.

Bs-mAb Targeted T Lymphocytes for Cancer Treatment

We and others have exploited the capacity of bs-mAbs to induce lymphocyte activation and to trigger the lytic and lymphokine-producing machineries of T cells for *in vivo* preclinical and clinical studies. Surprisingly, in mice much lower numbers of T lymphocytes were required to inhibit tumor growth *in vivo* than to induce complete lysis of all target cells *in vitro*. Detailed analysis of the underlying mechanisms for these observations revealed that lymphocytes during and after T cell activation by bs-mAb-mediated interaction with tumor cells produced lymphokines that inhibited growth of tumor cells even when these tumor cells were not recognized by the bs-mAb-targeted T cells, a phenomenon called inhibition of "bystander" tumor cell growth. This "bystander" effect did not require effector cell–target cell contact, as the supernatant, containing the lymphokines, itself inhibited tumor cell proliferation. The major lymphokine players identified in this growth arrest were tumor necrosis factor-α (TNF-α) and INF-γ. When these lymphokines were neutralized with relevant mAbs, their antitumor effects were blocked. A number of other inflammatory lymphokines were produced in addition to TNF-α and INF-γ, and these in turn recruited and acted on other cellular and humoral components of the immune system. The resulting inflammation process directed immune cells to the tumor site, and this localization of lymphokine production yielded a great advantage over systemic administration of the highly active biomolecules. After all, inflammatory lymphokines have pleiotropic effects on many normal cell types, and when injected they caused toxicity systemically. The tumor site-specific lymphokine production therefore favors its desired antitumor effect because lymphokines in general have a short half-life and as a consequence function only at short range. The target site-specific production and delivery of lymphokines generates signals to immune and target cells, thereby affecting their gene expression, proliferation, and differentiation profiles. Ultimately, these immune responses should cause target cell death.

The first international multicenter study involved locoregional (i.e., intraperitoneal) treatment of ovarian cancer in patients with advanced disease. These patients were selected because of their high frequency of relapse after induction chemotherapy; this high relapse rate called for an innovative treatment approach. Patients eligible for this study underwent laparotomy to reduce the tumor load surgically and to locate and document remaining lesions. Immunotherapy consisted of two 5-day cycles of treatment of daily intraperitoneal injections of *in vitro* activated and expanded autologous T cells targeted with bs-mAbs specific for CD3 on T cells and the folate receptor, which is overexpressed on ovarian carcinoma cells. Per infusion, 10^9 T lymphocytes that were targeted with bs-mAbs were administered into the peritoneal cavity. Patients received one additional infusion of IL-2 and bs-mAbs to maintain T cell survival, lytic activity, and bs-mAb-dictated specificity. Six to ten weeks following treatment patients with no sign of tumor progression underwent exploratory laparotomy for an objective assessment of the antitumor response by comparing the remaining tumor load with that documented during the pretreatment laparotomy. An impressive overall antitumor treatment intraperitoneal response of 27% was observed, with three patients showing complete remission in the intraperitoneal cavity. Although development of HAMA was observed, our *in vitro* studies showed that these HAMA did not block T lymphocyte activation activity in these patients during the treatment period.

It is important to note that the beneficial and significant antiovarian cancer effects of the bs-mAb-retargeted T lymphocytes were only locoregional. Extraperitoneal lesions were not affected by the immune treatment. One would expect that systemic administration of bs-mAb-retargeted activated T lymphocytes might be effective in producing systemic anticancer effects, as was earlier demonstrated in mice. So far there is only limited clinical experience with systemic treatment; and in the few instances that such systemic treatment was performed for ovarian cancer, it caused severe, acute toxicity within as short a time as 30 minutes after treatment. The patients developed chills, headache, and fever in combination with hypertension and fatigue; but all symptoms resolved immediately after cessation of treat-

ment. We concluded that this toxicity was most likely due to an increase in serum TNF-α levels because the bs-mAbs probably cross-reacted with antigens on the vascular endothelium. The activation of the bs-mAb-targeted T cells at the vascular bed may be responsible for the toxicity observed through cytokine production (37,38).

Other clinical pilot studies that involved infusion of bs-mAb-targeted T cells included patients with malignant ascites or plural effusions resulting from colon, mammary, ovarian, lung, or gastric carcinomas. In these patients strong biologic *in vivo* effects were observed within hours after infusion. The effects represented the formation of conjugates between tumor cells and T cells, a decrease in tumor cell number, an increase in granulocyte numbers, a decrease in serum levels of tumor markers, and elevated levels of cytokines. These clinical studies have provided "proof of concept" and have set the stage for further development of combined humoral and cellular anticancer treatments.

GENETIC PROGRAMMING OF T CELL IMMUNE SPECIFICITY FOR CANCER TREATMENT WITH SINGLE-CHAIN ANTIBODIES

The use of bs-mAb for cancer therapy may be hampered by the inaccessibility of solid tumors to mAb penetration (39). Moreover, bs-mAb-targeted CTLs retain the bs-mAb on their surface for only a limited time (i.e., 48–96 hours) owing to their dissociation (7,40). Finally, bs-mAb-targeted CTLs lose signal transducing and lytic capacity following target cell recognition and lysis (7).

To circumvent the limitations associated with bs-mAbs, we and others have adopted an approach in which T lymphocytes are genetically grafted with a permanent mAb-dictated specificity (41,42). To this end, the V_H and V_L domains of mAbs with tumor specificity were fused by a flexible linker. Such molecularly engineered Ab-based receptors have been shown to display antigen-binding affinities and specificities similar to those of the parental mAbs from which they are derived (43–45). Such single-chain Abs are juxtaposed to a signal transducing element such as the γ-chain of Fc(ε)RI molecules or the ζ-chain of CD3 molecules. These chimeric single-chain Ab/γ or ζ receptors have been functionally expressed in mouse T cell hybridomas and CTLs, TILs, and human CTLs. Stimulation of the chimeric receptors with the relevant target antigens results in full T cell activation (e.g., lymphokine production and T cell-mediated lysis of target cells) (41,42,44,46–49).

Gene cloning and viral vector-mediated gene transfer technologies have provided us the tools to develop clinically this next generation of "immuno-gene therapy." Cloning the antigen-binding regions of mAbs allows their direct molecular linkage to lymphocyte signaling elements (e.g., the γ- and ζ-chains; the result is a chimeric receptor).

Retroviral vectors are widely used for these gene transfers to proliferating somatic cells, including tumor cells and immune cells. Retroviral vectors transmit the genes to the recipient cells and to its progeny in a relatively stable fashion. However, no general applicable technology is yet available for *in vivo* target cell-specific gene transfer. As a consequence, the cells to be genetically programmed (e.g., for cancer specificity) are manipulated *ex vivo* because the efficacy of retroviral gene to human T cells is relatively low. *In vitro* gene transfer therefore needs to be followed by *in vitro* expansion of the gene-modified T cells to reach "therapeutic" lymphocyte numbers for clinical application (50).

T Lymphocytes Expressing Chimeric Single-Chain Ab/γ or ζ Receptor Specific for Renal Cell Cancer

We set out to construct one continuous molecule comprising the gene segments of the V regions of the renal cell carcinoma selective mouse mAb G250 (51) and the signal transducing transmembrane and intracellular regions of the human Fc(ε)RI-γ chain. The LXSN retroviral vector was used to generate

stable integration of the single-chain Ab/γ chimeric receptor gene into the genome (52). Co-cultivation of activated human T cells with irradiated, virus-producing packaging cells allowed transduction of the transgene. Indeed, DNA polymerase chain reaction (PCR) analysis demonstrated the presence of the chimeric single-chain Ab/γ viral construct in the genomic DNA of the recipient T lymphocytes. However, flow cytometric identification of the chimeric receptor in the membrane using antiidiotype Abs specific for the parental "G250" mAb from which the single-chain Ab/γ chimeric receptor was derived yielded negative results. Therefore the genetically modified T lymphocytes were tested for their capacity to secrete granulocyte/macrophage colony-stimulating factor (GM-CSF) and TNF-α during incubation with renal carcinoma cells expressing the G250 ligand compared to nonrelevant breast carcinoma cells and melanoma cells. The genetically modified T lymphocytes produced the lymphokines only when incubated with the relevant renal carcinoma cells, demonstrating that, although at low levels, the chimeric receptor was functionally expressed in the T cell membrane. The gene-modified T lymphocytes were also tested for their capacity to lyse the renal carcinoma cells. They were incubated with radioactive chromium 51 (^{51}Cr)-labeled G250 antigen-positive renal carcinoma cells and a G250 ligand$^-$ renal carcinoma; nonrenal carcinoma cells were used as controls. Only the relevant G250 ligand$^+$ renal carcinoma cells were lysed by the G250 gene-modified T lymphocytes: Renal carcinoma specificity was dictated by the chimeric transgene encoded chimeric G250 single-chain Ab/γ receptor. Additional proof of renal carcinoma specificity of the chimeric G250 single-chain Ab/γ receptor was obtained by showing that parental G250 mAbs completely inhibited renal carcinoma-specific lysis by shielding off the G250 antigens. An anti-MHC-I isotope mAb control had no effect on renal carcinoma-specific lysis. Continuous culture of the gene-modified lymphocytes showed that functional expression of the chimeric G250 single-chain Ab/γ receptor was maintained over a period of more than 4.5 months in culture. During this prolonged culture period a relative increase in the CD4$^+$ lymphocyte population was observed with a concomitant loss in lytic activity on a per-T lymphocyte basis. Depletion of CD4$^+$ T lymphocytes resulted in increased lytic activity on a per-lymphocyte basis, which demonstrates that tumor cell lysis is primarily exerted by the CD8$^+$ single-chain Ab/γ gene-transduced T lymphocytes. When the CD4$^+$ and CD8$^+$ gene-modified T lymphocyte populations were tested for lymphokine production, the CD4$^+$ T lymphocytes were found to produce approximately 5.5-fold more GM-CSF and 1.6-fold more TNF-α than CD8$^+$ T lymphocytes. T cell clones derived from the bulk culture of gene-modified T cells also showed G250 single-chain Ab/γ-dictated specific lysis of renal carcinoma. A proportion of the gene-modified T cell clones simultaneously exerted NK and AK lytic activities, as was already known to be the case for cloned "normal" T lymphocytes. It was surprising that high lytic activities were exerted by the T lymphocytes despite the fact that the G250 single-chain Ab/γ receptors could not be visualized using flow cytometric analysis (53).

To secure optimal effector cell–target cell interactions, the contribution of adhesion and co-activation molecules to the process of lymphocyte triggering is a critical factor. It even becomes limiting or a prerequisite when only low levels of antigens are expressed on the surface of target cells. We therefore determined the levels of expression of adhesion and accessory molecules on the single-chain Ab/γ$^+$ CTLs and renal carcinoma cells, respectively, by flow cytometry using fluorochrome-labeled mAbs. All gene-modified CTLs stained positive with Abs against CD2, CD3, CD8, and CD11a/CD18; the renal carcinoma cells from two renal carcinoma cell lines also stained positive with mAbs against CD54, CD58, and G250. We already stated that the CD2, CD3, CD11a/CD18, CD4, and CD8 molecules interact with the endogenous TCRs of T lymphocytes. Hence the question arises whether they can also interact with chimeric receptors that have been molecularly introduced into the T lymphocytes. The addition of mAbs specific for CD2, CD3, CD11a, and CD18 indeed inhibited lytic activity of the gene-modified CTLs but did not affect conjugate formation between the effector–target cells. These findings also showed that all of these CDs are functionally involved in target cell recognition and lysis, and that the mechanism of inhibition of target cell lysis involves delivery of a negative signal to the CTL cytoplasm, downstream of target cell binding. We know that MHC-presented antigen recognition by endogenous TCRs critically involves the CD8 receptor on T lymphocytes, whereas Ab binding to antigens is MHC-unrestricted. Therefore addition of anti-CD8 mAbs to the effector–target cell mixture was expected not to affect renal carcinoma-specific lysis by genetically modified CTLs through the single-chain Ab/γ chimeric receptor; and this was indeed the case. Proof that the single-chain Ab/γ chimeric receptors were functionally expressed in the T cell membrane was provided by experiments in which G250 antigen$^-$ melanoma cells were genetically programmed to express renal carcinoma in the G250 antigen. When gene-modified G250$^+$ melanoma cells were used as target cells, they now were identified as if they were G250 antigen$^+$ renal carcinoma cells (54).

It is also important to note that CTLs expressing single-chain Ab/γ receptors recognize the antigen in a MHC-unrestricted manner. Due to this feature chimeric single-chain Ab/γ or ζ receptor-engineered CTLs are able to recognize and lyse tumor target cells even when they have downregulated their MHC-I to escape T cell immune recognition.

Functional Balance Between Chimeric Single-Chain Ab/γ Receptor Density and Tumor Target Antigen Density

Now that we know that not only endogenous but genetically engineered chimeric receptors communicate with adhesion/co-activation receptor molecules on T lymphocyte surfaces, we need to answer the question of whether chimeric receptors can also be serially triggered by antigens. Moreover, if this is the case, how does triggering of these chimeric receptors depend on target cell antigen density. After all, when target cell antigen expression is low, the density of TCRs may become limiting, and not enough signal strength is accumulated to reach the threshold level for T cell activation.

To study these important questions regarding the functional relationship between TCRs and antigen densities it was necessary to have populations of CTLs available with varying densities of chimeric receptors on their membrane and renal carcinoma target cells with different G250 antigen densities. Knowing that gene transduction efficiencies obtained with the LXSN vector were always low and required repeated, laborious *in vitro* selection procedures, we constructed a retroviral vector facilitating the high expression of chimeric receptors following gene transduction. The "pSTITCH" vector we developed allows rapid screening for functional expression of chimeric receptors and T lymphocytes and facilitates (a) receptor structure/function analysis, (b) *in vivo* monitoring of T lymphocyte homing and assessment of the half life of gene modified T lymphocytes *in vivo,* (c) analysis of the physicochemical interaction of chimeric receptors (intracellularly, transmembrane, and extracellularly) with other signaling receptors and adhesion molecules in the membrane, and (d) biochemical characterization of the intracellular signaling pathways of genetically introduced chimeric receptors (55).

pSTITCH Retroviral Vector for Optimal Gene Transduction to Primary T Lymphocytes

The conventional LXSN viral gene transduction system has drawbacks: (a) low transduction efficiency (<1%), requiring co-transduction of a selection marker (e.g., neo-

mycin resistance) into the T cell, allowing repeated and prolonged lymphocyte culture in selection media containing the appropriate antibiotics; and (b) low membrane expression levels of the transgene, typically undetectable by flow cytometry. Therefore we developed a novel retroviral vector, called pSTITCH, and transfected this vector into two packaging cell lines. In brief:

1. pSTITCH contains the extended Moloney murine leukemia virus (MoMLV) packaging signal, a donor and acceptor splice site, a cloning site at the envelope gene position for optimal expression of the transgene, and the 5' and 3' MoMLV long terminal repeats (LTRs). The U3 region of the 5' LTR is replaced by the cytomegalovirus immediate early (CMV IE) promoter to upregulate expression of the transgene.

2. The presence of the SV40 origin of replication allows the vector to be used in both stable (i.e., PG13 packaging cell line) and transient transduction systems (i.e., co-transfection of the pSTITCH vector and packaging plasmids into the 293T packaging cell line, which results in the transient production of high-titered virus: 10^7 infectious units/ml).

3. PG13 and 293T have been chosen as packaging cell lines because they allow the production of pseudotyped MoMLV particles, which contain the gibbon ape leukemia virus (GALV) envelope instead of the envelope from MoMLV. Such pseudotyped virus particles infect human T lymphocytes much more efficiently owing to the high levels of the GALV envelope receptor on the cell membrane, whereas human T lymphocytes express only low levels of MoMLV envelope receptors.

4. The pSTITCH viral vector now allows high efficiency gene delivery to activated T lymphocytes from healthy donors as well as cancer patients (55). Because the efficacy of intracellular protein transport and functional expression of super immunoglobulin (Ig) family molecules in the

lymphocyte membrane critically depends on the receptor folding patterns, we also designed a number of chimeric receptor constructs (55).

Optimization of the Gene Structures of Single-Chain mAb Receptor Specific for G250 Antigen

We designed five chimeric receptor gene structures and subsequently compared their membrane expression on 293T cells and activated T lymphocytes. The aim was to study the effect of the chimeric receptor gene structure on the processes ultimately leading to functional T cell membrane expression. Flow cytometric analysis showed that distinct membrane expressions for the various chimeric receptor gene constructs were observed on 293T cells. Transduction of activated primary human T lymphocytes with four of the five chimeric receptor gene constructs resulted also in flow cytometrically detectable chimeric single-chain Ab/γ-receptor expression. These gene-modified T cells further demonstrated function, because they specifically recognized and lysed renal carcinoma cells.

We then studied the functional interaction between the density of single-chain Ab/γ-receptor expression on CTLs and the density of G250 ligands on renal carcinoma target cells. The low levels of single-chain Ab/γ-redirected lysis of renal carcinoma cells expressing G250 in low densities could be overcome by increasing the level of single-chain Ab/γ receptors on the CTLs. These combined results favor the use of T lymphocytes expressing single-chain Ab/γ receptors in high density for immunotherapy of renal carcinoma cells (55).

Further detailed studies of this kind can unravel the distinct phases of gene transduction: DNA transcription, protein folding, intracellular transport, functional membrane expression, affinity of antigen recognition, and signal transduction mechanisms. Such analysis may then finally allow definition of the basic gene structure requirements that

allow the engineering of functional chimeric receptors.

With the efficient pSTITCH retroviral gene transduction system and five optimal chimeric receptor gene constructs available, we now could study the functional balance between CTL chimeric receptor density and target cell antigen density. We already learned that individual TCRs on individual CTLs engage antigens and are serially triggered individually. The T cells then become activated as soon as a threshold signal has been accumulated. This serial use of sets of TCRs for antigen interaction on target cells underlies the mechanism by which CTLs lyse multiple target cells (7). Triggering TCRs below certain antigen densities therefore may not result in a full range of T cell functions. A good understanding of these parameters is of critical importance for the generation of gene-modified CTLs for immunogene therapy. To this end CTLs with relatively low and high chimeric receptor densities on the one hand and renal carcinoma cells with relatively low and high G250 antigen levels on the other were therefore mixed in all possible combinations. The following conclusions could be drawn: (a) triggering of the lytic machinery of single-chain Ab G250[LOW+] CTLs required a target G250 antigen threshold density on tumor cells, whereas (b) single-chain Ab G250[HIGH+] CTLs readily lysed target cells expressing G250 ligand below the threshold level.

Because we know that single-chain Ab/γ-mediated T lymphocyte lysis of tumor cells also involves adhesion/co-activation molecules, their expression was also determined by flow cytometry. Densities of CD54 and CD58 were identical for all renal carcinoma cell lines tested and therefore did not explain the lack of renal carcinoma cell lysis of G250 antigen[LOW+] renal carcinoma cells. When we employed single-chain Ab G250[HIGH+] CTLs in combination with G250 antigen[LOW+] target cells, even the G250 antigen[LOW] renal carcinoma cells were readily lysed. The same receptor–antigen relationship was found for lymphokine production. Our data show that the same set of rules apply to T cells expressing genetically introduced chimeric receptors that were earlier defined for T cells expressing endogenous TCRs. When neither receptor nor antigen density are limiting, the magnitude of the T lymphocyte response to antigen increases with increasing target cell antigen densities, possibly because the kinetics of the serial TCR triggering are enhanced, which may result in more frequent target cell lysis. The key point is that the quantity and quality of the T lymphocyte response depend on CTL receptor density as well as on target cell antigen density.

Chimeric TCR $\alpha\beta$ Gene Transfer into and Expression by Primary Human T Lymphocytes

We have seen that T lymphocyte specificity can be redirected by bs-mAbs or can be genetically reprogrammed by chimeric receptor gene transduction. We also noted that one of the reasons to take these approaches is the lack of technology that can reproducibly identify and clone T lymphocytes with MHC-restricted tumor specificity from individual patients. Despite the fact that the identification and cloning of MHC-presented tumor rejection antigens has been technically difficult, laborious, and unpredictable, the worldwide list of cloned tumor rejection

antigen-specific T lymphocyte clones and their relevant tumor rejection antigens (Table 30-1) has expanded.

Importantly, all of these recently identified and cloned tumor rejection antigens are not directly expressed at the tumor surface but are presented by MHC-I molecules following their intracellular degradation. Tumor rejection antigens can therefore be recognized only by TCRs on T lymphocytes and not by mAbs and so would escape immune recognition and destruction in mAb-based therapies. Obviously there is also an urgent need to be able to graft T lymphocytes from cancer patients with TCRs.

Studies involving HLA-typed cancer cells or cell lines transfected with MHC-I antigens have demonstrated that many T lymphocytes recognize shared tumor rejection antigens, restricted by a variety of MHC-I antigens (56–58). In principle, the knowledge is now available, which opens the way to apply a general strategy to graft any cancer patients' lymphocyte with a chimeric TCR-based tumor rejection antigen specificity, exactly as we have seen and for chimeric Ab-based receptor. To achieve this goal one has to construct chimeric TCRs comprising the α- and β-chains of tumor-specific TCRs by coupling them to the γ- and ζ-chain signaling transducing element. Then they must be tested to determine whether such chimeric TCRs re-

TABLE 30-1. *Overview of tumor rejection antigens associated with* in vivo *tumor regression*

Antigen	Other names	No. of amino acids	HLA restriction	Immunodominant	Characteristic
MART-I	Melan-A	118	A2	AAGIGILTV	Normal differentiation Ag
Gp 100	HMB-45 HMB-50 NKI/betab	661	A2	KTWGQYWQV ITDQVPFSV YLEPGPVTA	Normal differentiation Ag
Tyrosinase	—	529	A24	AFLPWHRLF	Normal differentiation Ag
P15	—	128	A24	AYGLDFYIL	Posttranscriptional control
TRP-I	gp75	527	A31	MSLQRQFLR	Translated from alternative ORF
β-Catenin	—	781	A24	SYLDSGIHF	Single base mutation

MAGE, GAGE, and BAGE gene families.
Ag, antigen; ORF, open reading frame.
Adapted from Rosenberg (36).

tain enough affinity and specificity to signal the T cell activation system following tumor rejection antigen stimulation. We used human CTLs specific for HLA-A1$^+$/MAGE-1$^+$ melanoma cells to pursue this goal.

Currently identified tumor rejection antigens comprise (a) proteins harboring tumor-specific mutations [e.g., β-catenin (59), CDK4 (60), and MUM-1 (61)]; (b) p15 protein and the MAGE, BAGE, and GAGE gene families, which are mainly expressed in the tumor and only in a few normal cell types (62,63); (c) normal differentiation antigens, such as MART-1, tyrosinase, or gp100, which are expressed in normal melanocytes and in malignant melanoma cells (62); and (d) proteins, which are expressed at a much higher level in the tumor than in the normal cells, such as wild-type p53 (64,65), carcinoembryonic antigen (CEA) (66), HER-2-neu (67), and the prostate-specific antigen (PSA) (68).

Construction and Expression of a Chimeric Two-Chain TCR with HLA-A1-Restricted Specificity for MAGE-1

Because only TCRs recognize tumor rejection antigen (56–58), we considered it necessary to extend our repertoire of tumor receptors for CTL gene targeting with HLA-restricted chimeric TCRs. As a model, we chose the TCR from the HLA-A1-restricted, MAGE-1-specific CTL clone MZ2-82/30 (69). This CTL clone has been derived from a patient with malignant melanoma; MAGE-1 is a peptide derived from the melanoma-associated antigen MZ2-E (69). MAGE-1 belongs to a family of closely related genes that are frequently expressed not only by melanomas but also by significant proportions of histologically distinct tumors, but not by normal tissues. The α- and β- chains of MZ2-82/30 belonged to the Vα12 and Vβ1 TCR families, for which family-type specific mAbs were available, allowing detection of gene-transduced chimeric TCRs on T lymphocytes by flow cytometry.

Construction and Transduction of the Chimeric TCR VαCα-ζ and VβCβ-ζ Genes

The extracellular domains from the TCRα- and β-chain were obtained by reverse transcriptase polymerase chain reaction (RT-PCR). RNA from the CTL clone MZ2-82/30 was amplified using α- and β-chain (Vα, Vβ, Cα, and Cβ) specific primers, which included appropriate restriction sites. To construct the chimeric VαCα-ζ and VβCβ-ζ genes, VαCα and VβCβ were ligated 5' to the ζ gene in pBluescript. The CD3 ζ-chain was isolated from a human T lymphocyte clone. The chimeric VαCα-ζ and VβCβ-ζ genes were then cloned into the pSTITCH retroviral vector.

For gene transduction, CD3 mAb-activated T lymphocytes were co-cultivated with the packaging cells producing pSTITCH-VαCα-ζ vectors, followed by co-cultivations with packaging cells producing pSTITCH-VβCβ-ζ vectors.

Using mAbs specific for the Vα12 and Vβ1 TCR gene families in a two-color immunofluorescence technique, we demonstrated the simultaneous and closely correlated membrane expression of the α and β transgenes on approximately 30% of the T lymphocytes. This result allowed us to enrich the chimeric two-chain TCR gene-transduced T lymphocytes by cell sorting. In parallel, we obtained T cell clones expressing both transgenes in a limiting dilution culture experiment.

The human, primary T lymphocytes expressing chimeric TCR$\alpha\beta$ genes indeed were shown, for the first time to our knowledge, to recognize and lyse melanoma cells with the relevant native HLA-A1-presented MAGE-1. HLA-A1$^+$, MAGE-1$^-$ melanoma cells were not lysed but became susceptible to lysis after peptide loading with MAGE-1. The efficacy of lysis by chimeric TCR$^+$ CTLs is, however, lower than that observed of the parental CTL clone.

In this context it is of importance to take

into account that progression of cancer is accompanied by a general reduction of immune functions such as NK activity, (cytolytic) lymphocyte functions, lymphokine production, and delayed-type hypersensitivity. Moreover, in mice and humans, altered patterns of protein tyrosine phosphorylations and significant reduction of the protein tyrosine kinases P56^{lck} and ζ-chain have been observed. These ζ-chains and protein tyrosine kinases fulfill pivotal functions in signal transduction and activation of T lymphocyte responses. These findings have been described in patients with cancer of several histologic types and in various stages of progression. The mechanisms involved in T cell inactivation have not yet been unraveled, but it is clear that one might consider first correcting the defect in lymphocyte signal transduction molecule expression. This may be achieved by an IL-2-based activation step in vaccination protocols or by genetically modifying autologous T lymphocytes that have been activated to exert immune functions following gene transduction.

Signaling molecules such as CD3-ζ can translate the variations in the half-lives of the TCR–ligand interactions into discrete phosphoforms resulting in distinct biologic outcomes: the translation of affinity into immune responses (70–72). Multistep ζ phosphorylation molecularly sets signaling thresholds that determine whether a TCR–ligand interaction is strong enough to result in a particular T cell function or in a full range of T cell functions. With this in mind, we could hypothesize that the putative lower affinity of a chimeric TCR versus the parental TCR results in a weaker triggering signal. This possibility calls for further identification and analysis of the signaling mechanisms and pathways. Such detailed knowledge would allow construction of chimeric TCRs that activate the full T cell response following target interaction in terms of quantity and quality: effective cancer cell kill, growth arrest, and antitumor T cell memory.

CONCLUSIONS

With the technology and the scientific advances of today combined with the cytokines and drugs available it is now possible to graft cancer patients with a specific anticancer active immune cell. Immune cells from the T, NK, or other myelolymphoid lineage can be programmed with any immune specificity for which an antibody on TCRs has been identified. To extend the list of TCRs one can exploit the fact that the use of immunodominant peptides derived from tumor rejection antigens can be pulsed into peripheral blood mononuclear cells. T lymphocytes can be generated *in vitro* with far greater antitumor potency (50 to 100 times) than that of the TILs. Once equipped with these chimeric signaling receptors, the immune cells produce cytokines, proliferate, and attack the tumor.

This chimeric receptor grafting approach is technology, rather than disease, oriented. Therefore it can also be instrumental for the clinical control and elimination of viral infections, autoimmune disease, and graft-versus-host disease. The use of these chimeric receptor-positive immune cells can be combined with cytokines and vaccination procedures in a combined therapeutic approach. A phase I/II clinical feasibility study in metastatic renal carcinoma using specific chimeric antibodies was to be initiated in 1999. The third wave of immune gene therapy has begun.

REFERENCES

1. Ehrlich P. Ueber den jetzigen Stand der Karzinomforschung. *Ned Tijdschr Geneeskd* 1901;35:273–290.
2. Burnett FM. The concept of immunological surveilance. *Prog Exp Tumor Res* 1970;13:1–27.
3. Ridge JP, Fuchs EJ, Matzinger P. Neonatal tolerance revisited: turning on newborn T cells with dendritic cells. *Science* 1996;271:1723–1726.
4. Bolhuis RLH, Hoogenboom HR, Gratama JW. Targeting of peripheral blood T lymphocytes. *Springer Semin Immunopathol* 1996;18:211–227.
5. Bolhuis RLH, Van de Griend RJ. Phytohemagglutinin-induced proliferation and cytolytic activity in T3$^+$ but not in T3$^-$ cloned T lymphocytes requires the involvement of the T3 antigen for signal transmission. *Cell Immunol* 1985;93:46–57.

6. Blank-Voorthuis CJAC, Braakman E, Ronteltap CPM, et al. Clustered CD3/TCR complexes do not transduce activation signals after bispecific monoclonal antibody-triggered lysis by cytotoxic T lymphocytes via CD3. *J Immunol* 1993;151:2904–2914.

7. Valitutti S, Müller S, Cella M, Padovan E, Lanzavecchia A. Serial triggering of many T-cell receptors by a few peptide-MHC complexes. *Nature* 1995; 375:148–151.

8. Van Seventer GA, Shimizu Y, Shaw S. Roles of multiple accessory molecules in T-cell activation. *Curr Opin Immunol* 1991;3:294–303.

9. Bolhuis RLH, Gravekamp C, Van de Griend RJ. Cell–cell interactions. *Clin Immunol Allergy* 1986;6:29–90.

10. Galandrini R, Albi N, Tripodi G, et al. Antibodies to CD44 trigger effector functions of human T cell clones. *J Immunol* 1993;150:4225–4235.

11. Seth A, Gote L, Nagarkatti PS. T-cell-receptor-independent activation of cytolytic activity of cytotoxic T lymphocytes mediated through CD44 and gp90[MEL-14]. *Proc Natl Acad Sci USA* 1991;88:7877–7881.

12. Kupfer A, Singer SJ, Janeway CA, Swain SL. Coclustering of CD34 (L3T4) molecule with the T-cell receptor is induced by specific direct interaction of helper T cells and antigen-presenting cells. *Proc Natl Acad Sci USA* 1997;84:5888–5892.

13. Hersey P, Bolhuis RLH. "Non-specific" MHC-unrestricted killer cells and their receptors. *Immunol Today* 1987;8:233–239.

14. Rodewald H-R, Moingeon P, Lucich JL, Dosiou C, Lopez P, Reinherz EL. A population of early fetal thymocytes expressing FctRII/III contains precursors of T lymphocytes and natural killer cells. *Cell* 1992;69:139–150.

15. Sanchez MJ, Spits H, Lanier LL, Philips JH. Human natural killer cell committed thymocytes and their relation to the T cell lineage. *J Exp Med* 1993; 178:1857–1866.

16. Kägi D, Ledermann B, Burki K, et al. Cytotoxicity mediated by T cells and natural killer cells is greatly impaired in perforin-deficient mice. *Nature* 1994; 369:31–37.

17. Arase H, Arase N, Saiti T. Fas-mediated cytotoxicity by freshly isolated natural killer cells. *J Exp Med* 1995;181:1235–1238.

18. Rouvier E, Lusiani MF, Golstein P. Fas involvement in Ca^{2+} independent T cell-mediated cytotoxicity. *J Exp Med* 1993;177:195–200.

19. Bennett M. Biology and genetics of hybrid resistance. *Adv Immunol* 1987;41:333–445.

20. Heslop BF. Allogeneic lymphocyte cytotoxicity (ALC) in rats: allogeneic recognition vs. failed self recognition. In Rolstad B (ed) *Natural Immunity to Normal Hemopoietic Cells.* Boca Raton, CRC Press, 1994, pp. 1–32.

21. Rolstad B, Wonigeit K, Vaage JT. 4. Alloreactive rat natural killer (NK) cells in vivo and in vitro: the role of the major histocompatibility complex (MHC). In Rolstad B (ed) *Natural Immunity to Normal Hemopoietic Cells.* Boca Raton, CRC Press, 1994, pp. 99–149.

22. Rolstad B, Ford WL. The rapid elimination of allogeneic lymphocytes: relationship to established mechanisms of immunity and to lymphocyte traffic. *Immunol Rev* 1983;73:87–113.

23. Moretta A, Bottino C, Pende D, et al. Identification of four subsets of human CD3$^-$ CD16$^+$ natural killer (NK) cells by the expression of clonally distributed functional surface molecules: correlation between subset assignment of NK clones and ability to mediate specific alloantigen recognition. *J Exp Med* 1990;172:1589–1598.

24. Ljunggren H-G, Kärre K. In search of the "missing self": MHC molecules and NK cell recognition. *Immunol Today* 1990;11:237–244.

25. Valiante NM, Lienert K, Shilling HG, Smits BJ, Parham P. Killer cell receptors: keeping pace with MHC class I evolution. *Immunol Rev* 1997; 155:155–164.

26. Moretta A, Tambussi G, Bottino C, et al. A novel surface antigen expressed by a subset of human CD3$^-$ CD16$^+$ natural killer cells. *J Exp Med* 1990;171:695–714.

27. Moretta A, Biassoni R, Bottino C, et al. Major histocompatibility complex class I-specific receptors on human natural killer and T lymphocytes. *Immunol Rev* 1997;155:105–117.

28. Litwin V, Gumperz J, Parham P, Philips JH, Lanier LL. NBK1: a natural killer cell receptor involved in the recognition of polymorphic HLA-B molecules. *J Exp Med* 1994;180:537–543.

29. Lanier LL, Corliss B, Philips JH. Arousal and inhibition of human NK cells. *Immunol Rev* 1997;155: 145–154.

30. Pende D, Biassoni R, Cantoni C, et al. The natural killer cell receptor specific for HLA-A allotypes: a novel member of the p58/p70 family of inhibitory receptors that is characterized by three immunoglobulin-like domains and is expressed as a 140-kD disulphide-linked dimer. *J Exp Med* 1996;184: 505–518.

31. Colonna M, Samaridis J. Cloning of immunoglobulin-superfamily members associated with HLA-C and HLA-B recognition by human natural killer cells. *Science* 1995;268:405–408.

32. Lanier LL, Philips JH. Inhibitory MHC class I receptors on NK cells and T cells. *Immunol Today* 1996;17:86–91.

33. Cella M, Döhring C, Samaridis J, et al. A novel inhibitory receptor (ILT3) expressed on monocytes, macrophages, and dendritic cells involved in antigen processing. *J Exp Med* 1997;185:1743–1751.

34. Romero P, Pannetier C, Herman J, Victor Jongeneel C, Cerottini J-C, Coulie PG. Multiple specificities in the repertoire of a melanoma patient's cytolytic T lymphocyte directed against tumor antigen MAGE-1.A1. *J Exp Med* 1995;182:1019–1028.

35. Bolhuis RLH, Schellekens H. Induction of natural killer cell activity and allocytotoxicity in human peripheral blood lymphocytes after mixed lymphocyte culture. *Scand J Immunol* 1981;13:401–412.

36. Rosenberg SA. Cancer vaccines based on the identification of genes encoding cancer regression antigens. *Immunol Today* 1997;4:175–182.

37. Bolhuis RLH, Lamers CHJ, Goey SH, et al. Adoptive immunotherapy of ovarian carcinoma with bsmAb targeted lymphocytes: a multicenter study. *Int J Cancer* 1992;7:78–81.

38. Canevari S, Stoter G, Arienti F, et al. Regression of advanced ovarian carcinoma by intraperitoneal treatment with autologous T lymphocytes retargeted by a bispecific monoclonal antibody. *J Natl Cancer Inst* 1995;87:1463–1469.

39. Jain RK. Delivery of novel therapeutic agents in tumors: physiological barriers. *J Natl Cancer Inst* 1989;81:570–576.

40. Lanzavecchia A, Scheidegger D. The use of hybrid hybridomas to target human cytotoxic T lymphocytes. *Eur J Immunol* 1987;17:105–111.

41. Eshhar Z, Waks T, Gross G, Schindler DG. Specific activation and targeting of cytotoxic lymphocytes through chimeric single-chains consisting of antibody binding domains and the γ or ζ subunits of the immunoglobulin and T cell receptors. *Proc Natl Acad Sci USA* 1993;90:720–724.

42. Stancovski I, Schindler DG, Waks T, Yarden Y, Sela M, Eshhar Z. Targeting of T lymphocytes to Neu/HER2-expressing cells using chimeric single-chain Fv receptors. *J Immunol* 1993;11:6577–6582.

43. Bird RE, Hardman KD, Jacobson JW, et al. single-chain antigen-binding proteins. *Science* 1988; 242:423–426.

44. Colcher D, Bird R, Roselli M, et al. In vivo tumor targeting of a recombinant single-chain antigen-binding protein. *J Natl Cancer Inst* 1990;82:1191–1197.

45. Wels W, Harwerth IM, Hynes NE, Groner B. Diminution of antibodies directed against tumor cell surface epitopes: a single-chain Fv fusion molecule specifically recognizes the extracellular domain of the c-erb B2 receptor. *J Steroid Biochem Mol Biol* 1992;43:1–7.

46. Brocker T, Peter A, Traunecker A, Karjalainen K. New simplified molecular design for functional T cell receptor. *Eur J Immunol* 1993;23:1435–1439.

47. Moritz D, Wels W, Mattern J, Groner B. Cytotoxic T lymphocytes with grafted recognition specificity for ERBB2-expressing tumor cells. *Proc Natl Acad Sci USA* 1994;91:4318.

48. Hwu P, Shafer GE, Treisman J, et al. Lysis of ovarian cancer cells by human lymphocytes redirected with a chimeric gene composed of an antibody V region and the Fc receptor γ chain. *J Exp Med* 1993;178:361–366.

49. Roberts MR, Qin L, Zhang D, et al. Targeting of human immunodeficiency virus-infected cells by CD8$^+$ T lymphocytes armed with universal T-cell receptors. *Blood* 1994;84:2878.

50. Bolhuis RLH, Gratama JW. Genetic re-targeting of T lymphocyte specificity. *Gene Ther* 1998;9:1153–1155.

51. Oosterwijk E, Debruyne FMJ, Schalken JA. The use of monoclonal antibody G250 in the therapy of renal-cell carcinoma. *Semin Oncol* 1995;22:34–41.

52. Braakman E, Van Beusechem VW, Van Krimpen BA, Fischer A, Bolhuis RLH, Valerio D. Genetic correction of cultured T cells from an adenosine deaminase-deficient patient: characteristics of nontransduced and transduced T cells. *Eur J Immunol* 1992;22:63–69.

53. Weijtens MEM, Willemsen RA, Valerio D, Stam K, Bolhuis RLH. Single-chain immunoglobin/γ gene redicted human T lymphocytes produce cytokines,

54. Weijtens MEM, Willemsen RA, van Krimpen BA, Bolhuis RLH. Chimeric scFv/γ receptor mediated T cell lysis of tumor cells is co-regulated by adhesion and accessory molecules. *Int J Cancer* 1998;77:181–187.

55. Weijtens MEM, Willemsen RA, Hart EH, Bolhuis RLH. A retroviral vector system "STITCH" in combination with an optimized single-chain antibody chimeric receptor gene structure allows efficient gene transduction and expression in human T lymphocytes. *Gene Ther* 1998;5:1195–1203.

56. Darrow TL, Slingluff CL, Seigler HF. The role of HLA class I antigens in recognition of melanoma cells by tumor-specific cytotoxic T lymphocytes: evidence for shared tumor antigens. *J Immunol* 1989;142:153–164.

57. Kawakami Y, Zakut R, Topalian SL, Stotter H, Rosenberg SA. Shared human melanoma antigens: recognition by tumor-infiltrating lymphocytes in HLA-A2.I-transfected melanomas. *J Immunol* 1992;148:638–643.

58. O'Neil BH, Kawakami Y, Restifo NP, Bennink JR, Yewdell JW, Rosenberg SA. Detection of shared MHC-restricted human melanoma antigens after vaccinia virus-mediated transduction of genes coding for HLA. *J Immunol* 1993;151:1410–1418.

59. Robbins PF, El-Gamil M, Li Y, et al. Cloning of a new gene encoding an antigen recognized by melanoma-specific HLA-A24-restricted tumor-infiltrating lymphocytes. *J Immunol* 1995;154:5944–5950.

60. Wölfel T, Hauer M, Schneider J, et al. A p16^{INK4a}-insensitive CDK4 mutant targeted by cytolytic T lymphocytes in human melanoma. *Science* 1995; 269:1281–1284.

61. Coulie PG, Lehmann F, Lethé B, et al. A mutated intron sequence codes for an antigenic peptide recognized by cytolytic T lymphocytes on a human melanoma. *Proc Natl Acad Sci USA* 1995;92:7976–7980.

62. Boon T, van der Bruggen P. Human tumor antigens recognized by T lymphocytes. *J Exp Med* 1996;183:725–729.

63. Böhm CM, Hanski M-L, Stefanovic S, et al. Identification of HLA-A2 restricted epitopes of the tumor-associated antigen MUC2 recognized by human cytotoxic T cells. *Int J Cancer* 1998;75:688–693.

64. Röpke M, Hald J, Guldeberg P, et al. Spontaneous human squamous cell carcinomas are killed by a human cytotoxic T lymphocyte clone recognizing a wild-type p53-derived peptide. *Proc Natl Acad Sci USA* 1996;93:14704–14707.

65. Theobald M, Bigg J, Dittmer D, Levine AJ, Scherman LA. Targeting p53 as a general tumor antigen. *Proc Natl Acad Sci USA* 1995;92:11993–11997.

66. Tsang KY, Zaremba S, Nieroda CA, Zhu MZ, Hamilton JM, Schlom J. Generation of human cytotoxic T cells specific for human carcinoembryonic antigen epitopes from patients immunized with recombinant vaccinia-CEA vaccine. *J Natl Cancer Inst* 1995;87:982–990.

67. Fisk B, Blevins TL, Wharton JT, Ioannides CG.

Identification of an immunodominant peptide of HER-2/neu protooncogene recognized by ovarian tumor-specific cytotoxic T lymphocyte lines. *J Exp Med* 1995;181:2109–2117.

68. Correale P, Walmsley K, Nieroda C, et al. In vitro generation of human cytotoxic T lymphocytes specific for peptides derived from prostate specific antigen. *J Natl Cancer Inst* 1997;89:293–300.

69. Van der Bruggen P, Traversari C, Chomez P, et al. A gene encoding an antigen recognized by cytolytic T lymphocytes on a human melanoma. *Science* 1991;254:1643–1647.

70. Neumeister Kersh E, Shaw AS, Allen PM. Fidelity of T cell activation through multistep T cell receptor ζ phosphorylation. *Science* 1998;281:572–575.

71. O' Rourke AM, Mescher MF. The roles of CD8 in cytotoxic T lymphocyte function. *Immunol Today* 1993;14:183–188.

72. Malissen B. Translating affinity into response. *Science* 1998;281:528–529.

Cytotoxic Cells: Basic Mechanisms and Medical Applications, edited by Michail V. Sitkovsky and Pierre A. Henkart. Lippincott Williams & Wilkins, Philadelphia © 2000.

Chapter 31

Cytotoxic T Lymphocyte Adoptive Immunotherapy for HIV Infection

Judy Lieberman

The Center for Blood Research and Department of Pediatrics, Harvard Medical School, Boston, Massachusetts 02115, USA

In most, if not all, untreated patients infected with the human immunodeficiency virus type 1 (HIV), a chronic infection is established that over time leads to destruction of lymphoid organs, progressive immunodeficiency, and eventual death. Antiretroviral drugs that target the viral reverse transcriptase and protease given in combination can generally control viral production to levels that are below detection of sensitive amplified polymerase chain reaction (PCR) assays and slow (or possibly prevent) the inexorable progression of immunodeficiency. Even under these circumstances, however, HIV infection persists in CD4 T cells and tissue macrophages, and infectious virus can be cultured and detected with sufficiently sensitive assays in lymphoid tissue (1). When antiretroviral drugs are discontinued, the virus typically rebounds to predrug levels. This suggests that protective immunosurveillance does not develop in most HIV-infected patients during the natural history of the infection or even after months of effective suppression of viral replication. The goal of immune-based therapy for HIV is to enhance the efficacy of highly active combination antiretroviral drug therapy (HAART) either to eradicate the virus or to induce a state of protective immunosurveillance that might enable drug withdrawal.

ANTIVIRAL CTLs: KEY COMPONENT OF PROTECTIVE IMMUNITY TO HIV INFECTION

Developing a successful strategy for immune-based therapy for HIV infection requires understanding which aspects of the immune response are protective, which are possibly harmful, and why the protective immune response ultimately fails. After more than a decade of intense investigation, no clear-cut consensus exists about the answers to these questions. In part this is because the virus infects key regulatory cells in the immune system, the CD4-expressing T-helper cells, and monocyte-derived macrophage antigen-presenting cells. The activation of these cells, required for their function in protective immunity, can also stimulate viral replication (2,3). The complex regulatory mechanisms that have evolved to contain a vigorous immune response also sometimes make it difficult to distinguish cause and effect in the immune response. Increased viral antigen can lead to a more pronounced immune response at low levels of virus but a dampened response at higher levels. Moreover, merely counting the number of activated or antigen-specific CD8 T cells can lead to misleading conclusions if cytolytic function does not correlate with the phenotypic activation state because of anergy. Similarly, although antigen-specific cells are likely to be protective, they may also (particularly CD4 T cells) provide excellent vehicles for enhanced viral replication. These factors together with the heterogeneity of HIV disease in a complex and varied human population and the absence of a good small animal model have made it difficult to develop a simple consensus about protective immunity. However, research focused at critical times in the infection, such as at the point of infection, and at subgroups of individuals with a widely differing disease course (long-term nonprogressors, or LTNPs, and rapid disease progressors) has begun to provide important information (Fig. 31-1).

Antiviral immunity can in some cases provide sterilizing protection from persistent infection. In studies of sex workers in two regions of Africa, homosexuals with multiple partners, the spouses of HIV-infected hemophiliacs, children born to HIV-infected mothers, and exposed health workers, some exposed individuals have vigorous T cell proliferative and cytotoxic T cell (CTL) responses to HIV proteins but have no evidence of ongoing viral infection or antiviral antibodies (5–8). It is uncertain whether these uninfected individuals were ever actively infected with replicating virus and cleared it, whether they were in effect immunized with defective virus, or whether they may harbor rare cells containing infection-competent virus. One case report of a child who appears to have cleared an active perinatally acquired infection suggests that it may indeed be possible for natural immunity to eradicate HIV infection or at least contain it to a level at which it escapes sensitive assays (9). The evidence from the uninfected exposed cohorts suggests that cellular immunity [by viral-specific T cells and probably natural killer (NK) cells] is likely critical for protection. In fact, some of the vaccination approaches that have been most successful in conferring protection in the

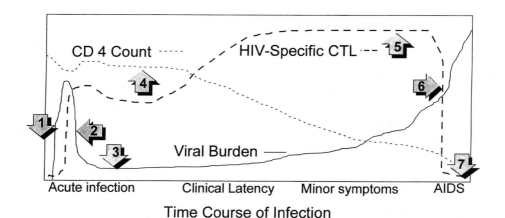

Time Course of Infection

FIG. 31-1. Clinical evidence that HIV-specific CTLs are protective.(1) Multiply exposed but uninfected individuals have HIV-specific T cell proliferation and CTLs. Vaccine strategies that are protective against SIV infection in macaques often induce antiviral CTLs. (2) Appearance of antiviral CTLs coincides with resolution of the viremia of primary infection. (3) The viral set-point (plasma viral level reached after resolution of primary infection) correlates with the frequency of viral-specific CTLs. (4) Neonates with immature cell-mediated immunity have a more rapid disease course. (5) Chronically infected individuals with gag-specific CTLs are less likely to progress to AIDS. (6) There is a decline in antiviral CTLs about the time of disease progression(4). (7) It is rare to detect antiviral CTLs in patients with a history of major opportunistic infections.

simian immunodeficiency virus (SIV) macaque model would be expected to induce antiviral CTLs (10,11).

In most patients natural immunity does not eradicate the virus but is able to control infection and maintain long-term clinical latency. At a certain point, however, the immune system loses control, the balance tips in favor of the virus, and the infected patient develops the complications of acquired immunodeficiency syndrome (AIDS). Circumstantial *in vitro* and epidemiological evidence supports the idea that HIV-specific CTLs play a key role in keeping HIV in check (Fig. 31-1). CD8 T cells are key effector cells in antiviral immunity against most viruses (12,13). CD8 T cells can suppress HIV replication *in vitro* by direct cytotoxicity and by secretion of soluble factors (14–17). These factors include the chemokines RANTES and MIP-1α, produced by effector CTLs. These chemokines bind to CCR5, the HIV co-receptor on monocytes, macrophages, and some T cells and block the fusion of HIV envelope protein gp160 to the cell membrane required for viral entry (17). Because the chemokines are stored in the cytotoxic granules (18), it is likely that direct cytotoxicity and viral suppression by chemokines work in parallel. In addition, the chemokines can stimulate cytolysis and lymphocyte proliferation (19). However, other CTL factors, including the distinct but uncharacterized CD8 T cell antiviral factor (CAF), interleukin-16 (IL-16), and interferon-γ (IFN-γ), may play a significant role in viral suppression by other mechanisms, including suppression of transcription from the HIV long terminal repeat (LTR) (20–23). CAF is probably produced by naive CD8 T cells that have not differentiated to CTLs, judged by the phenotype of cells that produce this activity (24). The relative importance of direct cytotoxicity versus indirect inhibition in controlling viral production is unclear (25).

Appearance of HIV-specific CTLs coincides with resolution of the viremia of the acute infection; neutralizing antibodies do not develop until weeks later (26,27). This is also true in primate models. An increased frequency of viral antigen-specific CD8 T cells, detected by their binding to HIV peptides attached to fluorescently-labeled HLA class I molecules (so-called tetramers) (28), correlates with lower plasma viremia in untreated patients (29). Recent studies of long-term nonprogressors suggest that these individuals have low viral burden in conjunction with high levels of anti-HIV precursor CTLs (30,31). Perinatal infection, at a time of incomplete maturity of cellular immunity, is generally associated with a weaker antiviral CTL response, higher levels of plasma viremia, and an accelerated disease course compared to adult infection. Moreover, infants who develop CD8 viral-suppressive activity and antiviral cytotoxicity tend to have a more benign course (32,33). In a cohort study of infected individuals, the likelihood of progressing to AIDS increases in patients who lack *gag*-specific CTLs (34,35). In another study less rapid disease progression after primary infection correlated with the presence of anti-gp160 CTLs (36). In studies of individual patients, virus-specific CTL activity declines just about the time that opportunistic infections appear (4,37). Once AIDS-defining opportunistic infections have occurred, it is unusual to detect virus-specific CTL activity.

When this evidence is taken together with the protective role CTLs play in animal infections with other pathogenic viruses, best demonstrated by adoptive transfer experiments or by generating protective antiviral immunity with a CTL epitope vaccine (12,38), it is likely that virus-specific CTLs are a key component of protective immunity. However, the protective versus pathologic role of CD8 T cells in HIV infection has been a subject of controversy (39,40). There are legitimate concerns that HIV-specific CTLs may contribute to the immunodeficiency of HIV infection by lysing HIV-infected CD4 cells or even CD4 cells that have bound and internalized serum gp120 via the CD4 receptor. Inflammatory changes induced by specific CTLs might also be involved in the neurologic manifestations of HIV infection or in HIV-related interstitial pneumonitis not attributable to any known infectious agent (41,42). These concerns have been reinforced by the association of increased numbers of activated CD38$^+$DR$^+$ CD8 T cells with increased plasma viral levels, decreased CD4 counts, and poor prognosis (43–46). In infections with nonpathogenic viruses, such as lymphochoriomeningitis virus or hepatitis B and C, viral-specific CTL contribute significantly to the immunopathology (39,47–53). However, HIV is a pathogenic virus. In these instances of CTL-induced immunopathology, CTLs induce apoptosis in bystander cells by activation of Fas- or tumor necrosis factor (TNF) receptor-mediated lysis (53–57). However, we have recently been able to show that neither CTL clones nor circulating CD8 T cells use the Fas pathway to any appreciable extent to lyse HIV-infected cells (58). Nor do they lyse uninfected bystander cells in the process of recognizing HIV-infected targets. Therefore, although the CTL response to HIV may have a role in some of the disease manifestations of HIV infection, such as nonspecific pneumonitis or central nervous system (CNS) symptoms, it is likely that their dominant effect is protective.

WHY DO VIRUS-SPECIFIC CTLs NOT PROVIDE BETTER PROTECTION?

There is a high frequency of HIV-specific CTLs in HIV-infected patients who have not yet developed major opportunistic infections [Centers for Disease Control (CDC) stages A and B]. Early estimates based on limiting dilution analysis suggested that as many as 1 in 1,000 circulating mononuclear cells were specific for HIV gag- or gp160-expressing targets (4,37). However, the assumptions of limiting dilution analysis were invalid, as the assays used in these studies were not sensitive enough to detect a single effector cell per well. We estimated that, in fact, as many as 1 in 12 mononuclear cells in some patients were specific for a particular HIV protein (59). Furthermore, assays that enumerated

HIV-specific precursor CTLs (pCTLs) gave underestimates because the clonogenic potential of CD8 T cells in infected patients was severely compromised (60). Studies that enumerated the frequency of CD8 T cells recognizing a particular HIV peptide epitope, using functional signs of antigen-specific activation or fluorescently-labeled tetramers of major histocompatibility complex class I (MHC-I) molecules folded with HIV epitopic peptides, suggest that up to a few percent of circulating CD8 T cells are specific for a particular HIV peptide epitope in patients with early- or moderate-stage disease (28,29,61,62). Because most patients recognize at least several dominant epitopes (63), the frequency of specific antiviral CD8 T cells comprises a substantial fraction (measured in the range of percents) of the expanded CD8 T cell pool. This number likely does not decline until late in disease, probably around the time of development of major opportunistic infections (4,61). The high frequency of antigen-specific CD8 T cells in HIV-infected donors simplifies the *ex vivo* generation of highly potent antiviral CTL lines or clones from infected donors (59,64–66).

Because the frequency of HIV-specific CTLs in most infected patients is high and these cells can suppress viral production by direct cytotoxicity and secreted soluble factors, the question arises why antiviral CTLs do not provide better protection. Even when viral production is relatively well controlled with HAART, protective immunosurveillance does not develop to prevent viral rebound on drug withdrawal. There are some recent clues to help answer this question. Many viruses have devised strategies to evade an immune response (67). During latent infection viral proteins are not expressed, and therefore latently infected cells are hidden from immune surveillance. Some reports indicate that HIV nef induces downmodulation of MHC-I molecules from the surface of the infected cell (68,69). Whether this is of sufficient extent to inhibit CTL recognition is not clear. Although we have found that many HIV-specific CTL clones recognize and lyse primary HIV-infected target cells as efficiently as artificial targets loaded with antigenic peptides (70), for some HIV-specific clones, perhaps those with lower-affinity T cell receptor or that recognize antigens produced in limiting amounts, the reduction of cell surface MHC expression may critically reduce recognition (69,71).

However, when freshly isolated blood mononuclear cells from HIV-infected donors who have not progressed to symptomatic disease are tested in short-term (4 hour) cytotoxicity assays, they generally do not demonstrate significant HIV-specific cytotoxicity (72) (Fig. 31-2). High levels of antiviral cytotoxicity (specific cytotoxicity of up to 30% at an effector/target ratio of 25:1) develop *in vitro*, however, after overnight culture in an IL-2-dependent manner. This suggests that circulating HIV-specific CD8 T cells are functionally anergic in lysing HIV-presenting targets (72–74). The molecular basis and etiology of the lack of cytotoxicity by freshly isolated cells is not certain. A large fraction of circulating CD8 T cells in HIV-infected donors are already activated, as evidenced by high levels of expression of CD38, HLA-DR, and CD57 and the cytolytic serine esterase granzyme A (44,74–82). Many of the CD8 T cells also do not express CD28 (76,83–85). In one study, 71% ± 12% of circulating CD8 T cells stained for granzyme A, compared to 41% ± 10% in normal donors (72). Moreover, there is a good correlation in circulating CD8 T cells between granzyme A and perforin expression (L. W. Kam and J. Lieberman, unpublished data). Therefore it seems likely that they are armed for cytolysis. However, anomalies of T cell signaling after activation have been described in CD8 T cells from HIV-infected donors (72,74,86–88). In fact, a large fraction of CD8 T cells in HIV-infected donors has downmodulated cell surface expression of CD3ζ, the key proximal signaling chain of the T cell receptor (72). Moreover, cells that have downmodulated CD3ζ also do not express the key co-stimulatory molecule CD28. CD8 T cells with downmodulated CD3ζ and CD28 are

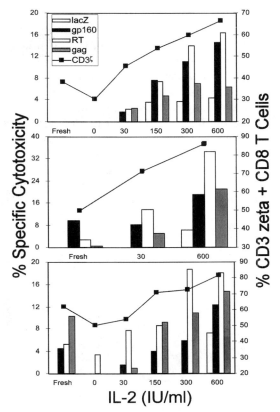

FIG. 31-2. HIV-specific cytotoxicity by freshly isolated lymphocytes is absent or barely detected in three HIV-infected donors but increases after overnight culture in an IL-2 dependent manner (72). Subject A has CDC stage B3 disease; subject B has stage C2 disease; and subject C has stage B2 disease. Cytotoxicity is measured against autologous B cells infected with recombinant vaccinia viruses expressing lacZ control (vSC8), gp160 (vPE16), RT (vCF21), and gag (vDK1). The percent of CD8 T cells that express CD3ζ increases concomitantly. (From ref. 72, with permission.)

relatively resistant to activation by the T cell receptor (L. Trimble and J. Lieberman, manuscript in preparation). A similar phenomenon has been described in tumor-infiltrating lymphocytes in mouse tumor models and human solid tumors, in circulating CD8 T cells in human lymphoma patients, in the blood of patients with systemic lupus erythematosus, and in the inflamed joints of rheumatoid arthritis (89–93)

CD3ζ downmodulation, which increases with disease progression and interferes with T cell activation, corrects within 6 to 10 hours of *in vitro* culture in an IL-2 dependent manner (72). Development of cytotoxic function *in vitro* requires a longer incubation time than that required for reexpression of CD3ζ. Therefore it is likely that the lack of cytolytic function is not simply due to CD3ζ and CD28 downmodulation and that other molecular events must occur *in vitro* to restore CTL function. Perforin expression has been found to be markedly reduced in lymph node CD8

T cells from samples taken after the acute infection (94) (Fig. 31-3). This defect is selective for perforin, as granzyme A is present and is specific to HIV infection because perforin and granzyme A are expressed in tandem in the lymph nodes during acute infectious mononucleosis. The lack of perforin in T cells at the site of infection is likely to interfere with the ability of CTLs to control HIV production.

Understanding why virus-specific CTLs are functionally anergic is critical to designing sustainable immunotherapy. Although

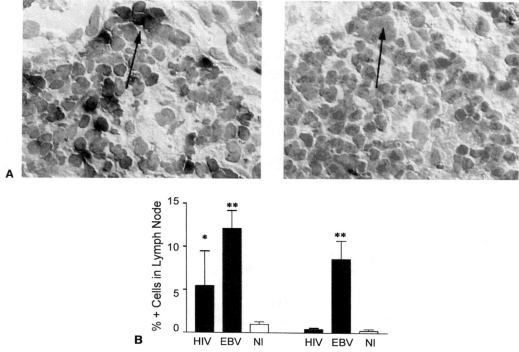

FIG. 31-3. **A:** Selective defect in perforin, but not granzyme A, expression is seen in immunohistochemically stained lymph node sections from a patient after primary HIV infection. Left (granzyme) and right (perforin) images are from the same tissue area. Perforin and granzyme A are stained brown with diaminobenzadine, and all cells are counterstained with hematoxylin. **B:** Bar graphs depict the mean area of perforin- and granzyme A-staining cells in lymph node biopsy specimens obtained from patients with recent HIV infection, acute Epstein-Barr virus (EBV) infection (infectious mononucleosis), and normal controls (NI). Quantitation is by *in situ* computer imaging. The proportion of granzyme A staining cells in the 16 HIV-infected samples differs significantly (* $p < 0.05$) from that of normal control samples, but perforin staining is comparable to that of normal controls. The lymph nodes from infectious mononucleosis patients had similar amounts of granzyme A and perforin staining, which was greatly increased compared to that in normal samples (** $p < 0.001$). (From ref. 94, courtesy of J. Andersson, Karolinska Institute.)

there are multiple plausible explanations for the ultimate loss of specific cellular immunity, the factors important in an infected person are not known. Along with the decline in CD4 T cell number and function with HIV infection, there is a notable absence of specific CD4 T cell proliferation to HIV in patients at all stages of disease (95). HIV-specific CD4 T cells may be selectively depleted early in infection because of the increased susceptibility of activated CD4 T cells to HIV infection (96). The consequent loss of second signals, ordinarily provided by the CD4 helper cell compartment and required for CTL proliferation and activation, surely contributes to the dysfunction and eventual demise of antiviral CD8 CTLs. In the lymphocytic choriomeningitis virus (LCMV) mouse model, CD4 T cells are required for antiviral CTLs during the chronic phase of infection (97,98). The requirement of CD4 T cells for antiviral CD8 T cell function can be supplied by exogenous IL-2 (99). Because CD8 T cell functional anergy can be reversed *in vitro* by exposure to IL-2, a lack of helper cell function and (especially of HIV-specific CD4 helper cells) may critically hamper the function of the abundant antiviral CD8 T cells.

Another probable contributing factor is antigen excess; T cells undergo programmed cell death when stimulated too frequently by the antigen they recognize (100). Moreover, they are more likely to undergo apoptosis when second-signal cytokines are low. Eventually in more advanced patients, even the number of CD8 T cells declines and viral-specific cytotoxicity, even after *in vitro* culture, becomes difficult to detect. As HIV disease progresses, increasing concentrations of cell-free virus and virus-infected cells, possibly initiated by a critical viral mutation, could reach a critical threshold that might induce the death of antiviral CTLs from repetitive antigenic activation. Such a scenario could positively feed back on itself, leading to ever more virus and further loss of protective immunity. Another contributing factor is the probable HIV-induced destruction of the thymus, the organ responsible for the production of most new T lymphocytes (101,102). Thymic destruction is not complete and irreversible, at least in early-stage and younger patients, who are capable of de novo thymopoiesis after HAART (103). Because CTLs are terminally differentiated cells, presumably capable of only a finite number of cell divisions, the available pool of viral-specific CTLs may become clonally exhausted in the absence of thymic production after about a decade of intense activation (104). It is also possible that in some cases the virus is able to mutate the sequences capable of triggering T cell recognition or to mutate to sequences that antagonize T cell activation (105,106).

STRATEGIES FOR IMMUNOTHERAPY

Because the host immune response is able to keep HIV infection under some sort of control for a decade in the average patient and the hallmark of the disease is loss of cellular immune function, therapies designed to bolster the cellular immune response to the virus are under investigation. Current thinking about immunotherapy is based on the following premises: Cellular immunity is the cornerstone of protection for intracellular pathogens, including viruses such as HIV-1. CTLs, mostly CD8, and NK cells are the final effectors of the cellular immune response; HIV-specific CTLs suppress HIV replication *in vitro* by direct cytotoxicity and by secretion of soluble factor(s). CD4 T cells, whose number and function are ravaged by HIV infection, are necessary to regulate and sustain the effective cellular response to HIV and other pathogens. Some of the functions of the CD4 compartment can be performed by exogenous cytokines, but with toxicity and loss of the exquisite control that local secretion provides. HIV-1 infection causes not only immunosuppression but also vigorous nonspecific immune stimulation, including secretion of inflammatory cytokines and an exaggerated humoral response (107). Chronic nonspecific immune activation may be harmful to the generation and maintenance of an effective immune response and may also increase viral replication. The intimate relation between viral replication and immune activation poses a challenge to the design of most immunotherapeutic approaches. Therefore ideal immunotherapy enhances the specific antiviral immune response with minimal nonspecific immune activation.

Immunotherapeutic intervention is most likely to be successful at the earliest stages of disease, in particular around the time of infection, when the viral burden is amenable to control, before HIV has mutated to more virulent forms and before destruction of the lymphoid organs. Most immunotherapeutic studies for HIV infection were performed before the advent of protease inhibitors and combination HAART therapy, which is capable of suppressing virus without the development of clinical resistance. No immune potentiation was ever demonstrated with vaccines or cytokine infusions in late-stage patients (defined roughly by CD4 counts < $250/mm^3$) with uncontrolled viral production (108). Although HAART therapy greatly enhances the chance of a response to immune-based therapy, it poses new challenges to clinical trial design. Because HAART reduces virus levels to below detection for all but the most sensitive assays in most patients and the incidence of HIV-related disease is also dramatically reduced, less direct measures of efficacy than prevention of opportunistic infections or reduction in viral load are required to determine whether an immune intervention is beneficial. Normalization of immune parameters, improved specific antiviral immune function, or reductions in the viral rebound on drug withdrawal are measurements being used in more recent immunotherapy trials.

Several approaches are possible to enhance anti-HIV cellular immunity. Early attempts focused on vaccination of infected individuals with HIV subunit vaccines (108).

Although these vaccines are not optimal at stimulating CD8 T cell-specific cellular immunity, subunit vaccination can enhance antiviral immunity, especially HIV-specific proliferation and antibody response, in patients who have not yet developed AIDS. Vaccination with inactivated viral particles, such as the Remune vaccine proposed by J. Salk, when given with HAART to early patients can induce substantial HIV-specific proliferative responses (109). Vaccines being developed to boost both CD4 and CD8 T cell immunity include polyvalent lipoprotein complexes, naked DNA vaccines, attenuated HIV or related viruses, recombinant attenuated viruses engineered to express HIV gene products, recombinant intracellular bacteria engineered to express HIV proteins, and recombinant toxin subunits or other pore-forming proteins to introduce whole proteins into the cytosol for degradation. A first-generation DNA vaccine of limited immunogenicity was the only one of these vaccines administered as an immunotherapeutic to HIV-infected recipients (110).

Virus-specific immunity can also be enhanced by administration of cytokines, but at the price of nonspecific immune activation and its counterpart—increased viral replication. In pioneering studies, Lane and his colleagues administered high doses of IL-2 to HIV-infected patients (111,112). After repeated infusions, a substantial fraction of patients without advanced disease experienced dramatic and sustained increases in CD4 counts. Whether these CD4 T cells truly enhance T cell function or affect the clinical course remains to be seen. This concern is reinforced by the transient increase in viral burden associated with the infusions and the lack of any improvement in viral burden over the long term as the CD4 counts improve. Other cytokines, including IL-7, IL-12, and IL-15, which are somewhat more specific than IL-2 at eliciting a TH1 and CTL response, may be more effective than IL-2 for HIV infection. IL-12 can enhance HIV replication in CD8-depleted mononuclear cells, but it does so in only a subset of patients (113,114).

ADOPTIVE TRANSFER OF ANTIVIRAL CTL

Viral-specific immunity can also be bolstered by the infusion of antiviral T cells. Early trials of infusion of autologous LAK-like T cells, generated from peripheral blood lymphocytes of HIV-infected subjects by stimulation with IL-2 and mitogen and with unknown anti-HIV cytolytic activity, showed no toxicity (115,116). Studies of infusion of genetically marked LAK-like T cells from HIV-seronegative donors into their HIV-infected identical twins also showed no toxicity and survived of the transduced infused cells for as long as 6 months (117).

In another study an advanced AIDS patient was infused with mononuclear cells from an HIV-uninfected identical twin who was vaccinated with recombinant vaccinia virus encoding HIV gp160 followed by a recombinant gp160 boost (118). The HIV-seronegative twin developed gp160-specific CTLs but not antibodies. When lymphocytes from the vaccinee were transferred, there was no improvement in clinical parameters. However, when the vaccinee's lymphocytes were stimulated *in vitro* with gp160 before infusion, there was an increase in CD4 count, development of a proliferative response to HIV, and a transient 3-log decline in plasma- and cell-associated viral burden in the infected twin.

Methods of generating autologous polyclonal CD8 T cell lines with potent anti-HIV cytolytic activity from infected individuals by *in vitro* stimulation with immunodominant peptides or autologous cells infected with recombinant vaccinia viruses expressing HIV genes have been developed (59,64,65). The outgrowth of viral-specific CTLs *in vitro* is not supported in serum-free media, which have been used to grow LAK cells for cancer and HIV therapy (119,120). In the absence of serum, antigen-specific cells undergo delayed apoptosis, whereas cytokine-stimu-

lated cells proliferate without difficulty. For clinical trial purposes, because of safety concerns with vaccinia in immunosuppressed subjects even after vaccinia inactivation with psoralen and ultraviolet (UV) treatment, peptide-stimulated T cell lines have been used. As seen by frequency analysis, as many as half of the T cells in peptide-specific lines were HIV-specific (59). Optimized methods to expand more than a billion progeny of HIV-specific CD8 T cell clones have also been developed and used in pilot clinical trials (66). Because polyclonal cell lines recognize multiple HIV-encoded peptide epitopes, the possibility of developing viral escape mutants to evade CTL recognition after CTL infusion is less of a concern than after the infusion of expanded CTL clones that recognize a single 8-11 aa viral peptide. However, treatment with T cell clones offers the advantages of a more well defined effector cell population and the possibility of following the trafficking and survival of infused cells by detecting the clonotypic receptor or a genetically transduced marker.

In a series of pilot trials 15 HIV-infected individuals with CD4 counts less than 400/mm^3 were treated with one to three infusions of 1 billion to 5 billion anti-HIV CTLs (121; J. Lieberman, unpublished results). There was no toxicity or clinical deterioration. During the first 2 weeks after infusion, the viral burden and CD4 counts of most subjects improved, and in some patients there have been substantial sustained improvements (Fig. 31-4). The subset of subjects with a log decline in cell-associated virus 6 months after the infusion had high circulating CD8 T cell counts (> 2,000/mm^3) at the time of therapy, suggesting that a sustained response requires a milieu favorable to CD8 T cell growth and development. All the mean study parameters in the initial trial were either unchanged or improved 6 months later, but none of the changes was statistically significant. One AIDS patient with recurrent atypical mycobacterial bursitis had a clinical response to the CTL infusion. Within 2 weeks of the infusion his infection cleared in the absence of

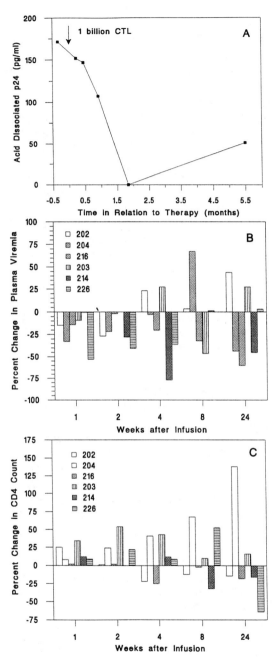

FIG. 31-4. In the initial pilot study of infusions of HIV-specific CD8 T cell lines by Lieberman et al. (121), improvements in plasma viral burden and CD4 T cell count were modest and mostly short-lived. **A:** Acid-dissociated p24 antigen was detectable only in subject 216. **B:** Plasma bDNA fell during the first 2 weeks for five of six subjects but only by small amounts. **C:** The absolute CD4 count rose for the first 2 weeks following infusion for all subjects. (From ref. 121, with permission.)

mycobacterial drug therapy and had not recurred 3 years later (J. Lieberman, unpublished results). These results support the hypothesis that antiviral CTLs are not harmful and suggest that they may be protective. However, treatment responses have been heterogeneous, generally short-lived, and not dramatic.

Several laboratories investigated the infusion of HIV-specific CTL clones in a small number of patients. Infusion of an anti-nef T cell clone was tested by Koenig et al. in one patient with advanced disease; there was no sign of improvement and possible worsening (122). However, that individual developed viral mutants that had deleted the targeted nef sequence. Viral escape from immune-based therapy could potentially become as much of a problem as viral escape from drug therapy (105). A clonal CTL approach with genetically marked cells has also been tested for HIV infection by Greenberg, Riddell, and colleagues, who had demonstrated in another viral system that cytomegalovirus (CMV)-specific CTL immunity can be transferred by infusion of CTL clones into bone marrow transplant recipients (123,124). In an early trial, infused patients developed a CTL response to the genetic marker (composed in part of a gene from a prevalent herpes virus) used to follow the life-span of the infused cells, which resulted in their early elimination (125). In a later study involving infusion of gag-specific CTL clones marked with the neo gene (which does not appear to elicit neo-specific CTLs), the genetically marked CTLs disappeared from the blood with a half-life of approximately 2 days and homed to the lymph nodes where they were detected in close proximity to HIV-infected cells 4 days later (126). Although there may have been a transient reduction in the circulating cell-associated virus shortly after the infusion, plasma viral levels did not decline and may have increased.

To circumvent the difficulties of cloning or selectively expanding virus-specific CTLs, an alternate approach has been developed to redirect the specificity of all CD8 T cells by transduction with chimeric receptors that target viral cell surface antigens. In one approach, the extracellular and transmembrane domains of CD4 were linked to the CD3ζ chain of CD3. Binding of gp120 on HIV-infected target cells to the extracellular domain of CD4 on this "universal receptor" would then be able to trigger T cell activation via the CD3ζ intracellular domain irrespective of the recipient's MHC background (127,128). In preliminary results from pilot trials with autologous or syngeneic gene-modified cells, transduced CD8 T cells rapidly disappeared from the circulation, falling by 1 to 4 logs within 4 weeks, but they persisted when CD4 T cells were transduced and infused in parallel (129,130). No antiviral activity of these treatments has been reported.

LESSONS FROM THE HUMAN ADOPTIVE THERAPY STUDIES

All the adoptive CD8 T cell therapy clinical experiments have been safe. This is probably the most direct evidence for the lack of any significant immunopathogenic effect induced by HIV-specific CD8 T cells. However, none of the studies resulted in dramatic benefits. For the one patient in whom a clinical benefit was seen (resolution of atypical mycobacterial infection), it is unclear whether it was due to infusion of HIV-specific CTLs or mycobacteria-specific T cells contained in the polyclonal cell line. The lack of substantial *in vivo* antiviral effect of HIV-specific CD8 T cell infusions could be due to infusing insufficient numbers of cells, their rapid demise, improper trafficking to the sites of infection, or eventual lack of function. Generally these trials have infused in the range of 10^9 to several times 10^{10} specific CD8 T cells. This is to be compared to approximately 5×10^9 total circulating CD8 T cells or approximately 10^{12} total body lymphocytes. If as many as 1% to 10% of CD8 T cells *in vivo* are HIV-specific, an estimate consistent with recent tetramer-staining data, an HIV-infected individual might contain as many as 10^{10} to 10^{11} HIV-specific CD8 T cells. The number of infused cells is then

comparable to or somewhat less than the number of HIV-specific T cells in asymptomatic HIV-infected hosts. In light of these numbers, it is perhaps not that surprising that these treatments have had little efficacy.

Marking studies have shown that the infused cells persist for at least several months and traffic to the lymph node, where they can be found juxtaposed to HIV-infected target cells (117,126). Therefore, it is likely that the infused cells do not control viral production for the same reasons the numerous *in vivo* generated CTLs do not. Even if *ex vivo* amplification in the presence of IL-2 improves viral suppression and cytotoxicity against infected target cells, the infused CTLs probably revert to their prior *in vivo* functional state sometime soon after being returned to the infected patient's milieu. The short-lived beneficial effects seen after adoptive transfer are consistent with the hypothesis that the *in vivo* function of HIV-specific CTLs is severely impaired.

The number of HIV-infected CD4 T cells is generally many orders of magnitude fewer than 1% of the total CD4 T cells. Therefore the number of infused CTLs in these studies and the number of native HIV-specific CTLs *in vivo* is many times the estimates of infected target cells in all but the most advanced patients. Therefore adoptive transfer therapies that only increase the numbers of antiviral CTLs are not likely to be of sustained benefit unless they also can reverse CTL functional defects.

Understanding the etiology of the *in vivo* dysfunction of antiviral CD8 is key to developing sustained immunotherapy. If the *in vivo* dysfunction is due to excessive viral antigen, ongoing adoptive transfer trials performed in the setting of HAART therapy may be more effective. If the *in vivo* functional defect arises from the absence of antiviral CD4 T cell help, strategies to replace or restore specific CD4 T cells are in order. Such measures may include vaccination to induce HIV-specific CD4 T cells, co-infusion of antigen-specific CD4 T cells [possibly rendered resistant to HIV infection by gene transfer (131)], treatment with exogenous cytokines [such as IL-2, IL-12 (132,133), or IL-15 (134–136)], that sustain CD8 T cell proliferation, or the use of genetic engineering to produce CD8 T cells that are independent of exogenous help (137). Methods to expand large numbers of CD4 T cells from HIV-infected donors have been developed that involve either expansion in the presence of antiretroviral drugs (138) or stimulation with cross-linked anti-CD3 and anti-CD28, a combination that does not induce the CCR5 chemokine co-receptor for HIV infection (139–141). Therapeutic infusions of the latter cells are currently being investigated in pilot trials (C. June, personal communication). In fact, adoptive transfer of CD8 T cells may prove unnecessary if antiviral or immunomodulatory therapies can restore *in vivo* function of antiviral CD8 T cells that are already present in abundant numbers in infected patients.

Acknowledgments

This work was supported in part by NIH grants AI36611 and AI42519. I thank Premlata Shankar and Linda Trimble for useful discussions and Jessica Fabry, Donna Fong, Paul Skolnik, Bob Parkerson, Miguel Perales, Heidi Sprang, Rachel Friedman, Susan Crockett, Sandra Burchett, Mark Patterson, and Ann Corbett for their help in developing and performing CTL adoptive immunotherapy trials.

REFERENCES

1. Finzi D, Hermankova M, Pierson T, et al. Identification of a reservoir for HIV-1 in patients on highly active antiretroviral therapy. *Science* 1997;278: 1295–1300.
2. McDougal JS, Mawle A, Cort SP, et al. Cellular tropism of the human retrovirus HTLV-III/LAV I: role of T cell activation and expression of the T4 antigen. *J Immunol* 1985;135:3151–3162.
3. Folks TM, Justement J, Kinter A, Dinarello CA, Fauci AS. Cytokine-induced expression of HIV-1 in a chronically infected promonocyte cell line. *Science* 1987;238:800–802.
4. Hoffenbach A, Langlade-Demoyen P, Dadaglio G, et al. Unusually high frequencies of HIV-specific cytotoxic T lymphocytes in humans. *J Immunol* 1989;142:452–462.

5. Cheynier R, Langlade-Demoyen P, Marescot MR, et al. Cytotoxic T lymphocyte responses in the peripheral blood of children born to human immunodeficiency virus-1-infected mothers. *Eur J Immunol* 1992;22:2211–2217.
6. Clerici M, Giorgi JV, Chou CC, et al. Cell-mediated immune response to human immunodeficiency virus (HIV) type 1 in seronegative homosexual men with recent sexual exposure to HIV-1. *J Infect Dis* 1992;165:1012–1019.
7. Langlade-Demoyen P, Ngo-Giang-Huong N, Ferchal F, Oksenhendler E. Human immunodeficiency virus (HIV) nef-specific cytotoxic T lymphocytes in noninfected heterosexual contact of HIV-infected patients. *J Clin Invest* 1994;93:1293–1297.
8. Rowland-Jones S, Sutton J, Ariyoshi K, et al. HIV-specific cytotoxic T-cells in HIV-exposed but uninfected Gambian women. *Nat Med* 1995;1:59–64.
9. Bryson Y, Pang S, Weil S, Dickover R, Diagne A, Chen IS. Clearance of HIV infection in a perinatally infected infant. *N Engl J Med* 1995;332: 833–838.
10. Daniel MD, Kirchoff F, Czajak SC, Sehgal PK, Desrosiers RC. Protective effects of live attenuated vaccine with a deletion in the nef gene. *Science* 1992;258:1938–1941.
11. Hu SL, Abrams K, Barber GN, et al. Protection of macaques against SIV infection by subunit vaccines of SIV envelope glycoprotein gp160. *Science* 1992;255:456–459.
12. Yap KL, Ada GL, McKenzie IF. Transfer of specific cytotoxic T lymphocytes protect mice inoculated with influenza virus. *Nature* 1978;273: 238–239.
13. Askonas BA, Taylor PM. T cell mediated immunity in virus infection. *Immunol Lett* 1987;16: 337–340.
14. Walker CM, Moody DJ, Stites DP, Levy JA. CD8⁺ lymphocytes can control HIV infection in vitro by suppressing virus replication. *Science* 1986;234: 1563–1566.
15. Walker BD, Chakrabarti S, Moss B, et al. HIV-specific cytotoxic T lymphocytes in seropositive individuals. *Nature* 1987;328:345–348.
16. Plata F, Autran B, Martins LP, et al. AIDS virus-specific cytotoxic T lymphocytes in lung disorders. *Nature* 1987;328:348–351.
17. Cocchi F, DeVico AL, Garzino-Demo A, Arya SK, Gallo RC, Lusso P. Identification of RANTES, MIP-1 alpha, and MIP-1 beta as the major HIV-suppressive factors produced by CD8⁺ T cells. *Science* 1995;270:1811–1815.
18. Wagner L, Yang OO, Garcia-Zepeda EA, et al. Beta-chemokines are released from HIV-1-specific cytolytic T-cell granules complexed to proteoglycans. *Nature* 1998;391:908–911.
19. Taub DD, Ortaldo JR, Turcovski-Corrales SM, Key ML, Longo DL, Murphy WJ. Beta chemokines costimulate lymphocyte cytolysis, proliferation, and lymphokine production. *J Leukoc Biol* 1996;59:81–89.
20. Mackewicz CE, Blackbourn DJ, Levy JA. CD8⁺ T cells suppress human immunodeficiency virus replication by inhibiting viral transcription. *Proc Natl Acad Sci USA* 1995;92:2308–2312.

21. Copeland KF, McKay PJ, Rosenthal KL. Suppression of activation of the human immunodeficiency virus long terminal repeat by CD8⁺ T cells is not lentivirus specific. *AIDS Res Hum Retroviruses* 1995;11:1321–1326.

22. Baier M, Werner A, Bannert N, Metzner K, Kurth R. HIV suppression by interleukin-16. *Nature* 1995;378:563.

23. Leith JG, Copeland KF, McKay PJ, Richards CD, Rosenthal KL. CD8⁺ T-cell-mediated suppression of HIV-1 long terminal repeat-driven gene expression is not modulated by the CC chemokines RANTES, macrophage inflammatory protein (MIP)-1 alpha and MIP-1 beta. *AIDS* 1997;11:575–580.

24. Barker E, Bossart KN, Fujimura SH, Levy JA. CD28 costimulation increases CD8⁺ cell suppression of HIV replication. *J Immunol* 1997;159:5123–5131.

25. Yang OO, Walker BD. CD8⁺ cells in human immunodeficiency virus type I pathogenesis:cytolytic and noncytolytic inhibition of viral replication. *Adv Immunol* 1997;66:273–311.

26. Koup RA, Safrit JT, Cao Y, et al. Temporal association of cellular immune responses with the initial control of viremia in primary human immunodeficiency virus type 1 syndrome. *J Virol* 1994;68:4650–4655.

27. Borrow P, Lewicki H, Hahn BH, Shaw GM, Oldstone MB. Virus-specific CD8⁺ cytotoxic T-lymphocyte activity associated with control of viremia in primary human immunodeficiency virus type 1 infection. *J Virol* 1994;68:6103–6110.

28. Altman JD, Moss PAH, Goulder PJR, et al. Phenotypic analysis of antigen-specific T lymphocytes. *Science* 1996;274:94–96.

29. Ogg GS, Jin X, Bonhoeffer S, et al. Quantitation of HIV-1-specific cytotoxic T lymphocytes and plasma load of viral RNA. *Science* 1998;279:2103–2106.

30. Rinaldo C, Huang XL, Fan ZF, et al. High levels of anti-human immunodeficiency virus type 1 (HIV-1) memory cytotoxic T-lymphocyte activity and low viral load are associated with lack of disease in HIV-1-infected long-term nonprogressors. *J Virol* 1995;69:5838–5842.

31. Harrer T, Harrer E, Kalams SA, et al. Strong cytotoxic T cell and weak neutralizing antibody responses in a subset of persons with stable nonprogressing HIV type 1 infection. *AIDS Res Hum Retroviruses* 1996;12:585–592.

32. Kourtis AP, Ibegbu C, Nahmias AJ, et al. Early progression of disease in HIV-infected infants with thymus dysfunction. *N Engl J Med* 1996;335:1431–1436.

33. Pollack H, Zhan MX, Safrit JT, et al. CD8⁺ T-cell-mediated suppression of HIV replication in the first year of life: association with lower viral load and favorable early survival. *AIDS* 1997;11: F9–13.

34. Buseyne F, McChesney M, Porrot F, Kovarik S, Guy B, Riviere Y. Gag-specific cytotoxic T lymphocytes from human immunodeficiency virus type 1-infected individuals: gag epitopes are clustered in three regions of the p24gag protein. *J Virol* 1993;67:694–702.

35. Riviere Y, McChesney MB, Porrot F, et al. Gag-specific cytotoxic responses to HIV type 1 are associated with a decreased risk of progression to AIDS-related complex or AIDS. *AIDS Res Hum Retroviruses* 1995;11:903–907.

36. Musey L, Hughes J, Schacker T, Shea T, Corey L, McElrath MJ. Cytotoxic T cell responses, viral load and disease progression in early human immunodeficiency virus type 1 infection. *N Engl J Med* 1997;337:1267–1274.

37. Carmichael A, Jin X, Sissons P, Borysiewicz L. Quantitative analysis of the human immunodeficiency virus type 1 (HIV-1)-specific cytotoxic T lymphocyte (CTL) response at different stages of HIV-1 infection: differential CTL responses to HIV-1 and Epstein-Barr virus in late disease. *J Exp Med* 1993;177:249–256.

38. Klavinskis LS, Whitton JL, Oldstone MB. Molecularly engineered vaccine which expresses an immunodominant T-cell epitope induces cytotoxic T lymphocytes that confer protection from lethal virus infection. *J Virol* 1989;63:4311–4316.

39. Zinkernagel RM, Hengartner H. T-cell-mediated immunopathology versus direct cytolysis by virus: implications for HIV and AIDS. *Immunol Today* 1994;15:262–268.

40. Zinkernagel RM. Are HIV-specific CTL responses salutary or pathogenic? *Curr Opin Immunol* 1995; 7:462–470.

41. Sethi KK, Naher H, Stroehmann I. Phenotypic heterogeneity of cerebrospinal fluid-derived HIV-specific and HLA-restricted cytotoxic T-cell clones. *Nature* 1988;335:178–181.

42. Autran B, Mayaud CM, Raphael M, et al. Evidence for a cytotoxic T-lymphocyte alveolitis in human immunodeficiency virus-infected patients. *AIDS* 1988;2:179–183.

43. Bofill M, Mocroft A, Lipman M, et al. Increased numbers of primed activated CD8⁺CD38⁺ CD45RO⁺ T cells predict the decline of CD4⁺ T cells in HIV-1-infected patients. *AIDS* 1996;10: 827–834.

44. Liu Z, Hultin LE, Cumberland WG, et al. Elevated relative fluorescence intensity of CD38 antigen expression on CD8⁺ T cells is a marker of poor prognosis in HIV infection: results of 6 years of follow-up. *Cytometry* 1996;26:1–7.

45. Liu Z, Cumberland WG, Hultin LE, Prince HE, Detels R, Giorgi JV. Elevated CD38 antigen expression on CD8⁺ T cells is a stronger marker for the risk of chronic HIV disease progression to AIDS and death in the Multicenter AIDS Cohort Study than CD4⁺ cell count, soluble immune activation markers, or combinations of HLA-DR and CD38 expression. *J Acquir Immune Defic Syndr Hum Retrovirol* 1997;16:83–92.

46. Mocroft A, Bofill M, Lipman M, et al. CD8⁺,CD38⁺ lymphocyte percent: a useful immunological marker for monitoring HIV-1-infected patients. *J Acquir Immune Defic Syndr Hum Retrovirol* 1997; 14:158–162.

47. Zinkernagel RM, Haenseler E, Leist T, Cerny A, Hengartner H, Althage A. T cell-mediated hepatitis in mice infected with lymphocytic choriomeningitis virus: liver cell destruction by H-2 class I-

restricted virus-specific cytotoxic T cells as a physiological correlate of the ^{51}Cr-release assay? *J Exp Med* 1986;164:1075–1092.

48. Cannon MJ, Openshaw PJ, Askonas BA. Cytotoxic T cells clear virus but augment lung pathology in mice infected with respiratory syncytial virus. *J Exp Med* 1988;168:1163–1168.

49. Barnaba V, Franco A, Alberti A, Balsano C, Benvenuto R, Balsano F. Recognition of hepatitis B virus envelope proteins by liver-infiltrating T lymphocytes in chronic HBV infection. *J Immunol* 1989;143:2650–2655.

50. Koziel MJ, Dudley D, Wong JT, et al. Intrahepatic cytotoxic T lymphocytes specific for hepatitis C virus in persons with chronic hepatitis. *J Immunol* 1992;149:3339–3344.

51. Ando K, Moriyama T, Guidotti LG, et al. Mechanisms of class I restricted immunopathology: a transgenic mouse model of fulminant hepatitis. *J Exp Med* 1993;178:1541–1554.

52. Ando K, Guidotti LG, Wirth S, et al. Class I-restricted cytotoxic T lymphocytes are directly cytopathic for their target cells *in vivo*. *J Immunol* 1994;152:3245–3253.

53. Ando K, Hiroishi K, Kaneko T, et al. Perforin, Fas/Fas ligand, and TNF-alpha pathways as specific and bystander killing mechanisms of hepatitis C virus-specific human CTL. *J Immunol* 1997;158:5283–5291.

54. Kagi D, Vignaux F, Ledermann B, et al. Fas and perforin pathways as major mechanisms of T cell-mediated cytotoxicity. *Science* 1994;265:528–530.

55. Kojima H, Shinohara N, Hanaoka S, et al. Two distinct pathways of specific killing revealed by perforin mutant cytotoxic T lymphocytes. *Immunity* 1994;1:357–364.

56. Lowin B, Hahne M, Mattmann C, Tschopp J. Cytolytic T-cell cytotoxicity is mediated through perforin and Fas lytic pathways. *Nature* 1994;370:650–652.

57. Walsh CM, Glass AA, Chiu V, Clark WR. The role of the Fas lytic pathway in a perforin-less CTL hybridoma. *J Immunol* 1994;153:2506–2514.

58. Shankar P, Xu Z, Lieberman J. Viral-specific cytotoxic T lymphocytes lyse HIV-infected primary T lymphocytes by the granule exocytosis pathway. *Blood,* in press, 1999.

59. Lieberman J, Fabry JA, Shankar P, Beckett L, Skolnik PR. Ex vivo expansion of HIV type 1-specific cytolytic T cells from HIV type 1-seropositive subjects. *AIDS Res Hum Retroviruses* 1995;11:257–271.

60. Pantaleo G, Koenig S, Baseler M, Lane HC, Fauci AS. Defective clonogenic potential of CD8$^+$ T lymphocytes in patients with AIDS: expansion in vivo of a nonclonogenic CD3$^+$CD8$^+$DR$^+$CD25$^-$ T cell population. *J Immunol* 1990;144:1696–1704.

61. Moss PA, Rowland-Jones SL, Frodsham PM, et al. Persistent high frequency of human immunodeficiency virus-specific cytotoxic T cells in peripheral blood of infected donors. *Proc Natl Acad Sci USA* 1995;92:5773–5777.

62. Lalvani A, Dong T, Ogg G, et al. Optimization of a peptide-based protocol employing IL-7 for in vitro restimulation of human cytotoxic T lymphocyte precursors. *J Immunol Methods* 1997;210:65–77.

63. Lieberman J, Fabry JA, Fong DM, Parkerson GR III. Recognition of a small number of diverse epitopes dominates the cytotoxic T lymphocyte response to HIV-1 in an infected individual. *AIDS Res Hum Retroviruses* 1997;13:383–392.

64. Lubaki MN, Egan MA, Siliciano RF, Weinhold KJ, Bollinger RC. A novel method for detection and ex vivo expansion of HIV type 1-specific cytolytic T lymphocytes. *AIDS Res Hum Retroviruses* 1994;10:1427–1431.

65. Shankar P, Fabry J, Lieberman J. A simple method to selectively expand HIV-1 specific cytotoxic T lymphocytes in vitro. *Immunol Invest* 1995;24:489–497.

66. Riddell SR, Greenberg, PD. The use of anti-CD3 and anti-CD28 monoclonal antibodies to clone and expand human antigen-specific T cells. *J Immunol Methods* 1990;128:189–201.

67. Wiertz EJ, Mukherjee S, Ploegh HL. Viruses use stealth technology to escape from the host immune system. *Mol Med Today* 1997;3:116–123.

68. Schwartz O, Marechal V, Le Gall S, Lemonnier F, Heard JM. Endocytosis of major histocompatibility class I molecules is induced by the HIV-1 Nef protein. *Nat Med* 1996;2:338–342.

69. Collins KL, Chen BK, Kalams SA, Walker BD, Baltimore D. HIV-1 Nef protein protects infected primary cells against killing by cytotoxic T lymphocytes. *Nature* 1998;391:397–401.

70. Shankar P, Sprang H, Lieberman J. Effective lysis of HIV-infected primary CD4 T cells by a cytotoxic T lymphocyte clone directed against a novel A2-restricted reverse transcriptase epitope. *J Acquir Immune Defic Syndr Hum Retrovirol* 1998;19:111–120.

71. Tsomides TJ, Aldovini A, Johnson RP, Walker BD, Young RA, Eisen HN. Naturally processed viral peptides recognized by cytotoxic T lymphocytes on cells chronically infected by human immunodeficiency virus type 1. *J Exp Med* 1994;180:1283–1293.

72. Trimble LA, Lieberman J. Circulating CD8 T lymphocytes in human immunodeficiency virus-infected individuals have impaired function and downmodulate CD3 zeta, the signaling chain of the T-cell receptor complex. *Blood* 1998;91:585–594.

73. Subramanyam M, Gutheil WG, Bachovchin WW, Huber BT. Mechanism of HIV-1 Tat induced inhibition of antigen-specific T cell responsiveness. *J Immunol* 1993;150:2544–2553.

74. Lewis DE, Tang DS, Adu-Oppong A, Schober W, Rodgers JR. Anergy and apoptosis in CD8$^+$ T cells from HIV-infected persons. *J Immunol* 1994;153:412–420.

75. Vanham G, Kestens L, Gigase P, et al. Evidence for circulating activated cytotoxic T cells in HIV-infected subjects before the onset of opportunistic infections. *Clin Exp Immunol* 1990;82:3–9.

76. Saukkonen JJ, Kornfeld H, Berman JS. Expansion of a CD8$^+$CD28$^-$ cell population in the blood and lung of HIV-positive patients. *J Acquir Immune Defic Syndr* 1993;6:1194–1204.

77. Watret KC, Whitelaw JA, Froebel KS, Bird AG.

Phenotypic characterization of CD8⁺ T cell populations in HIV disease and in anti-HIV immunity. *Clin Exp Immunol* 1993;92:93–99.

78. Ho HN, Hultin LE, Mitsuyasu RT, et al. Circulating HIV-specific CD8⁺ cytotoxic T cells express CD38 and HLA-DR antigens. *J Immunol* 1993; 150:3070–3079.

79. Zaunders J, Carr A, McNally L, Penny R, Cooper DA. Effects of primary HIV-1 infection on subsets of CD4⁺ and CD8⁺ T lymphocytes. *AIDS* 1995;9: 561–566.

80. Cossarizza A, Ortolani C, Mussini C, et al. Massive activation of immune cells with an intact T cell repertoire in acute human immunodeficiency virus syndrome. *J Infect Dis* 1995;172:105–112.

81. Roederer M, Dubs JG, Anderson MT, Raju PA, Herzenberg LA, Herzenberg LA. CD8 naive T cell counts decrease progressively in HIV-infected adults. *J Clin Invest* 1995;95:2061–2066.

82. Bouscarat F, Levacher-Clergeot M, Dazza MC, et al. Correlation of CD8 lymphocyte activation with cellular viremia and plasma HIV RNA levels in asymptomatic patients infected by human immunodeficiency virus type 1. *AIDS Res Hum Retroviruses* 1996;12:17–24.

83. Vingerhoets JH, Vanham GL, Kestens LL, et al. Increased cytolytic T lymphocyte activity and decreased B7 responsiveness are associated with CD28 down-regulation on CD8⁺ T cells from HIV-infected subjects. *Clin Exp Immunol* 1995;100: 425–433.

84. Kammerer R, Iten A, Frei PC, Burgisser P. Expansion of T cells negative for CD28 expression in HIV infection: relation to activation markers and cell adhesion molecules, and correlation with prognostic markers. *Med Microbiol Immunol* 1996; 185:19–25.

85. Lloyd TE, Yang L, Tang DN, Bennett T, Schober W, Lewis DE. Regulation of CD28 costimulation in human CD8⁺ T cells. *J Immunol* 1997;158:1551–1558.

86. Borthwick NJ, Bofill M, Gombert WM, et al. Lymphocyte activation in HIV-1 infection. II. Functional defects of CD28⁻ T cells. *AIDS* 1994;8:431–441.

87. Stefanova I, Saville MW, Peters C, et al. HIV infection–induced posttranslational modification of T cell signaling molecules associated with disease progression. *J Clin Invest* 1996;98:1290–1297.

88. Vingerhoets J, Kestens L, Penne G, et al. CD8⁺ cells and not CD4⁺ T cells are hyporesponsive to CD28- and CD40L-mediated activation in HIV-infected subjects. *Clin Exp Immunol* 1997;107: 440–447.

89. Mizoguchi H, O'Shea JJ, Longo DL, Loeffler CM, McVicar DW, Ochoa AC. Alterations in signal transduction molecules in T lymphocytes from tumor-bearing mice. *Science* 1992;258:1795–1798.

90. Finke JH, Zea AH, Stanley J, et al. Loss of T-cell receptor zeta chain and p56ˡᶜᵏ in T-cells infiltrating human renal cell carcinoma. *Cancer Res* 1993;53: 5613–5616.

91. Massaia M, Attisano C, Beggiato E, Bianchi A, Pileri A. Correlation between disease activity and

T-cell CD3 zeta chain expression in a B-cell lymphoma. *Br J Haematol* 1994;88:886–888.

92. Maurice MM, Lankester AC, Bezemer AC, et al. Defective TCR-mediated signaling in synovial T cells in rheumatoid arthritis. *J Immunol* 1997; 159:2973–2978.

93. Liossis SN, Ding XZ, Dennis GJ, Tsokos GC. Altered pattern of TCR/CD3-mediated protein-tyrosyl phosphorylation in T cells from patients with systemic lupus erythematosus. *J Clin Invest* 1998;101:1448–1457.

94. Andersson J, Behbahani H, Lieberman J, et al. Perforin is not co-expressed with granzymeA within cytotoxic granules in CD8 T-lymphocytes present in lymphoid tissue during chronic HIV infection. *AIDS* 1999;13:1295–1303.

95. Rosenberg ES, Billingsley JM, Caliendo AM, et al. Vigorous HIV-1-specific CD4⁺ T cell responses associated with control of viremia. *Science* 1997; 278:1447–1450.

96. Schnittman SM, Lane HC, Greenhouse J, Justement JS, Baseler M, Fauci AS. Preferential infection of CD4⁺ memory T cells by human immunodeficiency virus type 1:evidence for a role in the selective T-cell functional defects observed in infected individuals. *Proc Natl Acad Sci USA* 1990;87:6058–6062.

97. Matloubian M, Concepcion RJ, Ahmed R. CD4⁺ T cells are required to sustain CD8⁺ cytotoxic T-cell responses during chronic viral infection. *J Virol* 1994;68:8056–8063.

98. Zajac AJ, Blattman JN, Murali-Krishna K, et al. Viral immune evasion due to persistence of activated T cells without effector function. *J Exp Med* 1998;188:2205–2213.

99. Su HC, Cousens LP, Fast LD, et al. CD4⁺ and CD8⁺ T cell interactions in IFN-gamma and IL-4 responses to viral infections: requirements for IL-2. *J Immunol* 1998;160:5007–5017.

100. Boehme SA, Lenardo MJ. Propriocidal apoptosis of mature T lymphocytes occurs at S phase of the cell cycle. *Eur J Immunol* 1993;23:1552–1560.

101. Schnittman SM, Denning SM, Greenhouse JJ, et al. Evidence for susceptibility of intrathymic T-cell precursors and their progeny carrying T-cell antigen receptor phenotypes TCR alpha beta + and TCR gamma delta + to human immunodeficiency virus infection: a mechanism for CD4⁺ (T4) lymphocyte depletion. *Proc Natl Acad Sci USA* 1990;87:7727–7731.

102. Fauci AS, Pantaleo G, Stanley S, Weissman D. Immunopathogenic mechanisms of HIV infection. *Ann Intern Med* 1996;124:654–663.

103. Autran B, Carcelain G, Li TS, et al. Positive effects of combined antiretroviral therapy on CD4⁺ T cell homeostasis and function in advanced HIV disease. *Science* 1997;277:112–116.

104. Moskophidis D, Lechner F, Pircher H, Zinkernagel RM. Virus persistence in acutely infected immunocompetent mice by exhaustion of antiviral cytotoxic effector T cells. *Nature* 1993;362:758–761.

105. Phillips RE, Rowland-Jones S, Nixon DF, et al. Human immunodeficiency virus genetic variation that can escape cytotoxic T cell recognition. *Nature* 1991;354:453–459.

106. Klenerman P, Rowland-Jones S, McAdam S, et al. Cytotoxic T-cell activity antagonized by naturally occurring HIV-1 Gag variants [see comments]. *Nature* 1994;369:403–407.

107. Cohen OJ, Kinter A, Fauci AS. Host factors in the pathogenesis of HIV disease. *Immunol Rev* 1997; 159:31–48.

108. Redfield RR, Birx DL, Ketter N, et al. Phase I evaluation of the safety and immunogenicity of vaccination with recombinant gp160 in patients with early human immunodeficiency virus infection. *N Engl J Med* 1991;324:1677–1684.

109. Valentine FT, De Gruttola V, Kaplan M, et al. Effects of HAART compared to HAART plus an inactivated HIV immunogen on lymphocyte proliferative response (LPR) to HIV antigens. In: *Proceedings of the 12th World AIDS Conference,* Geneva, 1998, abstract 31227.

110. Kim JJ, Ayyavoo V, Bagarazzi ML, et al. Development of a multicomponent candidate vaccine for HIV-1. *Vaccine* 1997;15:879–883.

111. Kovacs JA, Baseler M, Dewar RJ, et al. Increases in CD4 T lymphocytes with intermittent courses of interleukin-2 in patients with human immunodeficiency virus infection: a preliminary study. *N Engl J Med* 1995;332:567–575.

112. Kovacs JA, Vogel S, Albert JM, et al. Controlled trial of interleukin-2 infusions in patients infected with the human immunodeficiency virus. *N Engl J Med* 1996;335:1350–1356.

113. Foli A, Saville MW, Baseler MW, Yarchoan R. Effects of the Th1 and Th2 stimulatory cytokines IL-12 and IL-4 on human immunodeficiency virus replication. *Blood* 1995;85:2114–2123.

114. Perales MA, Skolnik PR, Lieberman J. Effect of interleukin 12 on in vitro HIV type 1 replication depends on clinical stage. *AIDS Res Hum Retroviruses* 1996;12:659–668.

115. Ho M, Armstrong J, MacMahon, D, et al. A phase 1 study of adoptive transfer of autologous CD8+ T lymphocytes in patients with acquired immunodeficiency syndrome (AIDS)-related complex or AIDS. *Blood* 1993;81:2093–2101.

116. Whiteside TL, Elder EM, Moody D, et al. Generation and characterization of ex vivo propagated autologous CD8+ cells used for adoptive immunotherapy of patients infected with human immunodeficiency virus. *Blood* 1993;81:2085–2092.

117. Walker RE. A phase I/II pilot study of the safety of the adoptive transfer of syngeneic gene-modified cytotoxic T lymphocytes in HIV-infected identical twins. *Hum Gene Therapy* 1996;7:367–400

118. Bex F, Hermans P, Sprecher S, et al. Syngeneic adoptive transfer of anti-human immunodeficiency virus (HIV-1)-primed lymphocytes from a vaccinated HIV-seronegative individual to his HIV-1-infected identical twin. *Blood* 1994;84:3317–3326.

119. Trimble L, Perales M-A, Knazek R, Lieberman J. Serum enhances the ex vivo generation of HIV-specific cytotoxic T cells. *Biotech Bioeng* 1996; 50:521–528.

120. Trimble LA, Xu Z, Lieberman J. Clonal expansion of antigen-specific CD8+ cytotoxic T lymphocytes is regulated by delayed exposure to prevent apoptosis. *J Immunol Methods* 1999;225:39–52.

121. Lieberman J, Skolnik PR, Parkerson GR, et al. Safety of autologous, ex vivo-expanded human immunodeficiency virus (HIV)-specific cytotoxic T-lymphocyte infusion in HIV-infected patients. *Blood* 1997;90:2196–2206.

122. Koenig S, Conley AJ, Brewah YA, et al. Transfer of HIV-1-specific cytotoxic T lymphocytes to an AIDS patient leads to selection for mutant HIV variants and subsequent disease progression. *Nat Med* 1995;1:330–336.

123. Riddell SR, Watanabe KS, Goodrich JM, Li CR, Agha ME, Greenberg PD. Restoration of viral immunity in immunodeficient humans by the adoptive transfer of T cell clones. *Science* 1992;257: 238–241.

124. Walter EA, Greenberg PD, Gilbert MJ, et al. Reconstitution of cellular immunity against cytomegalovirus in recipients of allogeneic bone marrow by transfer of T-cell clones from the donor. *N Engl J Med* 1995;333:1038–1044.

125. Riddell SR, Elliott M, Lewinsohn DA, et al. T-cell mediated rejection of gene-modified HIV-specific cytotoxic T lymphocytes in HIV-infected patients. *Nat Med* 1996;2:216–223.

126. Brodie SJ, Lewinsohn DA, Patterson BK, et al. In vivo migration and function of transferred HIV-1-specific cytotoxic T cells. *Nat Med* 1999;5: 34–41.

127. Roberts MR, Qin L, Zhang D, et al. Targeting of human immunodeficiency virus-infected cells by CD8+ T lymphocytes armed with universal T-cell receptors. *Blood* 1994;84:2878–2889.

128. Yang OO, Tran AC, Kalams SA, Johnson RP, Roberts MR, Walker BD. Lysis of HIV-1-infected cells and inhibition of viral replication by universal receptor T cells. *Proc Natl Acad Sci USA* 1997; 94:11478–11483.

129. Hege KM, Deeks SG, Mitsuyasu RT, et al. Coinfusion of autologous HIV-1 specific gene-modified CD4 and CD8 T cells leads to improved T cell survival and tissue trafficking. In: *Proceedings of the 12th World AIDS Conference,* Geneva, 1998, abstract 42321.

130. Walker R, Bechtel CM, Natarajan V, et al. In vivo persistence of genetically modified HIV-1-specific syngeneic lymphocytes in HIV-1-discordant identical twins. In: *Proceedings of the 12th World AIDS Conference,* Geneva, 1998, abstract 42322.

131. Bridges SH, Sarver N. Gene therapy and immune restoration for HIV disease. *Lancet* 1995;345: 427–432.

132. Chouaib S, Chehimi J, Bani L, et al. Interleukin 12 induces the differentiation of major histocompatibility complex class I-primed cytotoxic T-lymphocyte precursors into allospecific cytotoxic effectors. *Proc Natl Acad Sci USA* 1994;91:12659–12663.

133. Aste-Amezaga M, D'Andrea A, Kubin M, Trinchieri G. Cooperation of natural killer cell stimulatory factor/interleukin-12 with other stimuli in the induction of cytokines and cytotoxic cell-associated molecules in human T and NK cells. *Cell Immunol* 1994;156:480–492.

134. Kanai T, Thomas EK, Yasutomi Y, Letvin NL. IL-

15 stimulates the expansion of AIDS virus-specific CTL. *J Immunol* 1996;157:3681–3687.

135. Agostini C, Trentin L, Sancetta R, et al. Interleukin-15 triggers activation and growth of the CD8 T-cell pool in extravascular tissues of patients with acquired immunodeficiency syndrome. *Blood* 1997;90:1115–1123.

136. Zhang X, Sun S, Hwang I, Tough DF, Sprent J. Potent and selective stimulation of memory-phenotype CD8+ T cells *in vivo* by IL-15. *Immunity* 1998;8:591–599.

137. Nelson BH, Lord JD, Greenberg PD. Cytoplasmic domains of the interleukin-2 receptor beta and gamma chains mediate the signal for T-cell proliferation. *Nature* 1994;369:333–336.

138. Wilson CC, Wong JT, Girard DD, et al. Ex vivo expansion of CD4 lymphocytes from human immunodeficiency virus type 1-infected persons in the presence of combination antiretroviral agents. *J Infect Dis* 1995;172:88–96.

139. Broder CC, Berger EA. Fusogenic selectivity of the envelope glycoprotein is a major determinant of human immunodeficiency virus type 1 tropism for CD4+ T-cell lines vs. primary macrophages. *Proc Natl Acad Sci USA* 1995;92:9004–9008.

140. Levine BL, Mosca JD, Riley JL, et al. Antiviral effect and ex vivo CD4+ T cell proliferation in HIV-positive patients as a result of CD28 costimulation. *Science* 1996;272:1939–1943.

141. Carroll RG, Riley JL, Levine BL, et al. Differential regulation of HIV-1 fusion cofactor expression by CD28 costimulation of CD4+ T cells. *Science* 1997;276:273–276.

Subject Index

Apoptosis
  in CTL memory, 335–339, 337*f*
  CTL-induced, *vs.* perforin-induced, 3–4
  granzyme/perforin-mediated, experimental
    models for, 157–159. *See also* Gran-
    zyme B (GrB)
  morphologic features of, 4
  vs. necrosis, 111–112
Arthritis, collagen-induced, Fas-dependent ly-
    sis in, 293, 294*t*
ATP. *See* Adenosine triphosphate (ATP)
Autoimmune diseases
  CTLs in, 249–252
  Fas-dependent lysis in, 293–295, 294*t*-295*t*
Autoimmune reactions, cytotoxic cells in, 2

B

B cell memory, definition of, 327
B cell response, T cell–dependent, Fas-depen-
    dent lysis in, 290–291, 292*f*
B cells
  communication with T helper cells, den-
    dritic cells and, 303. *See also* Dendritic
    cells
  in redirected cytotoxicity, 425
B6 mice, tumor surveillance in, by CTLs,
    284–286, 285*t*
Bacterial DNA. *See also* Oligodeoxynucleo-
    tide (ODN), CpG
  activity of, 395
  generation of CTLs by, 395–403
  as immunostimulant, 395–396
"Barrel stave" pore formation model, for
    activity of granulysin and NK-lysin,
    225
β-Catenin antigen, 371*t*, 372
Bispecific antibodies (bsAbs)
  animal studies of, 413–415
  clinical studies of, 415–417
    issues in, 417
  production of
    by chemical crosslinking, 409*f*–410*f*,
      409–410
    genetically engineered, 412*f*–413*f*,
      412–413
    hybrid hybridomas in, 410–412, 411*f*
  retargeting of T cells by, 415–416
  targeting of CTLs with, 428–429
  triggering molecules for, Fc receptors as,
    416–417
  for tumor antigens, 415
  types of, 409*f*–413*f*, 409–413
Bispecific-monoclonal antibodies (bs-mAbs),
    targeted at T cells, for cancer therapy,
    429–430
Bone marrow transplantation, use of NK cells
    during, 49, 49*t*
bsAbs. *See* Bispecific antibodies (bsAbs)

"Bystanders"
  lysis of
    by antigen-specific CTLs, 79–86
      LFA-1 and, 82–83
      regulation of, 83–85, 84*f*
      time sensitivity of, 82–83
    Fas-dependent, 295–298, 296*f*–298*f*
  stimulation of T cells by, during viral infec-
    tions, 334*f*, 334–335

C

C9-related protein. *See* Perforin
Calcium
  extracellular, and cytolysis, 2, 6
  and perforin polymerization, 148, 149*f*
Cancer-testis antigen, 364*t*, 364–366
Candidate antigens, epitopes on, identification
    of, 373–375
CASP-8 antigen, 372
Caspases
  activation of, in developmental cell death, 4,
    5*f*, 6, 8
  in granzyme B–mediated apoptosis, 166*t*,
    166–168, 167*f*, 184*f*
  maturation of, sites for, 167*f*
Cathepsin, in perforin-dependent cytotoxicity
    pathway, 117
Cbl, and tyrosine phosphorylation, 58*f*, 58–59
CD3–TCR complexes, and T cell activation,
    37–38
CD4 cell count, after adoptive immunother-
    apy, 449–451, 450*f*
CD4 cells
  as co-receptors in TCR signaling, 66–67
  in induction of CTL memory, 319–320
  in insulin-dependent diabetes mellitus,
    250–252
  lysis of, Fas in, 7–8
  in maintenance of T cell memory, 344–345
  perforin gene expression in, 125–126
CD8 cell memory, reduction of, after subse-
    quent viral infections, 348–350, 349*f*
CD8 cell repertoire, evolution of, in viral infec-
    tions, 339–343, 341*f*
  after clearing of infectious agent, 340–342,
    341*f*
  persistent, 342–343
  with secondary stimulation, 343
CD8 cells
  as adhesion molecules, 30–31
  on effector CTL, 67–68, 68*f*
    signals for activation of, 68–70, 69*f*
  antiviral activity of, 252–254, 257–258. *See
    also* specific viruses
  as co-receptor in TCR signaling, 66–67,
    70–71
  co-receptor of
    function of, 29–30